14th Edition

McCracken's REMOVABLE PARTIAL PROSTHODONTICS

McCracken's
REMOVABLE PARTIAL PROSTHODONTICS

Lisa A. Lang, DDS, MS, MBA, FACP
Professor of Prosthodontics
Executive Associate Dean
Associate Dean for Faculty Affairs
Indiana University School of Dentistry
Indianapolis, Indiana

Lily T. García, DDS, MS, FACP
Dean and Professor
James S. Cole Endowed Professorship
Texas A&M University College of Dentistry
Dallas, Texas

Ahmed Mahrous, DDS, MS, FACP
Associate Professor
Department of Prosthodontics,
Director of CAD CAM Dentistry
Arizona School of Dentistry and Oral Health
A.T. Stills University
Mesa, Arizona

ELSEVIER

Elsevier
3251 Riverport Lane
St. Louis, Missouri 63043

McCRACKEN'S REMOVABLE PARTIAL PROSTHODONTICS, 14TH EDITION ISBN: 978-0-323-83487-2

Senior Content Strategist: Kelly Skelton
Director, Content Development: Laurie K. Gower
Publishing Services Manager: Deepthi Unni
Project Manager: Nandhini Thanga Alagu
Design Direction: Patrick C. Ferguson

Printed in India

Last digit is the print number: 9 8 7 6 5 4 3 2 1

PREFACE

When approached by the publisher to update a highly regarded textbook, *McCracken's Removable Partial Prosthodontics* for the 14th edition, it takes a moment to consider the responsibility such a request entails. The 1960 copyright version found through a web search showed *Partial Denture Construction – Principles and Techniques* by William L. McCracken with the dedication page to "my [his] beloved wife Ruth." This 65-year legacy is remarkable, as well as the list of coauthors with Dr. McCracken and the editors that followed over the series of 13 editions; the names are a list of who's who in the history of removable prosthodontics.

So, when Dr. Lisa A. Lang was approached by the publisher to lead the revision of this textbook to produce the 14th edition, she sought to develop a revision with impact and relevance to our professional colleagues: practitioners, residents, and students. The premise of lifelong learning includes the perspective of how we learn today, including a gaming perspective through the eyes of our junior colleagues and a need for visualization as part of learning a treatment modality by which we improve the oral health of our patients.

Dr. Lang, along with her invited coeditors, Dr. Ahmed Mahrous and Dr. Lily T. García, is committed to engaging multiple colleagues throughout academic dentistry and practice, to provide the 14th edition that includes newer perspectives, animations, and video learning vignettes to help the lifelong learner both understand and implement the highest quality of care in removable partial prosthodontics. It is with the addition of updated information, visualization through animation, and video vignettes that support learning, regardless of advanced technologies developed or yet to be developed, that the fundamentals and principles in creating a removable prosthesis for a person are supported.

In addition, it is with the commitment to respect learning through the use of McCracken's textbook and building authorship capacity that the current editors and list of authors sustain a legacy of excellence that the 14th edition represents.

ABOUT THE AUTHORS

Dr. Lisa A. Lang is the Executive Associate Dean and tenured Professor of Prosthodontics at the Indiana University School of Dentistry. She received her DDS from the University of Michigan and a Certificate and Master of Science in Prosthodontics at the University of Texas Health Science Center, San Antonio. Her teaching and research focus on evidence-based prosthodontics and improving student learning through innovative curricular development in removable and implant prosthodontics. As author and coeditor of numerous publications, she has contributed to the prosthodontic scientific literature, resulting in awards for excellence in research and teaching. A Diplomate of the American Board of Prosthodontics, Dr. Lang has held leadership roles in various national and international dental organizations, including Past-President of the Academy of Prosthodontics.

Dr. Lily T. García serves as Dean of Texas A&M University College of Dentistry. She previously served as Dean of UNLV School of Dental Medicine and held leadership roles at the University of Iowa College of Dentistry, UTHSC San Antonio Dental School, the University of Colorado HSC Dental School, and the International Dental Academy in Japan. Dr. García is board-certified and a Diplomate of the American Board of Prosthodontics. She is also a Fellow of the American College of Prosthodontists and Academy of Prosthodontics, the Big 10 Academic Alliance Leadership, the *Hedwig van Ameringen* Executive Leadership in Academic Medicine, and the University of Texas System Leadership Institute.

Dr. Ahmed A. Mahrous, a Diplomate of the American Board of Prosthodontics, earned his BDS from Pharos University, a Certificate in Advanced Prosthodontics, and an MS in Oral Science from the University of Iowa. He has integrated digital technology into RPD workflows, developing tools like algorithm-based clasp selection and virtual surveying. Emphasizing clinical relevance, his work has enhanced educational frameworks and patient outcomes. Dr. Mahrous has directed RPD education at the University of Iowa and ASDOH, created online educational content, and contributed to the Dental Atlas. He also works in private practice and holds office in various scholarly venues.

ABOUT THE BOOK

NEW TO THIS EDITION

- **Updated Graphics and Visual Content**
  - Addition of 3D animations throughout the book to illustrate complex features such as biomechanics and attachments (available in the enhanced ebook version included with every new print purchase; see inside front cover for access information).
  - Replacement of low-resolution images with new high-resolution images.
- **Digital Workflow Integration**
  - Integration of digital workflows into RPD treatment planning and execution, featuring automated design, virtual surveying, and advanced fabrication techniques.
- **Content Updates and Additions**
  - Comprehensive update of content to reflect the latest standards of dental care and evidence-based research.
  - Addition of a new chapter on RPD framework materials, highlighting indications, considerations, and functions.
  - Updated coverage of implant use with RPDs, including treatment sequencing and planning.
  - Detailed descriptions of different impression techniques for RPDs, covering traditional and digital scanning methods.
  - Addition of a detailed description of framework try-in procedures and steps.
  - Inclusion of corrected cast techniques and their indications.
  - Update of the laboratory techniques chapter with a focus on digital fabrication techniques.
  - Consolidation of all laboratory-related content into a single chapter for improved clarity and organization.
- **Improved Flow and Consistency**
  - Removal of redundant material to streamline content.
  - Enhanced consistency of terminology and philosophies throughout the book.
  - Improved logical sequencing of topics for better understanding and learning.

KEY FEATURES

- Various philosophies and techniques are presented throughout, facilitating the selection and incorporation of the applicable techniques on a case-by-case basis
- Chapters are presented in three logically sequenced sections:
  - Part I: General Concepts/Treatment Planning
  - Part II: Clinical and Laboratory
  - Part III: Long-term Success: Patient and Prosthesis
  - Part IV: Maintenance

ACKNOWLEDGMENTS

As we embarked on the endeavor to revise this classic textbook, we engaged the expertise of our contributing authors to update its contents to include the state-of-the-art information from diagnosis to long-term care and maintenance for the partially edentulous patient. The task is to bring new content regarding the latest materials and procedures, in addition to improved images and videos to illustrate the content. Through the vision of Dr. Ahmed Mahrous' animations and video learning vignettes, the traditional two-dimensional prosthesis was brought alive. We would like to express our gratitude to Dr. William L. McCracken and all past editors upon whose shoulders we stand, along with the many contributors to this edition.

CONTRIBUTORS

Fatemeh Afshari, DMD, MS
Clinical Professor
Department of Restorative Dentistry
University of Illinois Chicago
College of Dentistry
Chicago, Illinois

David L. Botsko, DMD
Private Practice
Dental Software Developer
Davenport, Iowa

Wendy Clark, DDS, MS, FACP
Associate Professor of Prosthodontics
Department of Restorative Sciences
University of North Carolina Adams School of Dentistry
Chapel Hill, North Carolina

Russell J. Crockett, DMD
Assistant Professor of Prosthodontics
Arizona School of Dentistry and Oral Health
A.T. Stills University
Mesa, Arizona

Tamer El-Gendy, DMD, BDS, MS
Professor
Director of Prosthodontics
Arizona School of Dentistry and Oral Health
A.T. Stills University
Mesa, Arizona

Heba Elkassaby, BDS, DMD, MDSc, FACP
Assistant Professor
Department of Restorative Dentistry,
Director of Digital Dentistry
Rutgers Health School of Dental Medicine
Newark, New Jersey

Lily T. García, DDS, MS, FACP
Dean and Professor
James S. Cole Endowed Professorship
Texas A&M University College of Dentistry
Dallas, Texas

Craig Joseph Holland
Laboratory Technician
Adjunct Faculty, Pros
University of North Carolina Adams School of Dentistry
Chapel Hill, North Carolina;
President
General Dental Laboratory
3 Point Dental Studios Inc.
Middleburg Heights, Ohio

Leila Jahangiri, BDS, DMD, MMSc
Ira E. Klein Professor of Prosthodontics and Chair
Department of Prosthodontics
New York University College of Dentistry
New York, New York

Lisa A. Lang, DDS, MS, MBA, FACP
Professor of Prosthodontics
Executive Associate Dean
Associate Dean for Faculty Affairs
Indiana University School of Dentistry
Indianapolis, Indiana

Ahmed Mahrous, BDS, MS, FACP
Associate Professor
Department of Prosthodontics,
Director of Digital Dentistry
Arizona School of Dentistry and Oral Health
A.T. Stills University
Mesa, Arizona

Ramtin Sadid-Zadeh, DDS, MS
Professor
Head of Division of Prosthodontics
Associate Director for Advanced Education in Prosthodontics
University of Alabama – Birmingham School of Dentistry
Birmingham, Alabama

Berna Saglik, DDS, MS, D.ABDSM, FACP
Clinical Professor
Director
Graduate Prosthodontics Program
Department of Biologic Materials & Sciences and Prosthodontics
University of Michigan, School of Dentistry
Ann Arbor, Michigan

Audrey Marie Selecman, DDS, MDS
Associate Professor and Chair
Department of Prosthodontics
University of Tennessee Health Science Center College of Dentistry
Memphis, Tennessee

Patricia Swanson, DDS, FACP
Clinical Associate Professor
Director of Education in Prosthodontics
Department of Prosthodontics & Digital Technology
Stony Brook University School of Dental Medicine
Stony Brook, New York

Matt Tait, RDT BSc
Director of Technical Services, Customer Support – Product Development
Nobilium
Albany, New York;
Dental Applications Engineer, Support – Training
SenSable Technologies Inc.
Woburn, Massachusetts;
General Manager
Chromework Dental Laboratory
Chico, California;
Partner
European Dental Laboratory
Crediton
Devon, United Kingdom

Judy Chia-Chun Yuan, DDS, MS, MAS, FACP
Associate Professor
Department of Restorative Dentistry,
Interim Assistant Dean of Clinical Affairs
University of Illinois Chicago
College of Dentistry
Chicago, Illinois

CONTENTS

PART I

General Concepts/Treatment Planning

1

Partially Edentulous Epidemiology, Physiology, and Terminology

Judy Chia-Chun Yuan and Fatemeh Afshari

CHAPTER OUTLINE

The field of prosthodontics pertains to the restoration and maintenance of oral function, comfort, appearance, and health of the patient by the restoration of natural teeth and/or the replacement of missing teeth and craniofacial tissues with artificial substitutes (Fig. 1.1).[1,2] Removable prosthodontics is the branch of prosthodontics concerned with the replacement of teeth and contiguous structures for edentulous or partially edentulous patients by artificial substitutes that are readily removable from the mouth by the patient (Glossary of Prosthodontic Terms, 10th edition [GPT-10]). A removable partial denture (RPD) is a removable denture that replaces some teeth in a partially edentulous arch. This textbook focuses on what the clinician should know about partially edentulous patients to appropriately provide comfortable and useful tooth replacements in the form of RPDs.

Current practice in the management of partial tooth loss involves different types of prostheses (see Fig. 1.1). Each type of prosthesis varies in designing the use of remaining teeth, supporting soft tissues, and/or implants, and consequently demands appropriate application of knowledge and critical thinking to ensure the best possible outcome given the patient's needs and desires. Although more than one treatment modality can serve the needs of a patient, any prosthesis prescribed should be provided as part of overall management that meets the basic objectives of prosthodontic treatment: (1) the elimination of oral disease to the greatest extent possible; (2) the preservation of oral health and relationships of the teeth and various oral and paraoral structures, which will enhance the RPD design; and (3) the restoration of oral functions that are comfortable, esthetically pleasing, and do not interfere with the patient's speech. Ensuring the proper maintenance of RPDs is crucial for preserving overall health. To provide a perspective for understanding the impact of RPD prosthodontics, a review of tooth loss and its sequelae, functional restoration with prostheses, and prosthesis use and outcomes is in order.

Familiarity with accepted prosthodontic terminology related to RPDs is necessary. Chapters 5 to 9 will delve into details of the various components of an RPD. Fig. 1.2 provides an overview of the various components of RPDs. In a partially edentulous patient, the area of missing teeth is called an edentulous space or edentulous span. As seen in Fig. 1.2A, these spaces may be tooth bound (F) or not (G). The segment of the partial denture that holds the denture teeth (H) is known as the denture base. If the denture base is not tooth bound, it is referred to as the distal extension base (I). The metal support of the partial denture is called the metal framework (C). The RPD framework derives support, retention, and resistance to dislodgement from the remaining teeth. The teeth adjacent to an edentulous area that provide support to the RPD are known as the abutment teeth (J). Specific components of RPD framework are depicted in panels C–E. These components are the major connector, minor connector, the physical retention for the denture base material (latticework), occlusal rests, retentive clasp, the reciprocal clasp, and the proximal plate. (Fig. 1.2 , Video 1.2) Furthermore, Appendix A provides a review of selected prosthodontic terms. Additional terminology can be reviewed in *The Glossary of Prosthodontic Terms*[1] and a glossary of accepted terms in all disciplines of dentistry, such as *Mosby's Dental Dictionary*, fourth edition.[2]

DEMOGRAPHICS OF TOOTH LOSS

Despite advancements in health promotion and preventive dental care, it should come as no surprise that tooth loss and age are linked. A specific tooth loss relationship has been documented with increasing age as some teeth are retained longer than others. It has been suggested that, in general, an interarch difference in tooth

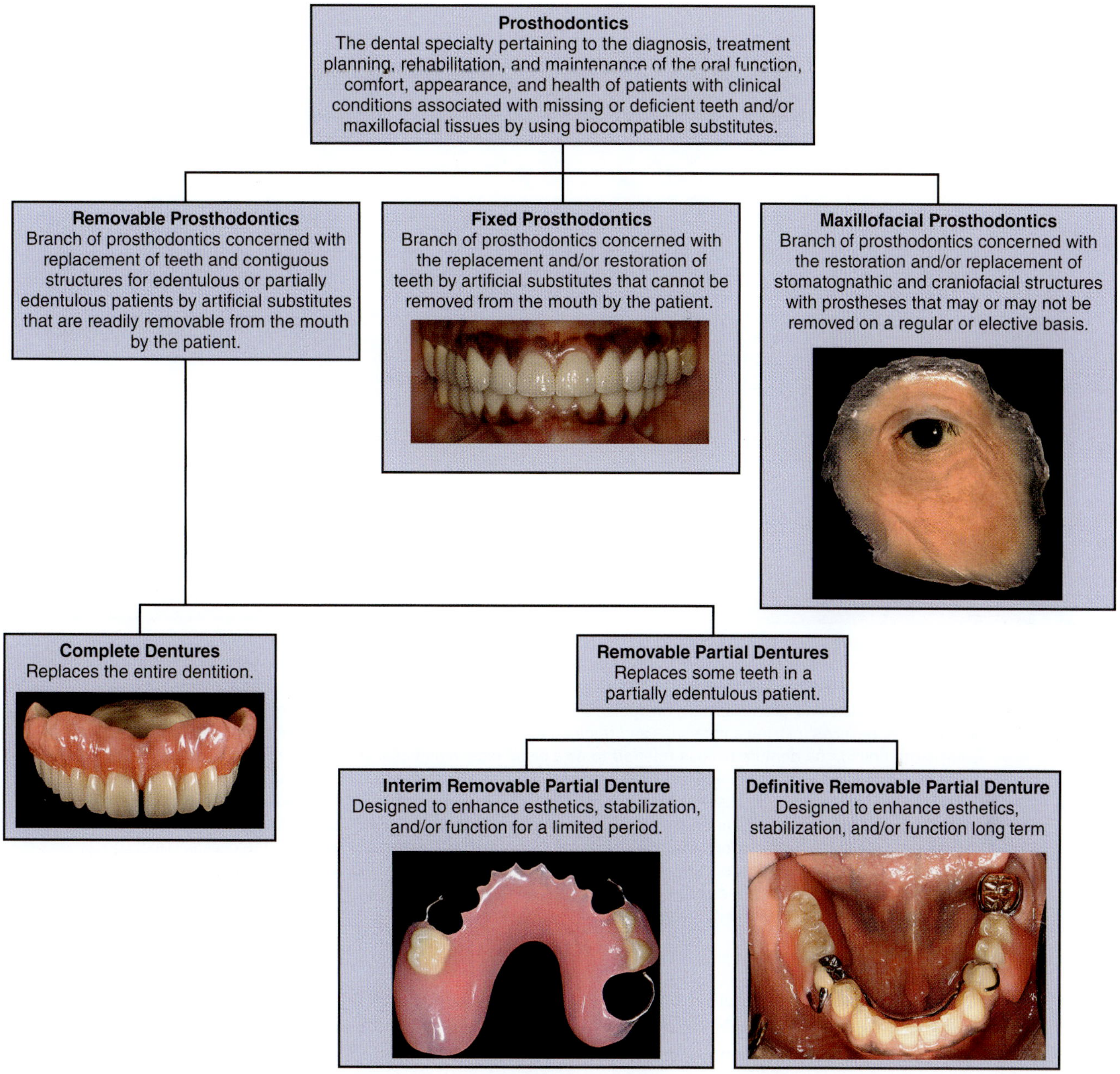

Fig. 1.1 Definitions[1] of breakdown of various branches of prosthodontics. (Courtesy of Lee Culp, Dr. Saad AlResayes, and Dr. Alvin Wee.)

loss occurs, with maxillary tooth loss prior to mandibular tooth loss. An intraarch difference has also been suggested, due to loss of posterior teeth before anterior teeth. These observations are related to respective caries susceptibilities, periodontal disease, as well as other multifactorial issues. Frequently, the last remaining teeth in the mouth are the mandibular anterior teeth, especially the mandibular canines. A frequent tooth loss outcome presents with an edentulous maxilla opposing mandibular anterior teeth.

If one accepts the premise that tooth loss and age are linked, how will this affect current and future dental practice? Replacement of missing teeth is a common patient need, and patients will demand restoration well into their elderly years. Current population estimates show that 16.8% of the US population is 65 years of age or older. By the year 2050, this percentage is projected to rise to 23%, with a significant increase expected worldwide.[3] These individuals are expected to be in better health, and health care strategies for this group focus on maintenance of active and productive lives. Optimal oral health care is expected to be a highly sought after need as a significant component of overall health.

Tooth loss patterns associated with age are also evolving. The proportion of edentulism in adults has been reported to be decreasing. However, the absolute number of edentulous patients who need care is increasing as the number of older individuals has been growing. On average, adults 20 to 64 years in age have 25.5 remaining teeth; older adults, non-Hispanic Black adults, current smokers, and those with lower incomes and less education have even fewer remaining teeth (Table 1.1).[4] Understanding and addressing social determinants of health may further improve access to oral health care and prevent future tooth loss.

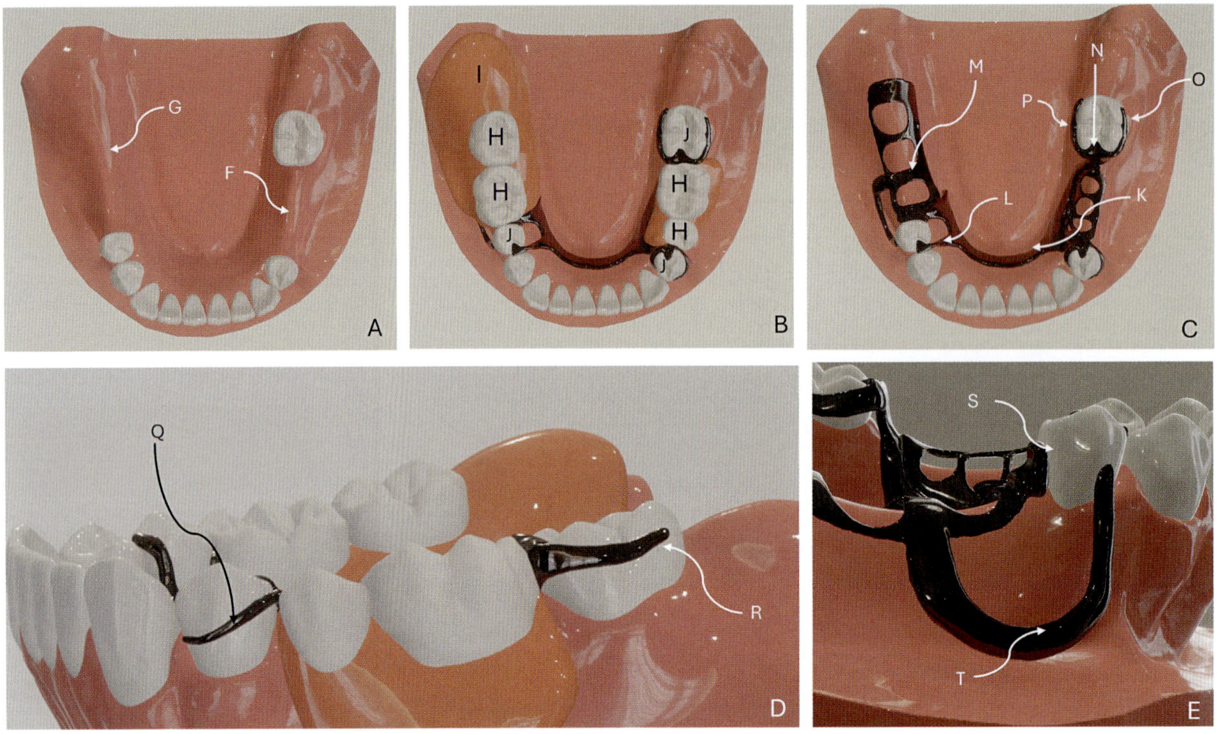

Fig. 1.2 **A,** A partially edentulous arch to be restored by a removable partial denture (RPD). The areas of missing teeth are called *(F)* and *(G)* edentulous spans. An edentulous span without a tooth at both ends of the space are also called a distal *extension*. **B,** RPD replacing missing mandibular right 1st and 2nd molars and mandibular left 2nd premolar and 1st molar. Denture teeth replace the missing teeth *(H)*, and *(I)* the denture base replaces missing soft tissues and rests on the patient's soft tissues. When the edentulous area is not tooth bound, the denture base is referred to as a distal extension base. The RPD derives its retention, resistance to dislodgement, and support from the adjacent remaining teeth *(J)* also called abutment teeth. **C**, The metal framework is an essential component of the RPD. It consists of *(K)* the major connector that connects both sides of the RPD and *(L)* minor connectors that connect the major connector to other smaller components like *(M)* the latticework which acts to retain the acrylic of the denture base, *(N)* the occlusal rest, *(O)* the retentive clasp, *(P)* the reciprocal clasp, and *(S)* the proximal plate which may be viewed in **(E)**. **D,** Retentive clasps can approach the abutment tooth from an occlusal direction *(Q, R)* or **E,** a gingival direction *(T)*. (Courtesy of Ahmed Mahrous Copyright © 2024. All rights reserved.)

Estimates suggest that the need for restoration of partially edentulous conditions is increasing as the population shifts from total edentulism to partial edentulism. The benefits offered by fluoridated water, effective preventive programs, and improved dental materials have resulted in a decrease in caries-associated tooth loss, thereby leading to an overall decline in total edentulism. The American College of Prosthodontists predicts that in the next 15 years, the number of partially edentulous patients will increase to more than 200 million in the United States alone because of rising life expectancy, growing aging population, and the retention of more teeth.[5] Consequently, the demand for prosthodontic care will continue to remain relevant and high. Furthermore, given the correlation between edentulism and lower socioeconomic status, RPDs will likely remain an affordable treatment modality for patients as compared to more costly fixed options.

CONSEQUENCES OF TOOTH LOSS

Anatomic

With the loss of teeth, the residual ridge no longer benefits from the functional stimulus it once experienced resulting in an expected loss of alveolar ridge volume—both height and width unless a dental implant is placed. The alveolar ridge volume loss is not predictable for all individuals with tooth loss because the change in anatomy is reported to be variable across patient groups. In general, bone loss is greater in the mandible than in the maxilla and more pronounced posteriorly than anteriorly, resulting in a broader mandibular arch while the maxillary arch appears constricted due to the differences in bone resorption patterns between the two arches. These anatomic changes can present challenges to fabrication of prostheses, including implant-supported prostheses and RPDs. Associated with a volumetric loss of bone is an accompanying alteration in the oral mucosa. The attached gingiva of the alveolar bone may appear to be replaced with less keratinized oral mucosa, which is more readily traumatized. Other consequences of tooth loss include positional changes of the remaining dentition, including drifting and/or rotation of adjacent teeth, supra-eruption of opposing teeth into the edentulous site, and subsequent jaw relation positional changes. The sequela can complicate future prosthodontic rehabilitation of the oral cavity.

Physiologic

Prosthodontics management of missing teeth includes consideration and replacement of both the physical anatomic means

TABLE 1.1 Mean Number of Permanent Teeth Remaining in Adults Aged 20 to 64 Years by Selected Characteristics

Characteristic	Mean Number of Permanent Teeth (1999–2004)	Mean Number of Permanent Teeth (2011–16)
Age		
20–34 years	26.9	27.0
35–49 years	25.0	25.5
50–64 years	22.2	23.4
Sex		
Male	25.0	25.5
Female	24.9	25.5
Race and Ethnicity		
White, non-Hispanic	25.2	25.7
Black, non-Hispanic	23.6	24.2
Mexican American	25.2	25.4
Poverty Status (Income Compared to Federal Poverty Level)		
Less than 100%	23.3	23.6
100%–199%	23.5	24.4
Greater than 200%	25.5	26.1
Education		
Less than high school	23.0	23.8
High school	24.3	24.5
More than high school	25.7	26.2
Smoking History		
Current smoker	23.3	23.5
Former smoker	25.1	25.5
Never smoker	25.6	26.1
Overall	24.9	25.5

From Centers for Disease Control and Prevention. *Oral Health Surveillance Reports: Trends in Dental Caries and Sealants, Tooth Retention, and Edentulism, United States 1999-2004 to 2011-2016.* Centers for Disease Control and Prevention, US Dept of Health and Human Services; 2019.

for mastication and physiologic oral capacity for neuromuscular functions to manipulate food. Chewing studies have shown that the oral sensory feedback involved in guiding mandibular movement during chewing comes from various sources. The most sensitive input, meaning the input that provides the most refined and precisely controlled movement, comes from periodontal mechanoreceptors (PMRs), with additional input coming from the gingiva, mucosa, periosteum/bone, and temporomandibular joint complex.

Chewing as a learned behavior has a basic pattern of movement generated from within the central nervous system. In typical function, masticatory movement is modulated inherently based on the food selected and physiologic task needs by oral sensory input from various sources. With loss of the finely tuned contribution from tooth PMRs, the resulting peripheral receptor influence is less precise in muscular guidance, producing more variable masticatory function. The type of prosthesis selected to replace missing teeth may potentially contribute to functional impediments.

Psychosocial

A person's facial appearance embodies a large portion of an individual's social identity. The esthetic impact of tooth loss can be highly significant and may be more of a concern to a patient than loss of function. It is generally perceived that societal norms convey significant social stigma with loss of visible teeth. With loss of teeth and diminishing residual ridge, facial features can change as the result of altered lip support and/or reduced facial height appearance caused by a reduction in occlusal vertical dimension. Restoring facial esthetics and function in a manner that helps maintain a patient's oral health-related quality of life can be a challenge and considered a major factor in the restorative and maintenance decisions made for various prosthetic treatments.

The Oral Health Impact Profile, based on a theoretical model by Locker,[6] is a metric used to determine the adverse effects of various oral conditions, such as tooth loss, on daily life. While both anterior and posterior missing teeth have an impact on the overall oral health–related quality of life, the location of the missing teeth and the number of occluding pairs of teeth have been shown to have a differential impact on patients. Although posterior teeth mainly impact function, anterior teeth have a broader impact on the patient in regard to pain, physical disability, and psychosocial domains. Furthermore, the prevalence of negative impact increases substantially when the remaining number of teeth present drops below 20 teeth.

FUNCTIONAL RESTORATION WITH PROSTHESES

Individuals with a full complement of teeth report some variation in their levels of masticatory function. The loss of teeth may lead patients to seek care for functional reasons if they notice diminished function to a level that is unacceptable to them. The level at which a patient finds function to be unacceptable varies among individuals. This variability increases with accelerating tooth loss. Comprehension of patient-perceived clinical outcomes may be confusing to clinicians, who perceive that they have provided prostheses of equal quality to different patients with the same tooth loss patterns, and yet have received different patient reports of success.

An understanding of variations among individuals with a full complement of teeth and those with prostheses can help clinicians formulate realistic treatment goals that can be communicated to the patient. A review of oral function, especially mastication, may help clinicians better understand issues related to the impact of RPDs.

Mastication

Although functionally considered a separate act, mastication as part of the feeding continuum precedes swallowing and is not an end in itself. The interaction of the two distinct but coordinated aspects of feeding suggests that some judgment of mastication termination or completeness precedes the initiation of swallowing. Although the mastication-swallowing sequence is obvious, the interaction of the two functions is not widely understood and may be important when considering RPDs as a treatment option.

Mastication involves two discrete but well-synchronized activities: (1) subdivision of food by applied force and (2) selective manipulation by the tongue and cheeks to sort out coarse particles and return to the occlusal surfaces of teeth for further breakdown. The initial subdivision or comminution phase involves the processes of selection, which refers to the chance that a particle is placed between the teeth in position to be broken, and breakage, which is the degree of fragmentation of a particle once selected. The size, shape, and texture of food particles provide the sensory input that influences the configuration and area of each chewing stroke. Larger particles are selectively reduced in size more rapidly than fine particles in efficient mastication. The process of mastication is therefore greatly influenced by factors that affect physical ability to reduce food and to monitor the reduction process by neurosensory means.

Food Reduction

Natural teeth or a prosthesis help reduce food to a point ready for swallowing. An index of food reduction is described as *masticatory efficiency*, or the ability to reduce food to a certain particulate size, in a given time frame. A strong correlation has been shown between masticatory efficiency and the number of occluding teeth in dentate individuals, which would suggest variability of particle selection related to contacting teeth. Performance measures reveal a great deal of functional variability in patients with similar numbers of opposing, contacting teeth, and even greater variability is seen within populations with greater tooth loss (increasing degrees of partial edentulism).

The loss of molar teeth would be expected to have a greater impact on performance measures in that the molar has a larger occlusal contact area, the latter being highly correlated with masticatory performance. This effect has been shown in individuals with missing molars, who require more chewing strokes and have a larger mean particle size before swallowing. The point at which an individual is prepared to swallow the food bolus is another measure of performance and is described as the *swallowing threshold*. Superior masticatory ability that is highly correlated with occlusal contact area which also achieves greater food particle reduction at the swallowing threshold. Conversely, a diminished ability to chew is reflected in larger particles at the swallowing threshold.

Functional Quality of Life

The objective measures described above, which demonstrate a benefit of molar contact in dentate individuals, may conflict with some subjective measures from patients who express no perceived functional problems associated with having only premolar occlusion. The *shortened dental arch* concept highlights that patient perceptions of functional compromise, as well as benefit, should be considered when it is decided whether to replace missing molars. When the loss of posterior teeth results in an unstable tooth position, such as distal or labial migration, or lack of posterior support of the jaws, tooth replacement should be carefully considered; the latter situation differs from the shortened dental arch concept.

It has been reported that prosthetic replacement of teeth provides function that is less optimal when compared to the complete, natural dentition state. Functional measures are closest to natural dentition when prosthodontic replacements such as fixed partial dentures are rigidly supported by teeth or implants, intermediate in function when replacements are removable and supported by teeth, lower in function when replacements are removable and supported by both teeth and edentulous ridges, and lowest in functional capacity when replacements are removable and supported by edentulous ridges alone.

Objective and subjective measures of a patient's oral function often are not in agreement. It has been shown that subjective measures of masticatory ability are often overrated compared with objective functional tests and that, for complete denture wearers, the subjective criteria may be more appropriate in monitoring perceived outcomes. Some literature reports that RPDs can be described by patients as adding very little benefit over not having a prosthesis. However, these findings may be multifactorial in nature including lack of maintenance of occluding tooth relationships, patient compliance level with follow-up visits, and intrinsic variation in patient response to prostheses.

CURRENT REMOVABLE PARTIAL DENTURE USE

Given an understanding of the relationship between tooth loss and age, the consequences of tooth loss, and the ability to restore function with removable partial prostheses, what is known about current prosthesis use and what are common clinical outcomes? Recent global market research suggests that approximately 19% of adults wear removable prostheses, of which 60% are RPDs (Fig. 1.3).[7,8] A retrospective study on factors influencing continual use and patient satisfaction with RPDs found that only 61% of prostheses were used 5 years postdelivery.[9] Patient age, location of the edentulous area(s), number of occluding teeth, and occlusal rest seat preparation significantly influenced patient compliance while pain and esthetics (denture teeth shade, tooth mold, and setup) were found to correlate with patient satisfaction. Of note, dentists typically emphasize the physical function of the prostheses whereas patients tend to focus more on the social aspects. As an affordable and noninvasive alternative, treatment with RPDs should ideally lead to improvements in overall oral health, patient satisfaction, and compliance.

NEED FOR REMOVABLE PARTIAL DENTURES

The implications from review of various factors associated with partial edentulism require knowledge of each factor when

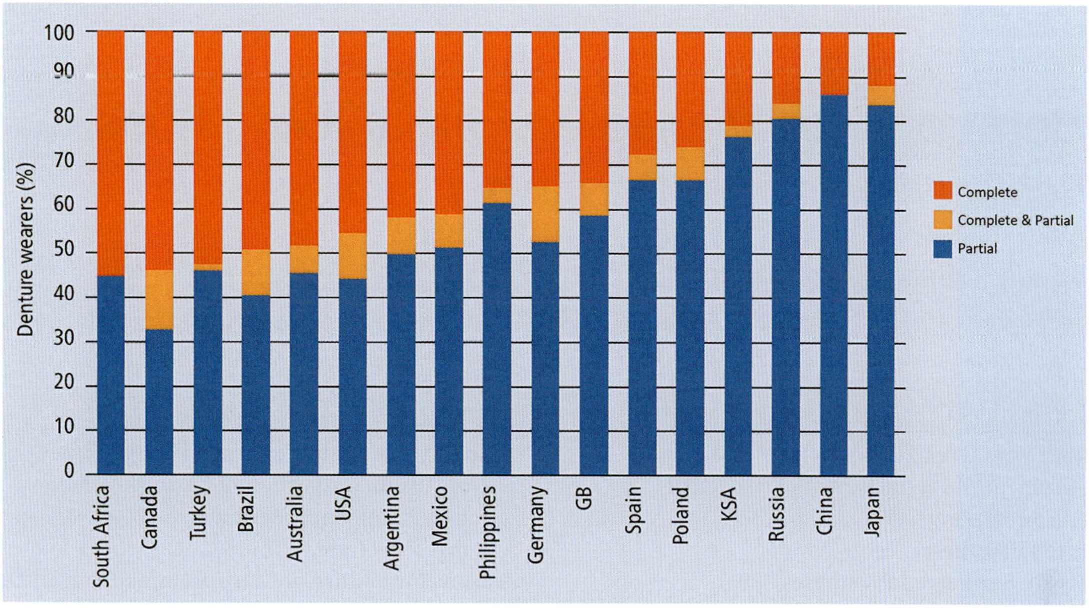

Fig. 1.3 Proportion of denture wearers with complete, complete and partial, and partial dentures. Data collected in a 2014 study[7] illustrates the large population of denture wearers (adults >18 years of age) who have partial dentures. $N = 1000$ per country, denture wearers only. (From Data on file. Oral Care Omnibus Study. 2014. Internal market research report; Shaha M, Varghese R, Atassi M. Understanding the impact of removable partial dentures on patients' lives and their attitudes to oral care. *Br Dent J*. 2021. https://doi.org/10.1038/s41415-021-2949-4.)

identifying the appropriate treatment modality for a patient. The need for prosthodontic management of partially edentulous patients will increase. Historically, patient use of RPDs has been high and is expected to continue with an increase in an aging population, who because they are retaining teeth longer, will present with more partially edentulous conditions. When discussing treatment options with partially edentulous patients, each patient must be educated regarding their treatment options for prosthesis that are entirely supported by teeth/implants, removable prostheses supported by teeth and/or the underlying residual ridge, or teeth and dental implants. Some patients, when given the choice between a prosthesis entirely supported by teeth/implants and an RPD, are not able to pursue fixed prosthodontic treatment options, which contributes to higher use of RPDs. It is important for patients to learn the benefit of dental implant placement to improve the performance of the RPD when making an informed decision regarding their treatment choice. Selective placement of an implant can be used to support an implant-supported fixed dental prosthesis in the event of future tooth loss.

Finally, studies suggest the need to maximize the opportunity for providing and maintaining stable prostheses while addressing patient needs and expectations. Consequently, throughout this text, the basic principles of diagnosis, abutment preparation, prosthesis design and fabrication, patient education, timely recall, and maintenance will be reinforced to improve the reader's understanding of RPD prostheses.

REFERENCES

1. The glossary of prosthodontic terms, ed 8. *J Prosthet Dent.* 2005;94(1):10–92. Available online http://www.sciencedirect.com/science/article/pii/S0022391305001757.
2. *Mosby's Dental Dictionary.* 3rd ed. Mosby/Elsevier.
3. <https://www.census.gov/data/tables/2023/demo/popproj/2023-summary-tables.html.> https://blogs.worldbank.org/en/opendata/worlds-population-will-continue-grow-and-will-reach-nearly-10-billion-2050.
4. Centers for Disease Control and Prevention. *Oral Health Surveillance Reports: Trends in Dental Caries and Sealants, Tooth Retention, and Edentulism, United States 1999-2004 to 2011-2016.* Centers for Disease Control and Prevention, US Dept of Health and Human Services; 2019.
5. American College of Prosthodontists. Facts and figures. Available at: https://www.gotoapro.org/facts-figures/.
6. Locker D, Allen F. What do measures of "oral health-related quality of life" measure? *Community Dent Oral Epidemiol.* 2007;35:401–411. https://doi.org/10.1111/j.1600-0528.2007.00418.x.
7. Data on file. Oral Care Omnibus Study. 2014. Internal market research report.
8. Shaha M, Varghese R, Atassi M. Understanding the impact of removable partial dentures on patients' lives and their attitudes to oral care. *Br Dent J.* 2021. https://doi.org/10.1038/s41415-021-2949-4.
9. Koyama S, Sasaki K, Yokoyama M, Sasaki T, Hanawa S. Evaluation of factors affecting the continuing use and patient satisfaction with removable partial dentures over 5 years. *J Prosthodont Res.* 2010;54:97–101.

2

Considerations for Managing Partial Tooth Loss

Tooth Replacements from the Patient's Perspective

Lisa A. Lang, Lily T. García, and Ahmed Mahrous

CHAPTER OUTLINE

MANAGING TOOTH LOSS OVER TIME

Patients who experience tooth loss also experience psychological impact on their well-being and quality of life.[1,2] It is important to understand how the practitioner interacts with patients in a manner that is considered how to treat versus how to manage tooth loss. Patients may require special consideration as an individual learns the implications of tooth loss both from the impact on their psychological well-being and a functional perspective. Patients may expect to comprehend outcomes both in the current state and in the future. It is helpful to make the distinction of "treating" partial edentulism as opposed to managing how to guide an individual in the treatment decision being made currently, which could have implications for future needs that may differ among choices between various prostheses.

Tooth Replacements from the Patient's Perspective

Tooth loss is a permanent outcome as a condition, similar to a chronic medical condition. For example, a chronic medical condition such as diabetes is not reversible and requires medical management to monitor care to ensure appropriate response over time. Similarly, tooth replacement utilizing a prosthesis must be managed to ensure appropriate response over time.

The term *management* suggests a focus on meeting needs that may change and evolve over time, some of which may be expected or unexpected. Expected outcomes are those that accompany the common clinical course for a type of prosthesis that is related to the tooth-tissue response. The biological response is heavily influenced by the type and design of the prosthesis chosen. Some needs can be due to prosthesis degradation over time, while other results are unexpected and require monitoring due to the interim time-to-retreatment concerns of life expectancy. Unexpected needs can involve factors related to tissue damage or abuse, material design flaws, or prosthesis design under the purview of the dentist or to those factors that cannot be controlled such as parafunctional habits or accidental trauma.

Understanding all factors is helpful when considering how best to educate patients about management of missing teeth over a lifetime. This perspective supports current decision-making, to be made with a long-term context, as well as allowing decisions to enhance future treatment options.

Treatment plan options for tooth replacement can include a full range of prosthetic designs including dental implant–supported prostheses, fixed prostheses, and removable prostheses. When a removable partial denture is offered as a treatment option, the prosthodontic treatment option may not be presented and described in detail similar to that in which fixed or implant prostheses are described. The distinction can be perceived as a less desirable tooth replacement option since it might be less like teeth. The desirability of a prosthesis is important from a patient's perspective. In addition, a discussion that includes strategic implant placement for use and support of a removable partial denture may be helpful for patients desiring options with implants.

In patients who have not experienced tooth loss before, it is important to discuss expectations with prosthetic replacements to describe, educate, and manage expectations. Treatment options presented to a patient are developed but may be biased based on professional judgment, practitioner's experience, and practitioner confidence and competence with certain treatments. Ultimately, seeking an option based on what is best for the patient and identifying whether a removable partial denture is a viable treatment option preclude bias. The patient-practitioner interaction is key to understanding expectations and capacity to experience and maximize treatment outcomes.

Shared Decision-Making

In order to achieve a state of oral health, a patient should be informed and understand their current oral health status, including recognition of behavioral issues related to plaque control, so that once active disease is controlled, they contribute to long-term good oral health. A shared decision-making approach addresses the need to fully inform patients about risks and benefits of care and ensures that the patient's values and preferences play a prominent role in the ultimate decision.

There is patient variability in their desire to participate in treatment decisions, so it is incumbent to engage through active inquiry during discussion. This becomes especially critical when discussing elective care, which involves a potentially high financial burden along with costly options vital for long-term maintenance requirements. It is essential to provide specific, relevant information that allows for an actively engaged patient to decide between treatment options. Educating a patient, including information relative to outcomes associated with a practitioner, is helpful in decision-making. Open discussion ideally relays data from one's own practice outcomes since it provides the patient with provider-specific effectiveness and describes exactly what aspects of care are important to the overall decision.

Educating a patient about the differences between different prosthetic options offers opportunities for patient education. Treatment outcomes include technical outcomes, physical outcomes, esthetic outcomes, various maintenance needs, initial and future costs, and even physiologic outcomes that suggest to what extent prostheses "feel" like teeth.

When tooth replacement prostheses are considered from a patient's perspective, a primary focus can be the desire to replace natural teeth with prosthetic options that serve functional and social roles in everyday life. In considering how well various types of prostheses may meet patients' specific needs, it is helpful to understand what features of the original dentition that the patient seeks to replicate. Existing extraoral and intraoral conditions may not easily allow complete restoration to a perceived original state in situations with poor oral health. Relative strengths and weaknesses for each of the prosthodontic options conveyed in a manner of educating the patient help develop realistic expectations.

For this textbook's purposes, the treatment option focuses on removable partial dentures as the choice for a replacement prosthesis in patients missing some but not all teeth. The replacement prosthesis should provide function with a level of comfort and functional stability. For the patient missing posterior teeth, a removable prosthesis replacing missing teeth is at risk for instability due to the edentulous ridge compressible support; therefore consideration of an implant in distalmost posterior position can be used to support the posterior segment—the distal extension—which can enhance functional stability.

If the prosthesis is visible during casual speaking, smiling, and/or laughing, it is obvious that the replacement should look as natural as the surrounding environment, which is a distinct challenge with removable partial dentures. In summary, tooth replacement prostheses should be acceptable in appearance, be comfortable and stable in function, and be designed to be cleaned and managed throughout the serviceable lifetime at a reasonable cost.

TOOTH-SUPPORTED PROSTHESES

For partially edentulous patients, available prosthetic options include natural tooth-supported fixed partial dentures, implant-supported fixed partial dentures, a combination of tooth- and implant-supported removable and/or fixed prostheses, and removable partial dentures. The extent to which the treatment options restore and maintain features similar to that of natural teeth depends largely on the number and location of the missing teeth. Categories that define presentation of tooth loss (see Chapter 3) follow the Kennedy classification for teeth present both anterior *and* posterior to an edentulous space (tooth supported) and for teeth either anterior *or* posterior to an edentulous space (tooth and tissue supported). All prosthetic options listed can be considered for the tooth-supported clinical scenario, although not necessarily indicated, but only removable partial dentures and implant-supported prostheses are available for a tooth- and tissue-supported scenario (distal extension).

Removable partial dentures can be designed in many ways that provide for incorporation of abutment teeth and supporting tissue for stability, support, and retention of the prosthesis. In terms of tooth-supported presentation, a removable partial denture is similar to a fixed partial denture because natural teeth alone provide direct resistance to functional forces. The design of the removable partial denture framework on the abutment teeth takes advantage of tooth support—similar to the relationship between a fixed partial denture retainer and a prepared tooth. The removable partial denture design transfers vertical support through rest seat preparations on abutment teeth and defines a restrictive angle of dislodgment through preparation of opposing guide planes. Removable partial denture clasps do not completely encircle the abutment tooth, as a fixed partial denture retainer does; the clasp is designed to engage more than half the abutment tooth circumference for prosthesis positional stability under horizontal chewing loads. The need for planning and natural tooth contour modifications are required to mitigate movement and improve functional stability for tooth-supported removable partial dentures. Tooth modification principles required to ensure stability for movement control in removable partial dentures are highlighted in detail (see Chapter 14).

TOOTH- AND TISSUE-SUPPORTED PROSTHESES

When a removable partial denture is planned for a tooth- and tissue-supported arch, the prosthesis must be designed to allow limited functional movement of the distal extension base on the residual alveolar ridge tissues. In this clinical scenario, the residual alveolar ridge helps support functional stability. Mucosal tissue displacement varies; a healthy residual ridge consisting of alveolar bone and attached keratinized mucosa is expected to have 1–3 mm of displacement. Unlike the tooth-supported design, the tooth- and tissue-supported framework design includes tooth modification for functional stability and compensates for vertical and/or horizontal movements of the distal extension base. Due to changes over time with tooth- and tissue-supported removable partial dentures, it is essential to carefully monitor patients to maintain support and ensure maximum prosthetic function.

The clasp-retained removable partial denture provides an accepted treatment option and is commonly used with a lower cost option as compared to a fixed or implant prosthodontics option (Fig. 2.1). There are several possible disadvantages of a clasp-retained partial denture:

- Stress loads on the abutment teeth may be caused by improper tooth preparation, poor clasp design, and/or loss of tissue support under the distal extension denture base.
- Clasps can be unesthetic, particularly when they are placed on visible tooth surfaces without consideration of esthetic impact.
- Caries may develop under framework components, especially if an appropriate hygiene maintenance protocol has not been implemented or the patient fails to understand the necessity to maintain the remaining teeth and tissues healthy and keep the prosthesis clean.

Despite these disadvantages, the use of removable prostheses may be preferred when tooth-bounded edentulous areas are extensive and cannot be restored predictably with fixed prostheses, or when cross-arch stabilization and wider distribution of forces are needed to support the remaining teeth and residual tissues.

A removable partial denture retained using prescribed internal attachments can eliminate some of the disadvantages of clasps but has higher costs associated. Use of prescribed attachments with a removable partial denture is indicated when alignment of the abutment teeth is favorable, periodontal health and bone support are adequate, the clinical crown is of sufficient length, the pulp morphology can accommodate the required tooth preparation, and the economic status of the patient permits. Under these clinical conditions, consideration

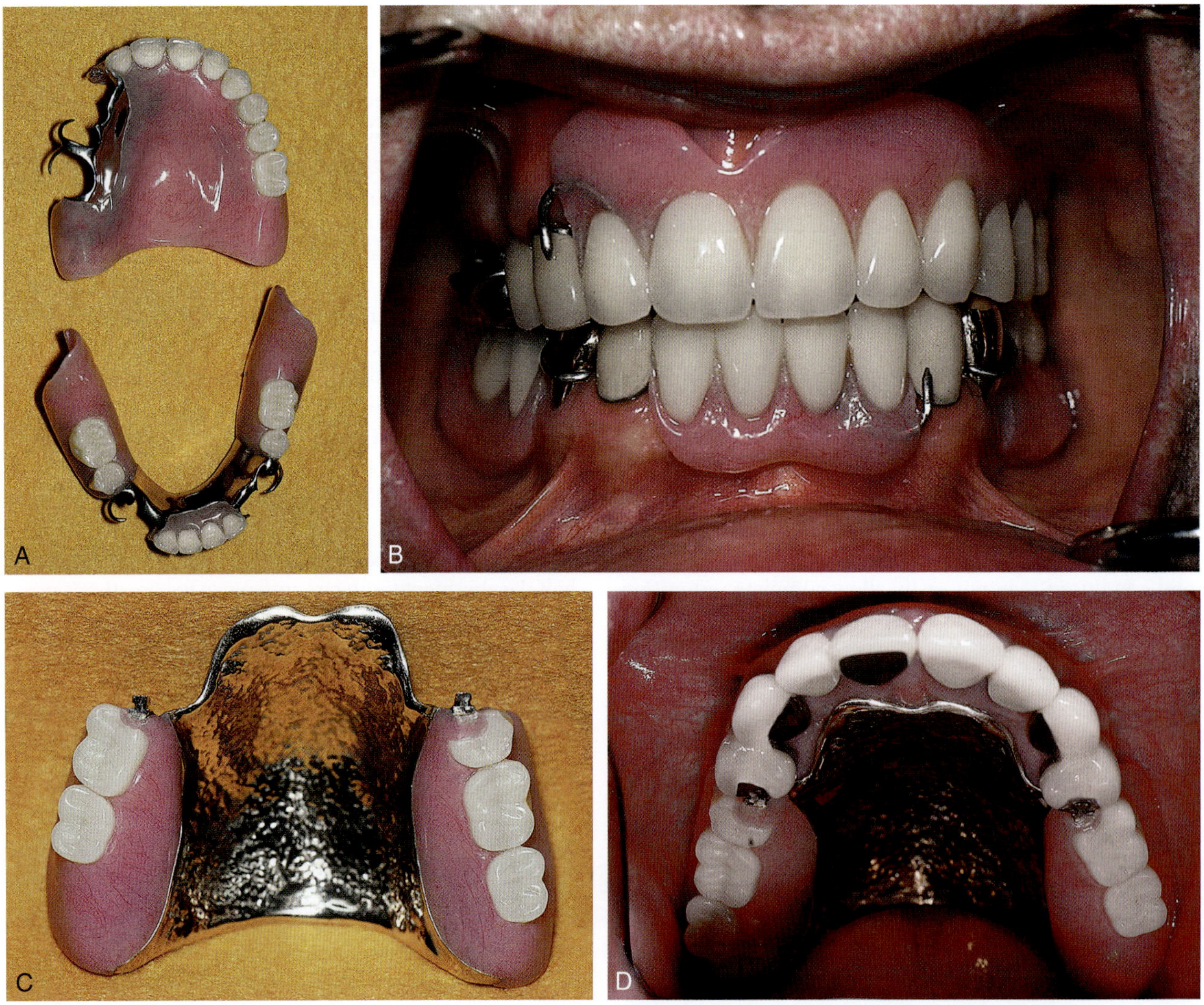

Fig. 2.1 **A,** Maxillary and mandibular clasp-retained removable partial dentures. All clasps are extracoronal retainers (clasps) on abutments. **B,** Prostheses from **(A)** shown intraorally in occlusion. **C,** Maxillary prosthesis using intracoronal retainers and full palatal coverage. The male portions of the attachments are shown at the mesial position of the artificial teeth and will fit into intracoronal rests. **D,** Internal attachment prosthesis in the patient's mouth. Note the precise fit of male and female portions of the attachments.

for a prescribed internal attachment can be compared to use of implants in design (see Chapter 25).

Indiscriminate use of internal attachments can lead to excessive torsional load on abutments supporting distal extension removable partial dentures, especially in the mandible. The use of hinges or other types of stress breakers is discouraged in these situations; although effective, they are often not used appropriately. For instance, use of a stress breaker in a mandibular distal extension partial denture does not provide for cross-arch stabilization and can result in excessive trauma from horizontal and torquing forces on the residual ridge. Therefore a rigid framework design that includes extracoronal clasp retainers is indicated and within the standard of care.

The goal in designing a removable partial denture is to ensure functional stability by using components to mitigate forces generated under normal function. This entails providing appropriate natural tooth preparation, accurate framework fit interface to tooth and tissue, and simultaneous occlusal relationship between natural and prosthetic opposing teeth and providing and maintaining optimum support from the soft tissue and teeth. It may also require strategic use of implants to control distal extension movement.

When functional movements are understood, use of appropriate components can be prescribed and designed to address biomechanics generated (see Chapter 4). There is a need to resist the removable partial denture movement on teeth and tissues and to resist a prosthesis from dislodgement, yet the more difficult scenario is to mitigate damaging movement forces during mastication and parafunction. It is important to control combined vertical (tissueward) and horizontal movements, which requires close attention to tooth modifications (rest and stabilizing component preparations) and verification of framework fit intraorally.

STEPS IN PATIENT CARE

There are multiple steps followed in patient care, and similarly, steps are followed in fabrication of a removable partial denture for a patient. Initially, the diagnosis, determination, and indication of the need for a removable partial denture and patient education regarding the prosthesis and expectations occur. Development of a treatment plan, design of the removable partial denture framework and following the design step treatment sequencing, and intraoral tissue (tooth and soft tissue) preparations are planned. The design considerations for support of a distal extension denture base should be reviewed as applicable to the tooth- and tissue-supported prosthesis. In designing and fabrication of a removable partial denture, occlusal relationships should be verified to avoid removable partial dentures creating interferences in function when complete. Following planning, designing, and fabrication, initial prosthetic intraoral placement and fitting procedures and patient education are reviewed to optimally maintain oral structures including restorations. On completion, follow-up services, including recall appointments for hygiene maintenance and periodic evaluation, are essential to ensure oral health and patient understanding of procedures to ensure success. Details pertaining to the various steps are presented in subsequent chapters.

Diagnosis and Patient Education

The term *patient education* is described in *Mosby's Dental Dictionary* as "the process of informing a patient about a health matter to secure informed consent, patient cooperation, and a high level of patient compliance."

The dentist and patient share responsibility for the ultimate success of a treatment intervention. A patient must understand the benefits of a removable partial denture as well as the required oral care and maintenance procedures to ensure success. Preservation of the oral structures, one of the primary objectives of prosthodontic treatment, is compromised without the patient's cooperation in oral hygiene and regular maintenance visits.

Patient education begins at the initial encounter and continues throughout treatment. This educational procedure is especially important when the treatment plan and prognosis are discussed with the patient. An informed patient accepts responsibility but must first learn about the care before definitive treatment is undertaken to improve prognosis. The information shared should also be available through written and oral presentations and can include sources from trusted organizations available through the internet.

Treatment Planning, Removable Partial Denture Framework Design, Treatment Sequencing, and Intraoral Tissue (Tooth and Soft Tissue) Preparations

Treatment planning and design begin with thorough medical and dental histories. A complete oral examination includes but is not limited to radiographic imaging and interpretation, diagnosis of caries, the condition of existing restorations, periodontal status, and evaluation of jaw relation and occlusal relations, which may require diagnostic mounting of full arch casts. After a complete diagnostic examination has been accomplished and a removable partial denture has been selected as the treatment of choice, a treatment plan is sequenced and the partial denture design is developed following design principles as prescribed by the licensed dentist, not the dental laboratory technician.

After treatment planning, a predetermined sequence of preparations (including crown procedures) is determined and reviewed to ensure the removable partial denture design has been properly sequenced. Intraoral preparations are sequenced to provide adequate support, occlusal function, stability, and retention for the removable partial denture. Diagnostic casts or images with the tentative framework design help guide the mouth preparations such as occlusal adjustments, abutment restorations, and abutment modifications.

Support for Distal Extension Denture Bases

For the distal extension removable partial denture, tooth- and tissue-supported prosthesis, the base is made to fit the residual alveolar ridge to provide adequate support under occlusal loading (Fig. 2.2). At times, an additional procedure, such as a corrected impression, can be accomplished to satisfy the need for appropriate border detail and extension. The primary supporting area should be recorded or related under functional load for support. This unique feature of a distal extension removable

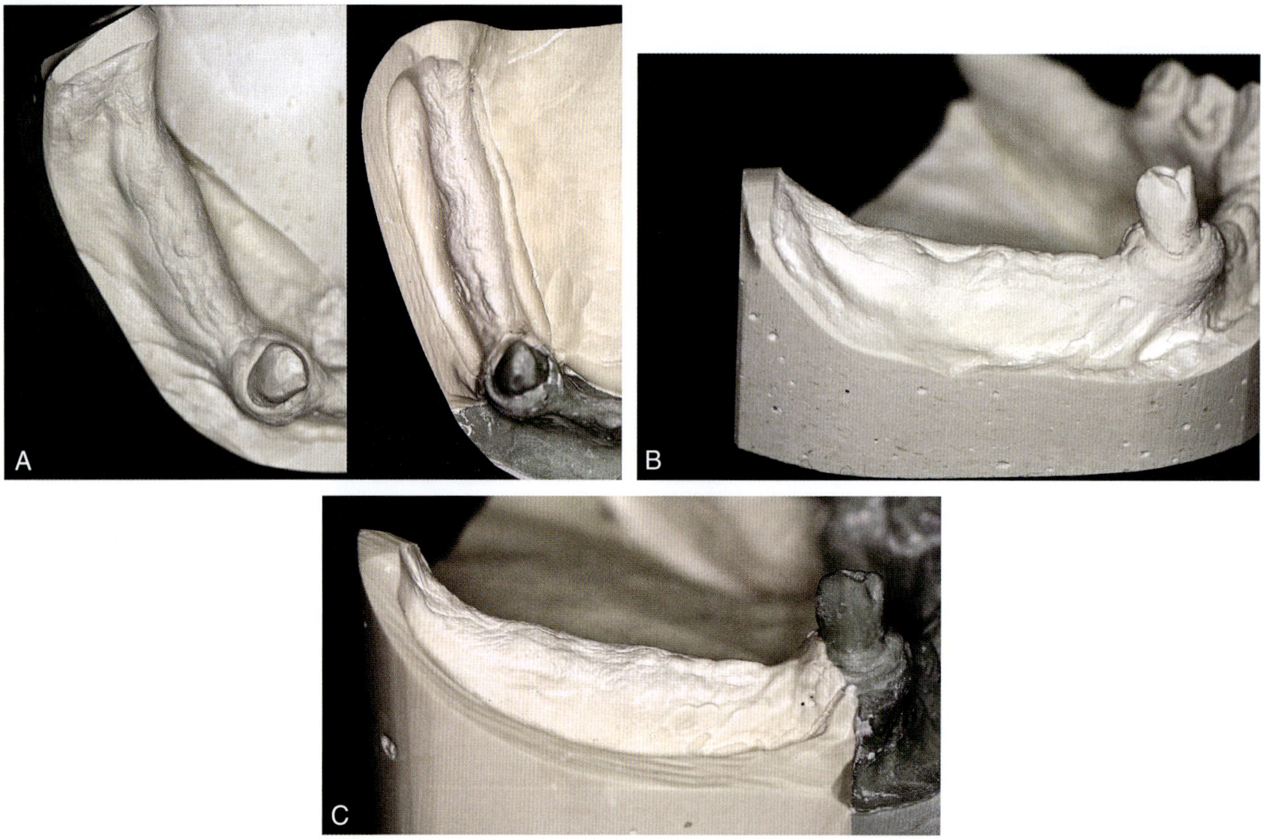

Fig. 2.2 **A,** Occlusal view of a cast from a preliminary impression, which produced an anatomic ridge form *(left)*, and an altered cast of the same ridge showing a functional or supportive form *(right)*. The altered cast impression selectively placed pressure on the buccal shelf region, which is the primary stress-bearing area of the mandibular posterior residual ridge. **B,** Buccal view of anatomic ridge form. **C,** Buccal view of functional or supportive ridge form. Note that the supportive form of the ridge clearly delineates the extent of coverage available for a denture base and is most different from the anatomic form when the mucosa is easily displaced.

partial denture attempts to achieve optimal support from the tissues underlying the distal extension base compatible with the tooth support to the extent possible.

A complete denture is entirely tissue supported, and the entire denture can move toward the tissue under function. In contrast, any movement of a removable partial denture base is inevitably a rotational movement that, if toward the tissue, may result in undesirable torquing forces to the abutment teeth and loss of planned occlusal contacts. Therefore every effort must be made to provide the best possible support for the distal extension base to minimize these forces.

Selecting an impression technique to record teeth, the residual alveolar ridge tissues, and adjacent structures is discussed in Chapter 16. A method should be used that can record these tissues in their supporting form or in a supporting relationship to the rest of the denture (see Fig. 2.2).

Design and Verification of Occlusal Relations

Whether the removable partial denture is tooth supported or is tooth and tissue supported, verification of occlusal relations is part of design. For the tooth-supported removable partial denture, ridge form is of less significance than it is for the tooth- and tissue-supported prosthesis since the former relies on support from abutment teeth only. For the distal extension base, jaw relation records are necessary to determine appropriate occlusal relations, usually recorded after the partial denture framework has been fitted and additional impressioning has been completed if indicated. Occlusal records for a removable partial denture may be made by the various methods described in Chapter 18.

Initial Placement Procedures

Initial placement of the prosthesis or "delivery" is accomplished by the dentist through fittng and adjustments of the prosthesis that are required for the patient to take possession. Refining fit of the denture base (tooth- and tissue-supported prosthesis) and occlusal adjustments are completed at the appointment. It must be ascertained that the patient understands home care instructions and expectations and demonstrates the ability to insert and remove the prosthesis comfortably. These facets of treatment are discussed in detail in Chapter 21.

Long-Term Care

Periodic reevaluation of the patient is critical for early recognition of intraoral changes. Routine examinations are necessary to monitor the condition of teeth and intraoral tissues, condition of the prosthesis, patient acceptance, and patient compliance in maintaining oral hygiene and cleanliness of the prosthesis. Although a 6-month recall period is adequate for most patients, more frequent evaluation may be required for some (see Chapter 21).

REASONS FOR FAILURE OF CLASP-RETAINED PARTIAL DENTURES

Clasp-retained removable partial dentures continue to be used in patient care. Objections to the visibility of retentive clasps can be minimized through clasp design and selection. Few contraindications for use of a properly designed clasp-retained removable partial denture are known. Concerns related to this type of removable partial denture can be attributed to deficiencies in each phase such as:

- Diagnosis: inadequate diagnosis, failure to assess tooth and tissue contours during framework design (lack of use of contour analytics tools).
- Intraoral preparation: improper intraoral sequencing, inadequate preparations, insufficient planning of the framework, failure to return supporting tissue to optimum health before impression procedures, inadequate impressions of hard and soft tissue.
- Framework design: failure to properly locate rest seats and poor rest seat preparations, flexible or incorrectly located major and minor connectors, incorrect use of clasp designs, poor clasp selection.
- Laboratory support: inaccurate impression, poor support for analog procedures, lack of verification of framework fit whether frame manufacture through technology or analog production, lack of doctor prescription for manufacture for accuracy.
- Distal extension design: inadequate coverage of residual soft and hard tissues, failure to record supporting tissue accurately.
- Jaw and occlusal relations: failure to verify occlusal relations, failure to prescribe appropriate materials for sustainable occlusal relations.
- Professional interactions: failure of the dentist to provide adequate dental health care information, including details on care and use of the prosthesis, failure to prescribe need for hygiene and recall maintenance appointment frequency, failure in patient education to comply with necessary oral health regimen for long-term success.

A removable partial denture designed and fabricated or manufactured can provide a reliable treatment option for patients who are partially edentulous. This prosthetic treatment option is considered one at a reasonable cost, can be made to fit comfortably, and can provide functional support as a definitive prosthodontic treatment.

REFERENCES

1. Settineri S, Rizzo A, Liotta M, Mento C. Clinical psychology of oral health: the link between teeth and emotions. *Sage Open*. 2017;7(3). https://doi.org/10.1177/2158244017728319.
2. Al-Sahan MM, MacEntee MI, Bryant SR. A metatheory explaining how patients manage tooth loss. *Gerontology*. 2020;37(3):258–270.

3

Classification of Partially Edentulous Arches

Lisa A. Lang, Lily T. García, and Ahmed Mahrous

CHAPTER OUTLINE

Although recent reports suggest a consistent decline in the prevalence of tooth loss during the past few decades, significant variation in tooth loss distribution remains. It is helpful to consider the most common tooth loss patterns and use common classifications for the purpose of communicating management of partially edentulous patients.

A classification system based on diagnostic criteria has been proposed for partial edentulism.[1] The purpose of this system is to facilitate treatment decisions on the basis of treatment complexity. Complexity is determined by four broad diagnostic categories that include location and extent of the edentulous spaces, position and condition of the abutments, occlusal characteristics and requirements, and residual ridge characteristics. The advantage of this particular classification system over others in standard use has yet to be documented.

The Kennedy classification system is widely accepted in the classification of partially edentulous arches. To encourage universal use of a classification system, the Kennedy classification system will be used in this textbook.

The Kennedy classification system provides descriptions for partially edentulous arches. A removable partial denture treatment planned to restore a particular distribution of remaining teeth and edentulous space(s) is referred to by the class of arch as described by the Kennedy classification system. For example, a removable partial denture that is designed to restore a partially edentulous Kennedy Class II arch is often referred to as a "Kennedy Class II removable partial denture."

Several classification systems of partially edentulous arches exist. The variations in systems led to some confusion and disagreement concerning which classification best describes all possible configurations. The most familiar classification systems are those originally proposed by Kennedy; however, Cummer and Bailyn, Beckett, Godfrey, Swenson, Friedman, Wilson, Skinner, Applegate, Avant, Miller, and others have also proposed classifications. It is evident that an attempt should be made to combine the best features of all classifications so that a universal classification can be adopted.

REQUIREMENTS OF AN ACCEPTABLE METHOD OF CLASSIFICATION

The classification of a partially edentulous arch should satisfy the following requirements:

- It should permit immediate visualization of the type of partially edentulous arch that is being considered.
- It should permit immediate differentiation between the tooth-supported and the tooth- and tissue-supported removable partial denture.
- It should be universally acceptable.

KENNEDY CLASSIFICATION

The Kennedy method of classification was originally proposed by Dr. Edward Kennedy in 1925. It attempts to classify the partially edentulous arch in a manner that suggests certain principles of design for a given situation (Fig. 3.1).

Kennedy divided all partially edentulous arches into four basic classes. Edentulous areas other than those that determine the basic class were designated as modification spaces (Fig. 3.2).

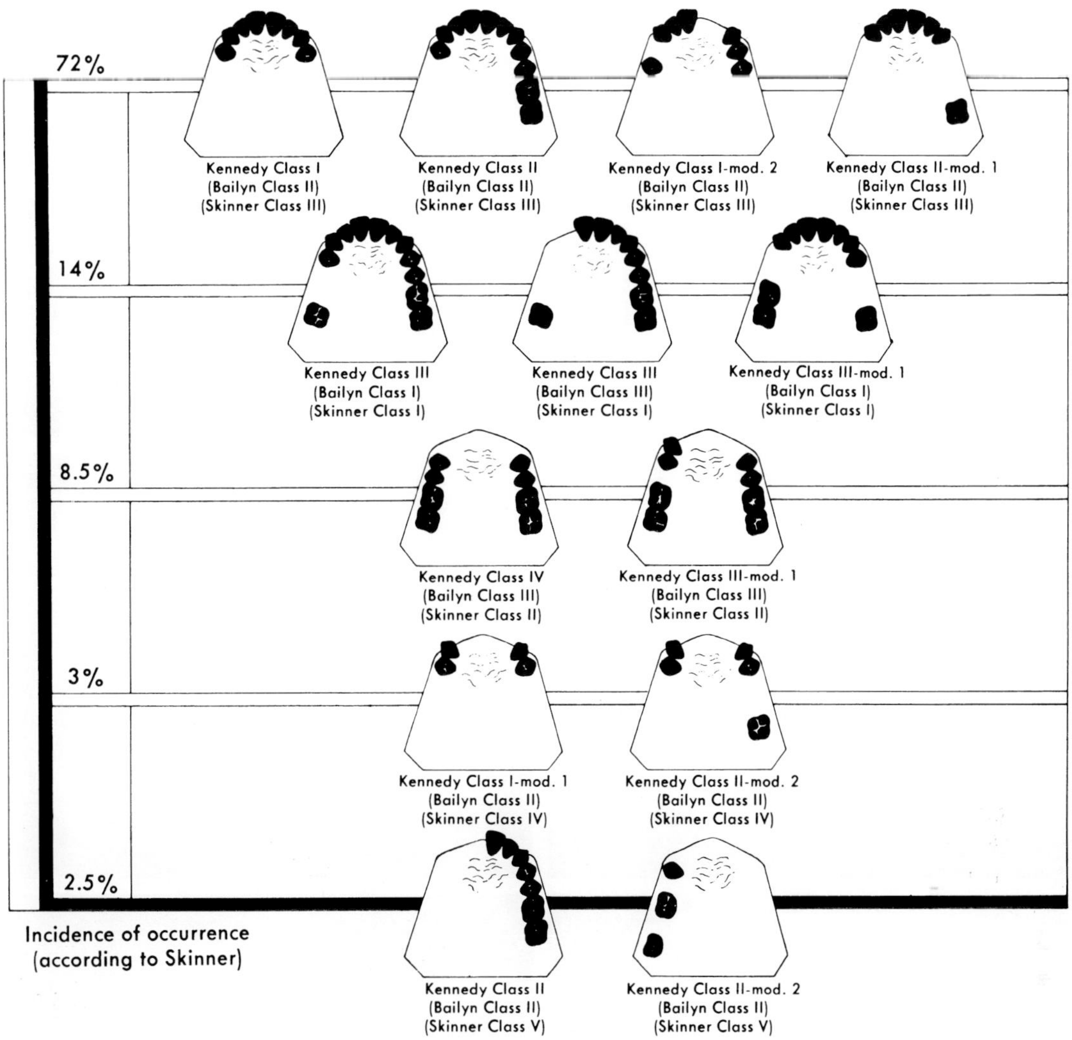

Fig. 3.1 Representative examples of partially edentulous arches classified by the Kennedy method. *mod.*, Modification.

The following is the Kennedy classification:

Class I	Bilateral edentulous areas located posterior to the natural teeth
Class II	A unilateral edentulous area located posterior to the remaining natural teeth
Class III	A unilateral edentulous area with natural teeth remaining both anterior and posterior to it
Class IV	A single, but bilateral (crossing the midline), edentulous area located anterior to the remaining natural teeth

One of the principal advantages of the Kennedy method is that it permits immediate visualization of the partially edentulous arch and allows easy distinction between tooth-supported versus tooth- and tissue-supported prostheses. Those schooled in its use and in the principles of removable partial denture design can readily relate the arch configuration design to be used in the basic removable partial denture. This method permits a systematic approach to the problems of design. It makes possible the application of sound principles of partial denture design and is therefore a logical method of classification. However, a classification system should not be used to stereotype or limit the concepts of design.

Additionally, implant placement can be used strategically to alter support in a distal extension base (the support similar to a tooth in a tooth-born segment). In this situation, understanding implant designations in future classifications, such as Kennedy Class Ii/i, Class IIi, and Class IVi, will improve communications.

APPLEGATE'S RULES FOR APPLYING THE KENNEDY CLASSIFICATION

The Kennedy classification is difficult to implement in every situation without certain rules for application. Applegate provided eight rules that govern the application of the Kennedy method (Box 3.1).

The principles of design are logical, although there is initial confusion why Class I refers to two edentulous spaces and Class II refers to one edentulous space. Kennedy placed the Class II unilateral edentulous space and unilateral distal extension type between the Class I bilateral distal extension classification and the Class III tooth-supported classification

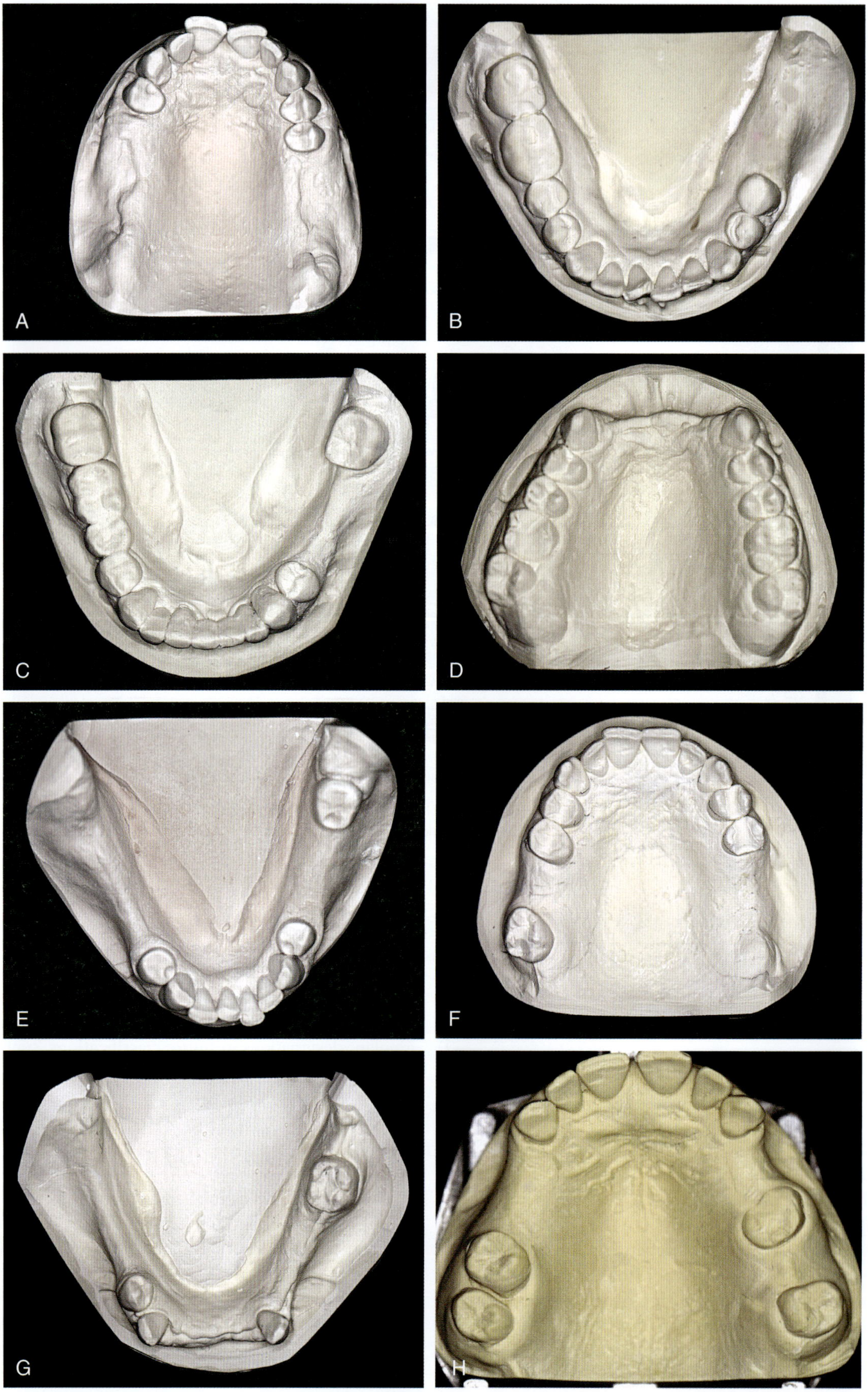

Fig. 3.2 Kennedy classification with examples of modifications. **A,** Class I maxillary arch. **B,** Class II mandibular arch. **C,** Class III mandibular arch. **D,** Class IV maxillary arch. **E,** Class II, modification 1 mandibular arch. **F,** Class II, modification 1 maxillary arch. **G,** Class II, modification 2 mandibular arch. **H,** Class III, modification 2 maxillary arch.

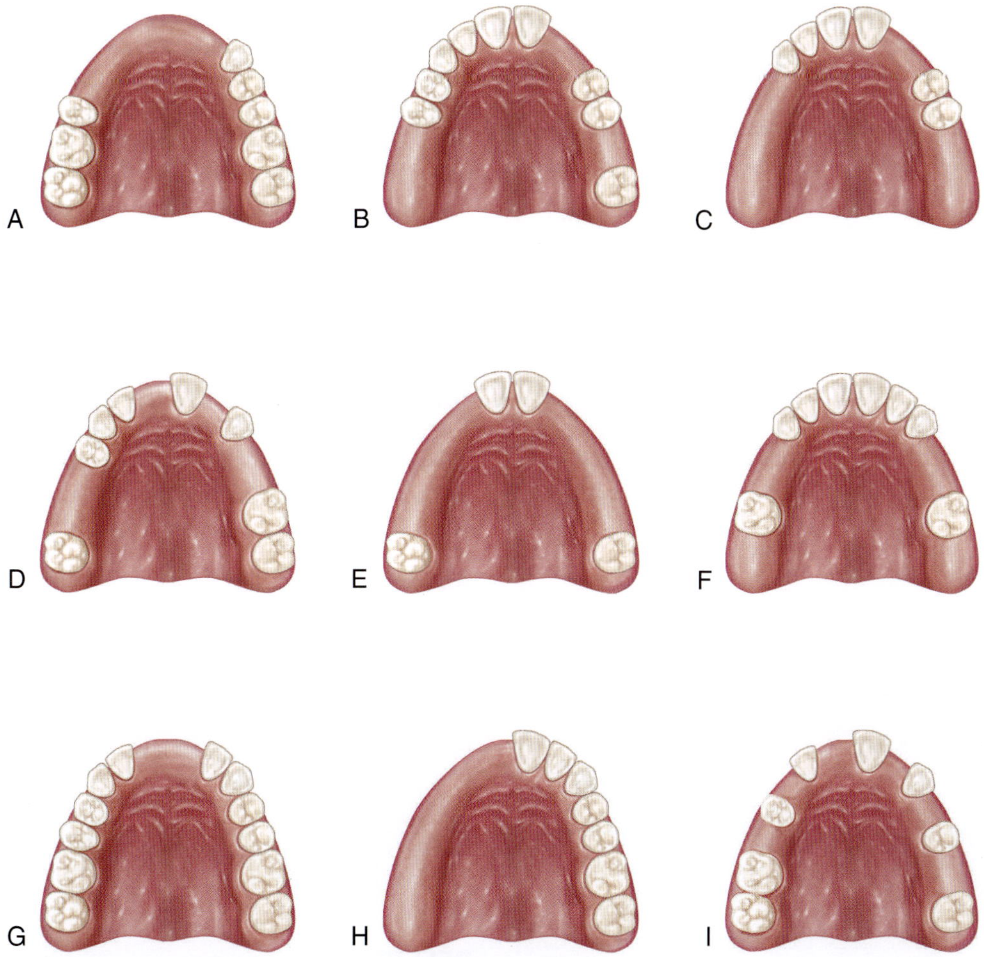

Fig. 3.3 A–I, Nine partially edentulous arch configurations. Identify each. Answers can be found at the end of this chapter.

BOX 3.1 Rules Governing Application of the Kennedy Method

Rule 1
Classification should follow rather than precede any extractions of teeth that might alter the original classification.

Rule 2
If a third molar is missing and is not to be replaced, it is not considered in the classification.

Rule 3
If a third molar is present and is to be used as an abutment, it is considered in the classification.

Rule 4
If a second molar is missing and is not to be replaced, it is not considered in the classification (e.g., if the opposing second molar is likewise missing and is not to be replaced).

Rule 5
The most posterior edentulous area (or areas) always determines the classification.

Rule 6
Edentulous areas other than those that determine the classification are referred to as *modifications* and are designated by their number.

Rule 7
The extent of the modification is not considered, only the number of additional edentulous areas.

Rule 8
No modification areas can be included in Class IV arches. (Other edentulous areas that lie posterior to the single bilateral areas crossing the midline would instead determine the classification; see Rule 5.)

because the Class II removable partial denture designation embodies features of both, especially when tooth-supported modifications are present. Since Class II has a tissue-supported, distal extension base, the removable partial denture must be designed similarly to a Class I removable partial denture. Often, however, Class III, a tooth-supported removable partial denture, has the component of an edentulous space present elsewhere in the arch. Thus the Class II removable partial denture design falls between Class I and Class III because it embodies design features common to both. In keeping with the principle that design is based on classification, the application of such principles of design is simplified by retaining the original classification of Kennedy.

Fig. 3.3 presents a chance to self-assess removable partial denture classification skills. Review the figure and classify the partially edentulous arches illustrated. The answers are provided at the end of this chapter.

Answers to Fig. 3.3

A. Class IV
B. Class II, modification 2
C. Class I, modification 1
D. Class III, modification 3
E. Class III, modification 1
F. Class III, modification 1
G. Class IV
H. Class II
I. Class III, modification 5

REFERENCE

1. McGarry TJ, Nimmo A, Skiba JF, et al. Classification system for partial edentulism. *J Prosthodont*. 2002;11(3):181–193.

4

Biomechanics of Removable Partial Dentures

Lisa A. Lang, Lily T. García, and Ahmed Mahrous

CHAPTER OUTLINE

To provide a patient with a functional removable partial denture (RPD) prosthesis, the design should maximize the stability of the prosthesis. RPDs are not rigidly attached to the teeth, so the control of potential movements under functional load is critical to prosthesis stability and patient accommodation. Prosthesis movement results from load stress applied to the teeth and tissues in contact with the prosthesis. It is important that the stress not exceed the level of physiologic tolerance, which is a range of mechanical stimulus that a system can resist without disruption or traumatic consequences. In the terminology of engineering mechanics, the prosthesis induces stress in the tissue equal to the force applied across the area of contact with the teeth and/or tissue. This same stress acts to produce strain in the supporting tissue, which results in load displacement in the teeth and tissue. The understanding of how mechanical phenomena act within a biological environment, unique to each patient, is discussed in terms of biomechanics (Box 4.1). In the design of RPDs, with a focus on the goal of providing and maintaining stable prostheses, consideration of basic biomechanical principles associated with the unique features of each mouth is essential. Oral hygiene and appropriate prosthesis maintenance procedures are required for continued benefit of optimum biomechanical principles. RPDs by design are intended to be removable—placed into and removed from the mouth since the prosthesis is not rigidly connected to the teeth or tissue. The removable feature subjects the prosthesis to movement in response to functional loads, such as those created by mastication. It is important for clinicians who provide RPD service to understand the potential for prosthesis movements under function and to be able to incorporate RPD components into the design to mitigate and control movement. In the masticatory cycle, the patient begins mastication (the mandible moves upward), the opposing teeth come into contact with the bolus (C), causing the mandibular denture base to move toward the residual ridge (Fig. 4.1, *A*). As the mandible completes the chewing stroke and opens (moving downward), the mandibular denture base moves upward away from the supporting tissue. This movement results in a rotational movement of the denture base with the proximal portion rotating in a downward movement toward the supporting ridge (see Fig. 4.1, *B*). Animation of this action may be seen in the Hyperlink to the Video 4.1.

BOX 4.1 Design Process for Removable Partial Dentures

Need
Tooth replacement

Definition of Problem
Provision of stable removable prosthesis

Objectives
Limited functional movement within tooth-tissue tolerance

Background Information
Forces of occlusion, tissue "load-displacement" character and potential for movement, biomechanical principles applied to specific features of this unique mouth, removable partial denture component parts assigned to control movement

Choice of a Solution (Among Alternatives) for Application
Based on prior experience, principles and concepts learned from school and textbooks, and applicable clinical research

BIOMECHANICAL CONSIDERATIONS

Biomechanical considerations provide background principles of movement associated with RPDs along with sequelae to the movement. Subsequent chapters cover the various components and describe how these components are incorporated into the design to control the resultant movements of prostheses.

The supporting intraoral structures for RPDs (abutment teeth and residual alveolar ridges) are dynamic elements that are subjected to mechanical forces. Biomechanical consideration of forces generated during function includes the direction, duration, frequency, and magnitude of the force. In the final analysis, it is the alveolar bone that provides the support for a removable prosthesis, that is, the alveolar bone by way of the periodontal ligament and the residual alveolar ridge through soft tissue

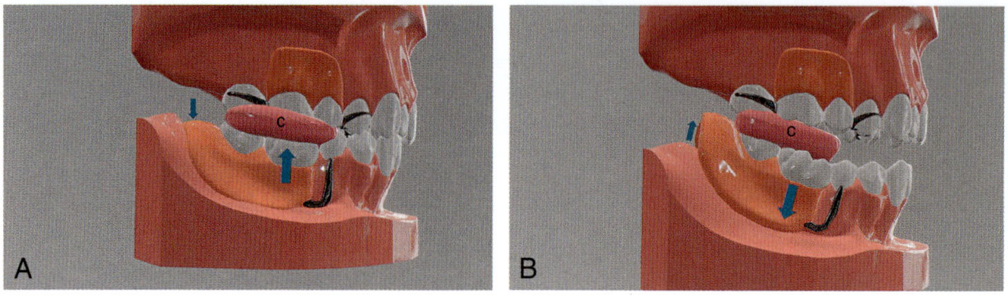

Fig. 4.1 Movement of the removable partial denture during mastication. **(A)** Large arrow represents mandibular movement upward toward the opposing arch, *C*= bolus, small arrow represents the movement of the prosthesis. This figure demonstrates the movement of the distal extension removable partial denture during function. The pink object *(C)* is a sticky food substance or bolus. **A,** During mastication as the patient bites into the object, forces are transmitted to the distal extension portion of the removable partial denture, and because of the compressible nature of the tissues in that area, the result is the downwards movement of the distal extension area. **B,** As the patient continues on the chewing stroke and opens the mouth, the sticky substance acts to "pull" the distal extension area upwards causing the distal extension area to lift off the tissues. It is worth noting that no such movement is seen on the maxillary tooth-supported removable partial denture as both sides of the removable partial denture are supported and retained by the abutment teeth.(Courtesy of Ahmed Mahrous Copyright © 2024. All rights reserved.)

covering. The forces that occur because of the removable prosthesis function can be distributed and directed broadly, resulting in minimizing the effect by appropriate design of the RPD. An appropriate design includes the selection and location of components in conjunction with a harmonious occlusion that will counteract those forces.

RPDs can move in a variety of directions under functional loads. Fig. 4.2 illustrates the movement of a mandibular RPD around the sagittal (A), the frontal (B), and the horizontal (C) planes. Distal extension RPDs will rotate when force is directed on the denture base. Differences in the displaceability of the periodontal ligament of the supporting abutment teeth and soft tissue covering the residual ridge permit this rotation, which occurs as a combination of various directions rather than in a unidirectional manner. The three possible movements of distal extension RPDs are (A) rotation around a fulcrum line passing through the most posterior abutments when the denture base moves vertically toward or away from the supporting residual ridges; (B) rotation around a longitudinal axis formed by the crest of the residual ridge; and (C) rotation around a vertical axis located near the center of the arch.

An understanding of simple machines applied to the design of RPDs helps when trying to mitigate movements to prevent unnecessary and potentially harmful forces on intraoral structures. The results of an improperly designed RPD can result in destructive forces and damage to intraoral support over the long term.

Machines may be classified into two general categories: simple and complex. The six simple machines are lever, wedge, screw, wheel and axle, pulley, and inclined plane. Of the simple machines, the lever form best represents the design of RPDs. In its simplest form, a lever is a rigid bar supported somewhere along its length. The support point of the lever is called the *fulcrum* (Fig. 4.3, *A*), and the lever can move around the fulcrum. There are three types of levers: first, second, and third class. This is determined based on the anteroposterior relationship of the fulcrum to the effort and resistance of the lever. Fig. 4.3, *B–D* describes each lever classification and the relationship of the fulcrum to the effort and resistance. To further understand how lever systems apply to RPD designs, Fig. 4.4 describes the three lever classifications as applied to edentulous spaces in RPDs.

RPDs that lack posterior tooth-borne support (Kennedy Class I and II) can mimic the dynamics of levers. In those configurations, the fulcrum is represented by a line that connects the most posterior rests around which the RPD may rotate (Fig. 4.5).

This line is called "the fulcrum line" and is the center of rotation as the extension base moves toward the supporting tissue when an occlusal load is applied. Fig. 4.6, *A* depicts this movement from the lateral view. Movement of the base in the opposite direction is caused by the effect of sticky foods when the mouth is opened (see Fig. 4.6, *B* Video 4.6). If the fulcrum line exists between the edentulous span and the clasp tip, it creates a first-class lever configuration. This is called "*a cantilever*" and should be avoided as it generates unnecessary stress onto the abutment tooth (Fig. 4.7, Video 4.7).

MANAGING STRESS WITH CLASP DESIGN

Even though the actual movement of the denture may be small, the lever force can be imposed on the abutment teeth. This is especially detrimental when prosthesis maintenance is neglected. The potential of a lever system to magnify a force is illustrated in Fig. 4.8. The most efficient mechanism to avoid that stress is to change the configuration of the first-class lever to a second-class lever. This is done by moving the fulcrum line to be ahead of both the clasp and the edentulous space. Fig. 4.9 (Video 4.9) illustrates how by placing the clasp tip between the fulcrum line and the edentulous span the lever becomes a Class II lever. This may be done by placing a rest seat on the mesial of the abutment tooth, thereby making the fulcrum anterior to the clasp tip. With this configuration, the distal denture base portion (cantilever) of the RPD rotates downward toward the supporting residual ridge and the anterior portion of the clasp

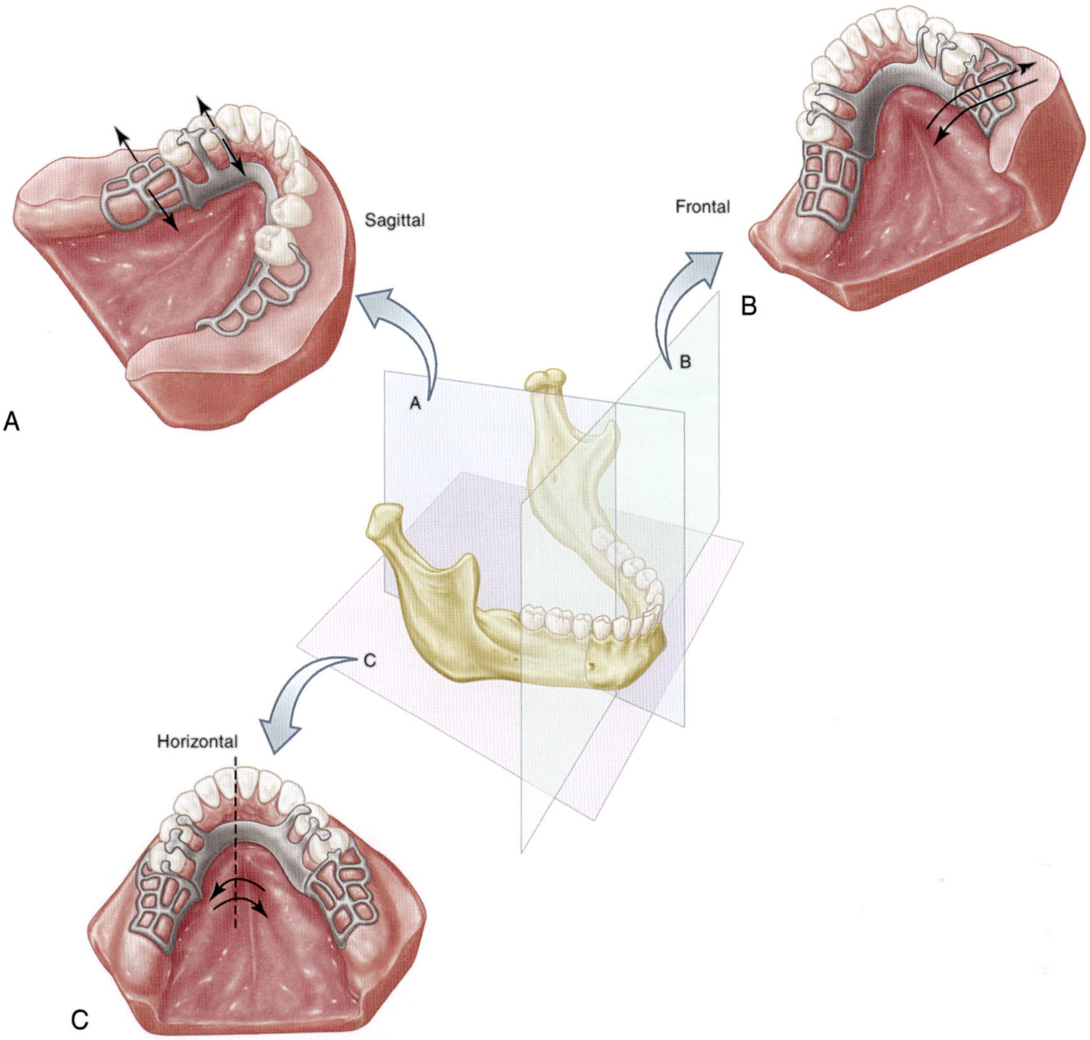

Fig. 4.2 Direction of removable partial denture around the planes. Sagittal **(A)**, frontal **(B)**, and horizontal **(C)** planes. Distal extension removable partial dentures will rotate when force is directed on the denture base. Differences in the displaceability of the periodontal ligament of the supporting abutment teeth and soft tissue covering the residual ridge permit this rotation. Rotation of the prosthesis occurs in a combination of directions rather than in a unidirectional way. The three possible movements of distal extension removable partial dentures are around the **(A)** sagittal, rotation around a fulcrum line passing through the most posterior abutments when the denture base moves vertically toward or away from the supporting residual ridges; **(B)** frontal, rotation around a longitudinal axis formed by the crest of the residual ridge; and **(C)** horizontal axis, rotation around a vertical axis located near the center of the arch.

tip also rotates downward. Additionally, placing a rest seat with a minor connector anterior to the fulcrum line is another way in which the design of the RPD can resist rotational movement around the fulcrum line.

Another design component used to reduce stress on the abutment tooth is accomplished by using a flexible clasp such as a wrought wire clasp. More information on managing stress with "stress-breaking" clasp designs will be discussed in Chapters 7 and 10.

Other possible partial denture movements include rotation about the longitudinal and vertical axes that occur under function because diagonal and horizontal occlusal forces are brought to bear on the RPD (see Fig. 4.2). Longitudinal forces are resisted by the rigidity of the major and minor connectors, while diagonal forces are resisted by reciprocal clasp arms and minor connectors that are in contact with vertical tooth surfaces. Stabilizing components on one side of the arch act to stabilize the partial denture against horizontal forces applied from the opposite side.

Horizontal forces always will exist to some degree because of lateral stresses that occur during mastication, bruxism, clenching, and other patient habits. These forces are accentuated by failure to consider the orientation of the occlusal plane, the influence of malpositioned teeth in the arch, and the effects of abnormal jaw relationships. Developing an occlusion that is in harmony with the opposing dentition and that is free of lateral interference during eccentric jaw movements may minimize the magnitude of lateral stress. The amount of horizontal movement occurring in the RPD, therefore, depends on the magnitude of the lateral forces

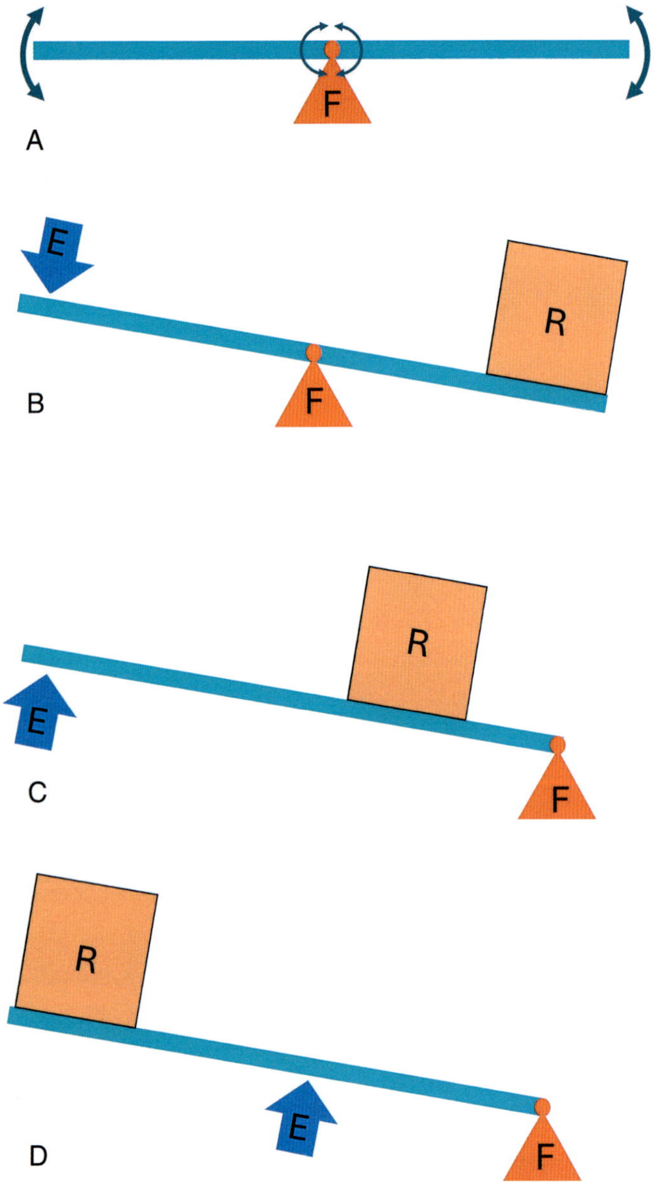

Fig. 4.3 Leverage classifications. **A,** In its simplest form, a lever is a rigid bar supported along its length. It is composed of an arm supported by a fulcrum. The support point *(F)* is the fulcrum. The fulcrum acts as a swivel around which the arm may rotate. **B,** A Class I lever is one where the fulcrum *(F)* exists between the force being exerted *(E)* and the resistance to movement *(R)*. Any movement of the effort arm will result in the movement of the resistance arm in an opposite direction. **C,** A Class II lever is one where the resistance *(R)* exists between the effort *(E)* and the fulcrum *(F)*. In this configuration, the resistance moves in the same direction as the effort being exerted. **D,** A Class III lever is one where the effort *(E)* exists between the resistance *(R)* and the fulcrum. Like the second-class levers, the resistance also moves in the same direction as the effort arm. (Courtesy of Ahmed Mahrous Copyright © 2024. All rights reserved.)

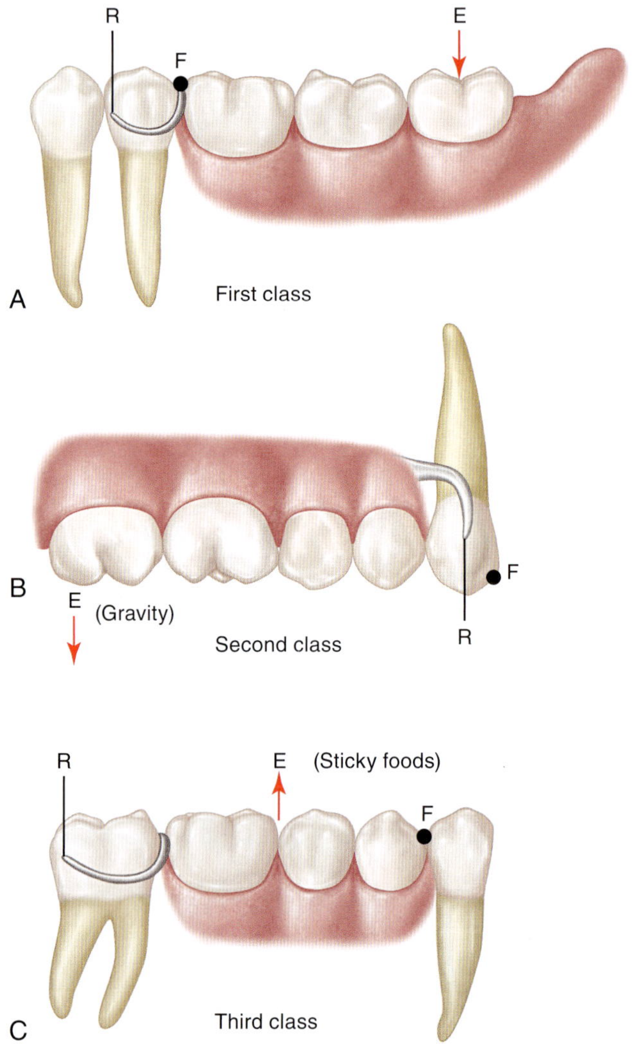

Fig. 4.4 **A** to **C,** The three classes of levers. Classification is based on the location of the fulcrum *(F)*, resistance *(R)*, and direction of effort (force) *(E)*. In dental terms, *E* can represent the force of occlusion or gravity, *F* can be a tooth surface such as an occlusal rest, and *R* is the resistance provided by a direct retainer or a guide plane surface.

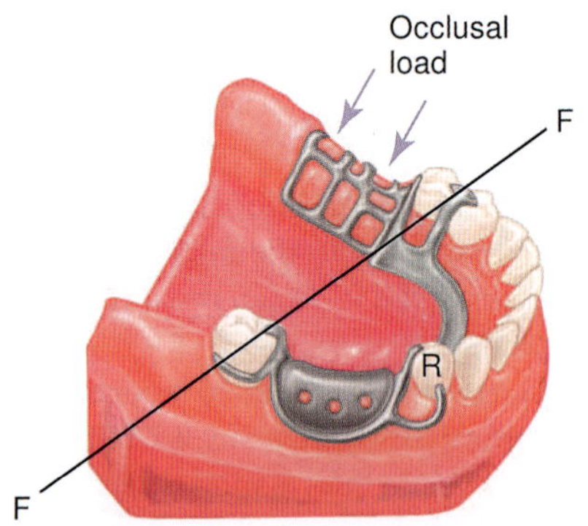

Fig. 4.5 The fulcrum line. On a removable partial denture, the fulcrum line *(F)* is an imaginary line that extends through the two terminal rests on an extension base removable partial denture around which the removable partial denture may rotate under function. When an occlusal load is directed on the extension base(s), there is movement toward the tissue resulting in rotation around the fulcrum line. Tissue support from the extension base area is important to minimize the lever action of the clasp. Additional direct or indirect retainer design could help accommodate minimizing force during the rotation of the denture base. This movement may be seen from the lateral view using this link (Video 4.5).

that are applied and on the effectiveness of the stabilizing components.

A tooth is better able to tolerate vertically directed forces than nonvertical, torquing, or horizontal forces. This characteristic is observed clinically, and it seems rational that more periodontal fibers are activated to resist the application of vertical forces to teeth than are activated to resist the application of nonvertical forces (Fig. 4.10). This statement holds true when

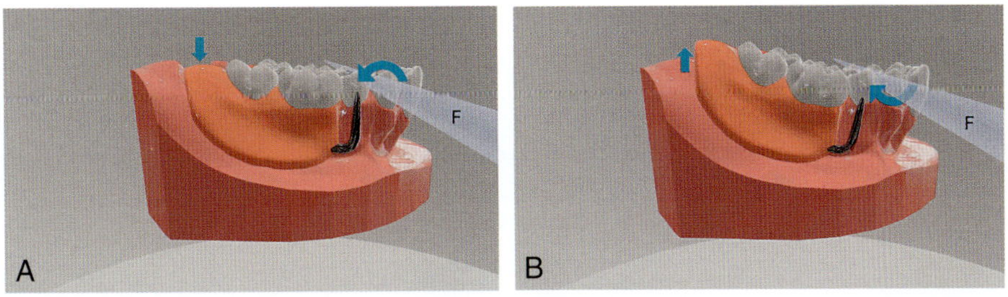

Fig. 4.6 Movement around the fulcrum line from the lateral view. The fulcrum line, an imaginary line that extends through the two terminal rests on an extension base removable partial denture (RPD) around which the removable partial denture may rotate under function, is depicted by *(F)* in this lateral view of an RPD. **A,** When the RPD is subjected to occlusal loads, the possible movements of the RPD extension base are counterclockwise and toward the supporting tissue. **B,** When the RPD is subjected to pulling forces, such as when eating sticky foods, the possible movements of the RPD extension base are clockwise and away from the supporting tissues. (Courtesy of Ahmed Mahrous Copyright © 2024. All rights reserved.)

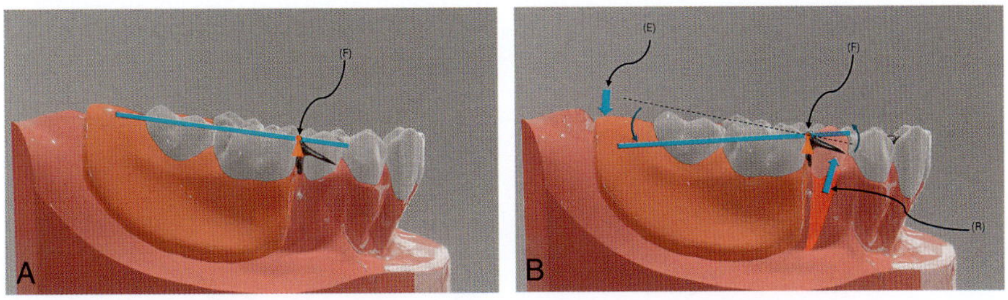

Fig. 4.7 Class I lever removable partial denture (RPD). A distal extension RPD can act as a Class I lever if the fulcrum line *(F)* connecting the terminal rests exists between the clasp and the edentulous span. The effort *(E)* represents the occlusal load being applied to the extension base. The result is a downwards movement of the denture base due to the compressibility of the tissues and a corresponding opposite movement of the resistance arm *(R)* representing the clasp. As the clasp moves upwards, it subjects the tooth to potentially damaging torquing forces. **A,** The fulcrum line is positioned between the clasp tip and the edentulous span, creating a cantilever (the edentulous span is distal to the fulcrum in this RPD design). **B,** As force is applied *(E)*, the distal denture base portion (cantilever) of the RPD rotates downward toward the supporting residual ridge and the anterior portion of the clasp tip rotates upward against the tooth. *E*, Effort/force; *F*, fulcrum; *R*, load. (Courtesy of Ahmed Copyright © 2024. All rights reserved.)

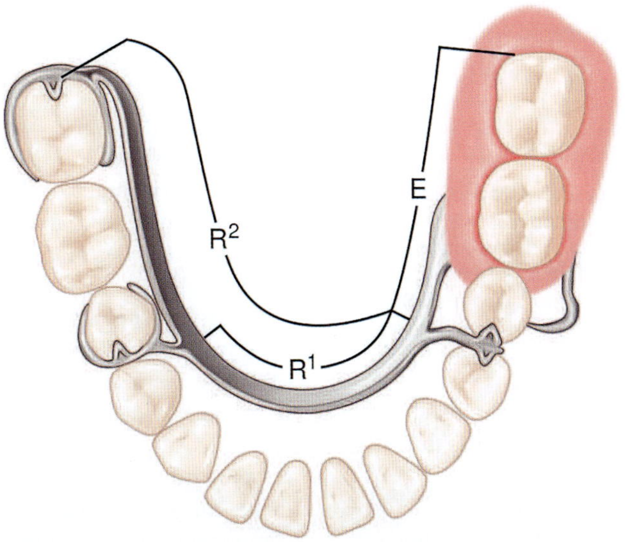

Fig. 4.8 The potential of a lever system to magnify force. In the removable partial denture pictured, the fulcrum support point occurs at the rest seat between the premolars (teeth #20 and #21). The fulcrum line is the line drawn between those premolars and the distal rest on tooth #31. The portion of the lever from the fulcrum to the point of application of force is called the *effort arm (E)*. The length of the lever from fulcrum to resistance *(R)* is called the *resistance arm*. Whenever the effort arm is longer than the resistance arm, the mechanical advantage favors the effort arm, proportionately to the difference in the length of the two arms. In other words, when the effort arm is twice the length of the resistance arm, a 25-lb weight on the effort arm will balance a 50-lb weight at the end of the resistance arm. The opposite is also true and helps illustrate cross-arch stabilization. When the resistance arm is lengthened (cross-arch clasp assembly placed on a second molar *[R^2]* vs. a second premolar *[R^1]*), the effort arm is more efficiently counteracted.

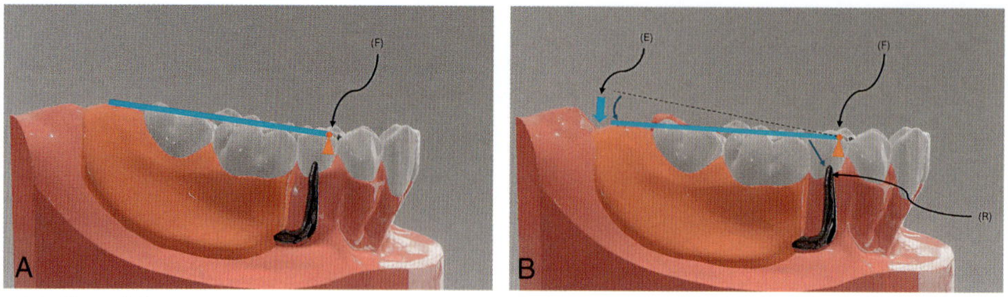

Fig. 4.9 Class II lever removable partial denture (RPD). **A,** Stress-breaking clasp assemblies on extension base RPD can reduce stress on the abutment tooth by transforming the lever system into a second-class lever. By placing the clasp tip between the fulcrum line *(F)* and the edentulous span (denture base), the lever becomes a Class II lever. This may be done by placing a rest seat on the mesial of the abutment tooth, thereby making the fulcrum anterior to the clasp tip. **B,** As the RPD is subjected to occlusal load, force is applied *(E)* depressing the distal denture base portion (cantilever) of the RPD rotating downward toward the supporting residual ridge, and the anterior portion of the clasp tip also rotates downward. Because the clasp moves in the same direction as the effort and disengages from the retentive undercut, it does not subject the tooth to excessive force. *E*, Effort/force; *F*, fulcrum; *R*, load. (Courtesy of Ahmed Mahrous Copyright © 2024. All rights reserved.)

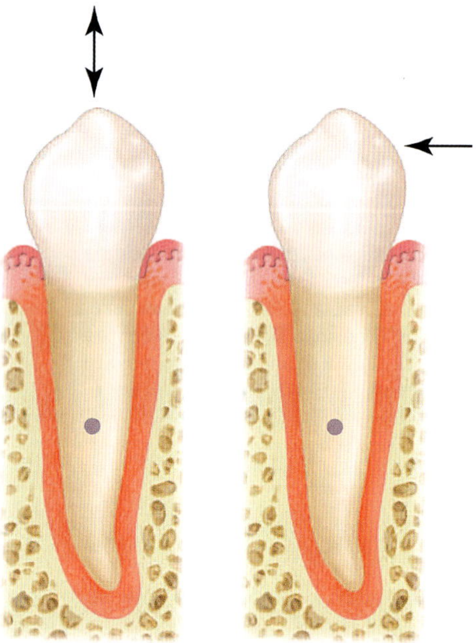

Fig. 4.10 When forces are applied vertically (down the long axis of the tooth), there are more periodontal fibers activated that can resist those vertically directed forces. When forces are applied horizontally (off-axis or lateral to the long axis of the tooth), fewer periodontal fibers are activated to resist the horizontally directed force. The horizontal axis of rotation is located somewhere in the root of the tooth.

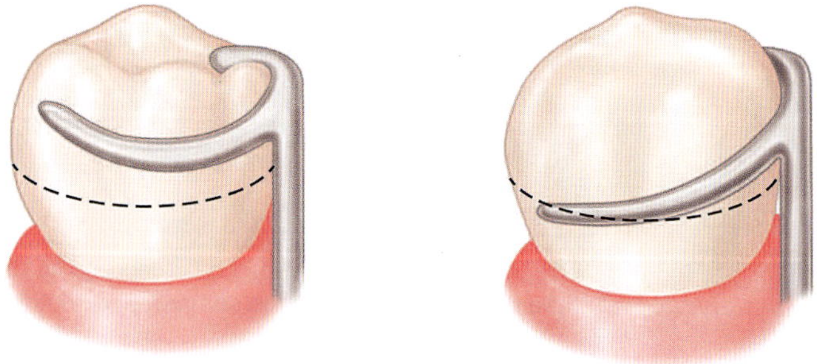

Fig. 4.11 Clasp assembly. The ideal location for the clasp to resist nonvertical forces is to place the clasp closer to the horizontal axis. The reciprocating arm, which is used to brace the tooth, is placed above the height of contour of the tooth on the lingual aspect of the tooth, where the tip of the clasp arm is placed below the height of contour of the tooth on the buccal aspect. Dotted line depicts the height of the contour of the tooth.

analyzing biomechanical forces applied to an abutment tooth. The abutment tooth will better tolerate vertical forces than nonvertical that may be rotational in nature.

However, an abutment tooth may tolerate nonvertical forces if these forces are applied as near as possible to the horizontal axis of rotation of the abutment. The nonvertical occlusal forces may be resisted by the reciprocating or bracing arm of the clasp assembly of the abutment tooth and by placing the clasp tip closer to the horizontal axis. The reciprocating arm is placed above the height of the contour of the tooth where the tip of the clasp arm is placed below the height of the contour of the tooth (Fig. 4.11). When the location of the height of the contour does not allow for ideal positioning of the clasp to be near the horizontal axis of rotation, the axial surface contours of the abutment teeth must be altered to locate the components of clasp assemblies more favorably in relation to the horizontal axis (Fig. 4.12).

In a tooth-supported RPD, the movement of the base toward the edentulous ridge is prevented primarily by the rests on the abutment teeth and to an extent by any rigid portion of the framework located occlusal to the height of contour.

For prostheses capable of movement in three planes, occlusal rests provide occlusal support only to resist tissue-ward movement. All other movements of the RPD should be resisted by components other than occlusal rests. Entrance of the occlusal rest into a stabilizing function would result in direct transfer of torque to the abutment tooth. Because movements around three different axes are possible in a distal extension RPD, occlusal rest seat preparation for such a removable partial denture should not have steep vertical walls or locking dovetails. This rest design is characterized by the lack of free movement,

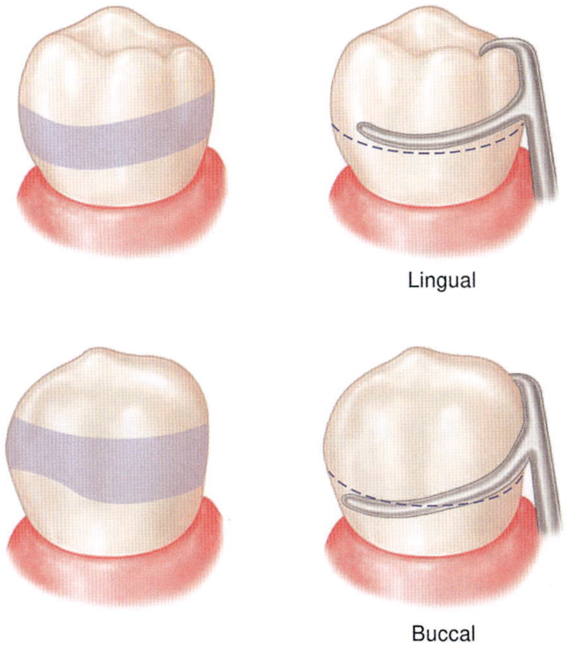

Fig. 4.12 The abutment tooth has been contoured *(see shaded region)* to allow for favorable locations of retentive and reciprocal stabilizing components *(mirror view)*.

which could cause horizontal and torquing forces to be applied intracoronally to the abutment tooth. In the tooth-supported RPD, the only movements of any significance are horizontal, and these may be resisted by the stabilizing effects of components placed on the axial surfaces of the abutments. Therefore in the tooth-supported RPD, the use of intracoronal rests is permissible. In these instances, the rests provide not only occlusal support, but also notable horizontal stabilization. In contrast, all Kennedy Class I and Class II RPDs, which have one or more distal extension bases, are not totally tooth supported. Neither are they completely retained by bounding abutments. Any extensive Kennedy Class III or Class IV RPD that does not have adequate abutment support falls into the same category. These latter dentures may derive some support from the edentulous ridge and therefore may have composite support from both teeth and ridge tissue.

5

Major and Minor Connectors

Lisa A. Lang, Lily T. García, and Ahmed Mahrous

CHAPTER OUTLINE

Selection of a major connector in the design of a removable partial denture is important to note since the role of the major connector is to join components on one side of the arch to those on the opposite side of the arch.[1] When the respective component parts of a removable partial denture are joined through an effective connection, the individual components contribute to the overall performance of a prosthesis.

Components of a typical removable partial denture are illustrated in Fig. 5.1.

1. Major connectors
2. Minor connectors
3. Rests
4. Direct retainers
5. Stabilizing or reciprocal components (as parts of a clasp assembly)
6. Indirect retainers (if the prosthesis has distal extension bases)
7. One or more bases, each supporting from one to several replacement teeth (see Fig. 5.1)

The chief functions of a major connector include unification of the components of the prosthesis, distribution of applied forces throughout the arch to selected teeth and tissue, and minimization of torque to individual teeth. A properly designed rigid major connector effectively distributes forces throughout the arch and acts to reduce the load to any one anatomical area while effectively controlling prosthesis movement.

A removable prosthesis by design allows for both insertion and removal from the mouth and must extend to both sides of the arch. The bilateral design enables the transfer of functional occlusal forces generated to all supporting teeth and tissues for optimum stability. It is through this cross-arch tooth contact, which occurs at some distance from the functional force, that optimum resistance can be achieved. This is most effectively accomplished when a rigid major connector joins the portion of the prosthesis receiving the function to selected regions throughout the arch.

The principles of leverage relate to the major connector. A rigid major connector limits movement possibilities by acting as a counteracting lever. This phenomenon is referred to as *cross-arch stabilization*. Cross-arch stability becomes more important in situations associated with a high potential for greater prosthesis movement (e.g., unilateral or bilateral distal extension bases).

Major and minor connectors are considered separately as to their function, location, and design criteria as follows. Other components are presented in separate chapters.

ROLE OF MAJOR CONNECTORS IN CONTROL OF PROSTHESIS MOVEMENT

The major connector component in a removable partial denture connects components of the prosthesis located on one side of the arch with those on the contralateral side, either directly or indirectly attached. By connecting all design components, the major connector provides cross-arch stability to help resist displacement caused by functional stresses.

The major connector may be compared with the frame of an automobile or with the foundation of a building. It is through the major connector that other components of the removable partial denture are unified. If the major connector is flexible under functional stresses, the other removable partial denture–connected components may be rendered ineffective. The ineffectiveness of connected components jeopardizes the health of supporting oral structures and can be a detriment to the comfort of the patient. Failure to design a rigid major connector can result in traumatic damage to the periodontal support of the abutment teeth, injury to residual alveolar ridges, or

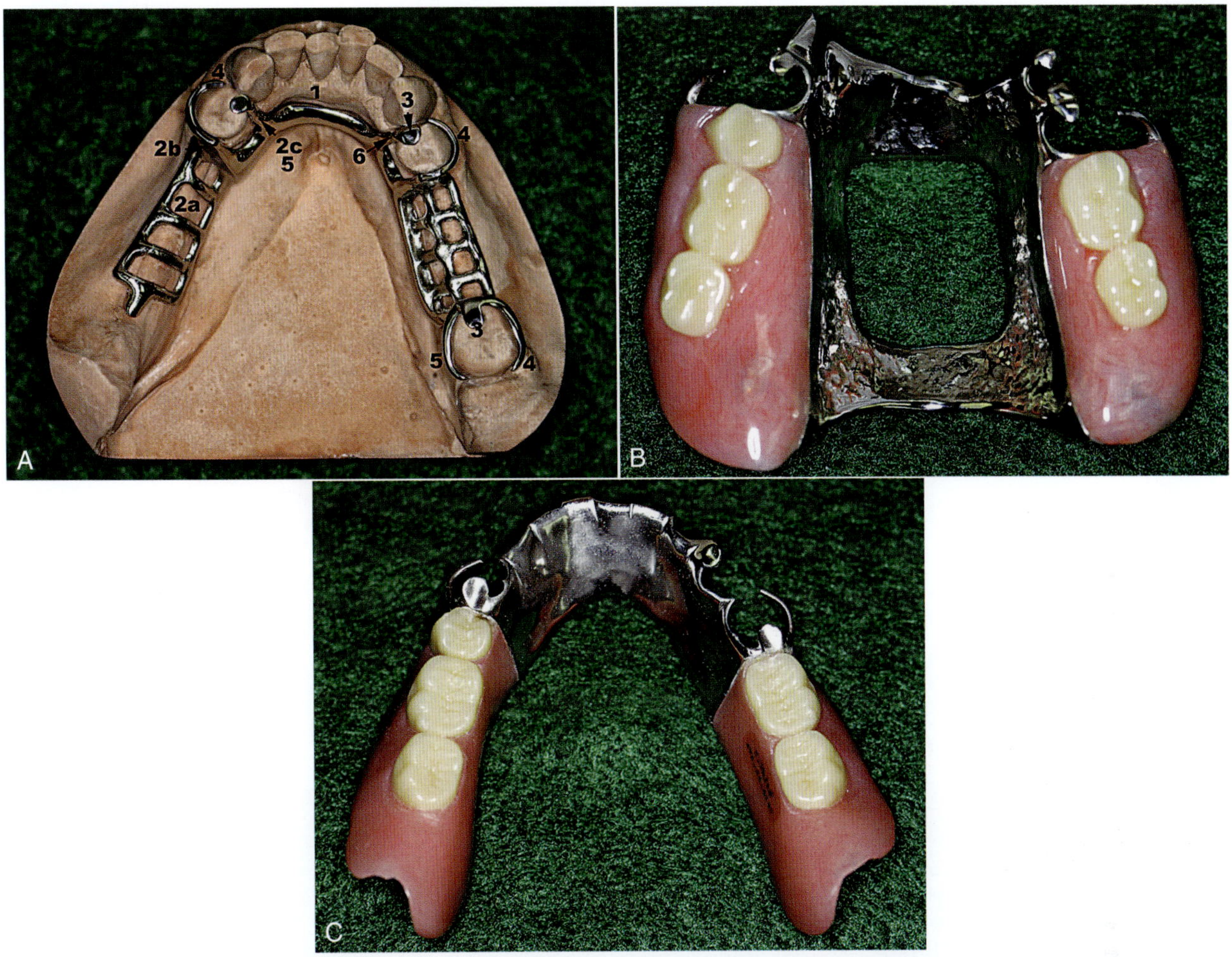

Fig. 5.1 A, Framework for mandibular removable partial denture with the following components: *1,* lingual bar major connector; *2a,* minor connector by which the resin denture base will be attached; *2b,* minor connector, proximal plate, which is part of the clasp assembly; *2c,* minor connector used to connect rests to major connectors; *3,* occlusal rests; *4,* direct retainer arm, which is part of the total clasp assembly; *5,* stabilizing or reciprocal components of clasp assembly (includes minor connectors); and *6,* an indirect retainer consisting of a minor connector and an occlusal rest. **B,** Maxillary removable partial denture with resin denture bases supporting artificial posterior teeth. Bases are attached to metal framework by ladderlike minor connectors similar to those seen in *2a.* **C,** Mandibular bilateral distal extension removable partial denture with resin denture bases supporting artificial posterior teeth.

impingement of underlying tissues. It is the dentist's responsibility to ensure that appropriate design and fabrication of the major connector are accomplished.

Location

Major connectors should be designed following the guidelines as listed:

1. Major connectors should be free of movable tissue.
2. Impingement of gingival tissue should be avoided.
3. Bony and soft tissue prominences should be avoided during placement and removal.
4. Relief should be provided beneath a major connector to prevent its settling into areas of possible interference, such as inoperable tori or elevated median palatal sutures.
5. Major connectors should be located and/or relieved to prevent impingement of tissue that occurs because the distal extension denture rotates in function.

Appropriate relief beneath the major connector prevents the need for its adjustment after tissue damage has occurred. If relief on the intaglio surface of the major connector is not incorporated into the design to relieve tissue impingement, postfabrication adjustment by grinding the intaglio surface of the major connector is both time consuming and can weaken the major connector, resulting in flexibility or possibly fracture. Major connectors should be carefully designed for proper shape, thickness, and location. Alteration of component dimensions after fabrication by grinding can be detrimental. Relief on the intaglio surface of a major connection is discussed further.

The margins of a major connector adjacent to gingival tissue should be located to avoid any possible tissue impingement. The distance recommended between the borders of a major connector and the soft tissue is based on the type of major connector designed. To accomplish this in the mandibular arch, the superior border of a lingual bar major connector should be located

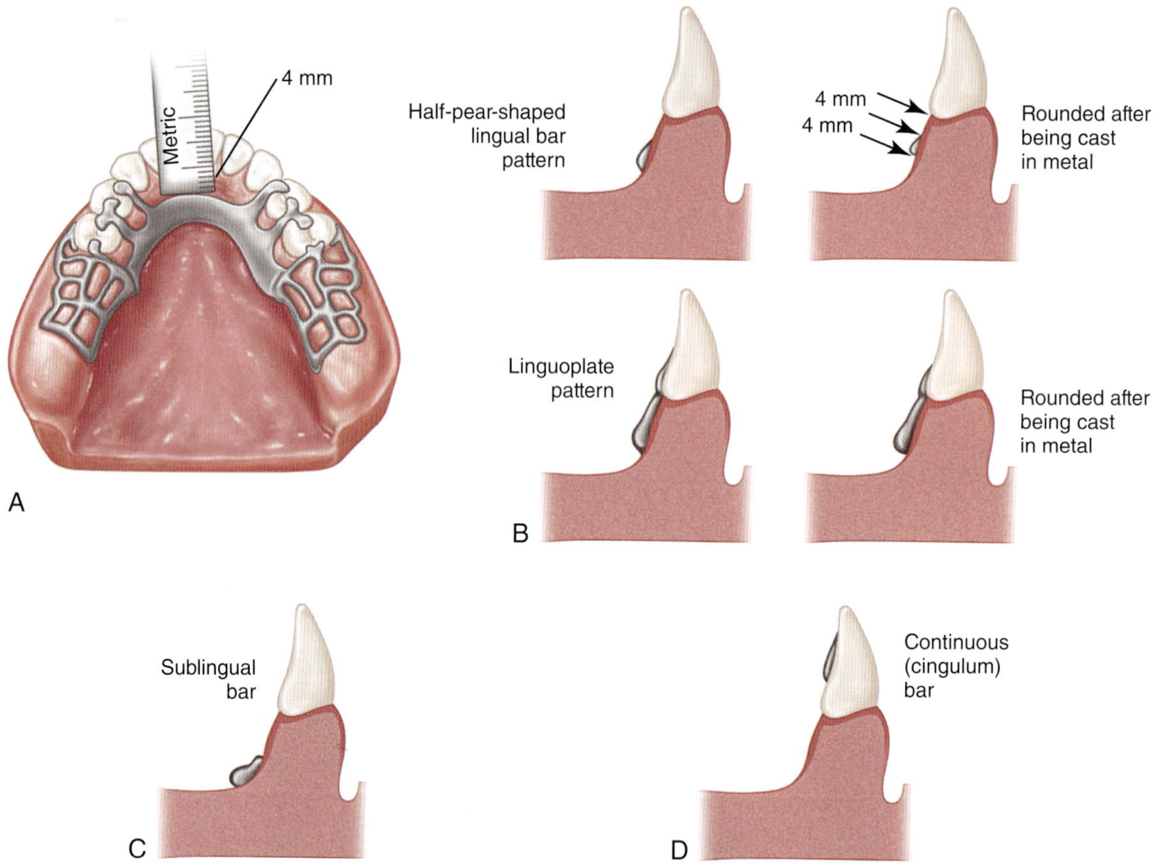

Fig. 5.2 A, Lingual bar major connector should be located at least 4 mm inferior to gingival margins and farther if possible. The vertical height of a finished lingual bar should be at least 4 mm for strength and rigidity. If less than 8 mm exists between gingival margins and the movable floor of the mouth, a lingual plate **(B)**, a sublingual bar **(C)**, or a continuous bar **(D)** is preferred as a major connector. Relief is provided for soft tissue under all portions of the mandibular major connector and at any location where the framework crosses the marginal gingiva. The inferior border of mandibular major connectors should be gently rounded after being cast to eliminate a sharp edge.

a minimum of 4 mm below the gingival margin(s) (Fig. 5.2). At the inferior border of the lingual bar major connector, the limiting factor is the height of the movable tissue in the floor of the mouth. Considering that the major connector must have sufficient width and bulk to provide rigidity, a linguoplate is commonly used when there is insufficient space, less than 8 mm between the gingival margin and the movable floor of the mouth is normally required for use of a lingual bar major connector.

In the maxillary arch, because there is less movable tissue present in the palate as compared to the floor of the mouth, the borders of a maxillary major connector may be placed well away from the gingival tissue. Structurally, the soft tissues covering the palate are well suited for the placement of the connector due to the presence of firm submucosal connective tissue and an adequate, deep blood supply. The soft tissue covering the palatal midline is less displaceable than the tissue covering the residual ridge, varying amounts of relief under the major connector must be provided to avoid tissue impingement. The amount of relief required is directly proportional to the difference in the displaceability of the tissue covering the midline of the palate and the tissue covering the residual ridges. The gingival tissue, on the other hand, must have an unrestricted superficial blood supply to remain healthy. To accomplish this, it is recommended that the borders of the palatal major connector be placed crossing perpendicular across the free gingival margins. The major connector should be designed at least a minimum of 6 mm away from and parallel to the gingival margins. Minor connectors that must cross the gingival tissue should do so abruptly, designed to connect with the major connector at nearly a right angle (Fig. 5.3). In this way, maximum effort to avoid impinging on the gingival tissues is accomplished.

Except for a palatal torus or a prominent median palatal suture area, palatal connectors ordinarily require no relief. Intimate contact between the connector and the supporting tissue adds much to the support, stability, and retention of the denture. Except for gingival areas, the intimacy of contact elsewhere in the palate is not detrimental to the health of the tissue if rests are provided on the abutment teeth to prevent tissueward movement during function.

An anterior palatal strap or the anterior border of a palatal plate also should be located as far as possible posteriorly to avoid interference with the tongue in the area of the rugae. It should be uniformly thin, and its anterior border should be located to follow the contours between the crests of the rugae.

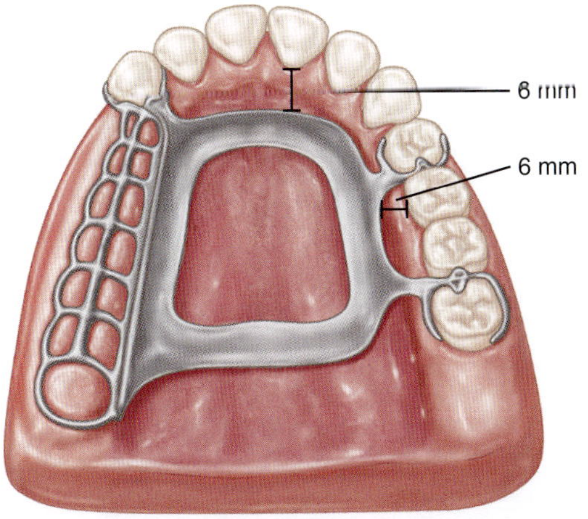

Fig. 5.3 Palatal major connector should be located at least 6 mm away from the gingival margins and parallel to their mean curvature. All adjoining minor connectors should cross the gingival tissues abruptly and should join major connectors at nearly a right angle.

BOX 5.1 Characteristics of Major Connectors Contributing to Health and Well-Being

1. Are made from a material compatible with oral tissue
2. Are rigid and provide cross-arch stability through the principle of broad distribution of stress
3. Do not interfere with and are not irritating to the tongue
4. Do not substantially alter the natural contour of the lingual surface of the mandibular alveolar ridge or of the palatal vault
5. Do not impinge on oral tissue when the restoration is placed, is removed, or rotates in function
6. Cover no more tissue than is absolutely necessary
7. Do not contribute to retention or trapping of food particles
8. Have support from other elements of the framework to minimize rotation tendencies in function
9. Contribute to the support of the prosthesis

The anterior borders of palatal major connectors therefore will be irregular in outline as they follow the contours between the rugae. The tongue may then pass from one rugae prominence to another without encountering the border of the connector if designed appropriately. When the connector border must cross a rugae crest, this should be done abruptly, while avoiding the crest as much as possible. The posterior limitation of a maxillary major connector should be slightly anterior to the vibrating line. A useful rule applied to major connectors and throughout removable partial denture design is to avoid adding any part of the denture framework to an already convex surface.

Characteristics of major connectors that contribute to the maintenance of the health of the oral environment and the well-being of the patient are listed as shown in Box 5.1.

Mandibular Major Connectors

There are six types of mandibular major connectors described historically. Of these, the lingual bar and the linguoplate are used the majority of the time.

1. Lingual bar (Fig. 5.4, *A*)
2. Linguoplate (see Fig. 5.4, *B*)
3. Sublingual bar (see Fig. 5.4, *C*)
4. Lingual bar with cingulum bar (continuous bar) (see Fig. 5.4, *D*)
5. Cingulum bar (continuous bar) (see Fig. 5.4, *E*)
6. Labial bar (see Fig. 5.4, *F*)

Lingual Bar

The basic cross-sectional form of a mandibular *lingual bar* major connector is a half-pear shape, located above the moving tissue but as far below the gingival tissue as possible. When the framework is fabricated using conventional laboratory techniques, it is usually made of reinforced, 6-gauge, half-pear–shaped wax or a similar plastic pattern (Fig. 5.5).

The major connector must be contoured so that it does not present sharp margins to the tongue and cause irritation or annoyance by an angular form. The superior border of a lingual bar connector should be tapered toward the gingival tissue superiorly, with its greatest bulk at the inferior border, resulting in a contour that has a half-pear shape. Lingual bar patterns, both wax and plastic, are made in this conventional shape. However, the inferior border of the lingual bar should be slightly rounded when the framework is polished. A rounded border will not impinge on the lingual tissue when the denture bases rotate inferiorly under occlusal loads. Frequently, additional bulk is necessary to provide rigidity, particularly when the bar is long or when a less rigid alloy is used. This is accomplished by lining the ready-made form underneath with a sheet of 24-gauge casting wax rather than altering the original half-pear shape which could weaken the shape after fabrication.

The inferior border of a lingual mandibular major connector must be located so that it does not impinge on the tissue in the floor of the mouth because it changes elevations during the normal activities of mastication, swallowing, speaking, licking the lips, and so forth. Yet at the same time, it seems logical to locate the inferior border of these connectors as far inferiorly as possible to avoid interference with the resting tongue and trapping of food substances when they are introduced into the mouth. In addition, the more inferiorly a lingual bar can be located, the farther the superior border of the bar can be placed from the lingual gingival crevices of adjacent teeth, thereby avoiding impingement on the gingival tissue.

At least two clinically acceptable methods may be used to determine the relative height of the floor of the mouth and locate the inferior border of a lingual mandibular major connector. The first method is to measure the height of the floor of the mouth in relation to the lingual gingival margins of the adjacent teeth with a periodontal probe (Fig. 5.6). When these measurements are taken, the tip of the patient's tongue should just lightly touch the vermilion border of the upper lip. Recording these measurements permits their transfer to both diagnostic and master casts, thus ensuring a rather advantageous location of the inferior border of the major connector. The second method is to use an individualized impression tray for which lingual borders are 3 mm short of the elevated floor of the mouth, and then to use an impression material that will permit the impression to be accurately molded as the patient

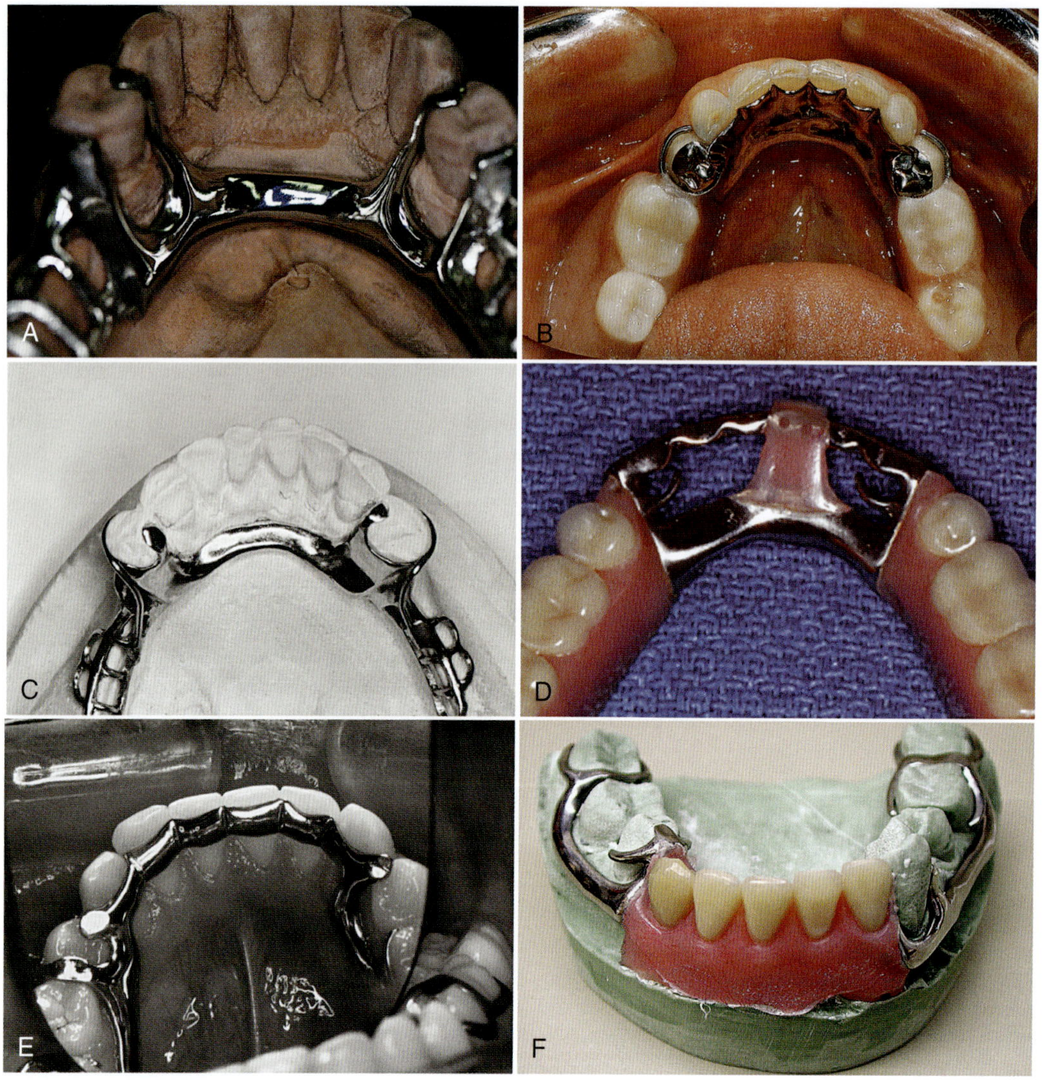

Fig. 5.4 Mandibular major connectors. **A,** Lingual bar. **B,** Lingual plate. **C,** Sublingual bar. **D,** Lingual bar with continuous bar (cingulum bar). **E,** Cingulum bar. **F,** Labial bar.

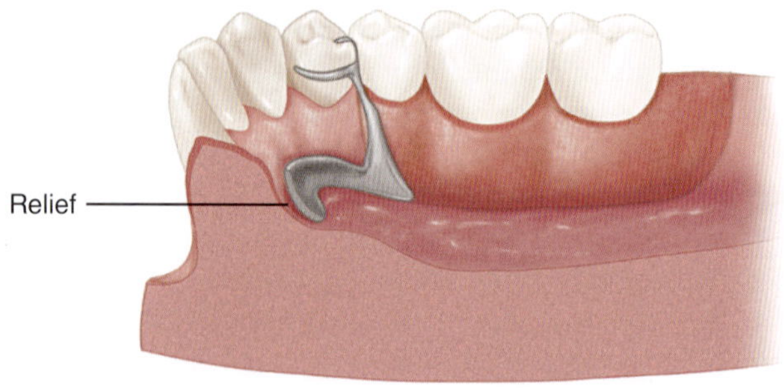

Fig. 5.5 Sagittal section showing half-pear shape of the lingual bar. A taper of the superior border of the bar to the soft tissues above minimizes interference with the tongue and is more acceptable to the patient than a dissimilar contour. Tissue relief is necessary to protect the soft tissue of the floor of the mouth.

licks the lips. The inferior border of the planned major connector can then be located at the height of the lingual sulcus of the cast resulting from such an impression. Of the two methods, we have found measuring the height of the floor of the mouth to be less variable and more clinically acceptable.

Lingual Plate (Linguoplate)

If the rectangular space is bounded by the lingual bar, the anterior tooth contacts, and the cingula and the bordering minor connectors are filled in resulting in a lingual plate (Fig. 5.7).

A lingual plate, referred to as linguoplate in some instances, should be made as thin as feasible and should be contoured to follow the contours of the teeth and the embrasures (Fig. 5.8). Patient awareness of this major connector can be mitigated by reducing bulk and minimizing variations in contour as much as possible. The upper border (border toward the incisal edges) should follow the natural curvature of the cingulum surfaces of the mandibular anterior teeth; the upper border should not extend above the middle-third of the lingual surface, except to cover interproximal spaces up to the location of the interproximal contacts. The half-pear shape of a lingual bar is unaltered to form the inferior border that provides the greatest bulk and rigidity. All gingival crevices and deep embrasures must be blocked out parallel to the path of insertion or placement to avoid impinging on gingival tissues resulting in gingival irritation and to avoid any wedging effect between the teeth. In many

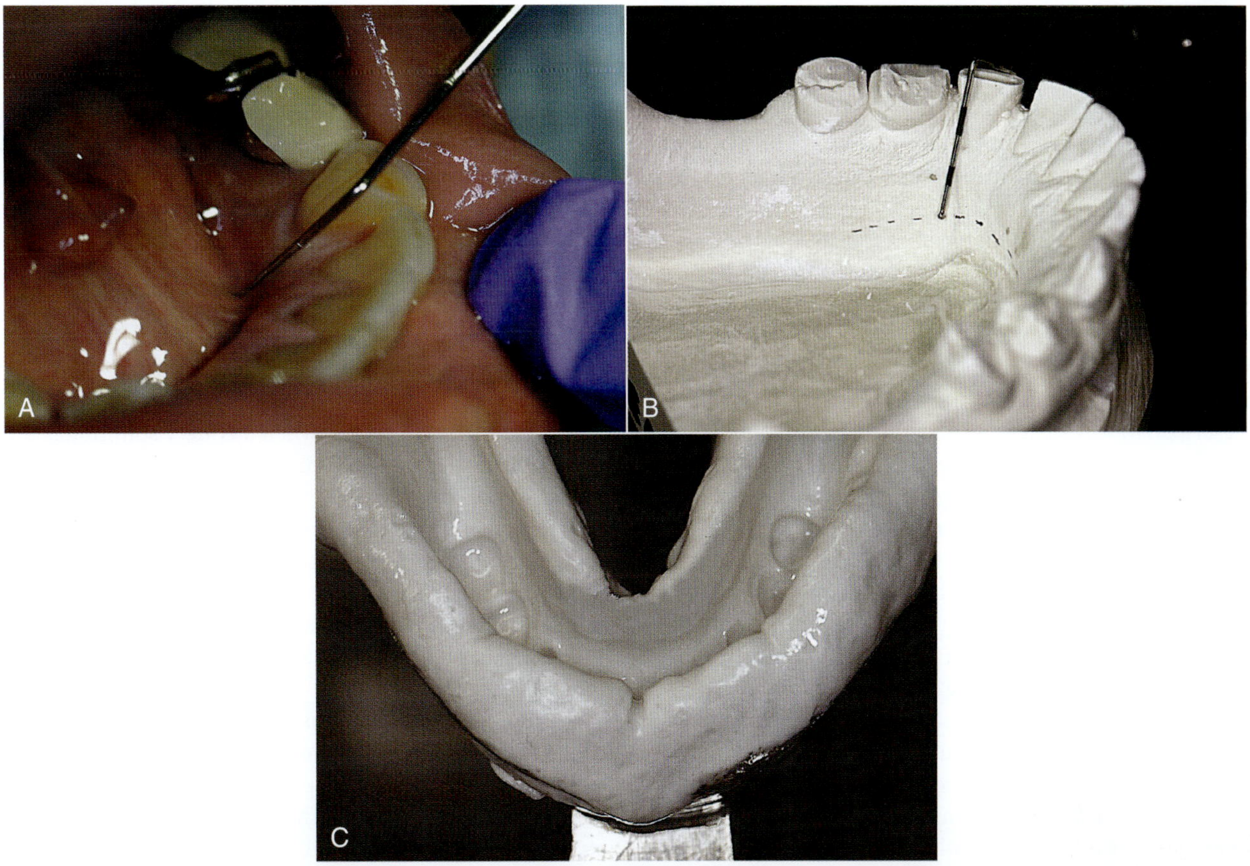

Fig. 5.6 A, Height of floor of the mouth (tongue elevated) in relation to lingual gingival sulci measured with a periodontal probe. **B,** Recorded measurements are transferred to a diagnostic cast and then to a master cast after mouth preparations are completed. The dotted line indicates the location of the inferior border of the major connector. If periodontal surgery is performed, the line on the cast can be related to the incisal edges of teeth and the measurements recorded for subsequent use. **C,** Impression made with functional movement of the tongue to demonstrate maximum shortening of the floor of the mouth. This allows visualization of the anatomic feature that establishes the inferior extent of a major connector. If a stock tray causes impingement on this functional position, an individualized or custom tray may be used for the same purpose.

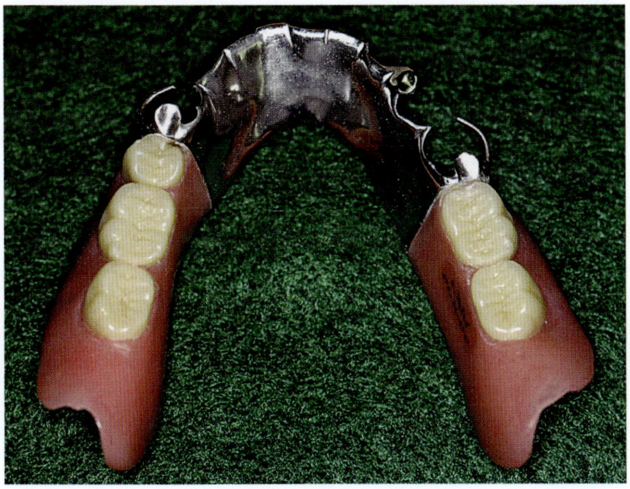

Fig. 5.7 View of mandibular Class I design with contoured lingual plate. The lingual plate is made as thin as possible and should follow the lingual contours of the teeth contacted. Doing so will often result in a scalloped superior margin. In this example, the straight superior margin can be bulky at the cingulum region, causing tongue discomfort.

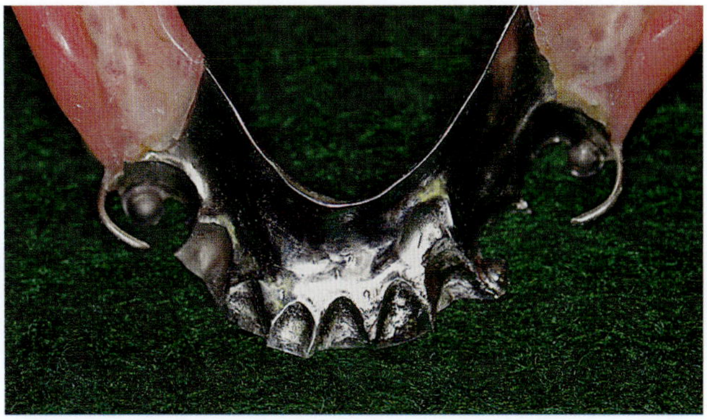

Fig. 5.8 Apron of the lingual plate (tissue side) is closely adapted to the teeth extending into nonundercut interproximal embrasures, resulting in a scalloped form. When well adapted, this form benefits from some anterior teeth acting together to help resist horizontal rotational tendencies of the prosthesis, especially if the posterior ridge form does not resist such movement.

instances, judicious and limited enamel recontouring of the lingual proximal surfaces of overlapped anterior teeth permits closer adaptation of the lingual plate major connector, eliminating otherwise deep interproximal embrasures to be covered (Fig. 5.9).

The lingual plate does not in itself serve as an indirect retainer. When indirect retention is required, definitive rest seats must be provided for this purpose. Both the lingual plate and the lingual bar ideally should have a terminal rest on either end, regardless of the need for indirect retention. However, when indirect retainers are necessary, the same rests described above may also serve as terminal rests for the lingual late or lingual bar.

Each component of a removable partial denture is selected and prescribed to serve a definite purpose in design. Indications for the use of a lingual plate may be listed as follows:

1. When the lingual frenum is high or the space available for a lingual bar is limited. In either instance, the superior border of a lingual bar would have to be placed too close to the gingival tissue. Irritation could be avoided only by generous relief, which might be annoying to the tongue and create an undesirable food trap. When a clinical measurement from the free gingival margins to the slightly elevated floor of the mouth is less than 8 mm, a lingual plate is indicated in lieu of a lingual bar. The use of a lingual plate permits the inferior border to be placed more superiorly without tongue and gingival irritation and without compromise of rigidity.
2. In Kennedy Class I situations where the residual ridges have undergone excessive vertical resorption. Flat residual alveolar ridges offer little resistance to horizontal rotational displacement of a distal extension base. The bracing effect provided by the remaining teeth must be depended upon to resist such rotation. A correctly designed lingual plate will engage the remaining teeth to help resist horizontal rotations.
3. For stabilizing periodontally weakened teeth, splinting with a lingual plate can be of some value when used with definite rests on sound adjacent teeth. In this instance, a cingulum bar may be used to accomplish the same purpose as it presents as the superior border of a linguoplate without the gingival apron that would be present for a lingual plate. The cingulum bar accomplishes stabilization along with the other advantages of a lingual plate. However, it is frequently objectionable to the patient's tongue and creates more of a food trap as compared to the contoured apron of a lingual plate.
4. When the future replacement of one or more incisor teeth will be facilitated by the addition of retention loops to an existing lingual plate. Mandibular incisors that are periodontally weak may thus be retained, with provisions for possible loss and future additions.

The same reasons for the use of a lingual plate anteriorly apply to its use elsewhere in the mandibular arch. If a lingual bar alone is to be used anteriorly, there is no reason to add an apron elsewhere. However, when auxiliary splinting is used for stabilization of the remaining teeth or for horizontal stabilization of the prosthesis, or for both, small rectangular spaces sometimes remain. Tissue response to limited spaces may be preferable when bridged with an apron as opposed to possible food traps when left open or uncovered. Generally, the apron is used to avoid gingival irritation or entrapment of food debris or to cover generously relieved areas that would be irritating to the tongue (Fig. 5.10).

In some clinical situations where a lingual plate is indicated as the major connector of choice, the patient may object strenuously if anterior teeth are spaced apart, allowing for metal to show through the spaces. The lingual plate can then be constructed to minimize metal appearance through the spaced anterior teeth (Fig. 5.11). This modified design for the lingual plate major connector can create a food trap similar to the cingulum (continuous) bar major connector.

Design of Mandibular Major Connectors

The following systematic approach to the design of a mandibular lingual bar and lingual plate major connectors can be readily used with diagnostic casts after considering the diagnostic data related to the basic principles of major connector design:

Step 1: Outline the basal seat areas on the diagnostic cast (Fig. 5.12, *A*).

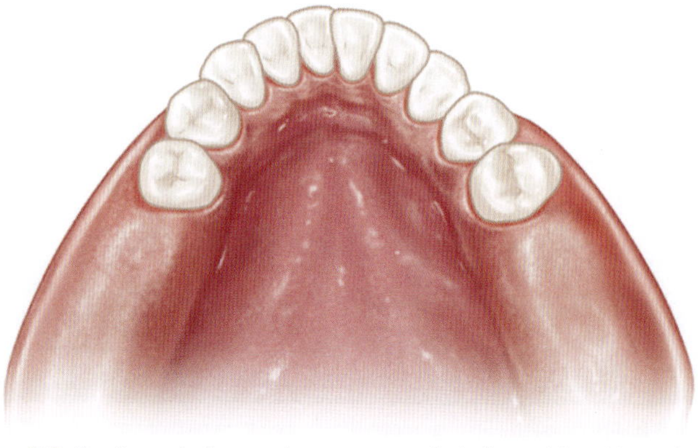

Fig. 5.9 If a lingual plate major connector is indicated for this patient with overlapped anterior teeth, judicious recontouring of the lingual proximal surfaces of right lateral, right central, and left lateral incisors eliminates excessive undercuts and permit closer adaptation of the lingual apron of the major connector.

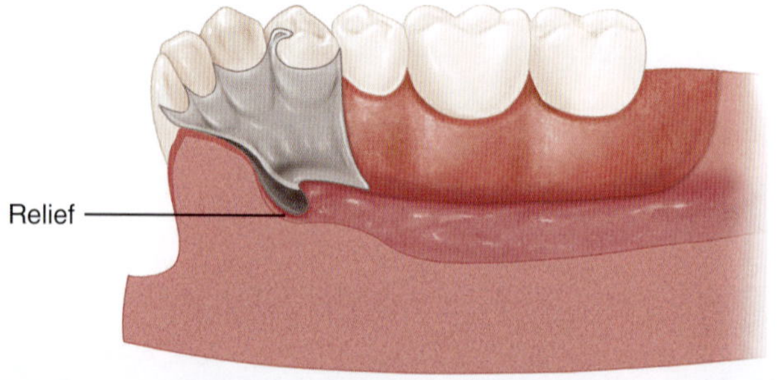

Fig. 5.10 Sagittal section through the lingual plate demonstrating a basic half-pear–shaped inferior border with the metallic apron extending superiorly. Extension of the lingual plate to the height of the contour on the premolar was accomplished to enclose a rather large triangular interproximal space inferior to the contact point between the canine and premolar. Such spaces may often be bridged to eliminate obvious food traps. Relief is provided for soft tissue under all portions of the mandibular major connector and at any location where the framework crosses the marginal gingiva.

Step 2: Outline the inferior border of the major connector (see Fig. 5.12, *B*).

Step 3: Outline the superior border of the major connector (see Fig. 5.12, *C*).

Step 4: Connect the basal seat area to the inferior and superior borders of the major connector, and add minor connectors to retain the acrylic resin denture base material (see Fig. 5.12, *D*).

Sublingual Bar

A modification of the lingual bar that has been demonstrated to be useful when the height of the floor of the mouth does not allow placement of the superior border of the bar at least 4 mm below the free gingival margin is the sublingual bar. The bar shape remains essentially the same as that of a lingual bar, but placement is inferior and posterior to the usual placement of a lingual bar, lying over and parallel to the anterior floor of the mouth. It is generally accepted that a sublingual bar can be used in lieu of a lingual plate if the lingual frenum does not interfere or in the presence of an anterior lingual undercut that would require considerable blockout for a conventional lingual bar. Contraindications include interfering lingual tori, high attachment of a lingual frenum, and interference with elevation of the floor of the mouth during functional movements.

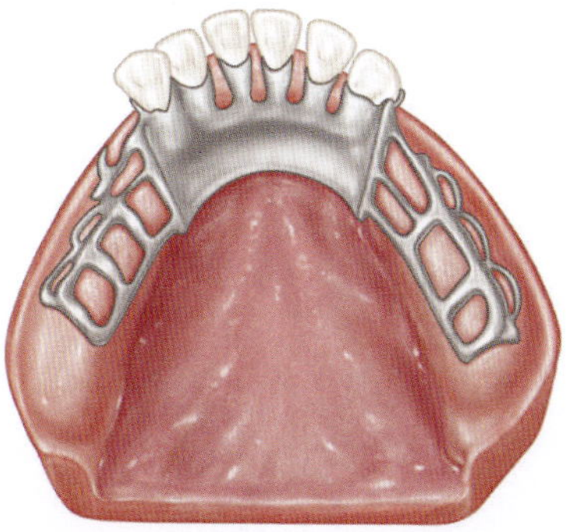

Fig. 5.11 Interrupted lingual plate in the presence of interproximal spaces.

Cingulum Bar (Continuous Bar)

When a lingual plate is the major connector of choice, but the axial alignment of the anterior teeth is such that excessive blockout of interproximal undercuts must be made, a cingulum bar may be considered. A cingulum bar, located on or slightly above the cingula of the anterior teeth, may be added to the lingual bar or can be used independently (Fig. 5.13). In addition, when wide diastemata exist between the mandibular anterior teeth, a cingulum bar retainer may be more esthetically acceptable than a lingual plate.

Labial Bar

The extreme lingual inclination of the remaining mandibular premolar and incisor teeth prevents the use of a lingual bar major connector in limited instances. With the use of

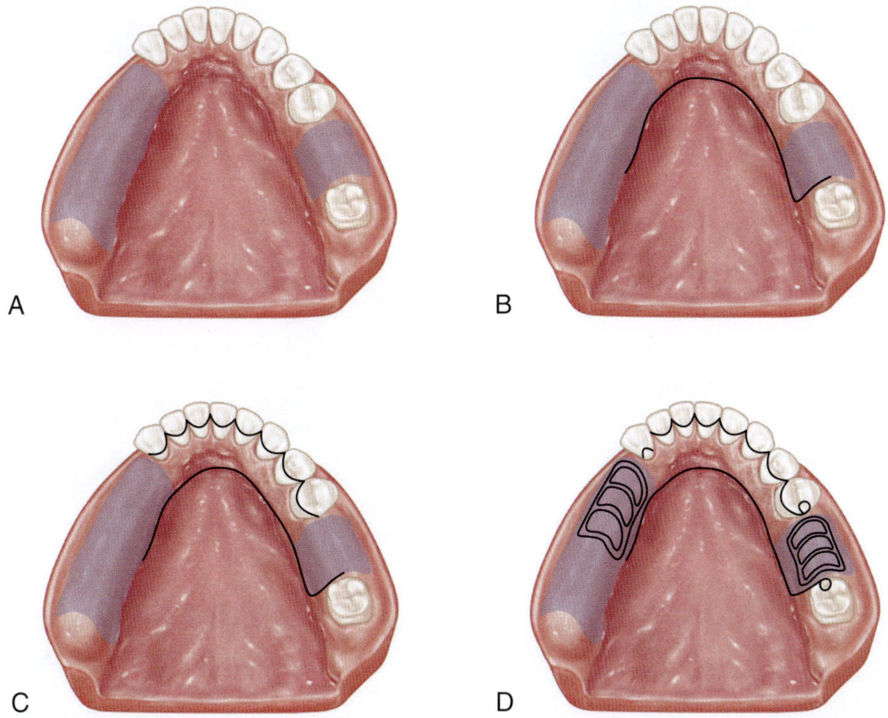

Fig. 5.12 Sequence of design considerations for a mandibular major connector. **A,** Diagnostic cast with basal seat areas outlined. **B,** Inferior border of the major connector is outlined. The location of the inferior border was determined as suggested in Fig. 5.6 and extends to the mesial of the mandibular right molar. **C,** Superior border of the major connector is outlined. Limited space for the lingual bar requires the use of the lingual plate major connector. The lingual plate requires that rest seats be used on canines and the first premolar for positive support. **D,** Rest seat areas on the posterior teeth are outlined, and minor connectors for retention of resin denture bases are sketched.

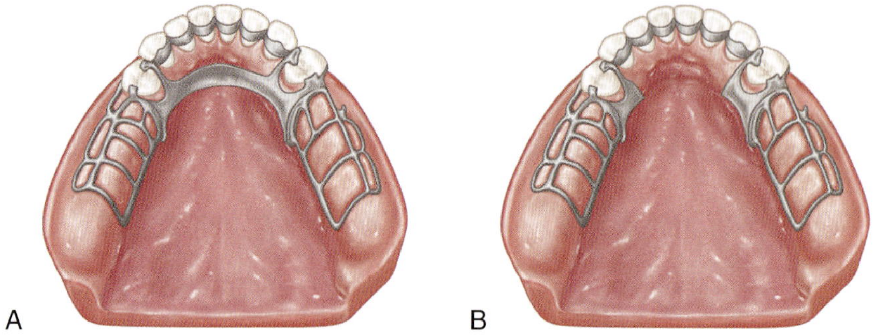

Fig. 5.13 **A,** Lingual bar and cingulum bar (continuous bar) major connector. The upper portion of this major connector is located on the cingula of the anterior teeth. The requirement of positive support by rest seats, at least as far anteriorly as the canines, is critical. Note that the superior border of the lingual bar portion is often placed objectionably close to the gingival margins if sufficient bulk for rigidity is to be obtained. This type of major connector easily traps food and is often more objectionable to patients than a lingual plate. **B,** Cingulum bar (continuous bar) major connector. Although this design may reduce the possibility of food entrapment, it may not provide adequate rigidity.

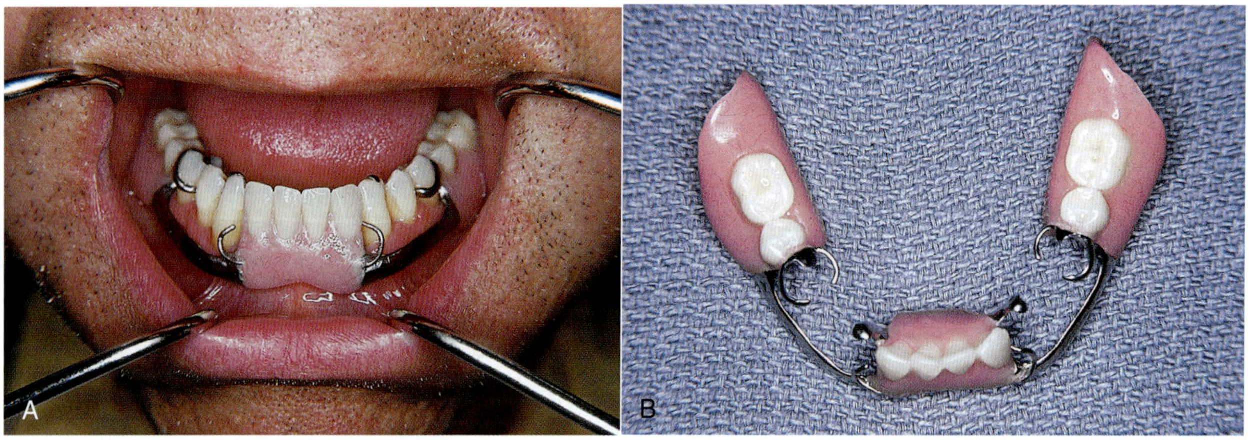

Fig. 5.14 **A,** Lingual inclination of patient's canines and premolars precludes the use of the lingual bar. **B,** Labial bar major connector was used in the treatment. Retention was obtained on terminal abutments. Support and stabilization were gained by using rests, minor connectors arising from the labial bar, and well-fitting denture bases.

conservative tooth preparations in the form of recontouring and blockout, a lingual major connector can almost always be used. Lingually inclined teeth may require full coverage crowns in order to create ideal contours. Although the use of a labial major connector may be necessary in rare instances, this should be avoided by considering additional tooth preparations rather than by accepting a condition that is otherwise correctable (Fig. 5.14). The same applies to the use of a labial bar when a mandibular torus interferes with the placement of a lingual bar. Unless surgery is contraindicated, interfering mandibular tori should be removed so that the use of a labial bar connector can be avoided.

A modification to the lingual plate is the hinged continuous labial bar. This concept is incorporated in the Swing-Lock[2] design, which consists of a labial or buccal bar that is connected to the major connector by a hinge at one end and a latch at the other end (Fig. 5.15).

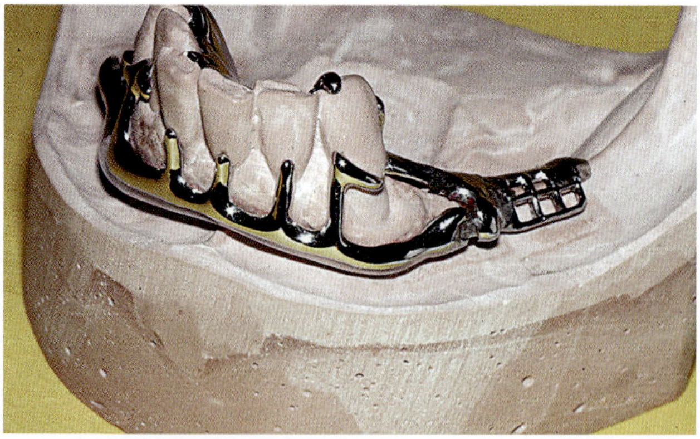

Fig. 5.15 The hinge for this continuous labial bar connector is located buccal and distal to the remaining dentition (area of tooth #21). The latching mechanism is opposite to the hinge, adjacent to tooth #28. In this location, it will be housed within the buccal flange of the denture.

Support is provided by multiple rests on the remaining natural teeth. Stabilization and reciprocation are provided by a lingual plate that contacts the remaining teeth and are supplemented by the labial bar with its retentive struts. Retention is provided by a bar type of retentive clasp with arms projecting from the labial or buccal bar and contacting the infrabulge areas on the labial surfaces of the teeth.

The use of the Swing-Lock concept can be considered as the primary choice when the following conditions are present:

1. Missing key abutments: When all remaining teeth are used for retention and stability, the absence of a key abutment (such as a canine) may not present as serious a treatment problem with this concept as with more conventional designs (Fig. 5.16).
2. Unfavorable tooth contours: When existing tooth contours (uncorrectable by recontouring with appropriate restorations) or excessive labial inclinations of anterior teeth prevent conventional clasp designs, the basic principles of removable partial design may be better implemented with the Swing-Lock concept.
3. Unfavorable soft tissue contours: Extensive soft tissue undercuts may prevent proper location of component parts of a conventional removable partial denture or an overdenture. The hinged continuous labial bar concept may provide an adjunctive modality to accommodate such unfavorable soft tissue contours.
4. Teeth with questionable prognoses: The possibility of losing a key abutment tooth with a guarded prognosis seriously affects the stability and retention of a conventional prosthesis. Because all remaining teeth function as abutments in the Swing-Lock denture, it seems that the loss of a tooth would not compromise retention and stability to such a degree. The hinged labial bar type of restoration can be used satisfactorily in certain clinically compromised situations. As is true with any type of removable restoration, good oral hygiene, maintenance, regular recall, and close attention to details of design are paramount to successful implementation of this treatment concept.

Clear contraindications to the use of a hinged-labial bar design concept include poor oral hygiene or lack of motivation for plaque control by the patient. Other contraindications include the presence of a shallow buccal or labial vestibule or a high frenal attachment. Any of these factors would prevent the proper placement of components in designing the Swing-Lock removable partial denture.

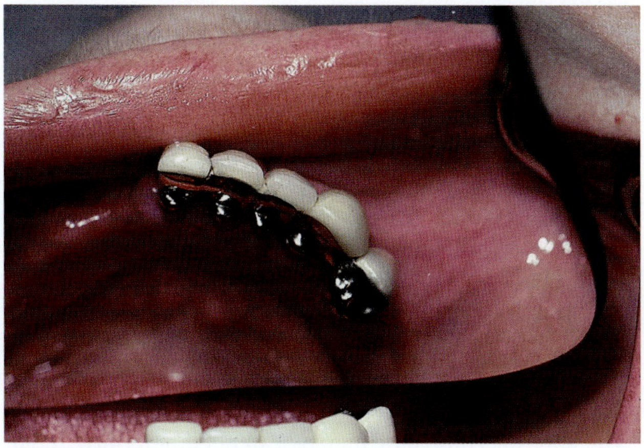

Fig. 5.16 Absence of the mandibular canine requires that all remaining anterior teeth be used for stabilization and retention of the replacement restoration. The Swing-Lock concept can be used to ensure that all remaining teeth share in the stabilization and retention of the prosthesis.

Maxillary Major Connectors

Six basic types of maxillary major connectors are considered:

1. Single palatal strap (Fig. 5.17, *A*)
2. Combination anterior and posterior palatal strap–type connector (see Fig. 5.17, *B*)
3. Palatal plate–type connector (see Fig. 5.17, *C*)
4. U-shaped palatal connector (see Fig. 5.17, *D*)
5. Single palatal bar (see Fig. 5.17, *E*)
6. Anterior-posterior palatal bars (see Fig. 5.17, *F*)

Whenever it is necessary for the palatal connector to contact the teeth for reasons of support, tooth preparation to support the teeth must be provided. This is best accomplished by establishing definitive rest seats on selected abutment teeth. Rest seat design requires that the tooth preparation should be located well above the gingival attachment to provide for bridging of the gingival crevice with blockout. At the same time, rest seat preparations should be located low enough gingivally on the tooth to avoid unfavorable leverage and low enough gingivally on the maxillary incisors and canine teeth to avoid incisal interference of the opposing dentition.

Major connector components resting on unprepared inclined tooth surfaces can lead to slippage of the denture or to orthodontic movement of the tooth or to both. In either situation, settling into gingival tissue is inevitable. In the absence of the required vertical support provided by rests, the health of the surrounding tissue is usually impaired. Similarly, interproximal projections of the major connector that rest on the gingival third of the tooth and on gingival tissues that are structurally unable to render support may be traumatized. To prevent these sequelae, one should support the major connector with definite rests on the teeth, provide adequate gingival relief, and/or locate the connector far enough away from the gingival margin to avoid any possible restriction of blood supply and entrapment of food debris. All gingival crossings should be abrupt and at right angles to the major connector. Creating a sharp, angular form on any portion of a palatal connector should be avoided, and all borders should be tapered toward the tissue.

Single Palatal Strap

Bilateral tooth-supported prostheses, even those with short edentulous spaces, are effectively connected with a single, broad palatal strap connector, particularly when the edentulous areas are located posteriorly (Fig. 5.18). Such a connector can be made rigid without objectionable bulk and interference with the tongue, provided the cast framework material is distributed in three planes. Suitable rigidity, without excessive bulk, may be obtained for a single palatal strap by the laboratory technician by casting a 22-gauge matte plastic pattern.

For reasons of torque and leverage, a single palatal strap major connector should not be used to connect anterior replacements with distal extension bases. To be rigid enough to resist torque and to provide adequate vertical support and horizontal stabilization, a single palatal strap would have to be objectionably bulky. When placed anteriorly, this bulk would

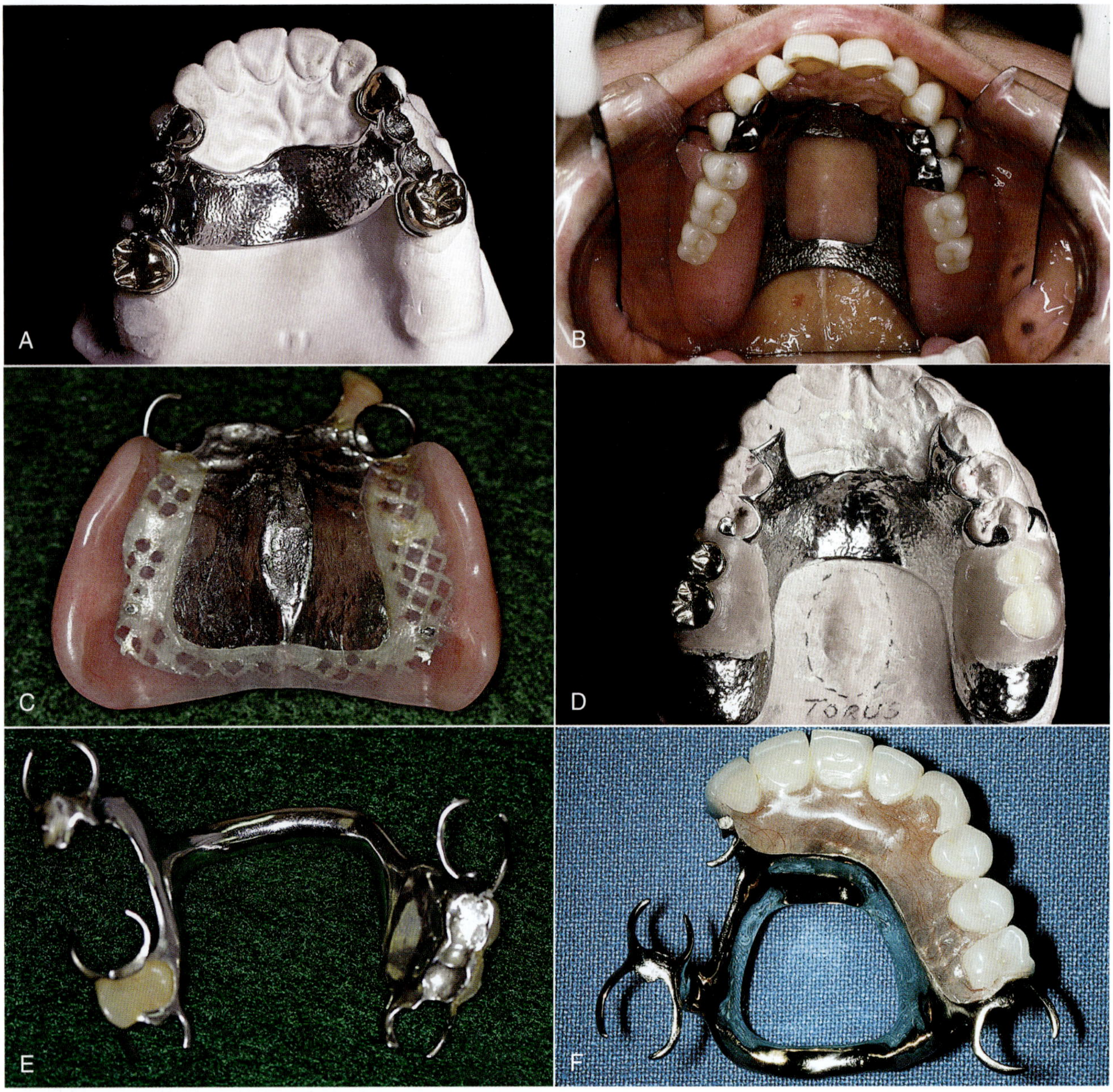

Fig. 5.17 Maxillary major connectors. **A,** Single palatal strap. **B,** Anterior-posterior palatal strap. **C,** Palatal plate. **D,** U-shaped. **E,** Single palatal bar. **F,** Anterior-posterior palatal bars.

become even more objectionable to the patient because it could interfere with speech.

Combination Anterior and Posterior Palatal Strap–Type Connector

Structurally, this is a rigid palatal major connector. The anterior and posterior palatal strap combination may be used in almost any maxillary removable partial denture design (Fig. 5.19).

A posterior palatal strap should be flat and a minimum of 8 mm wide, antero-posteriorly. Posterior palatal connectors should be located as far posterior as possible to avoid interference with the tongue but anterior to the vibrating line, a line of flexure formed by the junction of the hard and soft palates. The only condition that prevents their use is an inoperable maxillary torus that extends posterior to the soft palate. In this situation, a broad, U-shaped major connector may be used, as described elsewhere in this chapter.

The strength of this major connector design lies in the fact that the anterior and posterior components are joined together by longitudinal connectors on either side, which form a square or rectangular frame. Each component braces the others against possible torque and flexure. Flexure is practically nonexistent in such a design.

The anterior connector may be extended anteriorly to support anterior tooth replacements. In this form, a U-shaped connector is made rigid by the horizontal strap that has been added posteriorly. If a maxillary torus exists, it may be encircled by this type of major strap-type connector without reduced rigidity.

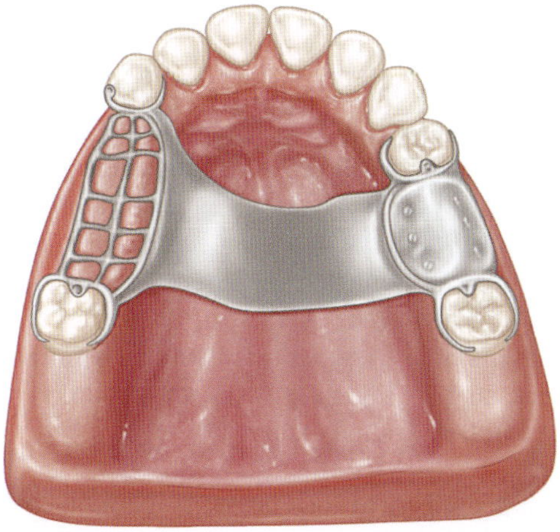

A

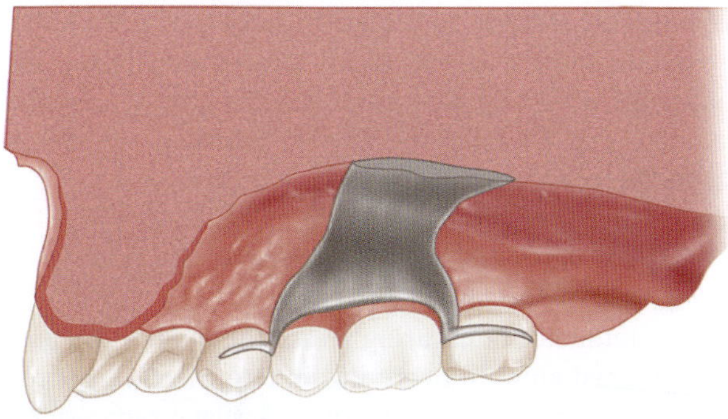

B

Fig. 5.18 A, This single palatal strap–type major connector is better suited for the restoration of short-span tooth-supported bilateral edentulous areas. It may also be used in tooth-supported unilateral edentulous situations with provision for cross-arch attachment by extracoronal retainers or internal attachments. The width of the palatal strap should be confined within the boundaries of supporting rests. **B,** Sagittal section. The midportion of the major connector demonstrates slight elevation to provide rigidity. The thickness of the major connector does not appreciably alter palatal contours.

The combination anterior-posterior connector design may be used with any Kennedy class of partially edentulous arch. It is used most frequently in Kennedy Class II and IV, whereas the single wide palatal strap is selected for use in Kennedy Class III situations. The palatal plate–type or complete palatal coverage connector is commonly used in Kennedy Class I situations for reasons to be explained subsequently. All maxillary major connectors should cross the midline at a right angle rather than at a diagonal. It has been suggested that the tongue will accept symmetrically placed components far more readily than those placed without regard for symmetry.

Palatal Plate–Type Connector

For lack of better terminology, the words *palatal plate* are used to designate any thin, broad, contoured palatal coverage used as a maxillary major connector and covering one-half or more of the hard palate (Fig. 5.20). Anatomic replica palatal castings have uniform thickness and strength by reason of their corrugated contours. Through the use of electrolytic polishing, uniformity of thickness can be maintained, and the anatomic contours of the palate are reproduced in the final removable partial denture.

The anatomic replica palatal major connector has several potential advantages:

1. It permits the making of a uniformly thin metal plate that reproduces faithfully the anatomic contours of the patient's own palate. Its uniform thinness and the thermal conductivity of the metal are designed to make the palatal plate more readily acceptable to the tongue and underlying tissue.
2. The corrugation in the anatomic replica adds strength to the casting; thus a thinner casting with adequate rigidity can be made.
3. Surface irregularities are intentional rather than accidental; therefore electrolytic polishing is all that is needed. The

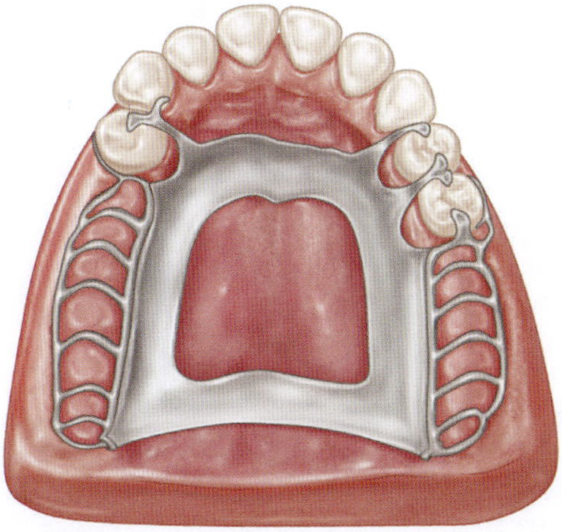

Fig. 5.19 Anterior-posterior palatal strap–type major connector. The anterior component is a flat strap located as far posteriorly as possible to avoid rugae coverage and tongue interference. The anterior border of this strap should be located just posterior to a rugae crest or in the valley between two crests. The posterior strap is thin, a minimum of 8 mm wide, and located as far posteriorly as possible, yet entirely on the hard palate. It should be located at right angles to midline rather than diagonally.

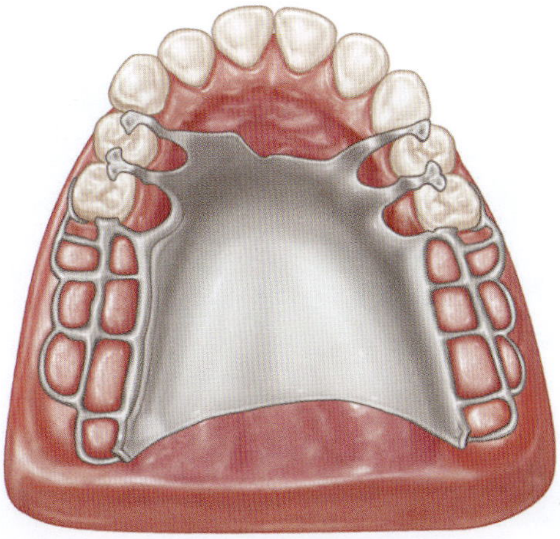

Fig. 5.20 Palatal major connector covering two-thirds of the palate. The anterior border follows valleys between rugae and does not extend anteriorly to indirect retainers on the first premolars. The posterior border is located at the junction of the hard and soft palates but does not extend onto the soft palate. In the bilateral distal extension situation illustrated, indirect retainers are necessary to aid in resisting horizontal rotation of the restoration. Note that provisions have been made for a butt-type joint joining the denture bases and framework as the denture base on each side passes through the pterygomaxillary notch.

original uniform thickness of the plastic pattern is thus maintained.

4. By virtue of intimate contact, interfacial surface tension between the intaglio surface of the metal and tissue provides the prosthesis with greater retention. Retention must be adequate to resist the pull of sticky foods, the action of movable soft tissues against the prosthesis, the forces of gravity, and the expelling forces generated through coughing and sneezing. Retention of the base interface itself can help resist many of the forces described, which is proportional to the total area of denture base contact with supporting tissue. The required amount of both direct and indirect retention will depend on the amount of retention provided by the denture base.

The palatal plate may be used in any one of three ways. It may be used as a plate of varying width that covers the area between two or more edentulous areas, as a complete or partial cast plate that extends to the junction of the hard and soft palates (Figs. 5.21 and 5.22), or in the form of an anterior palatal connector with a provision for extending an acrylic resin denture base in a posterior direction (Fig. 5.23).

The palatal plate should be located anterior to the posterior palatal seal area. A posterior palatal seal incorporated into a complete denture design is not necessary with the use of a maxillary removable partial denture palatal plate due to the accuracy and stability of the metal plate.

When the posterior most remaining abutment tooth on either side of a Kennedy Class I arch is the canine or first premolar tooth, complete palatal coverage is strongly advised, especially excessive vertical resorption of the alveolar ridges. This may be accomplished in one of two ways. One method is to use a complete cast plate that extends to the junction of the hard and soft palates (see Fig. 5.22). The other method is to use a cast major connector anteriorly, with retention posteriorly, for the attachment of an acrylic-resin denture base that extends posterior to the junction of the hard and soft palate anatomic landmark (see Fig. 5.23).

The advantages of a palatal plate make it preferable to using acrylic-resin full palatal coverage. However, the latter method may be used satisfactorily when relining is anticipated, or cost is a factor. The complete palatal plate major connector is considered to be a satisfactory major connector in designing maxillary removable partial dentures. In all circumstances, the portion contacting the teeth must have positive support from adequate rest seat preparation. The dentist should be familiar with selecting the palatal plate for use and know limitations when designing to maximize advantages.

Design of Maxillary Major Connectors

In 1953, Blatterfein[3] described a systematic approach to designing maxillary major connectors. His method involves five basic steps and is certainly applicable to most maxillary removable partial denture situations. When using a diagnostic cast and knowledge of the relative displaceability of the palatal tissue, including that covering the median palatal raphe, he recommends the following basic steps:

Step 1: Outline of primary bearing areas: The primary bearing areas are those that will be covered by the denture base(s) (Fig. 5.24, *A* and *B*).

Step 2: Outline of nonbearing areas: The nonbearing areas are the lingual gingival tissue within 5 to 6 mm of the remaining teeth, hard areas of the medial palatal raphe (including tori), and palatal tissue posterior to the vibrating line (see Fig. 5.24, *C*).

Step 3: Outline of connector areas: Steps 1 and 2, when completed, provide an outline or designate areas that are available to place components of major connectors (see Fig. 5.24,*C*).

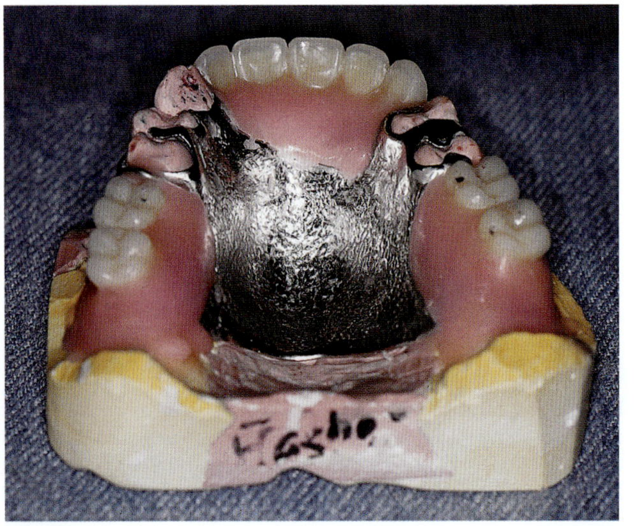

Fig. 5.21 Palatal plate major connector for a Kennedy Class I, modification 1 removable partial denture. The posterior border lies on the immovable hard palate and crosses the midline at a right angle. Total contact provides excellent support.

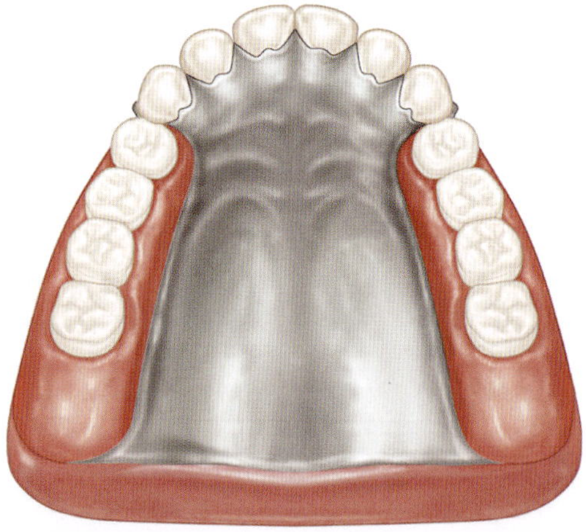

Fig. 5.22 Complete coverage palatal major connector. The posterior border terminates at the junction of the hard and soft palates. The anterior portion, in the form of the palatal lingual plate, is supported by positive lingual rest seats on canines. The location of the finish lines is most important in this type of major connector. Anteroposteriorly, they should be parallel to a line along the center of the ridge crest and located just lingual to an imaginary line contacting the lingual surfaces of missing natural teeth. Alteration of the natural palatal contour should be anticipated with its attendant detrimental effects on speech if these contours are not followed.

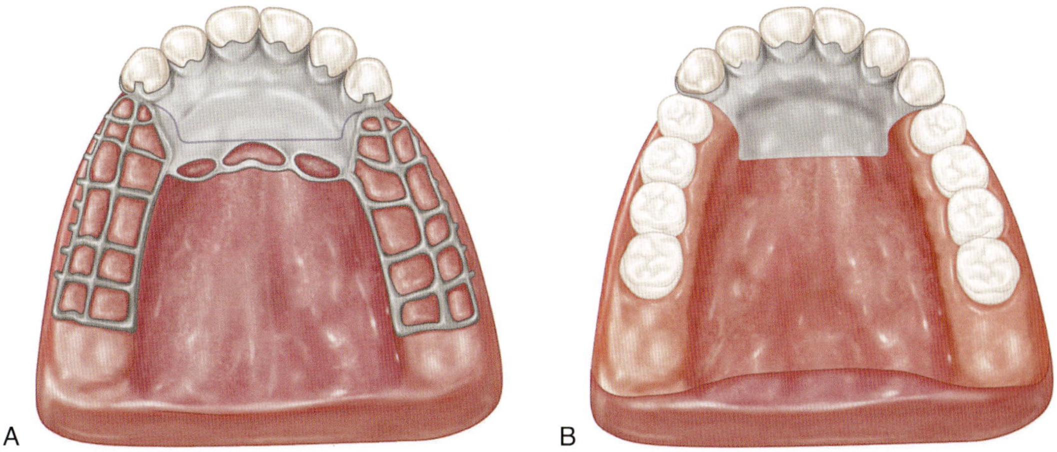

Fig. 5.23 A, Maxillary major connector in the form of a palatal lingual plate with provisions for attaching the full-coverage resin denture base. **B,** Completed removable partial denture with resin base. The palatal lingual plate is supported by rests occupying lingual rest seats prepared in cast restorations on canines. This type of removable partial denture is particularly applicable when (1) residual ridges have undergone extreme vertical resorption and (2) terminal abutments have suffered some bone loss and splinting cannot be accomplished.

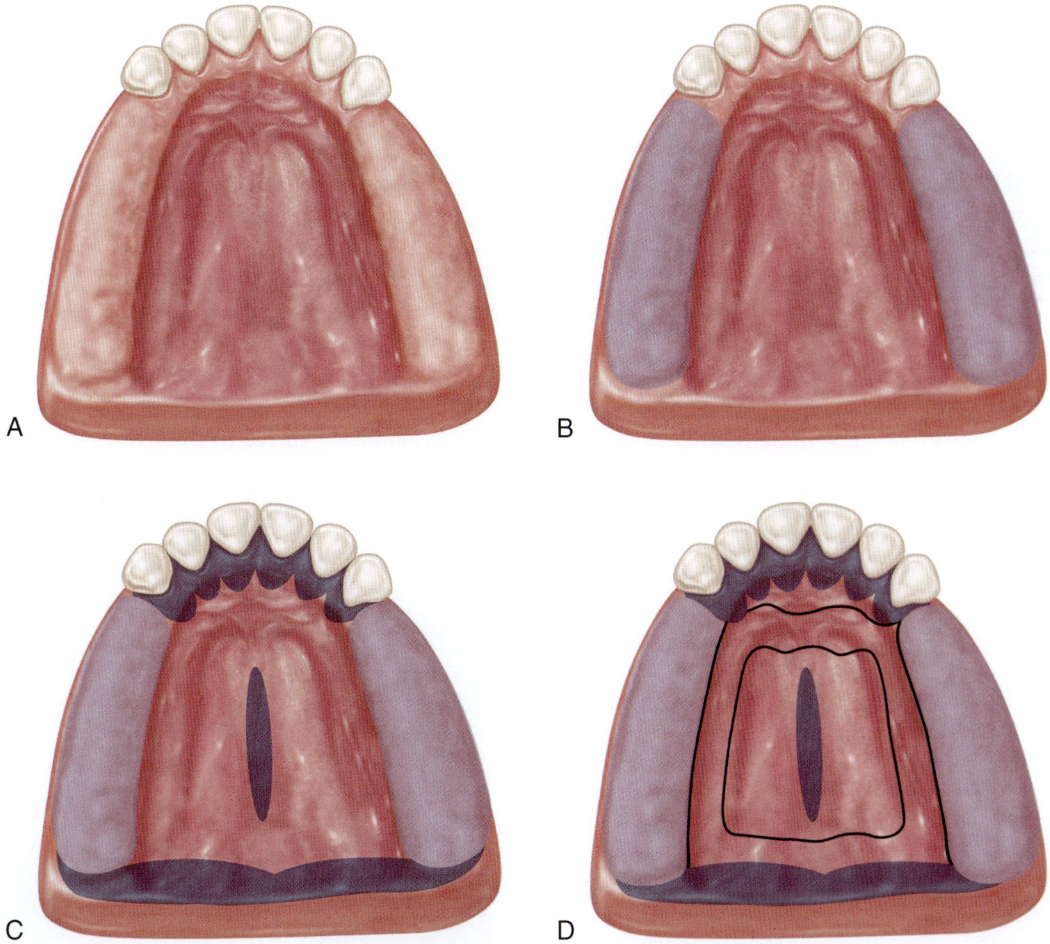

Fig. 5.24 A, Diagnostic cast of partially edentulous maxillary arch. **B,** The palatal extent of the denture base areas is located 2 mm from the palatal surface of the posterior teeth. **C,** Nonbearing areas outlined in black, which include lingual soft tissue within 5 to 6 mm of teeth, an unyielding median palatal raphe area, and the soft palate. The space bounded by bearing and nonbearing area outlines is available for placement of the major connector. **D,** The major connector selected will be rigid and noninterfering with the tongue and will cover a minimum of the palate.

Step 4: Selection of connector type: Selection of the type of connector(s) is based on four factors: (1) mouth comfort, (2) rigidity, (3) location of denture bases, and (4) indirect retention. Connectors should be of minimum bulk and should be positioned to minimize interference with the tongue during speech and mastication. Connectors must have a maximum rigidity to distribute stress bilaterally. The double-strap type of major connector provides the maximum rigidity without bulk and avoids full palatal tissue coverage. In many instances, the choice of a strap-type major connector is limited by the location of the edentulous ridge areas. When edentulous areas are located anteriorly, the use of only a posterior strap is not recommended. Conversely, when only posterior edentulous areas are present, the use of only an anterior strap is not recommended. The need for indirect retention influences the outline of the major connector. Provision must be made in the major connector so that indirect retainers may be attached.

Step 5: Unification: After the selection of the type of major connector based on considerations in Step 4, the denture base areas and connectors are joined (see Fig. 5.24, *D*).

Although many variations in palatal major connectors have been noted, a thorough comprehension of all factors that influence selection and design are considered to maximize patient benefit.

U-Shaped Palatal Connector

From both the patient's standpoint and biomechanical principles, the U-shaped palatal connector is the least desirable of maxillary major connectors from both the patient's perspective and biomechanical principles and should not be used arbitrarily. When a large inoperable palatal torus exists and occasionally when several anterior teeth are to be replaced, the U-shaped palatal connector may be indicated (Fig. 5.25). In most instances, however, other designs will serve more effectively.

The following are the disadvantages associated with the use of the U-shaped connector:

1. Lack of rigidity (compared with other designs) can allow lateral flexure under occlusal forces, which may induce torque or direct lateral forces to abutment teeth.
2. The design fails to provide good support characteristics and may permit impingement of underlying tissue when subjected to occlusal loading.
3. Bulk needed to enhance rigidity results in increased thickness in areas that may be objectionable to the patient as a hindrance to the tongue during speech and mastication.

Many maxillary removable partial dentures fail based on the excess flexibility of a U-shaped major connector (Fig. 5.26). To be rigid, the U-shaped palatal connector must have bulk where the tongue needs freedom the most—the rugae area. Without sufficient bulk, the U-shaped design leads to increased flexibility and movement at the open ends. In distal extension removable partial dentures, when tooth support posterior to the edentulous area is nonexistent, movement is particularly noticeable and can be traumatic to the residual ridge despite adequate support of distal extension(s) or harmonious occlusion.

The wider the coverage of a U-shaped major connector, the more it resembles a palatal plate–type connector with comparable advantages as opposed to a narrow U design which lacks rigidity. A U-shaped connector can be made more rigid by incorporating tooth support through additional definitive rests. A common error in the design of a U-shaped connector, however, is its proximity to, or actual contact with, gingival tissue. The principle that the borders of major connectors should be supported by rests in prepared rest seats or should be located well away from gingival tissue is a tenet in design. A common error with a U-shaped connector includes proximity to or contact with gingival tissues which can result in gingival irritation and periodontal damage to the tissues adjacent to remaining teeth.

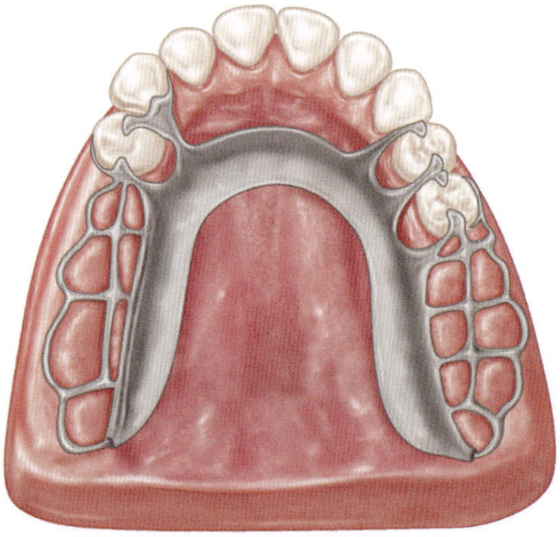

Fig. 5.25 U-shaped palatal connector is the least rigid type of maxillary major connector and should be used only when a large inoperable palatal torus prevents the use of palatal coverage or combination anterior-posterior palatal strap–type designed framework.

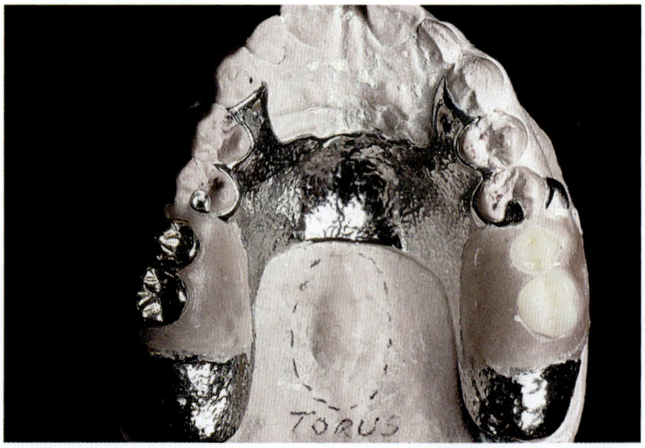

Fig. 5.26 Removable partial denture design that uses an objectionable U-shaped palatal major connector. Such a connector lacks necessary rigidity, places bulk where it is most objectionable to the patient, and impinges on gingival tissue lingual to remaining teeth.

Single Palatal Bar

To distinguish between a palatal bar and a palatal strap, a palatal connector component less than 8 mm in width is called a bar in this textbook. The single palatal bar is widely used and can be as objectionable as the selection of the U-shaped palatal connector.

For a single palatal bar to have the necessary rigidity for cross-arch distribution of stress, it must have concentrated bulk, a design element often missed. For a single palatal bar to be effective, it must be rigid enough to provide support and cross-arch stabilization and located centrally between the "halves" of the denture resulting in increasing patient objections due to the need to alter palatal contours.

The design of a removable partial denture using a single palatal bar major connector is often too thin and flexible or too bulky and objectionable to the patient's tongue. The decision to use a single palatal bar instead of a strap should be based on the size of the denture-bearing areas that are connected and on whether a single connector located between bilateral distal extensions would be rigid without objectionable bulk.

Combination Anterior and Posterior Palatal Bar–Type Connectors

Structurally, this combination of major connectors exhibits many of the same disadvantages as the single palatal bar (Fig. 5.27). To be sufficiently rigid and to provide needed support and stability, these connectors could be too bulky and could interfere with tongue function.

Beading of the Maxillary Cast

Beading is a term used to denote the scribing of a shallow groove (approximately half the depth of a size 4 round bur) on the maxillary master cast outlining the palatal major connector excluding rugae areas (Fig. 5.28). The purposes of beading are as follows:

1. To transfer the major connector design to the investment cast (Fig. 5.29)
2. To provide a visible finish line in the major connector (Fig. 5.30)
3. To ensure intimate tissue contact of the major connector with selected palatal tissue

Beading is readily accomplished by using an appropriate instrument, such as a cleoid carver. Care must be exercised to create a groove no deeper into the soft tissues than 0.5 mm in width or depth (Fig. 5.31).

MINOR CONNECTORS

Minor connectors are those components that serve as the connecting link between the major connector or the base of a removable partial denture and the other components of the prosthesis, such as the clasp assembly, indirect retainers, occlusal rests, or cingulum rests. In many instances, a minor connector may be continuous with some other component of the removable partial denture framework. For example, an occlusal rest at one end of a lingual plate is actually the terminus of a minor connector, such that it is continuous with the lingual plate. Similarly, the portion of a removable partial denture framework that supports the clasp and the occlusal rest is identified as a minor connector, which joins the major connector with the clasp proper.

The portions of a removable partial denture framework that retain the denture bases are also minor connectors. The denture base material is retained by one of three types of physical retention; open latticework, meshwork, and metal base (Fig. 5.32).

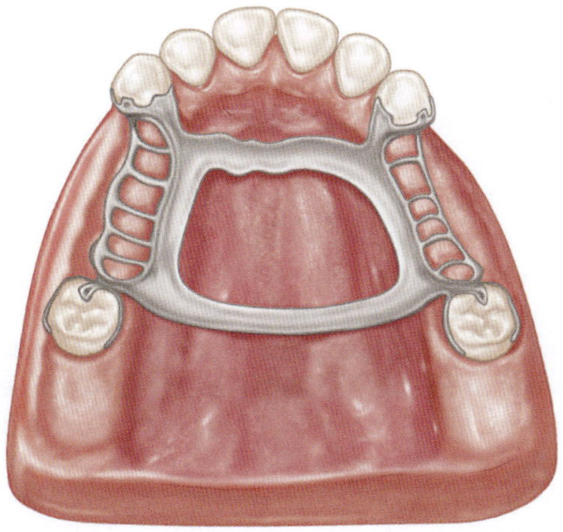

Fig. 5.27 Combination anterior-posterior palatal bar. To be sufficiently rigid to provide the required support and stability, these major connectors must be excessively bulky. Because of its bulk and location, the anterior bar often interferes with the tongue.

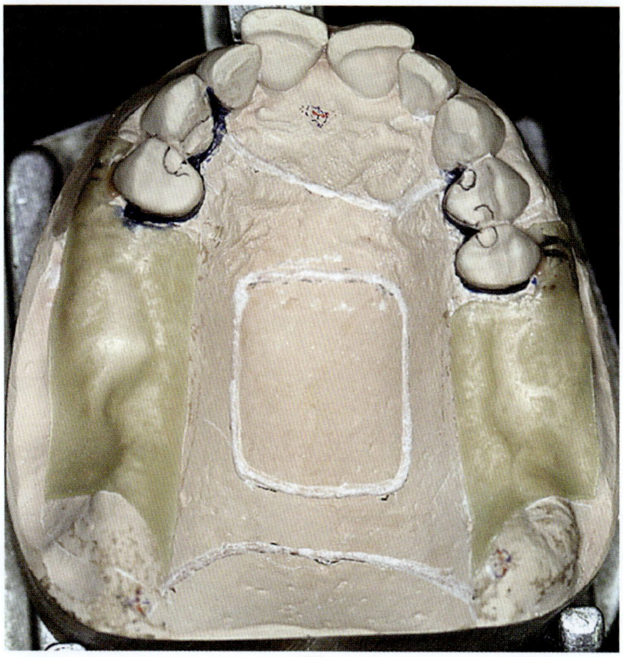

Fig. 5.28 Framework design on master cast before preparation for duplication in refractory investment. A shallow groove (0.5 mm) has been scribed on the outline of the anterior and posterior borders of the major connector. The anterior outline follows the valleys of rugae. Beading is readily accomplished with a cleoid carver. A slightly rounded groove is preferred to a V-shaped groove.

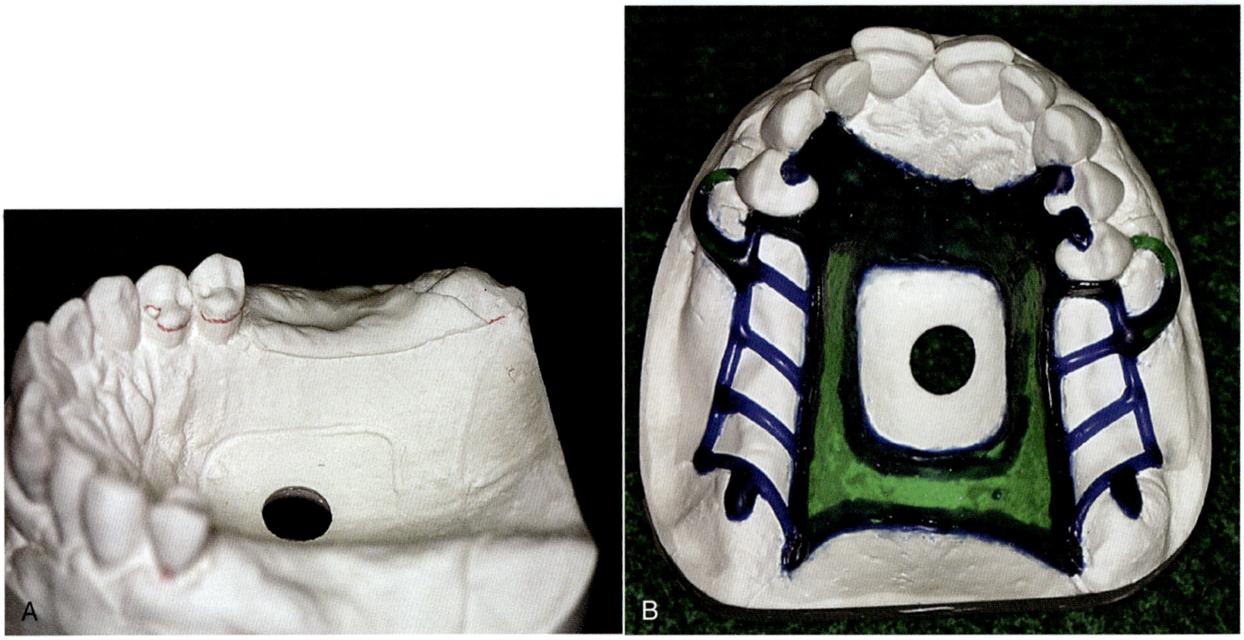

Fig. 5.29 A, Refractory cast. Note the definitive outline of the major connector indicated by beading lines that were transferred in duplicating the master cast. **B,** The wax pattern for the major connector is accurately executed by following the beading lines. The major connector is confined to previously scribed beading.

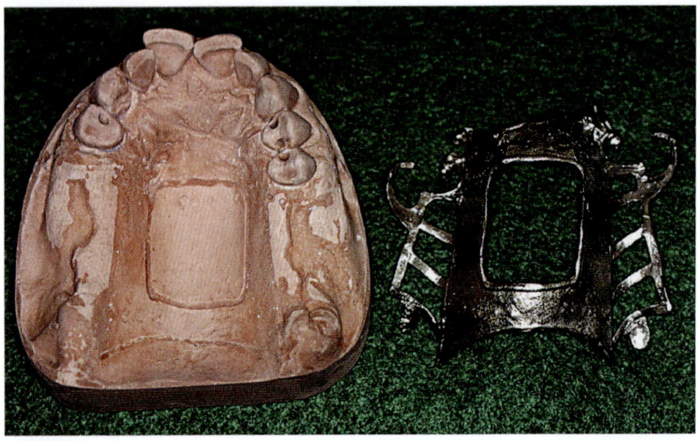

Fig. 5.30 Cast and framework showing metal margin produced by the 0.5-mm beading line scribed on the cast. Such a margin is easily finished in the lab and provides intimate tissue contact, preventing food from easily dislodging the prosthesis. Care should be exercised in adapting such a beaded margin to nondisplaceable tissue, such as the median palatal raphe.

For the open latticework and meshwork wax relief during processing of the denture base creates space for the denture resin to wrap around the framework. These types of denture bases may be relined. For the metal base framework, the metal base is fabricated to fit against the underlying supporting tissue with no relief beneath the framework. These denture bases cannot be relined.

When dental implants are placed, modifications can be required in the denture base area of physical retention for the acrylic base, which is a type of retaining minor connector. The need for and type of modification is dependent on how the implants will be engaged. Implants placed anteriorly to enhance retention by removing the need for a visible clasp must account for retentive device bulk and connection requirements for joining to the prosthesis (i.e., direct to the metallic frame or via embedding within the acrylic resin denture base). Modifications required for implants placed more distal for purposes of support typically require designing space for embedding an attachment housing within the denture base (Fig. 5.33).

Functions

In addition to joining denture parts, the minor connector serves two other purposes:

1. Transfers functional stress to the abutment teeth: This is a prosthesis-to-abutment function of the minor connector. Occlusal forces applied to the artificial teeth are transmitted through the base to the underlying ridge tissue if that base is primarily tissue supported. Occlusal forces applied to the artificial teeth are also transferred to abutment teeth through occlusal rests. The minor connectors arising from a rigid major connector make possible this transfer of functional stress throughout the dental arch.
2. Transfers the effects of the retainers, rests, and stabilizing components throughout the prosthesis: This is an abutment-to-prosthesis function of the minor connector. Thus forces applied on one portion of the denture may be resisted by other components placed elsewhere in the arch for that purpose. A stabilizing component on one side of the arch may be placed to resist horizontal forces that originate on the opposite side. This is possible only because of the transferring effect of the minor connector, which supports that stabilizing component, and the rigidity of the major connector.

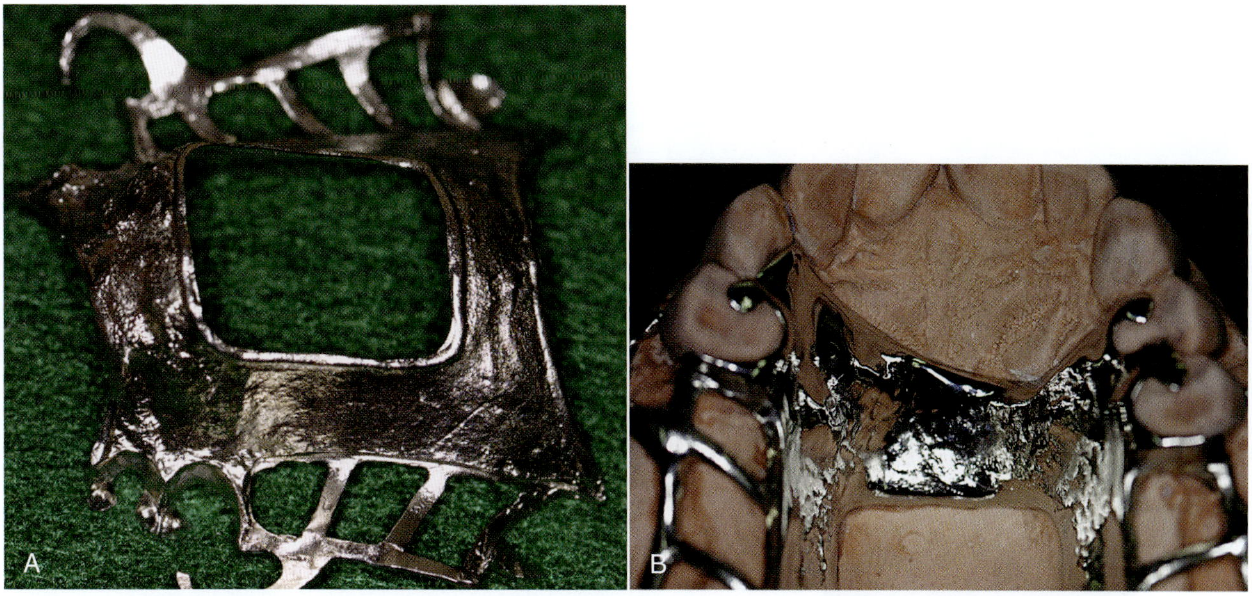

Fig. 5.31 A, Tissue side of casting. Note slightly elevated ridges outlining anterior, posterior, and midpalatal opening regions of this anterior-posterior palatal strap major connector. **B,** Casting finished to a demarcated outline and seated on the master cast showing intimate adaptation.

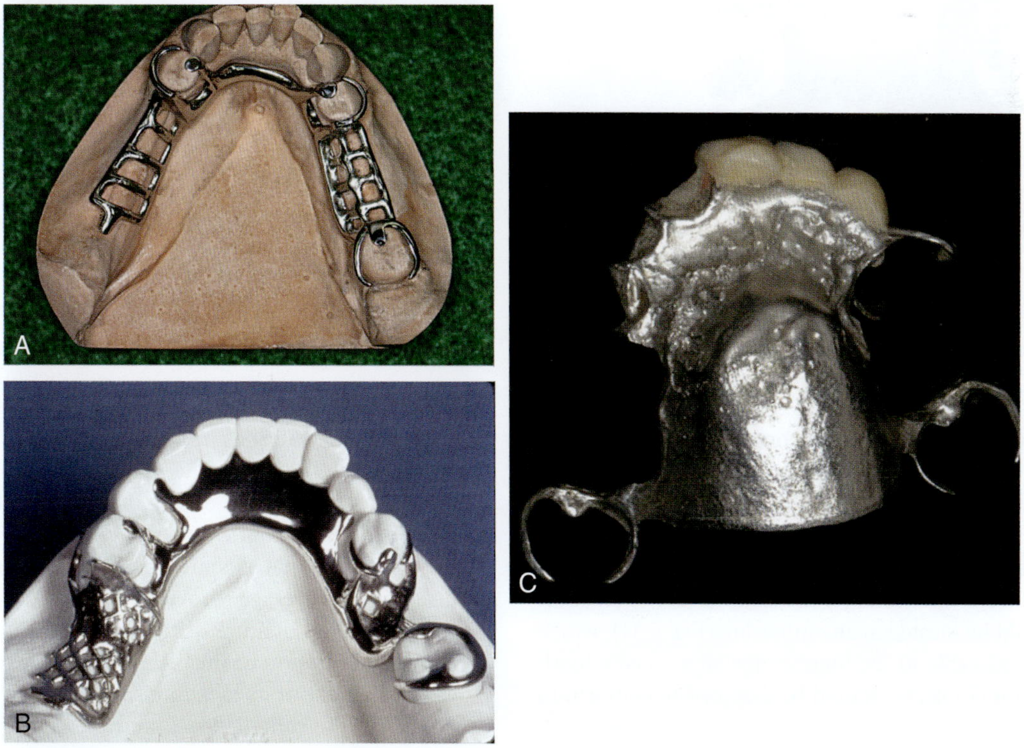

Fig. 5.32 Type of physical retention. **A,** The distal extension framework is using latticework physical retention. The longitudinal and transverse struts form a ladderlike design. The transverse struts are positioned to allow for the setting of denture teeth between the struts. The physical retention on the tooth-bound edentulous area is an example of meshwork. **B,** Both the distal extension and the modification space of this framework are examples of meshwork retention. The design is similar to a rigid metallic screen that will allow for penetration of the resin through the openings to provide encirclement of the resin and mechanical retention of the denture base. **C,** Metal base frameworks rest directly on the supporting tissue. The denture base is retained to the metal base using beads, nail heads, or wire components. (Photos courtesy of Lisa A. Lang and Lily T. Garcia.)

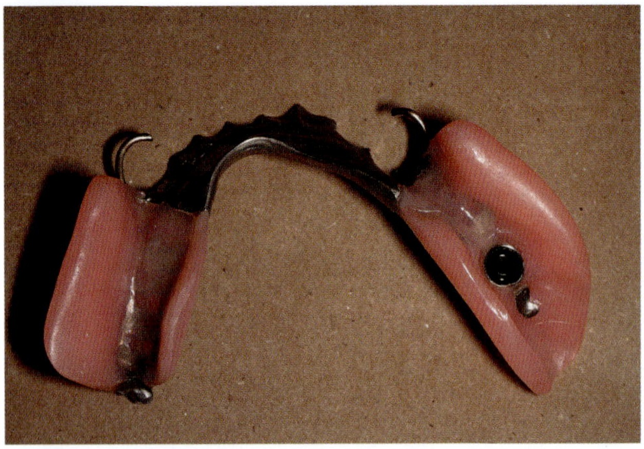

Fig. 5.33 The locator attachment in the posterior aspect of the distal extension base of the removable partial denture provides retention for the distal extension.

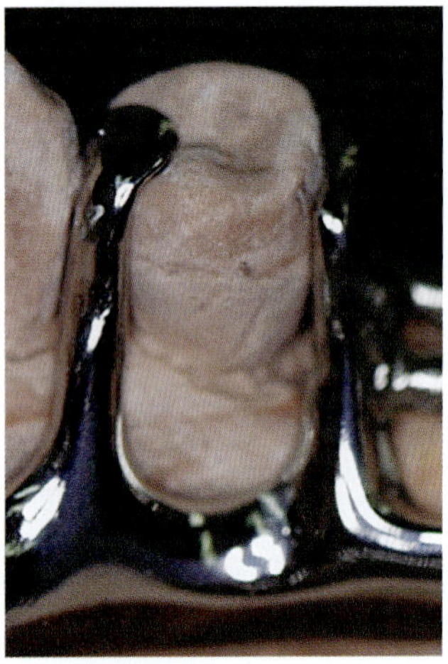

Fig. 5.34 In an embrasure space, the minor connector is tapered to the tooth to avoid bulk and to accommodate the tongue.

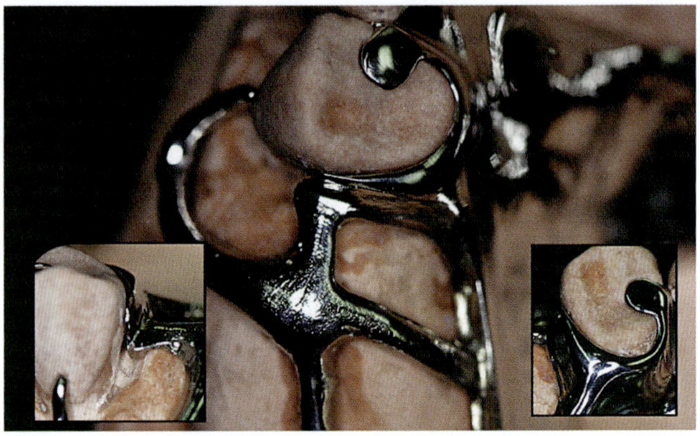

Fig. 5.35 The minor connector that contacts the guiding plane is part of a clasp assembly. It can be separated from the other parts, or, as in this case, it can be connected to the lingual stabilizing portion of the clasp assembly. The proximal plate minor connector contact is about one-half the distance between tips of adjacent buccal and lingual cusps of the abutment tooth, and it extends gingivally, contacting an area of the abutment from the marginal ridge to two-thirds the length of the enamel crown. Viewed from above, it is triangular, the apex of the triangle being located buccally, and the base of the triangle being located lingually. Less interference with the arrangement of the adjacent artificial tooth is encountered with minor connectors so shaped.

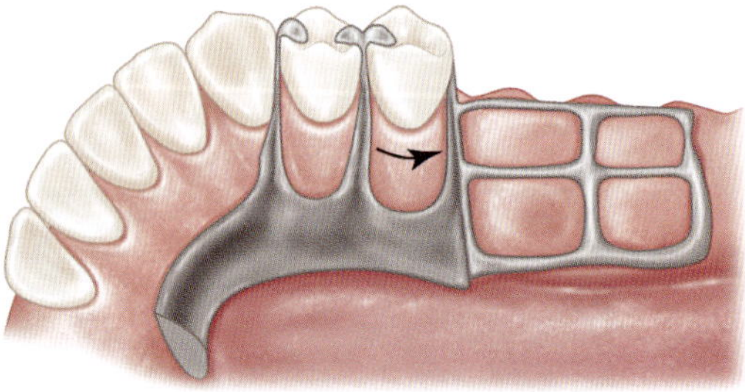

Fig. 5.36 Finish line at the junction of the ladderlike minor connector and the major connector blends smoothly into the minor connector contacting the distal guiding plane on the second premolar. The framework is feathered toward tissue anterior to the finish line to avoid as much bulk in this area as possible without compromising the strength of the butt-type joint.

Form and Location

Like the major connector, the minor connector must have sufficient bulk to be rigid; otherwise, the transfer of functional stresses to the supporting teeth and tissue will not be effective. At the same time, the bulk of the minor connector should not be objectionable.

A minor connector that contacts the axial surface of an abutment tooth should be located in an embrasure (Fig. 5.34), where it will be least noticeable to the tongue, not on a convex tooth surface. The minor connector should be designed to conform to the interdental embrasure, passing vertically from the major connector to minimize encroaching on gingival tissues. A tapering effect occurs from the major connector toward the contact area (Fig. 5.35).

The deepest part of the interdental embrasure does not fit into an undercut since the area should have been blocked out to avoid interference during placement and removal, and to avoid any wedging effect on the contacted teeth.

A modification of the conventional removable partial denture minor connector has been proposed. This application was suggested to be limited to the maxillary arch, with the minor connector located in the center of the lingual surface of the maxillary abutment tooth.

It is suggested that this modification reduces the amount of gingival tissue coverage, provides enhanced guidance for the removable partial denture during insertion and removal, and increases stabilization against horizontal and rotational forces. However, because of its location, such a design variation could encroach on the tongue space and create a greater potential space for food entrapment. The proposed variation should be used with careful application.

When a minor connector contacts tooth surfaces on either side of the embrasure in which it lies, it should be tapered as it approaches or toward the teeth. This avoids sharp angles, which could hinder tongue movement, and eliminates open spaces that could trap food (Fig. 5.36).

The minor connector referred to as the proximal plate contacts the guide plane surfaces of the abutment teeth, whether as a connected part of a direct retainer assembly or as a separate entity (see Fig. 5.35). The proximal plate must be wide enough—buccolingually such that the guide plane can be used to the fullest advantage. When it gives rise to a clasp arm, the connector should be tapered to the tooth below the origin of the clasp. If no clasp arm is formed (as when a bar clasp arm originates elsewhere), the connector should be tapered to a knife-edge the full length of its buccal aspect.

When an artificial tooth is placed against a proximal minor connector, the minor connector design has the largest bulk located toward the lingual aspect of the abutment tooth. In this manner, there is sufficient bulk located to ensure the least interference with the placement of the artificial tooth. Ideally, the artificial tooth should contact the abutment tooth with only a thin layer of metal intervening buccally. Lingually the bulk of the minor connector should lie in the interdental embrasure—the same as between two natural teeth.

As was stated previously, those portions of a denture framework by which acrylic-resin denture bases are attached are minor connectors. This type of minor connector should be so designed that it will be completely embedded within the denture base.

The junctions of these mandibular minor connectors with the major connectors should be strong butt-type joints but without appreciable bulk (see Fig. 5.36). Angles formed at the junctions of the connectors should not be greater than 90 degrees, thus ensuring the most advantageous and the strongest mechanical connection between the acrylic-resin denture base and the major connector.

An open latticework or ladder type of design is preferable and managed in the dental laboratory using preformed 12-gauge half-round and 18-gauge round wax strips. The minor connector for the mandibular distal extension base should extend posteriorly about two-thirds the length of the edentulous ridge and overlaps lingual and buccal slopes of the residual ridge surfaces. The design of the minor connector support for denture base material adds support for the denture base and may minimize the distortion of resin that occurs during processing. The minor connector design must be planned to avoid interfering with the arrangement of artificial teeth (Fig. 5.37).

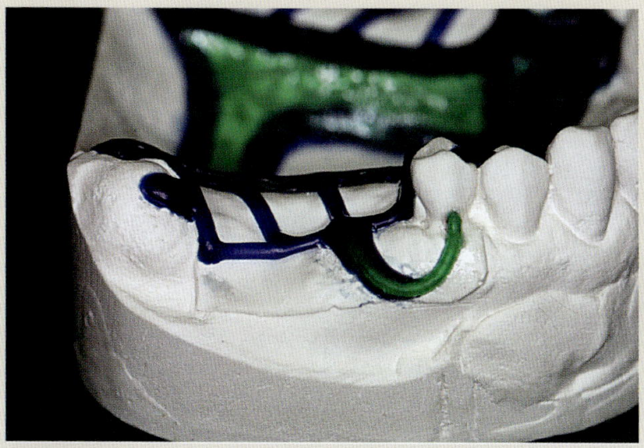

Fig. 5.37 The minor connector for attaching the resin denture base should be designed so that denture tooth placement is not compromised. The minor connector design should not include a main lattice strut at the ridge crest or in a desired tooth location.

The framework design can include a means to attach resin extensions as impression trays to the mandibular framework when a corrected impression is planned. Incorporating "nailhead" minor connectors fabricated as part of the distal extension minor connector can help support impressioning for a corrected cast or the resin trays can detach or loosen during impression-making procedures. Minor connectors for maxillary distal extension denture bases should extend the entire length of the residual ridge and can be a ladderlike and loop design (Fig. 5.38).

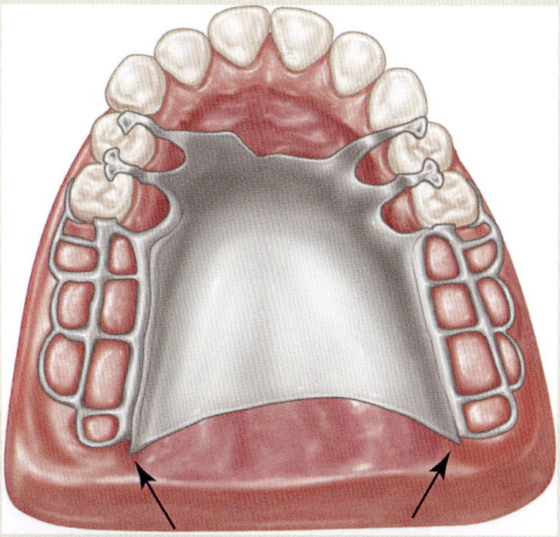

Fig. 5.38 Extension of the finish line to the area of the pterygomaxillary notch provides a butt-type joint for attachment of the border portion of the resin base through the pterygomaxillary notch *(arrows)*.

Tissue Stops

Tissue stops are integral parts of minor connectors which can aid in the retention of resin bases. Tissue stops are designed to allow a defined spacer between the minor connector and supporting tissues and provide additional framework stability to the framework during the stages of transfer and processing. Tissue stops can engage buccal and lingual slopes of the residual ridge for stability (Fig. 5.39).

FINISH LINES

Another integral part in the design of the minor connector used to retain denture base material is similar to a tissue stop but serves a different purpose is the *finish line*. It is located distal to the terminal abutment and is a continuation of the minor connector contacting the guiding plane. Its purpose is to establish a definitive finishing index tissue stop for the denture base material after processing.

The finish line of the removable partial denture framework is the junction between the metal framework and the denture base material. The two materials form a butt joint to create a smooth, distinct border between dissimilar materials (Fig. 5.40). There are two types of finish lines: an internal and external finish line. The internal finish line is located on the intaglio surface of the framework, where the external finish line is on the nontissue side of the framework (Fig. 5.41). The finish line junction with the major connector forms an angle not greater than 90 degrees, possibly undercut (Fig. 5.42).

In the maxillary arch, the medial extent of the minor connector depends on the lateral extent of the major palatal connector.

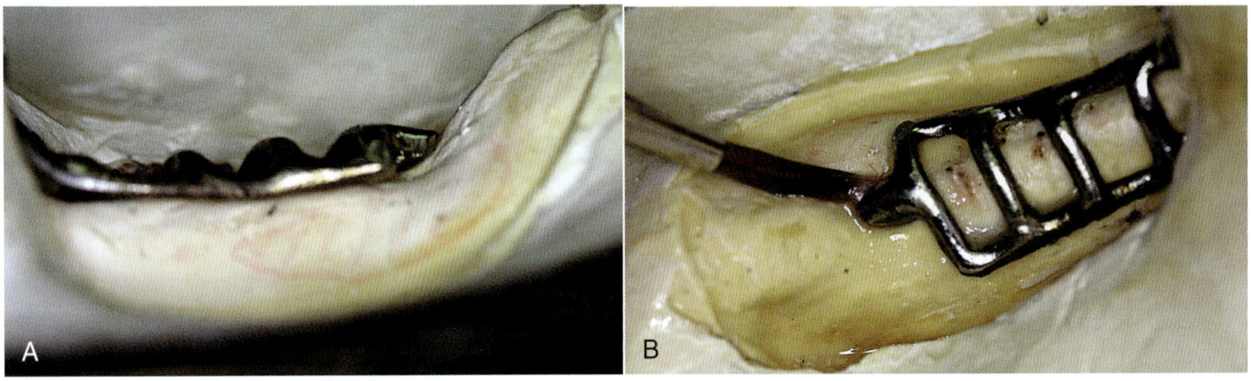

Fig. 5.39 Note the location of the tissue stops at the terminal portion of the minor connector elevated from the residual ridge. The framework was developed on the cast, with the tissue stop designed to provide stability of the framework during processing of the acrylic and facilitate finishing of the denture base resin at the region of the terminal abutment. The residual ridge was later recorded in its functional form by a corrected impression, thus the elevated tissue stop. The tissue stop as seen from the lateral view **(A)** and the occlusal view **(B)**.

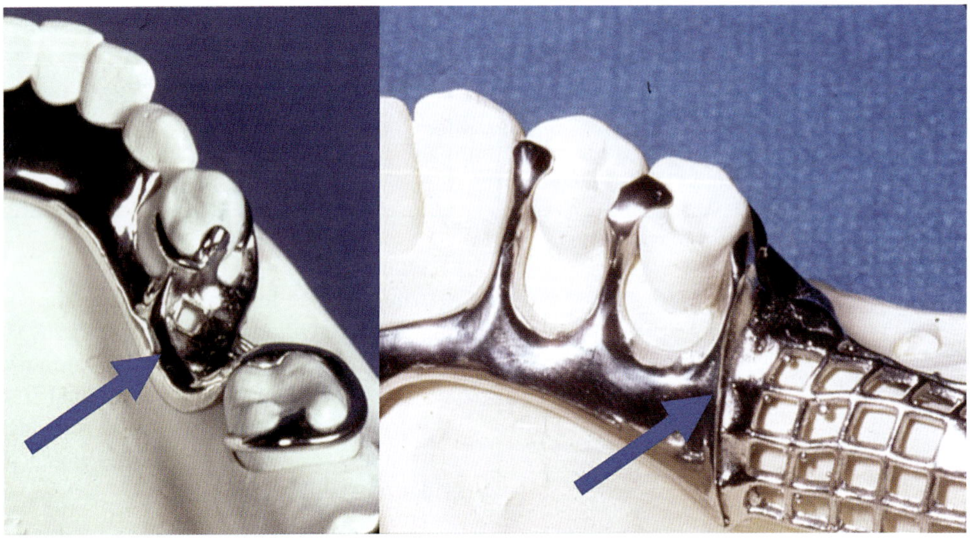

Fig. 5.40 Removable partial denture framework illustrating external finish lines. The arrows identify the butt joint of the finish line. (Photo courtesy of Lisa A. Lang.)

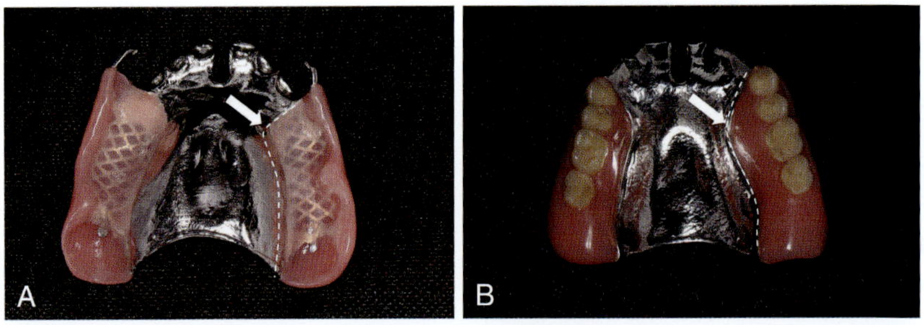

Fig. 5.41 The *arrows* point to a dotted outline of the maxillary removable partial denture finish lines. **A,** The intaglio surface of a maxillary removable partial denture with its *internal finish line*. **B,** The polished surface of a maxillary removable partial denture with its *external finish line*. (Photo courtesy of Ahmed Marous Copyright © 2024. All rights reserved.)

If the finish line is located too far medially, the natural contour of the palate will be altered by the thickness of the framework junction and the resin supporting the artificial teeth (Fig. 5.43). On the contrary, if the finish line is located too far buccally, it will be difficult to create a natural contour in resin material mimicking the palatal slope adjacent to artificial teeth. The location of the finish line at the junction of the major and minor connectors should be planned as creating the natural palatal shape.

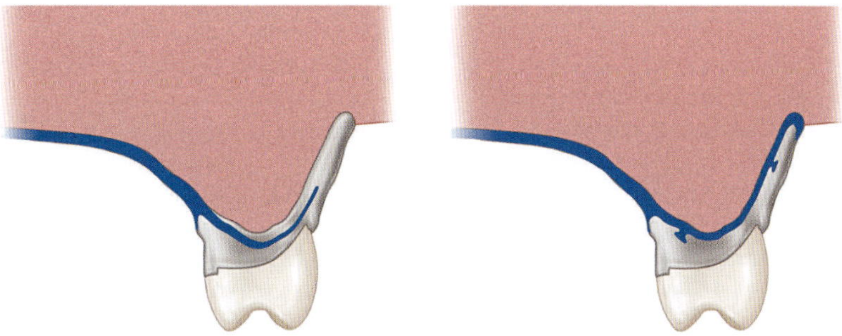

Fig. 5.42 Frontal sections through lingual finish lines of palatal major connectors. The *right image* is through the full-cast metal base major connector; the *left image* is through the resin denture base. In both situations, the location of finish lines minimizes the bulk of resin attaching to the artificial teeth. Palatal contours are restored, enhancing speech, and contributing to a natural feeling for the patient.

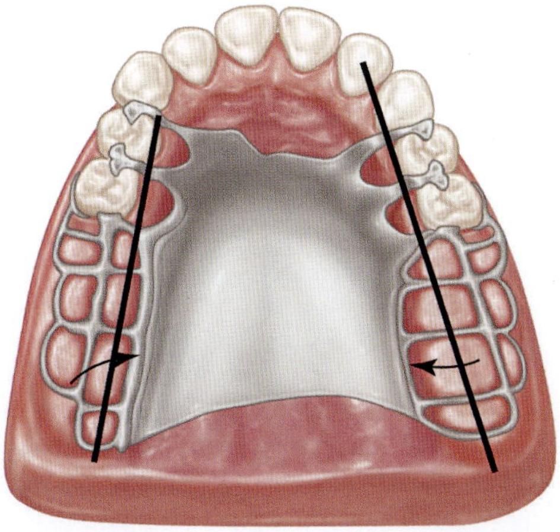

Fig. 5.43 Junction of the major connector and the minor connector at palatal finish lines should be located 2 mm medial from an imaginary line that would contact the lingual surfaces of missing posterior teeth. The finish line on the right is too far toward the midline of the palate. The natural contours of the palate will be altered.

Equal consideration must be given to the junction of minor connectors and bar-type direct retainer arms. These junctions are 90-degree butt-type joints and should follow the guidelines for base contour and clasp length.

REACTION OF TISSUE TO METALLIC COVERAGE

The reaction of tissue to coverage by the metallic components of a removable partial denture has been the subject of significant controversy, particularly in regions of marginal gingiva and broad areas of tissue contact. These tissue reactions can result from pressure caused by lack of support, lack of adequate hygiene measures, and prolonged contact through continuous use of a prosthesis.

Pressure areas can occur if the design does not incorporate components to mitigate movement of the prosthesis. Tissue impingement can occur due to loss of tooth and/or tissue support. Impingement can also be caused by fracture and loss of rests, or improper rest design, caries involvement, or intrusion of abutment teeth under occlusal loading. It is important to maintain adequate relief and support from both teeth and tissue as changes in support can also produce pressure elsewhere in the arch, such as beneath major connectors. Routine maintenance appointments should evaluate the prosthesis for "settling" which necessitates intervention or corrective procedures since if unnoticed can cause damage to supporting teeth and/or tissues.

Lack of adequate oral hygiene measures can result in tissue reactions caused by an accumulation of food debris and bacteria. The physical coverage of tissues by the prosthesis requires hygiene maintenance of the prosthesis itself to avoid compounding factors that compromise intraoral health.

Patients may become so accustomed to wearing a removable prosthesis restoration that they neglect to remove it frequently to allow for tissue health maintenance. Continuous wearing of a removable prosthesis can contribute to poor tissue health including inflammation. This can occur more frequently when a removable partial denture includes replacement of anterior teeth; an individual should plan time that allows the prosthesis to be out of the mouth for example, in the privacy of the bathroom during toothbrushing. Patients should be instructed to remove their removable partial denture for several hours each day so that the negative effects of tissue contact can subside, and the tissue can return to a normal state.

Clinical experience with the use of linguoplates and complete metal palatal major connectors in removable partial dentures has shown that when factors of pressure, cleanliness, and time are controlled, tissue coverage is not solely detrimental to the health of intraoral tissues.

MAJOR CONNECTORS IN REVIEW

Mandibular Lingual Bar

Indications for Use: The lingual bar should be used for mandibular removable partial dentures when sufficient space exists between the slightly elevated alveolar lingual sulcus and the lingual gingival tissue.

Characteristics and Location: The design is half-pear shaped with the bulkiest portion inferiorly located and the superior border tapered toward the soft tissue. It is recommended when there is a minimum of 8 mm between the gingival margin and the movable floor of the mouth. The superior border of a lingual bar connector should be located a minimum of 4 mm below the gingival margin(s).

Mandibular Linguoplate

Indications for Use: (1) When the alveolar lingual sulcus so closely approximates the lingual gingival crevices that adequate width for a rigid lingual bar does not exist. (2) In those instances, in which the residual ridges in Kennedy Class I arch have undergone such vertical resorption that they will offer only minimal resistance to horizontal rotations of the denture through its bases. (3) In situations where periodontally weakened teeth need to function together to furnish support to the prosthesis and to help resist horizontal (off-vertical) rotation of the distal extension type of denture. (4) When the future replacement of one or more incisor teeth will be facilitated by the addition of retention loops to an existing linguoplate.

Characteristics and Location: The design is a half-pear shaped with bulkiest portion inferiorly located with a thin metal apron extending superiorly to contact cingula of anterior teeth and lingual surfaces of involved posterior teeth at their height of contour. The apron extends interproximally to the height of contact points (i.e., closing interproximal spaces). The scalloped contour of the apron is dictated by interproximal blockout. The superior border is finished to a continuous plane with contacted teeth. The inferior border at the ascertained height of the alveolar lingual sulcus when the patient's tongue is slightly elevated.

Mandibular Sublingual Bar

Indications for Use: The sublingual bar should be used for mandibular removable partial dentures when the height of the floor of the mouth in relation to the free gingival margins will be less than 6 mm. It also may be indicated whenever it is desirable to keep the free gingival margins of the remaining anterior teeth exposed and the depth of the floor of the mouth is inadequate to place a lingual bar.

Contraindications for Use: Remaining natural anterior teeth severely tilted toward the lingual.

Characteristics and Location: The sublingual bar is essentially the same half-pear shape as a lingual bar, except that the bulkiest portion is located to the lingual and the tapered portion is toward the labial. The superior border of the bar should be at least 3 mm from the free gingival margin of the teeth. The inferior border is located at the height of the alveolar lingual sulcus when the patient's tongue is slightly elevated. Mandibular lingual bar with continuous bar (cingulum bar).

Indications for Use: (1) When a lingual plate is otherwise indicated but the axial alignment of anterior teeth is such that excessive blockout of interproximal undercuts would be required. (2) When wide diastemata exist between mandibular anterior teeth and a lingual plate would objectionably display metal in a frontal view.

Characteristics and Location: The conventionally shaped bar is located the same as lingual bar major connector component when possible. A thin, narrow (3 mm) metal strap is located on the cingula of anterior teeth, scalloped to follow interproximal embrasures with inferior and superior borders tapering to tooth surfaces. The major connector originates bilaterally from incisal, lingual, or occlusal rests of adjacent principal abutments.

Mandibular Continuous Bar (Cingulum Bar)

Indications for Use: When a lingual plate or sublingual bar is otherwise indicated but the axial alignment of the anterior teeth is such that excessive blockout of interproximal undercuts would be required.

Contraindications for Use: Anterior teeth severely tilted to the lingual and/or when there are wide diastemata that exist between the mandibular anterior teeth and the cingulum bar that would objectionably display metal in a frontal view are rationale to not use this major connector.

Characteristics and Location: A thin, narrow (3 mm) metal strap is located on the cingula of anterior teeth, scalloped to follow interproximal embrasures with inferior and superior borders tapering to tooth surfaces. The major connector originates bilaterally from incisal, lingual, or occlusal rests of adjacent principal abutments.

Mandibular Labial Bar

Indications for Use: (1) When lingual inclinations of remaining mandibular premolar and incisor teeth cannot be corrected, preventing placement of a conventional lingual bar connector. (2) When severe lingual tori cannot be removed and prevent the use of a lingual bar or lingual plate major connector. (3) When severe and abrupt lingual tissue undercuts make it impractical to use a lingual bar or a lingual plate major connector.

Characteristics and Location: The design is a half-pear shaped with bulkiest portion inferiorly located on the labial and buccal aspects of the mandible. Its superior border is tapered toward the soft tissue. The superior border is located at least 4 mm inferior to labial and buccal gingival margins and farther if possible. The inferior border is located in the labial-buccal vestibule at the juncture of attached (immobile) and unattached (mobile) mucosae.

Single Palatal Strap–Type Major Connector

Indications for Use: Bilateral edentulous spaces of short span in a tooth-supported restoration.

Single Broad Palatal Major Connector

Indications for Use: (1) Kennedy Class I partially edentulous arches with residual ridges that have undergone little vertical resorption and will lend excellent support. (2) V- or U-shaped palates. (3) Strong abutments (single or made so by splinting). (4) More teeth in arch than six remaining anterior teeth. (5) Direct retention not a problem. (6) No interfering tori.

Characteristics and Location: The design form replicates that anatomic form of the palate. Its anterior border follows valleys of rugae as near right angle to median suture line as possible and not extending anterior to occlusal rests or indirect retainers. Additionally, the posterior border is located at the junction of hard and soft palate but not extended onto the soft palate and at right angles to the median suture line and extended to pterygomaxillary notches.

Anterior-Posterior Strap–Type Major Connector

Indications for Use: (1) Kennedy Class I and II arches in which excellent abutment and residual ridge support exist, and direct retention can be made adequate without the need for indirect retention. (2) Long edentulous spans in Kennedy Class II, modification 1 arches. (3) Kennedy Class IV arches in which anterior teeth must be replaced with a removable partial denture. (4) Inoperable palatal tori that do not extend posteriorly to the junction of the hard and soft palates.

Characteristics and Location: The design of this major connector is parallelogram shaped and open in center portion. (2) The width should be relatively broad (8–10 mm) anterior and posterior palatal straps. (3) Lateral palatal straps (7–9 mm) narrow and parallel to the curve of arch; minimum of 6 mm from gingival crevices of remaining teeth. (4) Anterior palatal strap: Anterior border should not be placed farther anteriorly than anterior rests and never closer than 6 mm to lingual gingival crevices; it should follow the valleys of the rugae at right angles to the median palatal suture. If the posterior border is in the rugae area, it should follow valleys of the rugae at right angles to the median palatal suture. (5) Posterior palatal connector: Posterior border should be located at the junction of hard and soft palates and at right angles to median palatal suture and extended to hamular notch area(s) on distal extension side(s). (6) Anatomic replica or matte surface.

Complete Palatal Coverage Major Connector

Indications for Use: (1) In most situations in which only some or all anterior teeth remain. (2) Kennedy Class II arch with a large posterior modification space and some missing anterior teeth. (3) Kennedy Class I arch with one to four premolars and some or all anterior teeth remaining, when abutment support is poor and cannot otherwise be enhanced; residual ridges have undergone extreme vertical resorption; direct retention is difficult to obtain. (4) In the absence of a pedunculated torus.

Characteristics and Location: (1) Anatomic replica form for full palatal metal casting supported anteriorly by positive rest seats. (2) Palatal linguoplate supported anteriorly and designed for attachment of acrylic-resin extension posteriorly. (3) Contacts all or almost all of the teeth remaining in the arch. (4) Posterior border: Terminates at the junction of the hard and soft palates; extended to hamular notch area(s) on distal extension side(s); at a right angle to the median suture line.

U-Shaped Palatal Major Connector

This connector should be used only in those situations in which inoperable tori extend to the posterior limit of the hard palate.

The U-shaped palatal major connector is the least favorable design of all palatal major connectors because it lacks the rigidity of other types of connectors. When it must be used, indirect retainers must support any portion of the connector that extends anteriorly from the principal occlusal rests. Anterior border areas of this type of connector must be kept at least 6 mm away from adjacent teeth. If for any reason the anterior border must contact the remaining teeth, the connector must again be supported by rests placed in properly prepared rest seats. It should never be supported even temporarily by inclined lingual surfaces of anterior teeth.

REFERENCES

1. The glossary of prosthodontic terms, ed 9. *J Prosthet Dent.* 2005;94(1):10–92. Available online: http://www.sciencedirect.com/science/article/pii/S0022391305001757.
2. Swing-Lock Inc., Milford, Texas.
3. Blatterfein L. A systematic method of designing upper partial denture bases. *J Am Dent Assoc.* 1953;46(5):510–525. https://doi.org/10.14219/jada.archive.1953.0085.

6

Rests and Rest Seats

Lisa A. Lang, Lily T. García, and Ahmed Mahrous

CHAPTER OUTLINE

Although the major connector joins all removable partial denture (RPD) component parts, engaging the remaining teeth through appropriate use of rest seats and rests affords efficient resistance to functional chewing forces. The capacity for teeth to resist functional forces and remain stable over time is provided through their sophisticated support mechanisms. Studies have shown that displacement and recovery following loading are far better for natural teeth than for oral mucosa. Similarly, the capacity of implants to resist the functional forces of chewing may exceed that of teeth.

Consequently, appropriate use of the teeth to help resist functional forces in removable prostheses is a critical strategy to control prosthesis movement and achieve functional stability. When situations of multiple missing teeth are seen in conjunction with less-than-ideal soft tissue support opposing natural dentition, implant use should be strongly considered.

ROLE OF RESTS IN CONTROL OF PROSTHESIS MOVEMENT

Appropriate use of teeth requires consideration as to how best to engage teeth for the supportive qualities they provide. Because the most effective resistance can be provided if the tooth is stressed along its long axis, the prosthesis framework should engage the tooth in a manner that encourages axial loading. The various forms of rests have as a main goal a form that allows for axial loading. It is important to realize that this goal can be achieved only through some form of tooth modification.

Vertical support must be provided for an RPD. Any component of an RPD on a tooth surface that provides vertical support is called a *rest* (Fig. 6.1). Rests should always be located on properly prepared tooth surfaces. The prepared surface of an abutment to receive the rest is called the *rest seat*. Rests are designated by the surface of the tooth prepared to receive them (occlusal rest, lingual rest, and incisal rest). The topography of any rest should generally restore the topography of the tooth that existed before the rest seat was prepared.

The primary purpose of the rest is to provide vertical support for the partial denture. In doing so, it also:

- Maintains components in their planned positions
- Maintains established occlusal relationships by preventing settling of the denture
- Prevents impingement of soft tissue
- Directs and distributes occlusal loads to abutment teeth

Thus rests serve to support the position of a partial denture and to resist movement toward the tissue. They serve to transmit vertical forces to the abutment teeth and to direct those forces along the long axes of the teeth. In this respect, tooth-supported RPD rests function in a manner similar to fixed abutment retainers. It is obvious that for this degree of stability to exist, the rests must be rigid and must receive positive support from the abutment teeth, which means that under occlusal loading, the rest and the tooth remain in stable contact and no independent movement or slippage occurs.

In an RPD that has one or more distal extension bases, the denture base becomes increasingly tissue supported as the distance from the abutment increases. Closer to the abutment, however, more of the occlusal load is transmitted to the abutment tooth by means of the rest. The load is thereby distributed between the abutment and the supporting residual ridge tissue.

When rests prevent movement of the removable partial denture in an apical direction, the position of the retentive portion of the clasp arms can be maintained in designated relation to the tooth undercuts. Although passive when it is in its terminal position, the retentive portion of the clasp arm should remain in contact with the tooth, ready to resist a vertical dislodging force. Then, when a dislodging force is applied, the clasp arm should immediately become actively engaged to resist vertical displacement. If settling of the denture base results in clasp arms that

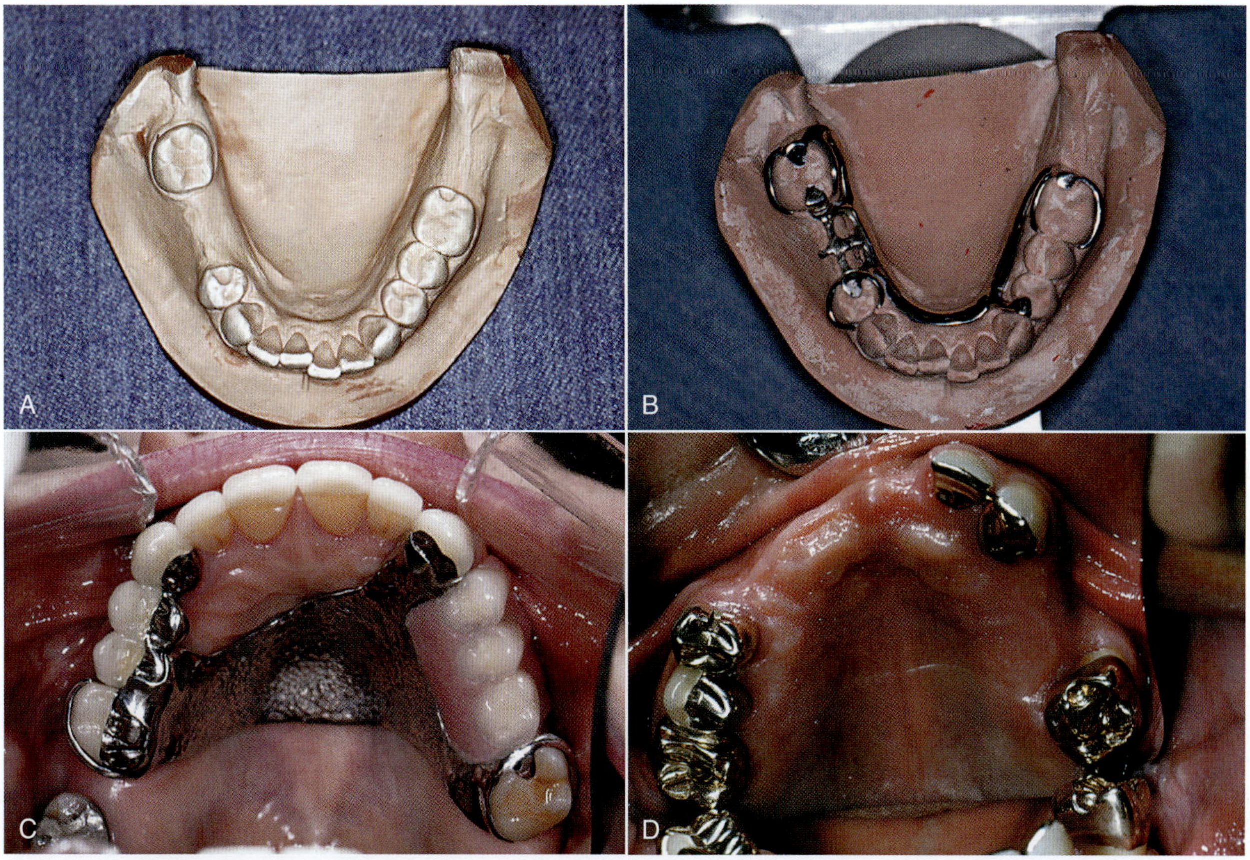

Fig. 6.1 A, Occlusal rest seats have been prepared on molar and premolar teeth to provide vertical support for the removable partial denture. **B,** Framework for tooth-supported removable partial denture. Rests on patient's right provide vertical support to the replacement dentition; rests on patient's left provide cross-arch support and stabilization. **C,** Tooth support for this prosthesis is provided by rests that occupy definite, prepared, rest seats on the canine and occlusal surfaces of selected posterior teeth. **D,** Kennedy Class III, modification 1, maxillary arch with rest seats prepared on the lingual surfaces of the canine, and lateral incisor and on the occlusal surfaces of the premolar and molar.

stand away from the tooth, some vertical displacement is possible before the retainer can become functional. The rest prevents such settling, thereby helping maintain the vertical stability of the removable partial denture.

The use of an implant as a rest can also be considered. In this application, the implant eliminates compression of supporting soft tissues, controls vertical movement of the denture base, eliminates or alters fulcrum lines, and serves to increase support and stability of the prosthesis.

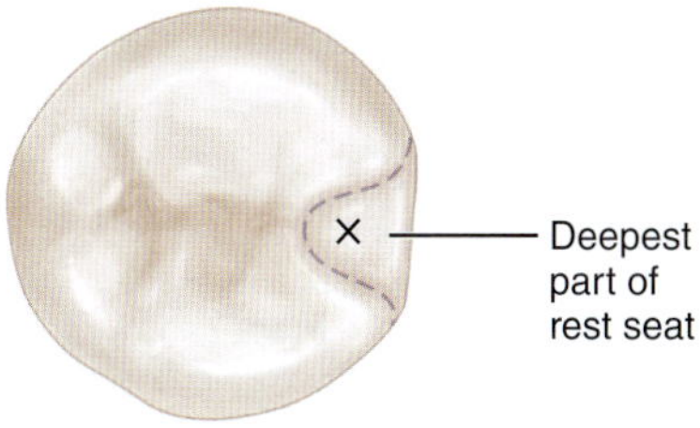

Fig. 6.2 The deepest part of an occlusal rest preparation should be inside the lowered marginal ridge at X. The marginal ridge is lowered to provide bulk and to accommodate the origin of the occlusal rest with the least occlusal interference.

FORM OF THE OCCLUSAL REST AND REST SEAT

The form of the occlusal rest seat should be designed and located with the following guidelines in mind:

- The outline form of an occlusal rest seat should be a rounded triangular shape with the apex toward the center of the occlusal surface (Fig. 6.2).
- It should be as long as it is wide, and the base of the triangular shape (at the marginal ridge) should be at least 2.5 mm for both molars and premolars. Rest seats of smaller dimensions do not provide an adequate bulk of metal for rests, especially if the rest is contoured to restore the occlusal morphology of the abutment tooth.
- The marginal ridge of the abutment tooth at the site of the rest seat must be lowered to permit a sufficient bulk of metal for strength and rigidity of the rest and the minor connector. This means reduction of the marginal ridge of approximately 1.5 mm is usually necessary.
- The floor of the occlusal rest seat should be apical to the marginal ridge and the occlusal surface and should be concave or

spoon shaped (Fig. 6.3). Caution should be exercised in preparing a rest seat to avoid creating sharp edges or line angles in the preparation.

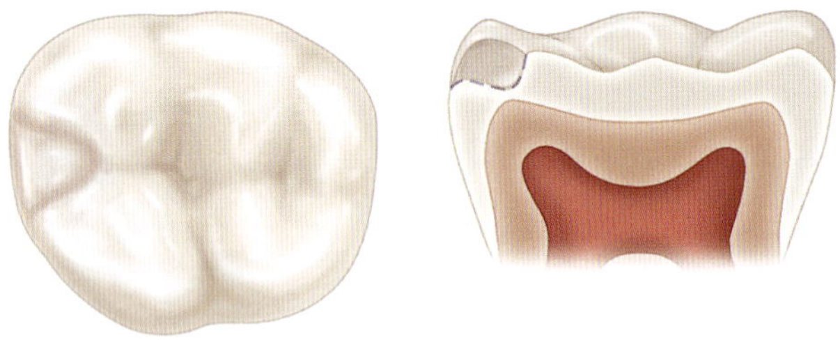

Fig. 6.3 Occlusal rest seat preparation on molar. The preparation is rounded, and the triangular concavity has smooth margins on the occlusal surface and a lowered, rounded marginal ridge.

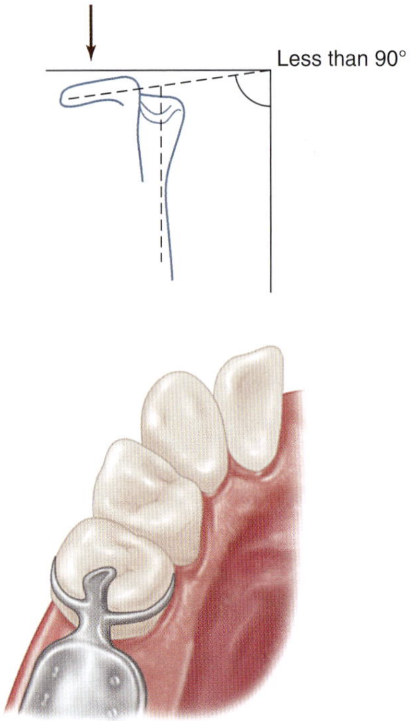

Fig. 6.4 The occlusal rest should be spoon shaped and slightly inclined apically from the marginal ridge. The rest should restore the occlusal morphology of the tooth that existed before preparation of the rest seat.

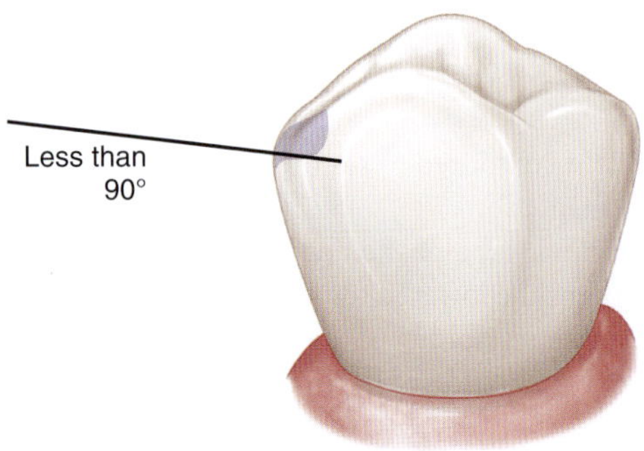

Fig. 6.5 The floor of the occlusal rest seat should be inclined apically from the lowered marginal ridge. Any angle less than 90 degrees is acceptable if the proximal surface preparation and lowering and rounding of the marginal ridge precede completion of the rest seat.

- The angle formed by the occlusal rest and the vertical minor connector from which it originates should be less than 90 degrees (Figs. 6.4 and 6.5). Only in this way can the occlusal forces be directed along the long axis of the abutment tooth. An angle greater than 90 degrees fails to transmit occlusal forces along the supporting vertical axis of the abutment tooth. This also permits slippage of the prosthesis away from the abutment, which can result in orthodontic-like forces being applied to an inclined plane on the abutment, with possible tooth movement (Fig. 6.6).

When an existing occlusal rest preparation is inclined apically toward the reduced marginal ridge and cannot be modified or deepened because of fear of perforation of the enamel or restoration, then a secondary occlusal rest must be employed to prevent slippage of the primary rest and orthodontic movement of the abutment tooth (Fig. 6.7). Such a rest should pass over the lowered marginal ridge on the side of the tooth opposite the primary rest and should, if possible, be inclined slightly apically from the marginal ridge. However, two opposing occlusal rests on diverging tooth inclines will function to

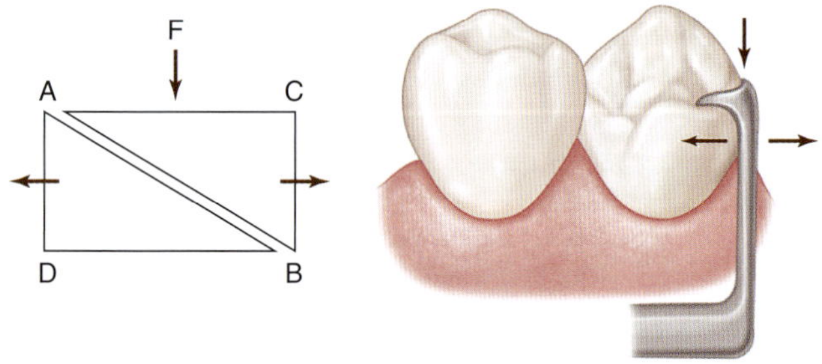

Fig. 6.6 The result of force applied to an inclined plane when the floor of the occlusal rest preparation inclines apically toward the marginal ridge of the abutment tooth. *F*, Occlusal force applied to the abutment tooth. *AB*, Relationship of the occlusal rest to the abutment tooth when the angle is greater than 90 degrees. *ABC*, Removable partial denture framework. *ABD*, Abutment tooth.

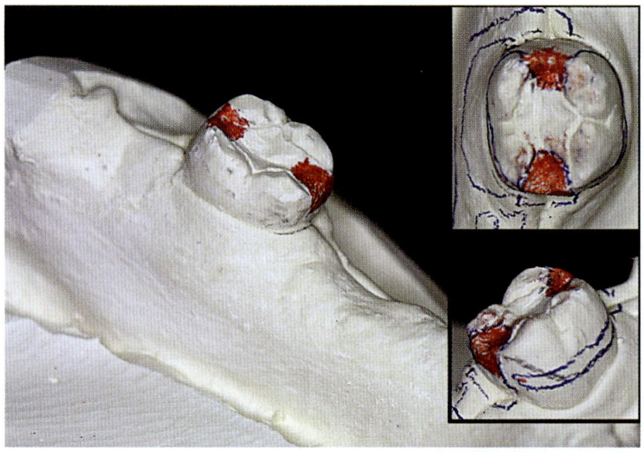

Fig. 6.7 Diagnostic cast evaluation of mesially tipped molar abutment. The anterior tilt of molar precludes preparation of acceptable rest seat on the mesio-occlusal surface. The patient could not afford a crown to improve axial alignment or orthodontic treatment to upright the molar. Occlusal rests will be used on mesio-occlusal and disto-occlusal surfaces to support restoration and direct forces over the greatest root mass of the abutment. The proposed ring clasp design is outlined.

prevent unfavorable forces if all related connectors are sufficiently rigid. In any tooth-tissue–supported RPD, the relation of the occlusal rest to the abutment should be that of a shallow ball-and-socket joint, to prevent a possible transfer of horizontal stresses to the abutment tooth. The occlusal rest should provide only occlusal support. Stabilization against horizontal movement of the prosthesis must be provided by other components of the RPD rather than by any locking effect of the occlusal rest, which will cause the application of leverages to the abutment tooth.

EXTENDED OCCLUSAL REST

In Kennedy Class II, modification 1, and Kennedy Class III situations in which the most posterior abutment is a mesially tipped molar, an extended occlusal rest should be designed and prepared to minimize further tipping of the abutment and to ensure that the forces are directed down the long axis of the abutment. This rest should extend more than one-half the mesiodistal width of the tooth, should be approximately one-third the buccolingual width of the tooth, and should allow for a minimum of 1-mm thickness of the metal; the preparation should be rounded with no undercuts or sharp angles (Fig. 6.8).

In situations in which the abutment is severely tilted, the extended occlusal rest may take the form of an onlay to restore the occlusal plane (Fig. 6.9). The tooth preparation for this type of extended rest must include removing or restoring pits, fissures, and grooves; placing a 1- to 2-mm bevel on the buccal and lingual occlusal surfaces to allow the extended rest (onlay) to provide stabilization; allowing the rest to restore the contour and occlusion of the natural tooth; and ensuring that the rest directs the forces down the long axis of the tooth. Tooth preparation must also include a 1- to 2-mm guiding plane on the mesial surface of the abutment.

INTERPROXIMAL OCCLUSAL REST SEATS

The design of a direct retainer assembly, such as an embrasure clasp, may require the use of interproximal occlusal rests (Fig. 6.10). These rest seats are prepared as individual occlusal rest seats, with the exception that the preparations must be extended farther lingually than is ordinarily accomplished (Fig. 6.11). Adjacent rests, rather than a single rest, are used to prevent interproximal wedging by the framework. In addition, the joined rests are designed to shunt food away from contact points.

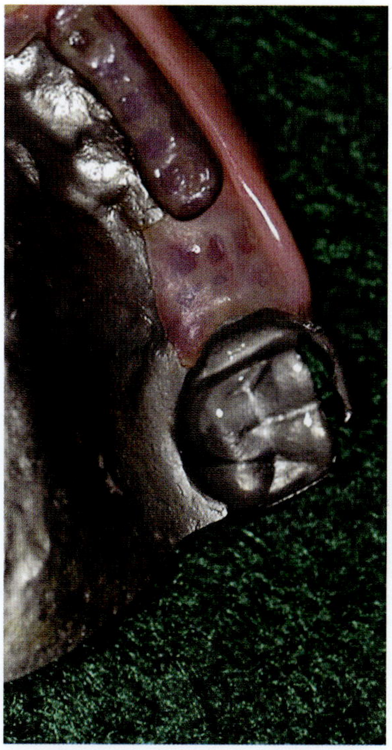

Fig. 6.9 The intaglio surface of an onlay occlusal rest restoring contour and occlusion for this maxillary molar.

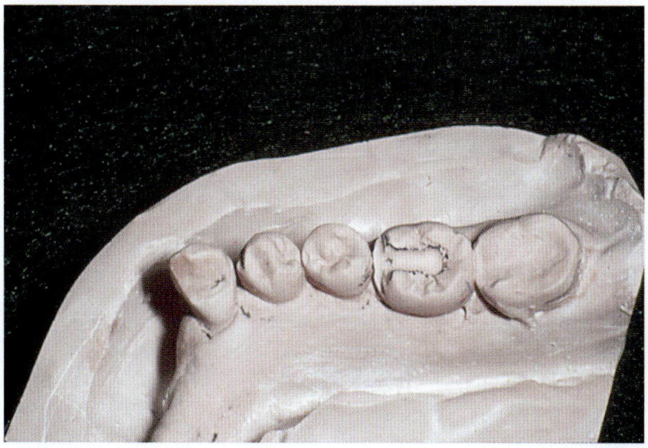

Fig. 6.8 Cast shows extended occlusal rest on the mandibular first molar, designed to ensure maximum bracing from the tooth. If placed on a mesially inclined molar next to a modification space (as in Fig. 6.7), the extended rest would ensure that the forces are directed down the long axis of the abutment, and therefore the disto-occlusal rest would not have been needed.

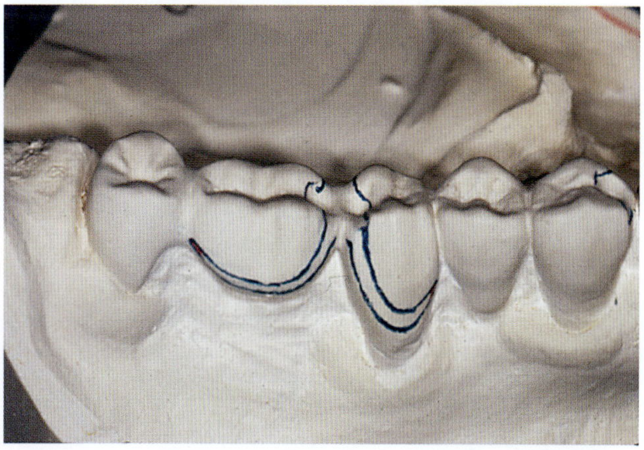

Fig. 6.10 Drawing on cast shows the desired design of a direct retainer assembly on mandibular premolar and molar abutments that incorporates interproximal occlusal rests. The direct retainers on the distobuccal undercut of the molar and on the mesiobuccal undercut of the premolar are extended from the joined occlusal rests, which occupy specifically prepared adjoining rest seats.

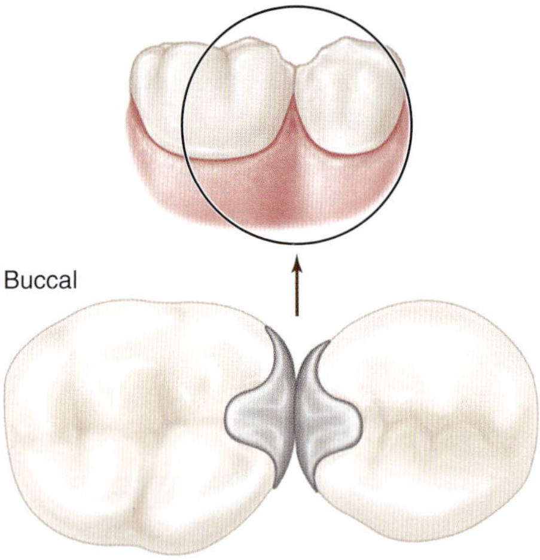

Fig. 6.11 Rest seat preparations on the premolar and molar fulfill requirements of properly prepared rest seats. Preparations are extended lingually to provide strength (through bulk) without overly filling the interproximal space with a minor connector. This type of preparation is challenging for natural tooth modification, and care must be exercised to avoid violation of contact points—yet the marginal ridge of each abutment should be sufficiently lowered (1.5 mm).

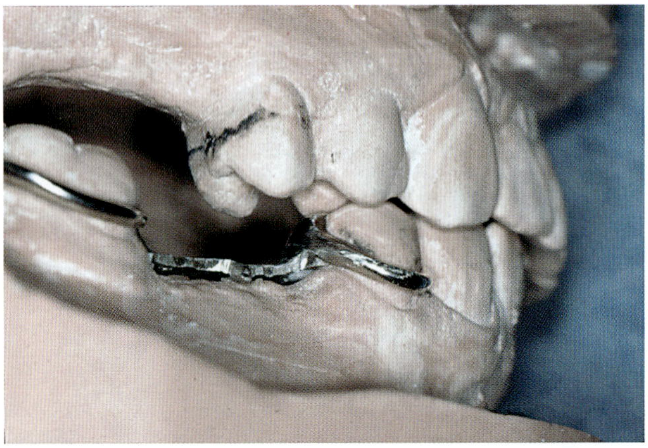

Fig. 6.12 View of mounted casts with the framework fully seated illustrates that interocclusal space was made available by a properly prepared rest seat.

When such rest seats are prepared, care must be exercised to avoid reducing or eliminating contact points of abutment teeth. However, sufficient tooth structure must be removed to allow adequate bulk of the component for strength and to permit the component to be so shaped that occlusion will not be altered. Therefore analysis of mounted diagnostic casts is mandatory for assessment of interocclusal contact areas in which rests are to be placed. Sufficient space must be present or created to avoid interference with the placement of rests (Fig. 6.12).

The lingual interproximal area requires only minor preparation. Creation of a vertical groove must be avoided to prevent a torquing effect on the abutments by the minor connector.

INTERNAL OCCLUSAL RESTS

An RPD that is totally tooth supported by means of cast retainers on all abutment teeth may use intracoronal rests for both occlusal support and horizontal stabilization (Fig. 6.13).

An intracoronal rest is not a retainer and should not be confused with an attachment. Occlusal support is derived from the floor of the rest seat. Horizontal stabilization is derived from the near-vertical walls of this type of rest seat. The form of the rest should be parallel to the path of placement, slightly tapered occlusally, and slightly dovetailed to prevent dislodgment proximally.

The main advantages of the internal rest are that it facilitates the elimination of a visible clasp arm buccally and permits the location of the rest seat in a more favorable position in relation to the tipping axis (horizontal) of the abutment. Retention is provided by a lingual clasp arm, either cast or of wrought wire, lying in a natural or prepared infrabulge area on the abutment tooth.

Internal rests are carved in wax or spark eroded in abutment castings. Ready-made plastic rest patterns are readily available and can be waxed into crown or partial-veneer patterns, invested, and cast after having been positioned parallel to the path of placement with a dental cast surveyor. Future developments and techniques promise more widespread use of the internal occlusal rest but only for tooth-supported partial dentures.

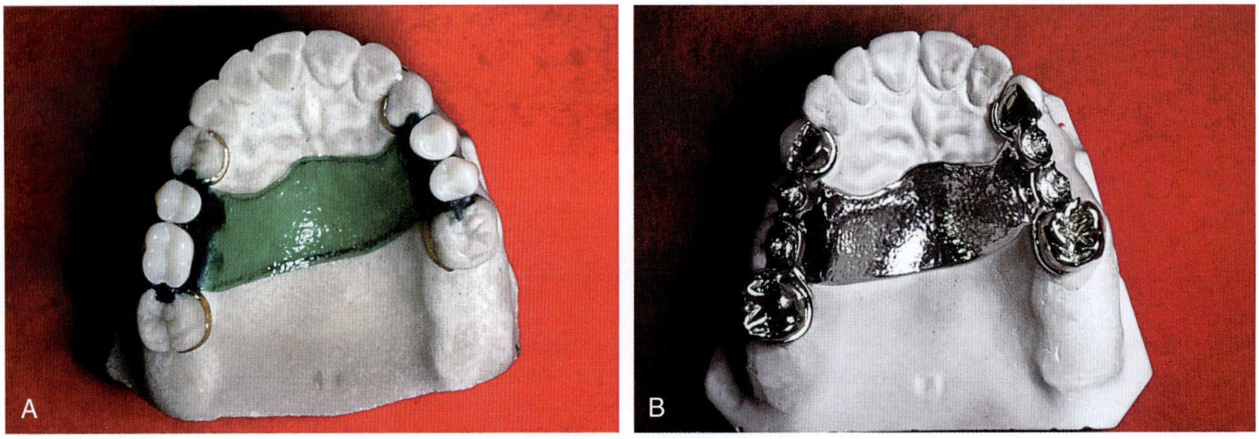

Fig. 6.13 Maxillary tooth–supported removable partial denture utilizing internal occlusal rests. **A,** Wax pattern developed utilizing internal rests on canine, premolar, and molars. **B,** Maxillary framework on cast with the internal rests fitted within surveyed crowns.

IMPLANTS AS A REST

Implants can be considered to serve as a rest when one takes advantage of the vertical stiffness characteristic they possess. In this application, they can serve to resist tissue-ward movement alone but may be considered useful for retentive needs as well. When a dual role is considered, selection of the retentive element requires consideration of how much stress from vertical movement resistance (the rest function) will affect the retentive function of the attachment mechanism.

When used as a rest, implants can serve to efficiently resist vertical movement and provide positive support. This use allows a low-profile connection (i.e., close to the ridge), imparting less torque to the implant. Location can be prescribed for maximum advantage, and the implants can effectively alter rotation around a fulcrum line—eliminating it if applied to an unsupported end of a denture base or reducing the effects by decreasing the effective lever arm. Because its position can be selected, it is important to consider (1) future use as a support to a fixed implant prosthesis and (2) current placement at the distal-most tooth position to resist functional forces of occlusion most effectively.

SUPPORT FOR RESTS

Rests may be placed on sound enamel or on any restoration material that has been proven scientifically to resist fracture and distortion when subjected to applied forces.

Rests placed on sound enamel are not conducive to caries in a mouth with a low-caries index, provided good oral hygiene is maintained. Proximal tooth surfaces are much more vulnerable to caries attack than are the occlusal surfaces supporting an occlusal rest. The decision to use abutment coverage is usually based on needed mouth preparation, determined from the survey of diagnostic casts, to accommodate modifications of abutment teeth necessary to fabricate an RPD (see Chapter 11). When precarious fissures are found in occlusal rest areas in teeth that are otherwise sound, they may be removed and appropriately restored without resorting to more extensive abutment protection. Although it cannot be denied that the best protection from caries for an abutment tooth is a full-coverage crown, such crowns must be contoured properly to provide support, stabilization, and retention for the removable partial denture.

When the decision of whether to use unprotected enamel surfaces for rests is made, the future vulnerability of each tooth must be considered because it is not easy to fabricate full-coverage crowns to accommodate rests and clasp arms after the removable partial denture has been made. In many instances, sound enamel may be used safely for the support of occlusal rests. In such situations, the patient should be advised that future susceptibility to caries is not predictable and that much depends on oral hygiene and potential future changes in caries susceptibility. Although the decision to use unprotected abutments logically should be left up to the dentist, economic factors may influence the final decision. The patient should be informed of the risks involved and of their responsibility for maintaining good oral hygiene and for returning periodically for observation.

Rest seat preparations should be made in sound enamel. In most instances, preparation of proximal tooth surfaces is necessary to provide proximal guide planes and to eliminate undesirable undercuts that rigid parts of the framework must pass over during placement and removal. The preparation of occlusal rest seats always must follow proximal surface preparation, never precede it. Only after the alteration of proximal tooth surfaces is completed may the location of the occlusal rest seat in relation to the marginal ridge be determined. When proximal preparation follows occlusal rest seat preparation, the inevitable consequence is that the marginal ridge is too low and too sharp, with the center of the floor of the rest seat too close to the marginal ridge. Therefore it is often impossible to correct the rest preparation without making it too deep, which causes irreparable damage to the tooth.

Occlusal rest seats in sound enamel may be prepared with burs and polishing points that leave the enamel surface as smooth as the original enamel (Fig. 6.14). The larger round bur is used first to lower the marginal ridge and to establish the outline form of the rest seat. The resulting occlusal rest seat is

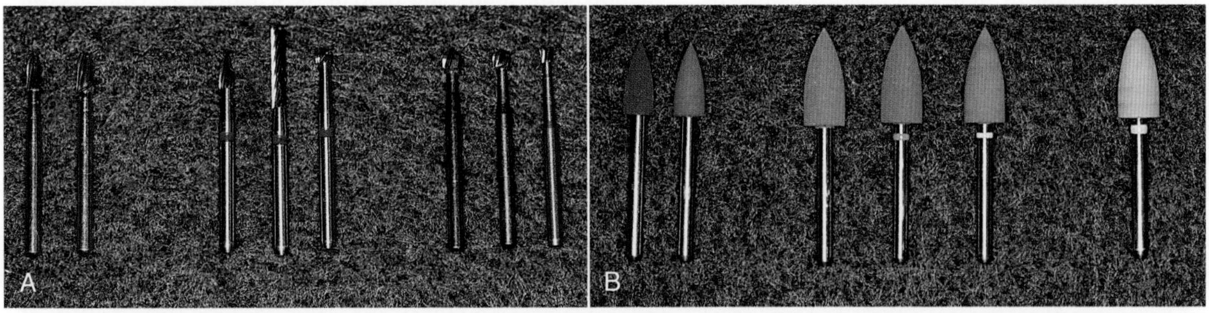

Fig. 6.14 Recontouring of axial surfaces and rest seat preparations in enamel may be readily accomplished with selected use of accessories. **A,** The two pear-shaped, multi-fluted burs *(two burs on the left)* can be used for cingulum rests and rounding marginal ridges; the longer straight, multifluted enameloplasty bur *(middle bur)* is ideal for height of contour adjustments and guide plane preparation; round multifluted or carbide burs *(three burs at right of middle)* are used for occlusal rest preparation; and the inverted cone *(far right bur)* can be used for cingulum rests as well. **B,** Various abrasive rubber polishing points are necessary to ensure a smooth surface finish following any enameloplasty procedure. Following the manufacturer's recommended sequence of abrasives should return the surface to smoothness comparable with the original condition. Diamonds are not recommended for this type of tooth reduction.

then complete except that the floor is not sufficiently concave. A slightly smaller round bur is then used to deepen the floor of the occlusal rest seat. At the same time, it forms the desired spoon shape inside the lowered marginal ridge. The preparation is smoothed by a polishing point of suitable size and shape.

When a small enamel defect is encountered in the preparation of an occlusal rest seat, it is usually best to ignore it until the rest preparation has been completed. Then, with small burs, the remaining defect should be prepared to receive a small restoration. This may be finished contiguous with the floor of the previous rest preparation.

A fluoride gel should be applied to abutment teeth following enamel recontouring. If the master cast will be fabricated from an irreversible hydrocolloid impression, application of the gel should be delayed until after impressions are made because some fluoride gels and irreversible hydrocolloids may be incompatible.

Occlusal rest seat preparations in existing restorations are treated the same way as those in sound enamel. Any proximal preparations must be done first, for if the occlusal rest seat is placed first and then the proximal surface is prepared, the outline form of the occlusal rest seat sometimes is irreparably altered.

The possibility that an existing restoration may be perforated in the process of preparation of an ideal occlusal rest seat is always present. Although some compromise is permissible, the effectiveness of the occlusal rest seat should not be jeopardized for fear of perforating an existing restoration. The rest seat may be widened to compensate for shallowness, but the floor of the rest seat should still be slightly inclined apically from the marginal ridge. When this is not possible, a secondary occlusal rest should be used on the opposite side of the tooth to prevent slipping of the primary rest.

When perforation does occur, it may be repaired, but occasionally the making of a new restoration is unavoidable. In such a situation, the original preparation should be modified to accommodate the occlusal rest, thereby avoiding the risk of perforating the completed restoration or fabricating a restoration with an inadequate rest seat.

Occlusal rest seat location in new restorations should be known when the tooth is prepared so that sufficient clearance may be provided for the rest seat within the preparation. The final step in the preparation of the tooth should be to make sure such clearance exists and, if not, to make a depression to accommodate the depth of the rest (Fig. 6.15).

Occlusal rest seats in crowns and inlays generally are made somewhat larger and deeper than those in enamel. Those made in abutment crowns for tooth-supported RPDs may be made slightly deeper than those in abutments that support a distal extension base; thus they approach the effectiveness of boxlike internal rests.

Internal rest seats also should be created first in wax, either with suitable burs in a handpiece holder or by waxing around a lubricated mandrel, which is held in the surveyor. In either situation, the rest preparation must be finished on the casting with burs in a handpiece holder or with a precision drill press. Plastic and metal shoes that fit over a mandrel are also

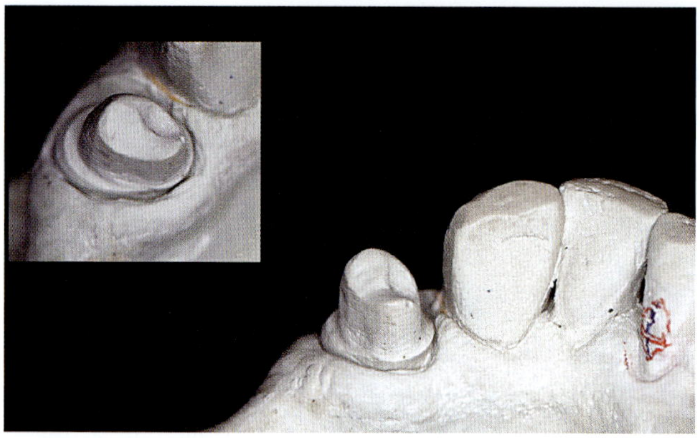

Fig. 6.15 Preparation on mandibular premolar for surveyed crown incorporates space for mesio-occlusal rest seat. Adequate occlusal reduction was accomplished to accommodate the depth of the rest seat in the abutment crown. The modification for the rest seat is performed following the standard crown preparation.

available for this purpose. Thus a smooth casting is ensured, and the need for finishing the inside of the internal rest with burs is eliminated. Sufficient clearance must be provided in the preparation of the abutment to accommodate the depth of the internal rest.

LINGUAL RESTS ON CANINES AND INCISOR TEETH

Analysis of mounted diagnostic casts is mandatory in assessment of incisal and lingual contact areas where rests are to be placed. Sufficient space must be present or created to avoid interference with placement of rests.

Although the preferred site for an external rest is the occlusal surface of a molar or a premolar, an anterior tooth may be the only abutment available for occlusal support of the denture. Also, an anterior tooth occasionally must be used to support an indirect retainer or an auxiliary rest. A canine is much preferred over an incisor for this purpose. When a canine is not present, multiple rests that are spread over several incisor teeth are preferable to the use of a single incisor. Root form, root length, inclination of the tooth, and ratio of the length of the clinical crown to the alveolar support must be considered when the site and form of rests placed on incisors are determined.

A lingual rest is preferable to an incisal rest because it is placed closer to the horizontal axis of rotation (tipping axis) of the abutment and therefore will have less of a tendency to tip the tooth. In addition, lingual rests are more esthetically acceptable than incisal rests.

If an anterior tooth is sound and the lingual slope is gradual rather than perpendicular, a lingual rest sometimes may be placed in an enamel seat at the cingulum or just incisally to the cingulum (Fig. 6.16). This type of lingual rest is usually confined to maxillary canines that have a gradual lingual incline and a prominent cingulum. In a few instances, such a rest also may be placed on maxillary central incisors. The lingual slope of the mandibular canine is usually too steep for an adequate lingual rest seat to be placed in the enamel, and some other provision for rest support must be made. Lingual rest seat preparations

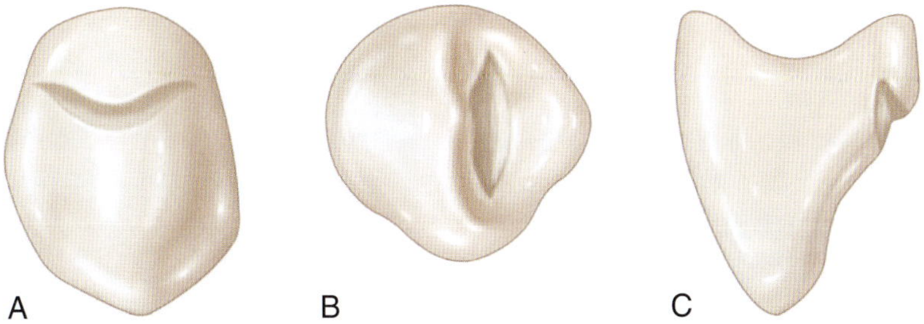

Fig. 6.16 Three views of lingual rest seat prepared in enamel of the maxillary canine. **A,** The rest seat, from the lingual aspect, assumes the form of a broad inverted V, maintaining the natural contour sometimes seen in a maxillary canine cingulum. An inverted V notch form is self-centering for the rest and at the same time directs forces favorably in an apical direction. **B,** From the incisal view, it will be noted that the rest seat preparation is broadest at the most lingual aspect of the canine. As the preparation approaches the proximal surface of the tooth, it is less broad than at any other area. **C,** The proximal view demonstrates correct taper of the floor of the rest seat. It also should be noted that the borders of the rest seat are slightly rounded to avoid line angles in its preparation. The mesiodistal length of the preparation should be a minimum of 2.5–3 mm, labiolingual width about 2 mm, and incisal-apical depth a minimum of 1.5 mm. It is a risky preparation and should not be attempted on lower anterior teeth.

in enamel are rarely satisfactory on mandibular anterior teeth because of a lack of thickness of the enamel in which a seat of adequate form to be truly supportive is prepared.

The preparation of an anterior tooth to receive a lingual rest may be accomplished in one of two ways:

1. A slightly rounded chevron or V-shape rest seat is prepared on the lingual surface at the junction of the gingival and the middle one-third of the tooth. The apex of the V is directed incisally. This preparation may be started by using an inverted, cone-shaped diamond stone and progressing to smaller, tapered stones with round ends to complete the preparation. All line angles must be eliminated, and the rest seat must be prepared within the enamel and must be highly polished. Shaped, abrasive rubber polishing points, followed by flour of pumice, produce an adequately smooth and polished rest seat. A predetermined path of placement for the RPD must be kept in mind when the rest seat is prepared. The lingual rest seat must not be prepared as though it was going to be approached from a direction perpendicular to the lingual slope. The floor of the rest seat should be toward the cingulum rather than the axial wall. Care must be taken not to create an enamel undercut, which interferes with placement of the denture (see Fig. 6.16).
   In a similar manner and if there is adequate clearance anteriorly noted after evaluating space available with teeth in maximum intercuspation, a cingulum rest seat can be created using composite resin on the lingual or palatal surface of an anterior tooth. Following clinic protocol in tooth preparation for composite resin, the same chevron or V-shape rest seat can be created and refined to accommodate the rest for the RPD. This is a viable option when the natural tooth anatomy does not appear to have a prominent cingulum or there is a lack of adequate enamel thickness that can be prepared without exposing tooth dentin.
2. The most satisfactory lingual rest from the standpoint of support is placed as an ideally designed rest seat in a cast restoration (Fig. 6.17). This is done most effectively by planning and executing a rest seat in the wax pattern rather than by attempting to cut a rest in a cast restoration in the mouth. This also requires additional tooth surface reduction to accommodate the rest seat depth within the confines of the cast restoration. The rest contour as part of the framework restores the lingual form of the tooth.

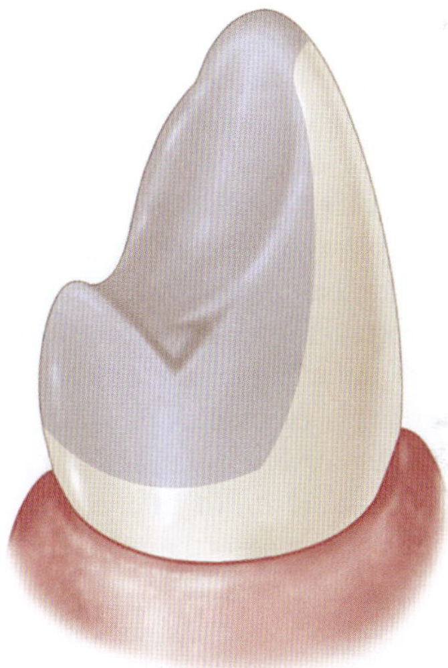

Fig. 6.17 Rest seat preparation can be exaggerated for better support when it is prepared in cast restoration.

When the cingulum in the wax pattern is accentuated, the floor of the rest seat is readily carved to be the most apical portion of the preparation. A saddle-like shape, which provides a positive rest seat located favorably in relation to the long axis of the tooth, is formed. The framework of the RPD is made to fill out the continuity of the lingual surface so that the tongue contacts a smooth surface without the patient being conscious of excessive bulk or surface irregularities.

The lingual rest may be placed on the lingual surface of a cast veneer crown (Fig. 6.18), a three-quarter crown, an inlay, a laminate veneer, a composite restoration, or an etched metal restoration. The latter displays less metal than the three-quarter crown, especially on the mandibular canine, where the lingual

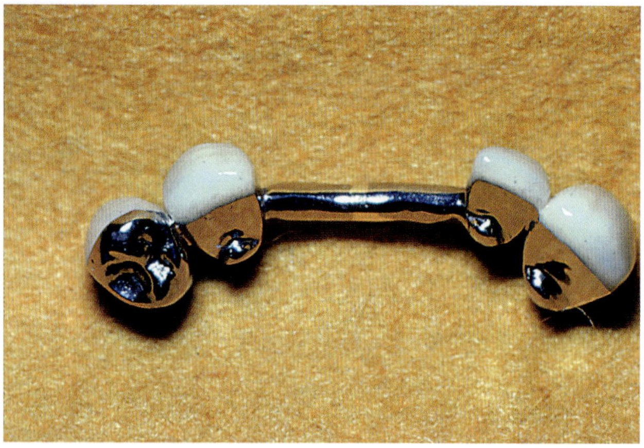

Fig. 6.18 Positive vertical support for a prosthesis is furnished by rest seats prepared in splinted metal ceramic crowns. The cingulum rest seats are optimally placed as near the horizontal axis of rotation as possible to minimize tipping forces.

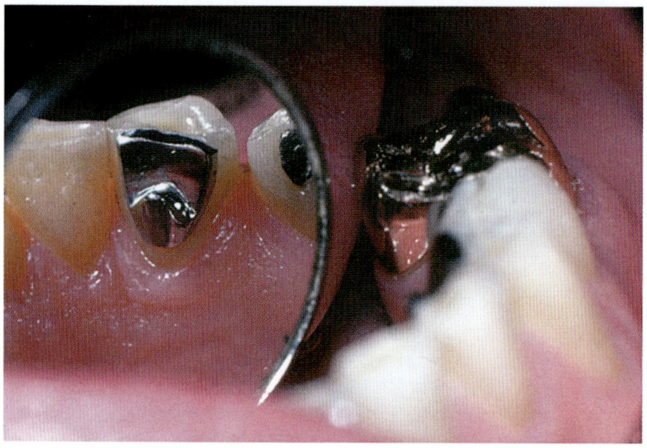

Fig. 6.19 Chromium-cobalt lingual rest seat on mandibular canine retained by resin cement with acid-etched tooth preparation.

rest that was placed on a cast restoration is frequently used, and it is a more conservative restoration. The three-quarter crown may be used if the labial surface of the tooth is sound and if the retentive contours are satisfactory. However, if the labial surface presents inadequate or excessive contours for placement of a retentive clasp arm or if gingival decalcification or caries is present, a veneered complete coverage restoration should be used.

In some instances, ball types of rests may be used in prepared seats. Such rest seats may be cautiously prepared in tooth surfaces with overly sufficient enamel thickness or may be prepared in restorations placed in teeth in which enamel thickness is inadequate. Conservative restorations (e.g., silver amalgam, pin inlays, or composite resin) in anterior teeth may be better suited for ball types of rest seats than are the less conservative inverted chevron types of rest seats.

Some scientific evidence demonstrates that individually cast chromium-cobalt alloy rest seat forms (attached to lingual surfaces of anterior teeth by the use of composite resin cements with acid-etched tooth preparation), laminates, and composite resins have been successfully used as conservative approaches to forming rest seats on teeth with unacceptable lingual contours (Fig. 6.19). Sapphire ceramic orthodontic brackets have also been bonded to the lingual surfaces of mandibular canines and shaped as rest seats. These have advantages over the metal acid-etched retained rests in that a laboratory step is avoided and increased bond strengths are achieved. The major disadvantage of using orthodontic brackets is that removal of the rest seat would necessitate that they be ground off with the potential of heat generation and possible pulpal damage.

INCISAL RESTS AND REST SEATS

Incisal rests are placed at the incisal angles of anterior teeth and on prepared rest seats. Although this is the least desirable placement of a rest seat for reasons previously mentioned, it may be used successfully for selected patients when the abutment is sound and when a cast restoration is not otherwise indicated. Therefore incisal rests generally are placed on enamel (Fig. 6.20). Incisal rests are used predominantly as auxiliary rests or as indirect retainers.

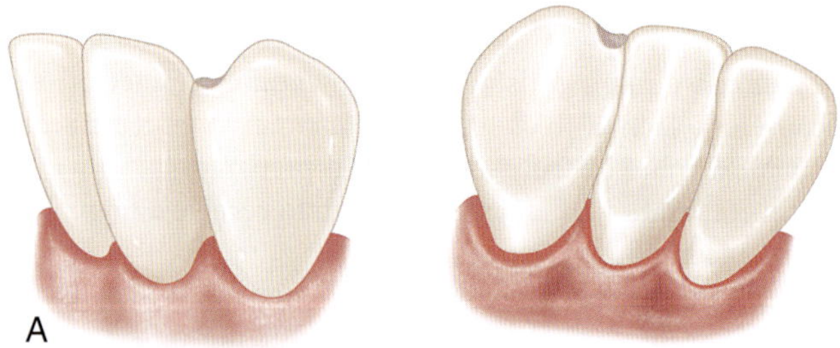

A

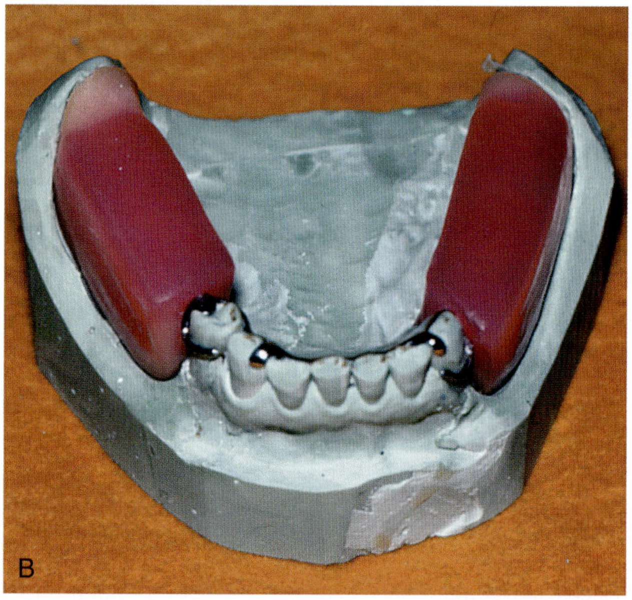

B

Fig. 6.20 **A,** Incisal rest seat placed in the mesial incisal edge of the lower canine. Note that the contact point is not involved in preparation of the rest seat. **B,** Mesial incisal rests on the canines furnish excellent vertical support and indirect retention for this prosthesis upon completion. The incisal rest on tooth #27 also provides a third point of reference when frame orientation is established during maintenance reline procedures.

Although the incisal rest may be used on a canine abutment in either arch, it is more applicable to the mandibular canine.

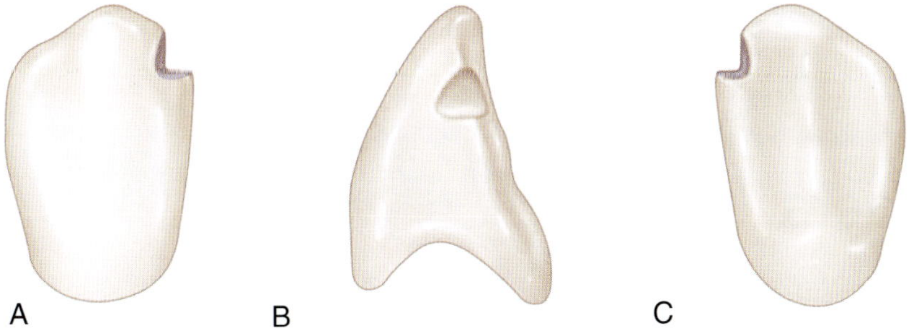

Fig. 6.21 Three views of an incisal rest seat preparation on the mandibular canine adjacent to a modification space. **A,** The labial view demonstrates inclination of the floor of the rest seat, which allows forces to be directed as near as possible along the long axis of the tooth. Note that the floor of the rest seat has been extended slightly onto the labial aspect of the tooth. **B,** As can be seen from a proximal view, the proximal edge of the rest seat is rounded rather than straight. **C,** The lingual view shows that all borders of the rest seat are rounded to avoid sharp line angles. It is especially important to avoid a line angle at the junction of the axial wall of the preparation and the floor of the rest seat. The rest that occupies such a preparation should be able to move slightly in a lateral direction to avoid torquing of the abutment tooth.

This type of rest provides definite support with relatively little loss of tooth structure and little display of metal. Esthetically it is preferable to the three-quarter crown. The same criteria may be applied when one is deciding whether to use unprotected enamel for an occlusal rest on a molar or premolar. An incisal rest is more likely than a lingual rest to lead to some orthodontic movement of the tooth because of unfavorable leverage factors.

An incisal rest seat is prepared in the form of a rounded notch at the incisal angle of a canine or on the incisal edge of an incisor, with the deepest portion of the preparation apical to the incisal edge (Fig. 6.21). The notch should be beveled both labially and lingually, and the lingual enamel should be partly shaped to accommodate the rigid minor connector connecting the rest to the framework. An incisal rest seat should be about 2.5 mm wide and 1.5 mm deep so that the rest will be strong without having to exceed the natural contour of the incisal edge (Fig. 6.22).

In the absence of other suitable placements for incisal rests and rest seats, incisal rests on multiple mandibular incisors may be considered. Use of such rests may be justified by the following factors:

1. They may take advantage of natural incisal faceting.
2. Tooth morphology does not permit other designs.
3. Such rests can restore defective or abraded tooth anatomy.
4. Incisal rests provide stabilization.
5. Full incisal rests may restore or provide anterior guidance.

If full incisal rests are considered, the patient should be thoroughly informed regarding their location, form, and esthetic impact.

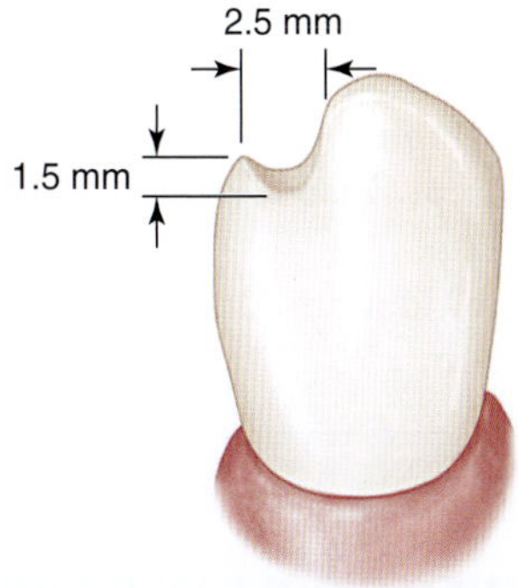

Fig. 6.22 Dimensions given in the illustration for an incisal rest seat preparation will provide adequate strength of the framework at the junction of the rest and the minor connector. Rest seats of smaller dimensions have proved unsatisfactory regardless of the metal alloy from which the framework is made.

It is, of course, essential that both the master cast and the casting be accurate if rests are to seat properly. The incisal rest should be overcontoured slightly to allow for labial and incisal finishing to the adjoining enamel, in much the same manner as a three-quarter crown or inlay margin is finished to enamel. In this way, minimal display of metal is possible without jeopardizing the effectiveness of the rest.

Care taken in selecting the type of rest seat to be used, in preparing it, and in fabricating the framework casting does much to ensure the success of any type of rest. The topography of any rest should be such that it restores the topography of the tooth that exists before the rest seat is prepared.

7

Direct Retainers

Lisa A. Lang, Lily T. García, and Ahmed Mahrous

CHAPTER OUTLINE

DIRECT RETAINER'S ROLE IN CONTROL OF PROSTHESIS MOVEMENT

Retention of a removable prosthesis is a unique concern when compared with other prostheses. When one is dealing with a crown or fixed partial denture, the combined use of preparation geometry (i.e., resistance and retention form) and a luting agent can fix the prosthesis to the tooth in a manner that resists all forces to which the teeth are subjected. As was mentioned in Chapter 4, the direction of forces acting on a prosthesis can be toward, across, or away from the tissue. In general, the forces acting to move prostheses toward and across the supporting teeth and/or tissue are the greatest in intensity. This is because most often they are forces of occlusion.

Forces acting to displace the prosthesis from the tissue can consist of gravity acting against a maxillary prosthesis, the action of adherent foods acting to displace the prosthesis on the opening of the mouth in chewing, or functional forces acting across a fulcrum to unseat the prosthesis. The first two directional forces are seldom at the magnitude of functional forces, and the latter is minimized through the use of adequate support. The component part applied to resist this movement away from the teeth and/or tissue provides retention for the prosthesis and is called the *direct retainer*.

A direct retainer is any unit of a removable dental prosthesis that engages an abutment tooth or implant to resist displacement of the prosthesis away from basal seat tissue. The direct retainer's ability to resist this movement is greatly influenced by the stability and support of the prosthesis provided by major and minor connectors, rests, and tissue bases. This relationship of the supportive and retentive components highlights the relative importance of these component parts. Although the forces working against a removable partial denture (RPD) to move it away from the tissue generally are not as great as the functional forces causing stress toward the tissue, the RPD must have retention appropriate to resist reasonable dislodging forces. Sufficient retention is provided by two means. Primary retention for the RPD is accomplished mechanically by placing retaining elements (direct retainers) on the abutment teeth. Secondary retention is provided by the intimate relationship of the minor connector contact with the guide planes and denture bases and of the major connector (maxillary) with underlying tissue. The latter is similar to the retention of a removable complete denture. It is proportionate to the accuracy of the impression registration, the accuracy of the fit of the denture bases, and the total involved area of contact. Retention can also be provided through the engagement of an attachment mechanism on a dental implant.

Direct retainers can be in the form of "clasp assemblies" or "attachments." Clasp assemblies are the most common form. Clasp assemblies are made of four components that provide many of the essential functions of the RPD: retentive clasp, reciprocal element, rest, and the proximal plate (guide plate). Clasp assemblies come in a variety of configurations that cater to many situations. Attachments also come in a variety of configurations and will be discussed later in this chapter.

It is important to make the distinction between the different terms *direct retainer*, *clasp assembly*, and *retentive clasp* (Fig. 7.1).

REQUIREMENTS OF CLASP ASSEMBLIES

The clasp assembly of a RPD serves the function of (1) retention of the prosthesis, (2) support for the prosthesis, (3) reciprocation or bracing of the abutment tooth, (4) cross-arch stabilization of the prosthesis and the teeth, (5) guidance of the insertion pathway, (6) encirclement, and (7) stress breaking of tipping and rotational forces to the abutment. Retention is provided through a retentive clasp component of the clasp assembly. The amount of retention should always be the minimum necessary to resist reasonable dislodging forces. Additionally, retentive clasps should be passive when fully seated and only engage the undercut when the RPD is subjected to a dislodging force (Fig. 7.2) (Video 7.2). The terminal end of the retentive arm is optimally placed in the gingival third of the crown (Figs. 7.3–7.5). These locations permit better resistance to horizontal and torquing forces caused by a reduction in the effort arm as described in Chapter 4.

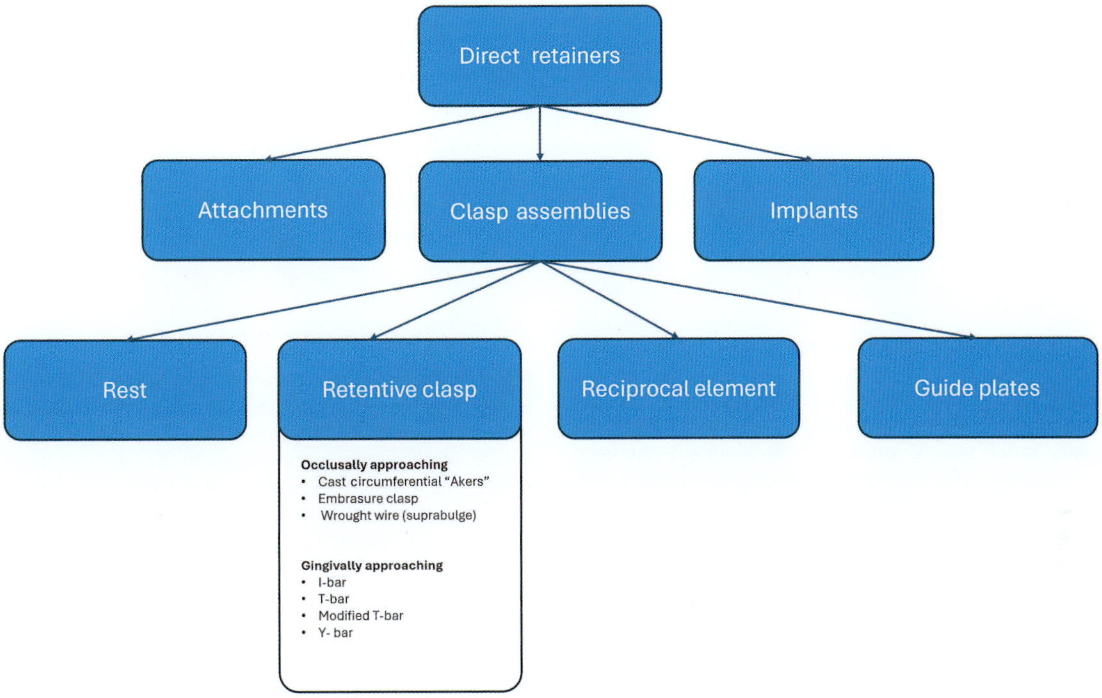

Fig. 7.1 There are various methods of categorizing and organizing clasps, clasp assemblies, and direct retainers. Thus before further discussion in the chapter, it is important to keep in mind different terms used to describe the different components or combinations of components used.

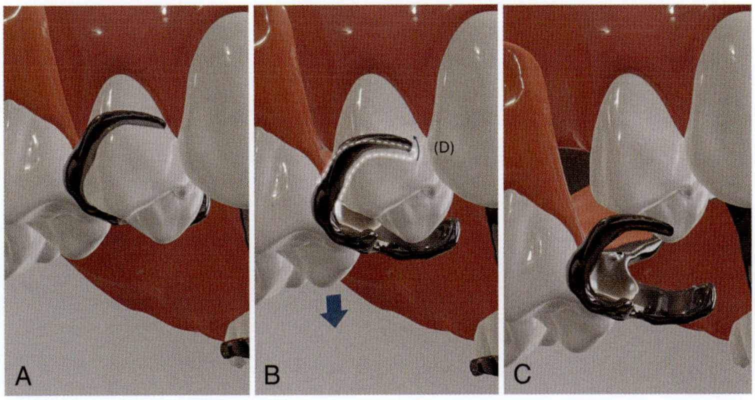

Fig. 7.2 When the removable partial partial denture is fully seated **(A)**, the clasp arm should be passive and should not induce any pressure onto the abutment tooth. When a dislodging force is applied to the partial denture **(B)**, the retentive clasp arm engages the retentive undercut. As more force is applied, the retentive arm elastically deforms **(C)**. **(D)** represent the flexing of the clasp in and out of the rete ntive undercut; this force acts to resist the removal of the partial from the mouth. If subjected to enough force, the clasp will deform enough to be removed from the mouth and the clasp will elastically return to its original form. The process is also reversed as the partial is being seated.

1. Support is provided by rests. A rest must be designed to prevent movement of the clasp arms cervically.
2. Reciprocation is provided by any rigid component capable of resisting any transient pressures exerted by the retentive clasp arm during placement and removal (Fig. 7.6). For this to occur, the reciprocal element must be in contact during the time of retainer arm deformation. In some instances, the reciprocal clasp arm will not contact the tooth until the denture is fully seated. Reciprocal elements of the clasp assembly should be at the junction of the gingival and middle thirds of the crowns of the abutment teeth, creating a bracing effect for the abutment tooth. Cast restorations permit a parallel surface to be contacted by the reciprocal arm at the same time as the retentive clasp engages the retentive undercut. This is discussed in Chapter 15.

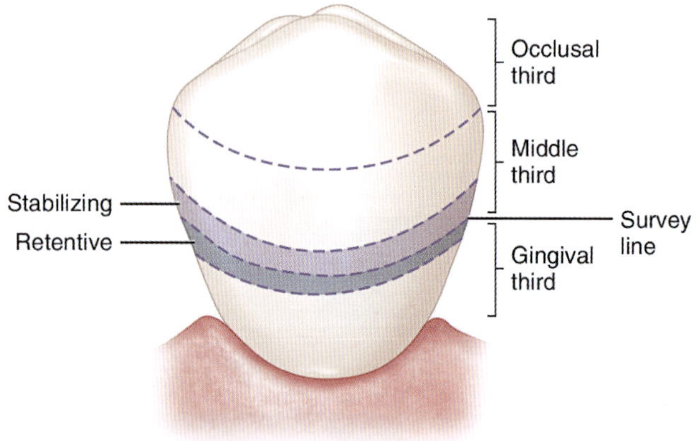

Fig. 7.3 Simple mechanical laws demonstrate that the nearer stabilizing-reciprocal and retentive elements of direct retainer assemblies are located horizontally to the axis of rotation of the abutment, the less likely it is that physiologic tolerance of the periodontal ligament will be exceeded. The horizontal axis of rotation of the abutment tooth is located somewhere in its root.

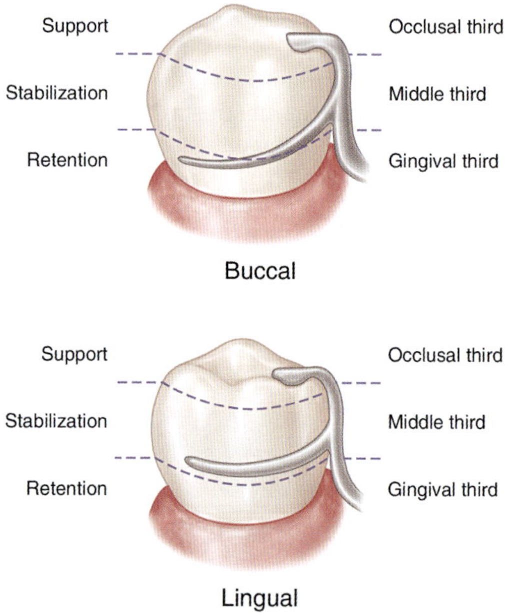

Fig. 7.4 Circumferential clasp on the mandibular premolar. Support is provided by the occlusal rest; stabilization is provided by the occlusal rest, proximal minor connector, lingual clasp arm, and rigid portion of the buccal retentive clasp arm occlusal to the height of contour. Retention is realized by the retentive terminal of the buccal clasp arm; reciprocation is provided by the nonflexible lingual clasp arm. Assembly engages more than 180 degrees of the abutment tooth's circumference.

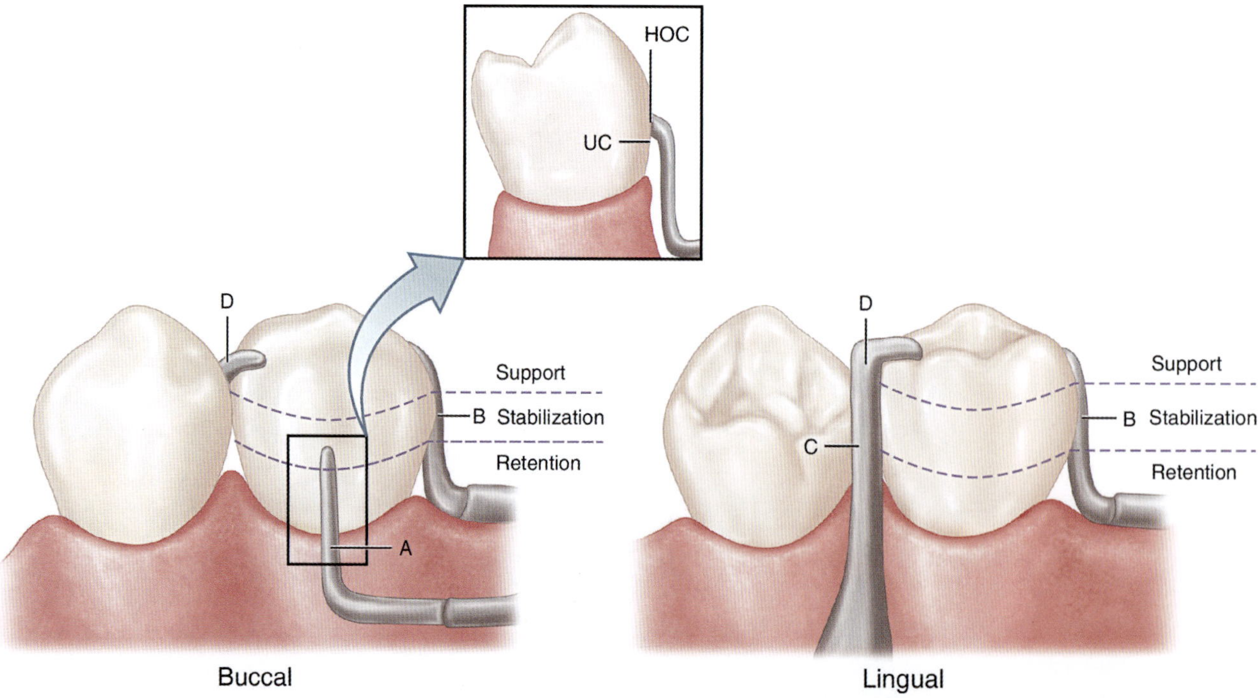

Fig. 7.5 A bar-type clasp assembly consists of the buccal retentive arm engaging the measured undercut **(A)** (with slight occlusal extension for stabilization [see magnified insert]); the stabilizing (reciprocal) elements, with the proximal plate minor connector on the distal **(B)**; the lingually placed mesial minor connector for the occlusal rest, which also serves as a stabilizing (reciprocal) component **(C)**; and the mesially placed supporting occlusal rest **(D)**. Assembly remains passive until activated. *HOC*, Height of contour; *UC*, undercut.

3. Cross-arch stabilization. Stabilizing and reciprocal components must be rigidly connected bilaterally (cross-arch) to realize the reciprocation of the retentive elements. Retentive clasp arms should be bilaterally opposed (i.e., buccal retention on one side of the arch should be opposed by buccal retention on the other or lingual retention on one side opposed by lingual on the other). In Kennedy Class II situations, the third abutment may have buccal or lingual retention. In Kennedy Class III situations, retention may occur bilaterally or may be diametrically opposed (Fig. 7.7).

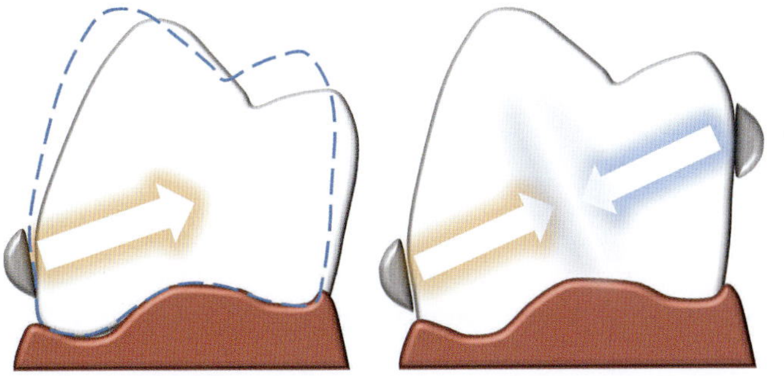

Fig. 7.6 **A,** Flexing action of the retentive clasp arm initiates lingually directed pressure on the abutment teeth as its retentive tip springs over the height of the contour. **B,** Reciprocation to medially directed pressure is counteracted by rigid lingually placed bracing arms contacting the abutments simultaneously with the buccal arms or by rigid stabilizing components of the framework contacting the lingual surface when the buccal arms begin to flex.

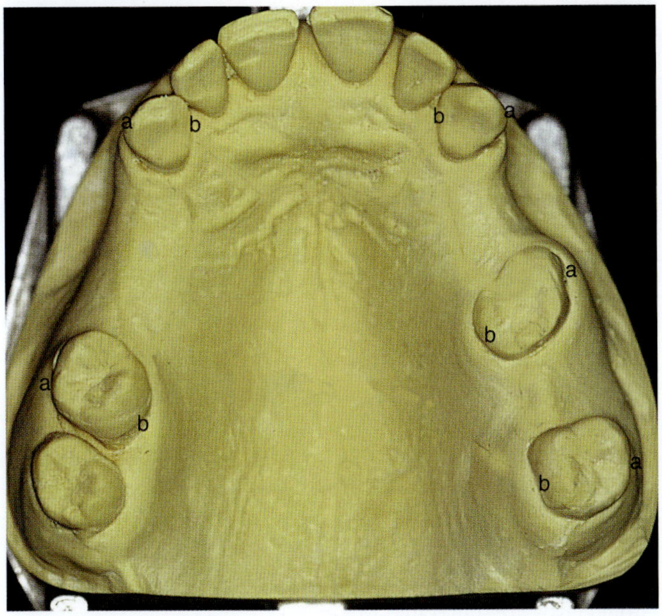

Fig. 7.7 Retentive clasp arms should be bilaterally opposed. This means bilateral buccal or bilateral lingual undercuts should be used, as shown on this Kennedy Class III, modification 2 arch, in which the retention may be *(a)* bilaterally buccal or *(b)* bilaterally lingual.

4. Guidance is provided by proximal guide plates that guide the path of escapement for each retentive clasp terminal of the RPD that is engaging with the planned retentive undercut.
5. Encirclement occurs as the clasp assembly must contact 180 degrees of the tooth (Fig. 7.8). This ensures the stability of both the tooth, clasp assembly, and the RPD. The engagement can occur in the form of continuous contact, such as in a circumferential clasp, or discontinuous contact, such as in the use of a bar clasp. Both provide tooth contact in at least three areas encircling the tooth: (1) the occlusal rest area, (2) the retentive clasp terminal area, and (3) the reciprocal clasp terminal area.
6. Stress breaking occurs as clasp retainers on the abutment teeth adjacent to distal extension bases should be designed so that they avoid direct transmission of tipping and rotational forces to the abutment. In effect, they must act as stress breakers, either by their design or by their construction. This is accomplished through the proper location of the retentive terminal relative to the rest or by a more flexible clasp arm in relation to the anticipated rotation of the denture under functional forces.

CRITERIA FOR SELECTING A GIVEN CLASP DESIGN

When a particular clasp design is selected for a given situation, its function and limitations must be carefully evaluated. Clasp assemblies should be considered as components of a RPD framework. They should be designed and located to perform the specific functions of support, stabilization, reciprocation, and retention. It does not matter whether the clasp assembly components are physically attached to each other or originate from

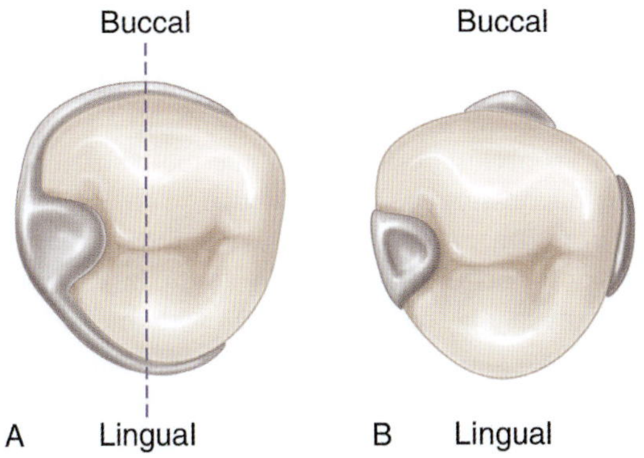

Fig. 7.8 **A,** *Dashed line* drawn through the illustration represents 180 degrees of the greatest circumference of abutment tooth from the occlusal rest. Unless portions of the lingual reciprocal arm and the retentive buccal arm are extended beyond the line, the clasp would not provide the appropriate amount of encirclement and therefore would not accomplish its intended purpose. If the respective arms of the retainer were not extended beyond the line, the abutment tooth could be forced away from the retainer through torquing action of the clasp or the removable partial denture could move away from the abutment. **B,** Bar-type clasp assembly engagement of more than 180 degrees of the circumference of the abutment is realized by the minor connector for the occlusal rest, the minor connector contacting the guide plane on the distal proximal surface, and the retentive bar arm.

major and minor connectors of the framework. If attention is directed to the separate function of each component of the clasp assembly, then the selection of a clasp assembly is simplified.

Although some rather complex designs are used for retentive clasps, they all may be classified into one of two basic categories. One is the *occlusally approaching* or *suprabulge clasps* which approach the retentive undercut from an occlusal direction like a circumferential clasp arm. The other is the *gingivally approaching* or *infrabulge* clasps, which approach the retentive undercut from a cervical direction like the bar clasp arm. A clasp assembly may comprise various retentive arms (i.e., a cast circumferential, a bar clasp arm, or a wrought-wire retainer), depending on the specific requirement for retainer construction, given the necessary adjustability, clasp approach position, and survey line location.

No confusion should exist between the choice of clasp arm and the purpose for which it is used. Either type of cast clasp arm (bar or circumferential) may be made tapered and retentive or nontapered (rigid) and nonretentive. The choice depends on whether it is used for retention, stabilization, or reciprocation.

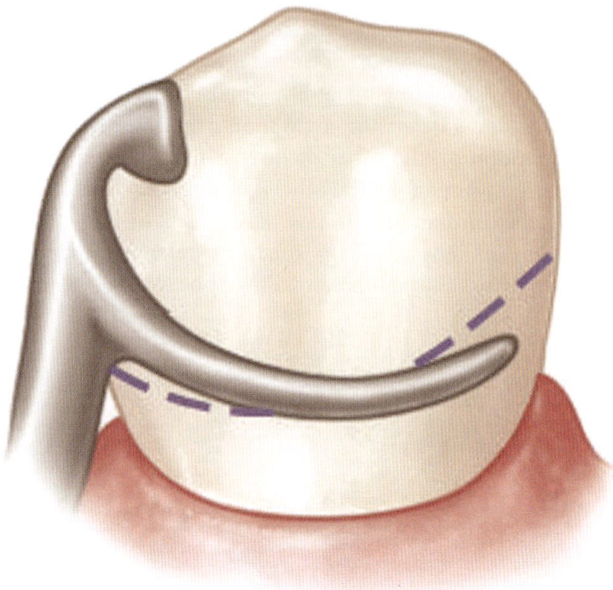

Fig. 7.9 The typical appearance of a cast circumferential clasp arm.

Occlusally Approaching "Suprabulge" Clasps

This group of clasps approaches the undercut of a tooth from an occlusal direction. Those clasps are generally simpler to apply to different situations and provide adequate retention. However, their main disadvantage is that they cover a large segment of the axial surface of the tooth, making them both unesthetic and potentially plaque harboring.

Cast Circumferential Clasp "Akers"

The cast circumferential clasp is usually the simplest clasp to use with all tooth-supported partial dentures (Kennedy Class III) because of its retentive and stabilizing ability (Fig. 7.9). Only when the retentive undercut may be approached better with a bar clasp arm or when esthetics will be enhanced should the latter be used for a Kennedy Class III. The cast circumferential clasps cover more tooth surface than with a bar clasp arm because of its occlusal origin. On some tooth surfaces, particularly the buccal surfaces of mandibular teeth and the lingual surfaces of maxillary teeth, its occlusal approach may increase the width of the occlusal surface of the tooth. In the mandibular arch, more metal may be displayed than with the bar clasp arm. As with all cast clasps, its half-round form makes adjustment challenging. Despite its disadvantages, the cast circumferential clasp arm may be used effectively, and many of these disadvantages may be minimized by mouth preparation. Adequate mouth preparation will permit its point of origin to be placed far enough below the occlusal surface to avoid poor esthetics and increased tooth dimension (Fig. 7.10). Although some of the disadvantages listed imply that the bar-type clasp may be preferable, the circumferential clasp is superior to a bar clasp arm that is improperly used or poorly designed. Experience has shown that faulty application and design too often negate the possible advantages of the bar clasp arm, whereas the circumferential clasp arm is not as easily misused.

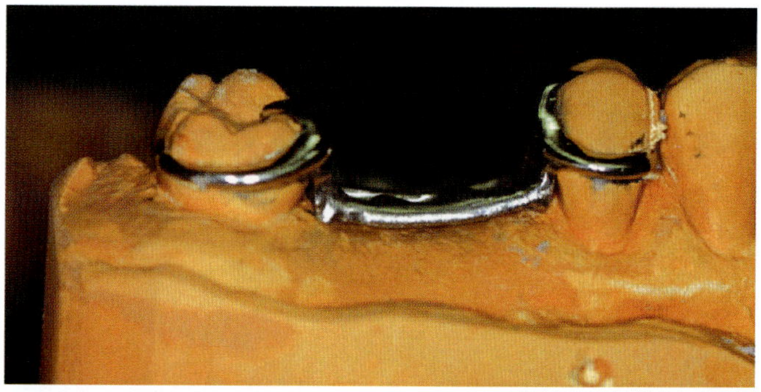

Fig. 7.10 Cast circumferential retentive clasp arms are properly designed. They originate on or occlusal to the height of contour, which they then cross in their terminal third, and engage retentive undercuts progressively as their taper decreases and their flexibility increases.

The basic form of the circumferential clasp is a buccal and lingual arm originating from a common body (Fig. 7.11). This clasp is used improperly when two retentive clasp arms originate from the body and occlusal rest areas and approach bilateral retentive areas on the side of the tooth away from the point of origin. The correct form of this clasp has only one retentive clasp arm, opposed by a nonretentive reciprocal arm on the opposite side. A common error is to use this clasp improperly by making both clasp terminals retentive. This not only is unnecessary but also disregards the need for reciprocation and bilateral stabilization. Other common errors in the design of circumferential clasps are illustrated in Fig. 7.12.

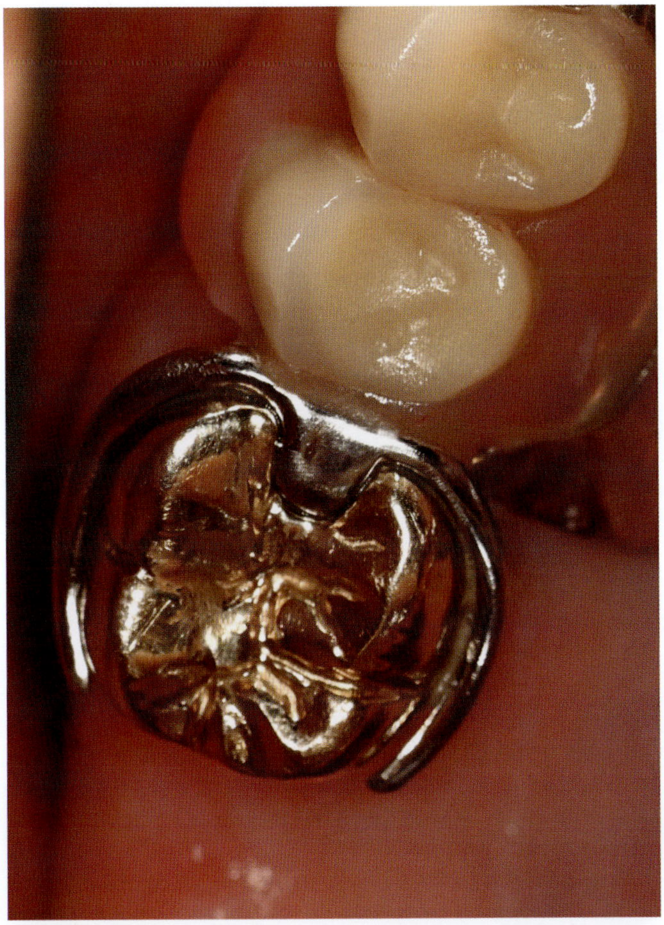

Fig. 7.11 A Cast circumferential clasp engaging the distobuccal undercut along with a lingual cast reciprocal arm and a mesial rest and proximal guide plate.

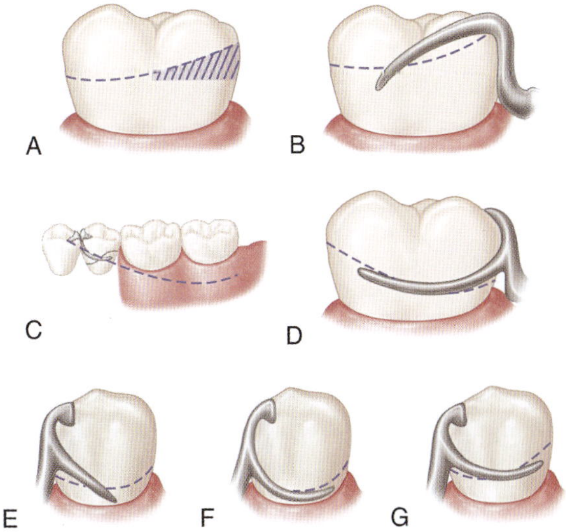

Fig. 7.12 Some improper applications of circumferential clasp design and their recommended corrections. **A,** Tooth with an undesirable height of contour in its occlusal third. **B,** Unsuitable contour and location of retentive clasp arm on an unmodified abutment. **C,** More favorable height of contour achieved by modification of the abutment. **D,** Retentive clasp arm is properly designed and located on a modified abutment. **E,** Unsuitable contour and location of the retentive arm in relation to the height of contour (straight arm configuration provides a poor approach to the retentive area and is less resistant to dislodging force). **F,** The terminal portion of the retentive clasp arm located too close to the gingival margin. **G,** Clasp arm that is properly designed and located.

Ring Clasp

The ring clasp encircles nearly all of a tooth from its point of origin (Fig. 7.13). It is used when a proximal undercut cannot be approached by other means. For example, when a mesiolingual undercut on a lower molar abutment cannot be approached directly because of its proximity to the occlusal rest area and cannot be approached with a bar clasp arm because of lingual inclination of the tooth, the ring clasp encircling the tooth allows the undercut to be approached from the distal aspect of the tooth.

If a long ring clasp is designed as an unsupported ring, its potential to open and close as a ring increases and its ability to provide reciprocation or stabilization decreases. Instead, a long ring clasp could be used with a supporting strut on the nonretentive side, with or without an auxiliary occlusal rest on the opposite marginal ridge. The advantage of an auxiliary rest is that further movement of a mesially inclined tooth is prevented by the presence of a distal rest. In any event, the supporting strut should be regarded as a minor connector from which the flexible retentive arm originates. Reciprocation then comes from the rigid portion of the clasp lying between the supporting strut and the principal occlusal rest.

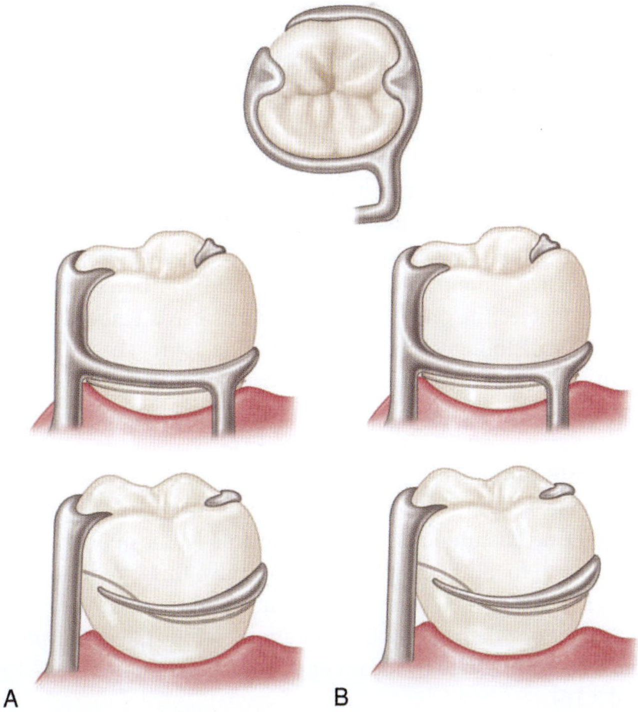

Fig. 7.13 Ring clasp(s) encircling nearly all of the tooth from its point of origin. **A,** Clasp originates on the mesiobuccal surface and encircles the tooth to engage the mesiolingual undercut. **B,** Clasp originates on the mesiolingual surface and encircles the tooth to engage the mesiobuccal undercut. In either example, a supporting strut is used on the nonretentive side (*drawn both as a direct view of the near side of the tooth and as a mirror view of the opposite side*).

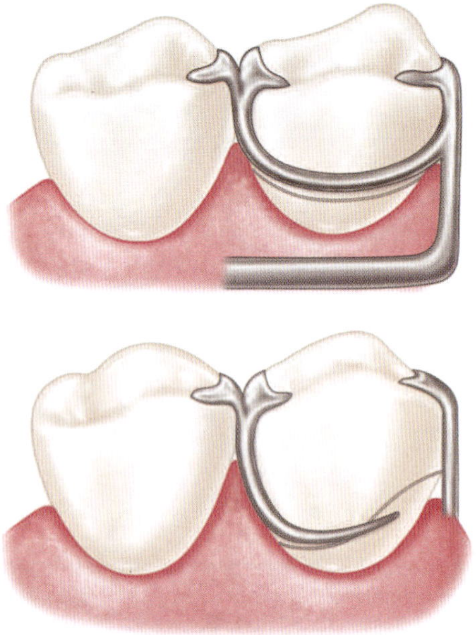

Fig. 7.14 The auxiliary occlusal rest (*mirror view*) may be used rather than the reciprocal clasp arm without violating any principle of clasp design. Its greatest disadvantages are that the second rest seat must be prepared and that enclosed tissue space at the gingival margin can result in a food trap. The auxiliary occlusal rest is also sometimes used to prevent slippage when the principal occlusal rest seat cannot be inclined apically from the marginal ridge. Minor connectors used to close the interproximal space most often require rests on adjacent teeth to avoid a wedging effect when force is placed on the denture.

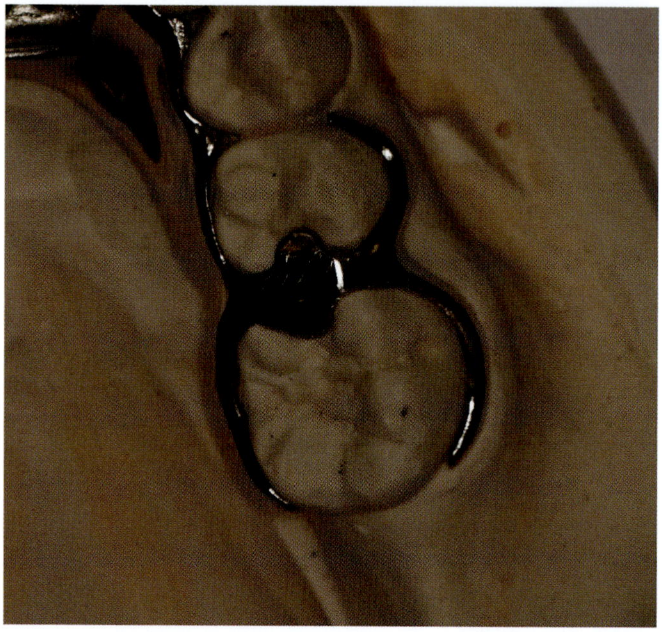

Fig. 7.15 An embrasure clasp on a master cast.

The ring-type clasp should be used on protected abutments, whenever possible because it covers such a large area of the tooth surface. Esthetics need not be considered on such a posteriorly located tooth.

A ring-type clasp may be used in reverse on an abutment located anterior to a tooth-bounded edentulous space (Fig. 7.14). Although potentially an effective clasp, this clasp covers an excessive amount of tooth surface and can be esthetically objectionable. The only justification for its use is when a distobuccal or distolingual undercut cannot be approached directly from the occlusal rest area and/or tissue undercuts prevent its approach from a gingival direction with a bar clasp arm.

Embrasure Clasp

In the fabrication of an unmodified Kennedy Class II or Class III RPD, no edentulous spaces are available on the opposite side of the arch to aid in clasping. Mechanically, this is a disadvantage. However, when the teeth are sound and retentive areas are available, or when multiple restorations are justified, clasping can be accomplished by means of an embrasure clasp (Figs. 7.15 and 7.16)

Historically, this clasp assembly demonstrates a high percentage of fracture caused by inadequate tooth preparation in the contact area. Because vulnerable areas of the teeth are involved, abutment protection with inlays or crowns is recommended. The decision to use unprotected abutments must be made at the time of oral examination and should be based on the patient's age, caries index, and oral hygiene, as well as on whether existing tooth contours are favorable or can be made favorable by tooth modification. Preparation of adjacent, contacting, uncrowned abutments to receive any type of embrasure clasp of adequate interproximal bulk is difficult, especially when it is opposed by natural teeth.

The embrasure clasp always should be used with double occlusal rests, even when definite proximal shoulders can be established. This is done to avoid interproximal wedging by the prosthesis, which could cause separation of the abutment teeth, resulting in food impaction and clasp displacement. In addition to providing support, occlusal rests serve to shunt food away from contact areas. For this reason, occlusal rests should always be used whenever food impaction is possible.

Embrasure clasps should have two retentive clasp arms and two reciprocal clasp arms that are bilaterally or diagonally opposed. An auxiliary occlusal rest or a bar clasp arm can be substituted for a circumferential reciprocal arm, as long as definite reciprocation and stabilization are achieved. A lingually placed retentive bar clasp arm may be substituted if a rigid circumferential clasp arm is placed on the buccal surface for reciprocation, provided lingual retention is used on the opposite side of the arch.

Reverse action clasp

The reverse action clasp, also known as a hairpin clasp, is a specific type of direct retainer used in RPDs. This clasp design features a unique shape that allows it to engage an undercut on the same side of the tooth as the origin of the clasp arm, making it particularly useful in certain clinical scenarios.

The reverse action clasp is primarily indicated in situations where the undercut is located on the same side of the tooth as the retentive arm's origin, which may occur in teeth with lingual or buccal tilts. It is also suitable for the design of unilateral removable partial dentures, where retention on one side of the tooth is needed.

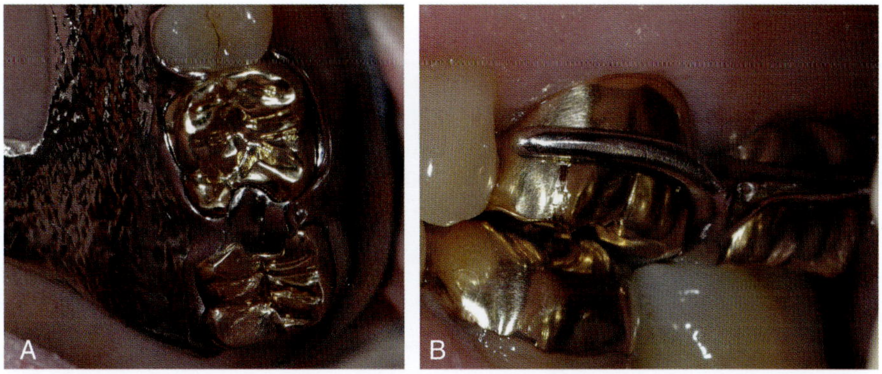

Fig. 7.16 Example of the use of an embrasure clasp for a maxillary Kennedy Class II partially edentulous arch. arch (**A**, lingual view, **B**, buccal view). Embrasure clasp on the two left molar abutments was used due to the absence of posterior modification space on the countralateral side. In this case, a lingual plate (**B**) was used as the reciprocal element for both retentive clasp arms.

However, the reverse action clasp has several contraindications. It should not be used on teeth with short clinical crowns, as it requires sufficient vertical height to accommodate the loop on the facial surface. The design of the reverse action clasp can sometimes generate excessive forces on the tooth during insertion and removal, which may lead to discomfort or damage to the abutment tooth over time. Generally, a clinical crown needs to be at least 5–7 mm tall to properly support the reverse action clasp, ensuring enough space for the clasp to function effectively.

In summary, the reverse action clasp is a versatile option in the prosthodontist's toolkit, offering specific advantages in terms of retention under certain conditions. However, careful consideration of its indications and contraindications is essential to ensure optimal outcomes in RPD design and patient satisfaction.

Wrought-wire suprabulge clasp

This clasp design mimics the structure of an "Akers" clasp as it traverses the axial surface of the abutment tooth diagonally and engages the undercut from an occlusal direction. Wrought as a material is discussed in detail in Chapter 12. The wrought wire is usually soldered to the cast framework and incorporated into a cast clasp assembly called the "combination clasp assembly" (Fig. 7.17). The wrought-wire clasp offers several advantages, which include (1) its flexibility; (2) its adjustability; (3) its esthetic advantage over cast circumferential clasp arms; (4) coverage of a minimum tooth surface as a result of its line contact with the tooth, rather than having the surface contact a cast clasp arm; and (5) a less likely occurrence of fatigue failure in service with the tapered wrought-wire retentive arm versus the cast, half-round retentive arm.

However, the wrought-wire clasp also has several disadvantages: (1) it involves extra steps in fabrication, particularly when high-fusing chromium alloys are used; (2) it may be distorted by careless handling on the part of the patient; (3) because it is bent by hand, it may be less accurately adapted to the tooth and therefore may provide less stabilization in the suprabulge portion; and (4) it may distort with function and not engage the tooth.

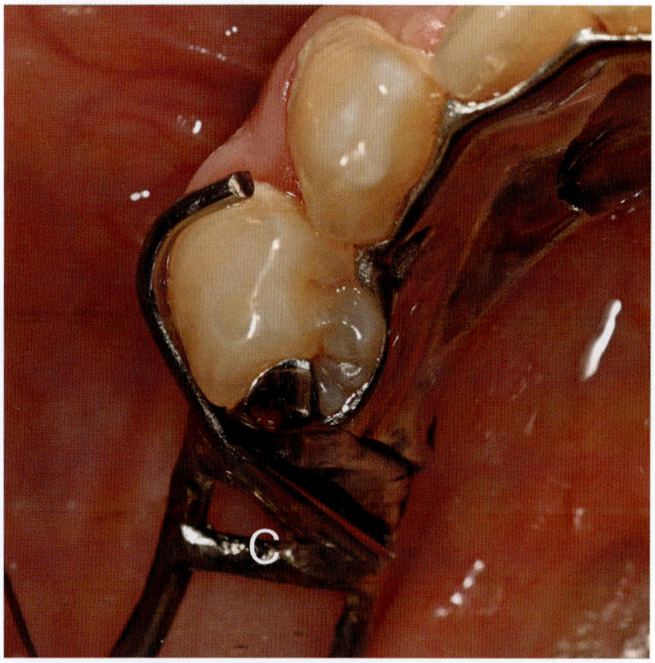

Fig. 7.17 A wrought-wire clasp is attached by solder to the framework after the framework is completed, and the wire is formed to the proper contour. *C* designates the soldered wire to the framework.

Gingivally approaching "infrabulge" clasps

This group of clasps approaches the undercut of a tooth from a gingival direction. This classification of clasps is generally referred to as *bar clasps*. The term bar clasp is generally preferred over the less descriptive historical term *Roach clasp arm*. Reduced to its simplest term, the *bar clasp arm* arises from the denture framework or a metal base and approaches the retentive undercut from a gingival direction (see Fig. 7.18). The bar clasp arm has been classified by the shape of the retentive terminal. Thus it has been identified as an I-bar, T-bar, modified T-bar, or Y-bar. The form the terminal takes is of little significance if it is mechanically and functionally effective, covers as little tooth surface as possible, and displays as little metal as possible.

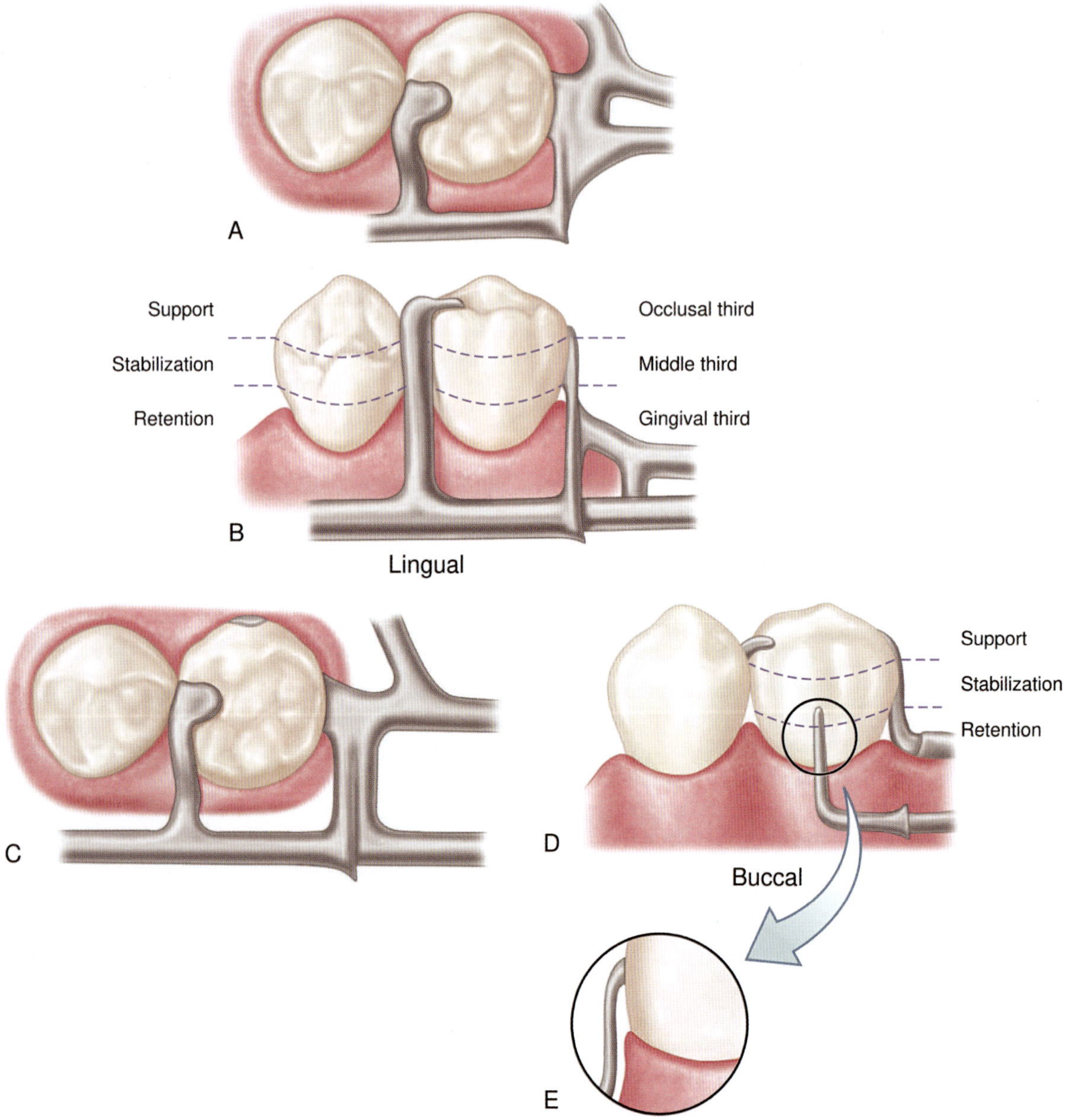

Fig. 7.18 Bar-type clasp assembly. **A,** Occlusal view. Component parts (proximal plate minor connector, rest with minor connector, and retentive arm) tripod the abutment to prevent its migration. **B,** The proximal plate minor connector extends just far enough lingually so that it combines with the mesial minor connector to prevent lingual migration of the abutment. **C,** On narrow or tapered abutments (mandibular first premolars), the proximal plate should be designed to be as narrow as possible but still sufficiently wide to prevent lingual migration. **D,** I-bar retainer located at greatest prominence of the tooth in the gingival third. **E,** Mesial view of I-bar illustrating the retentive tip relationship to the undercut and a region superior to the height of contour, which serves a stabilization function in encirclement.

In most situations, the bar clasp arm can be used with tooth-supported partial dentures, with tooth-supported modification areas, or when an undercut that can be logically approached with a bar clasp arm lies on the side of an abutment tooth adjacent to a distal extension base (Fig. 7.19). If a tissue undercut prevents the use of a bar clasp arm, a mesially originating ring clasp, a cast, or a wrought-wire clasp or reverse-action clasp may be used. Preparation of adjacent abutments (natural teeth) to receive any type of interproximal direct retainer, traversing from lingual to buccal surfaces, is most difficult to adequately accomplish. Inevitably, the relative size of the occlusal table is increased, contributing to undesirable and additional functional loading.

Specific indications for use of a bar clasp arm include (1) when a small degree of undercut (0.01 inch) exists in the cervical third of the abutment tooth, which may be approached from a gingival direction, (2) on the abutment teeth for tooth-supported RPDs or tooth-supported modification areas (Fig. 7.20), and (3) in situations in which esthetic considerations must be accommodated and a cast clasp is indicated. Thus the use of the bar clasp arm is contraindicated when a deep cervical undercut exists or when a severe tooth and/or tissue undercut exists, either of which must

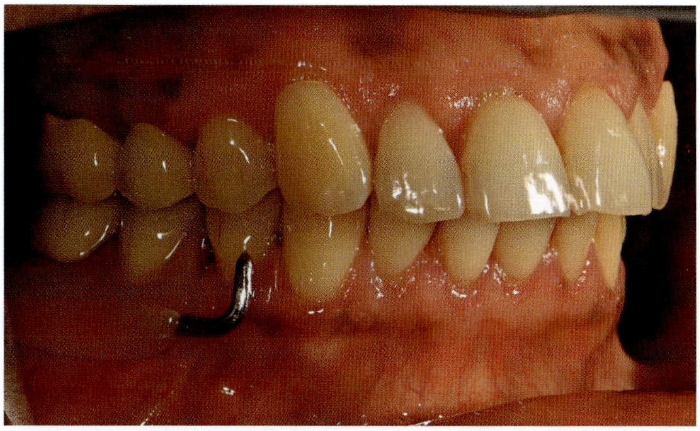

Fig. 7.19 Bar clasp arm is properly positioned on the terminal abutment. The combination of rest, proximal plate, and bar clasp contacting the abutment tooth provides more than 180 degrees of encirclement. A uniform taper to the bar ensures proper flexibility and internal stress distribution. Taper can originate from the minor connector junction or at a finishing line indicating the anterior extent of the denture base. Encirclement does not require that retentive tip modification (in the form of a T) be provided, and such a modification adds little to the clasp assembly.

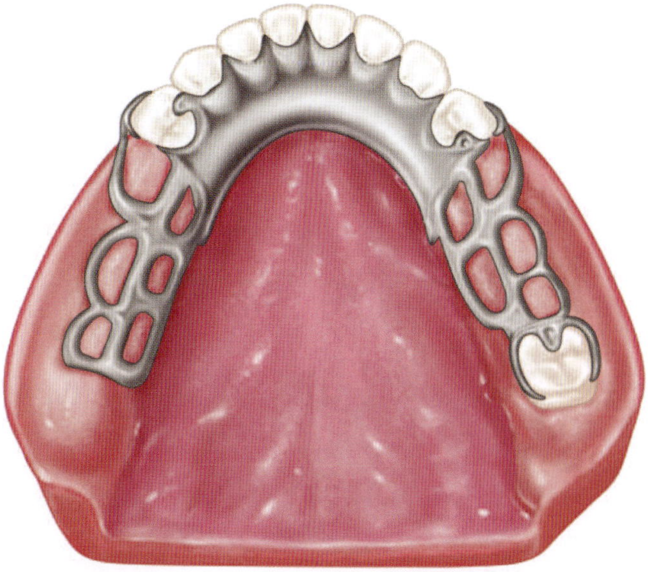

Fig. 7.20 A bar retainer (T-bar) is used on the anterior abutment of the modification space, and its terminus engages the distobuccal undercut. The denture is designed to rotate around the terminal abutments when force is directed toward the basal seat on the left. Such rotation would impart force on the right premolar directed superiorly and anteriorly. However, this direction of force is resisted in great part by mesial contact with the canine. A direct retainer on the right premolar engaging the mesiobuccal undercut would tend to force the tooth superiorly and posteriorly.

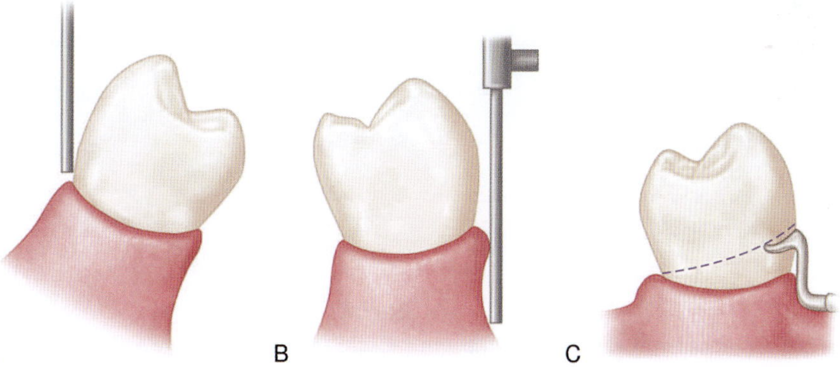

Fig. 7.21 Contraindications for selection of bar-type clasps. **A,** Severe buccal or lingual tilts of abutment teeth. **B,** Severe tissue undercuts. **C,** Shallow buccal or labial vestibules.

be bridged by excessive blockout. When severe tooth and tissue undercuts exist, a bar clasp arm usually is an annoyance to the tongue and cheek and may trap food debris. Other limiting factors in the selection of a bar clasp assembly include a shallow vestibule or an excessive buccal or lingual tilt of the abutment tooth (Fig. 7.21). Some common errors in the design of bar-type clasps are illustrated in Fig. 7.22. The bar clasp arm is not a particularly flexible clasp arm because of the effects of its half-round form and its several planes of origin.

Some advantages attributed to the infrabulge clasp are (1) its interproximal location, which may be used to esthetic advantage; (2) increased retention without tipping action on the abutment; and (3) less chance of accidental distortion resulting from its proximity to the denture border. The wearer should be meticulous in the care of a removale partial denture not only for reasons of oral hygiene but also to prevent cariogenic debris from being held against tooth surfaces.

The T and Y clasp arms are the most frequently misused. It is unlikely that the full area of a T or Y terminal is ever necessary for adequate clasp retention. Although the larger area of contact would provide greater frictional resistance, this is not true clasp retention, and only that portion engaging an undercut area should be considered retentive; any portion of the clasp above the height of contour provides only limited stabilization. Only one terminal of such a clasp arm should be placed in an undercut area (Fig. 7.23).

TYPES OF CLASP ASSEMBLIES

A clasp assembly should consist of four component parts. First, one or more minor connectors should be present, from which the clasp components originate. In most cases, the proximal guide plate is incorporated into the minor connector. Second, a principal rest should be designed to direct stress along the long axis

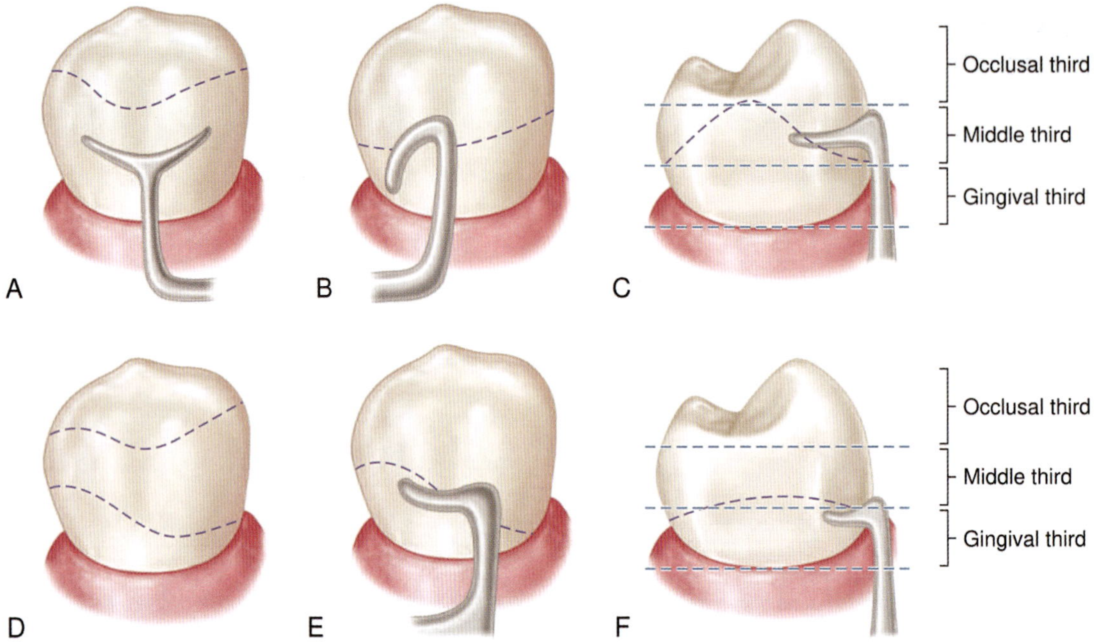

Fig. 7.22 Common errors and recommended corrections in the design of bar-type clasp assemblies. **A,** Survey line is unsuitable for the bar clasp (too high). **B,** Retentive portion of the bar clasp arm is improperly contoured to resist dislodging force in the occlusal direction. **C,** Retentive tip is not located in the gingival third of abutment. **D,** Contour of abutment is correctly altered to receive bar clasp. **E** and **F,** The correct position of bar clasp assembly.

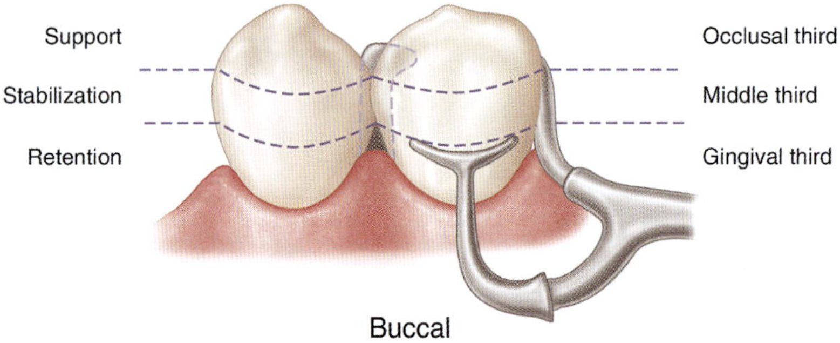

Fig. 7.23 Only one terminal of the retentive arm engages the undercut in the gingival third of the abutment. The suprabulge portion of the retentive clasp arm provides only limited stabilization and may be eliminated.

of the tooth. Third, a retentive arm should engage a tooth undercut. Fourth, a nonretentive arm (or other component) should be present on the opposite side of the tooth for stabilization and reciprocation against horizontal movement of the prosthesis (reciprocation) (Table 7.1). A wide variety of clasp assemblies are available to adapt to different oral situations. Some clasp assemblies are designed to accommodate prosthesis functional movement discussed in Chapter 4. Those clasp assemblies are described as "stress breaking." Although it has been demonstrated by Kapur et al.[1] that adverse outcomes are not always associated with the use of nonstress-breaking clasp assemblies in distal extension base classifications, it is advised to use stress-breaking clasp assemblies in extension base situations to reduce any unnecessary stress on the abutment tooth.

Stress-breaking clasp assemblies are designed to address the concern of a Class I lever. The concern is that the distal extension acts as a long "effort arm" across the distal rest "fulcrum" to

TABLE 7.1 Function and Position of Clasp Assembly Parts

Component Part	Function	Location
Rest	Support	Occlusal, lingual, incisal
Minor connector	Stabilization	Proximal surfaces extending from a prepared marginal ridge to the junction of the middle and gingival one-third of the abutment crown
Clasp arms	Stabilization (reciprocation)	Middle one-third of crown
	Retention	Gingival one-third of crown in measured undercut

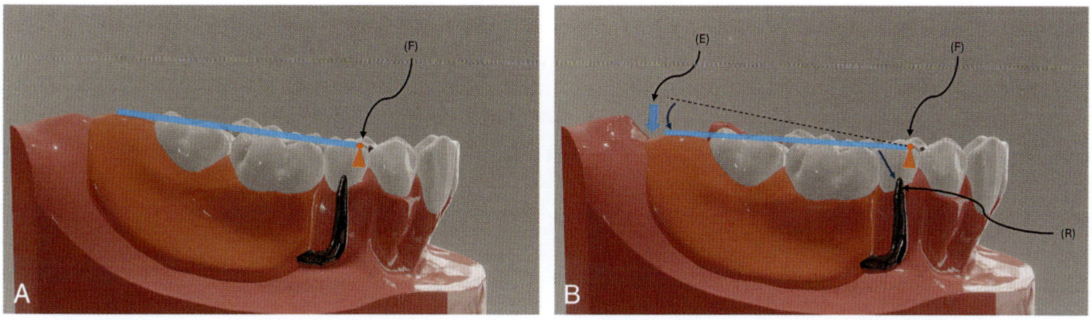

Fig. 7.24 Stress-breaking clasp assemblies on extension base partials can reduce stress on the abutment tooth by transforming the lever system into a second-class lever **(A)**; this is usually done by keeping the clasp arm between the fulcrum *(F)* and the extension base. As the partial is subjected to occlusal load **(B)**, the effort *(E)* acts to depress the extension base. Because the clasp or resistance arm *(R)* exists between the fulcrum *(F)* and the effort *(E)*; the clasp moves in the same direction as the effort and disengages from the retentive undercut and therefore does not subject the tooth to excessive force.

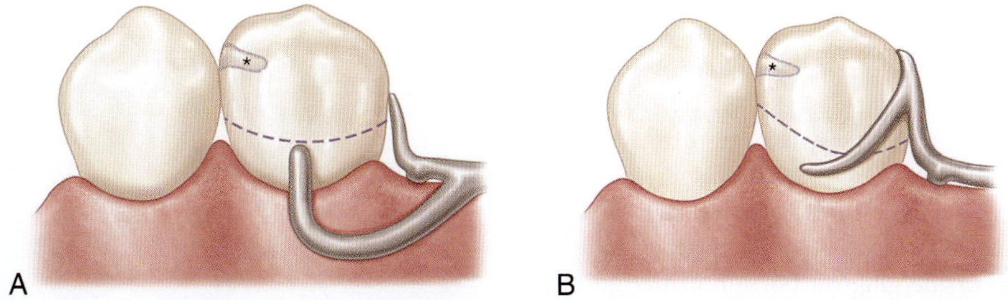

Fig. 7.25 **A,** RPI clasp assembly is composed of a mesial rest, a distal proximal plate, and I -bar clasp. **B,** RPA clasp assembly is composed of a mesial rest, a distal proximal plate, and Akers clasp. Notice the *asterisk* indicating the center of rotation on both clasp assemblies is anterior to the clasp tip, thereby creating a second-class lever and breaking possible stress.

cause the clasp tip "resistance arm" to engage the tooth undercut (Fig. 7.24). This results in harmful tipping or torquing of the tooth, which is greater with rigid clasps and increased denture base movement. Two strategies may be adopted: change the fulcrum location and subsequently the "resistance arm" engaging effect (mesial rest concept clasp assemblies) or minimize the effect of the lever using a flexible arm (combination clasp assembly).

Mesial Rest Concept Clasp Assemblies

Mesial rest concept clasps have been proposed to accomplish movement accommodation by changing the fulcrum location. This concept includes the rest, proximal plate, I-bar (RPI) and rest, proximal plate, and Akers (RPA) clasps (Fig. 7.25). The RPI clasp assembly consists of a mesio-occlusal rest with the minor connector placed into the mesiolingual embrasure, but not contacting the adjacent tooth (see Fig. 7.18, *A*). A distal guide plate extends from the marginal ridge to the junction of the middle and gingival thirds of the abutment tooth (see Fig. 7.18, *B*). The buccolingual width of the guide plane is determined by the proximal contour of the tooth (see Fig. 7.18, *A* and *C*). The proximal plate, in conjunction with the minor connector supporting the rest, provides the stabilizing and reciprocal aspects of the clasp assembly. The I-bar should be located in the gingival third of the buccal or labial surface of the abutment in a 0.01-inch undercut (see Fig. 7.18, *D*). The whole arm of the I-bar should be tapered to its terminus, with no more than 2 mm of its tip contacting the abutment. The retentive tip contacts the tooth from the undercut to the height of contour (see Fig. 7.18, *E*). This area of contact, along with the rest and proximal plate contact, provides encirclement (see Fig. 7.18, *C*). The horizontal portion of the approach arm must be located at least 4 mm from the gingival margin and even farther if possible.

An occlusal rest, such as in the RPI component parts of the clasp assembly concept, may be used rather than a reciprocal clasp arm to satisfy the need for encirclement, provided it is located in such a way that it can accomplish the same purpose (see Fig. 7.5). The addition of a lingual apron to a cast reciprocal clasp arm alters neither its primary purpose nor the need for proper location to accomplish that purpose.

Three basic approaches to the application of the RPI system may be used. The location of the rest, the design of the minor connector (proximal plate) as it relates to the guide plane, and the location of the retentive arm are factors that influence how this clasp system functions. Variations in these factors provide the basis for differences among these approaches. All advocate the use of a rest located mesially on the primary abutment tooth

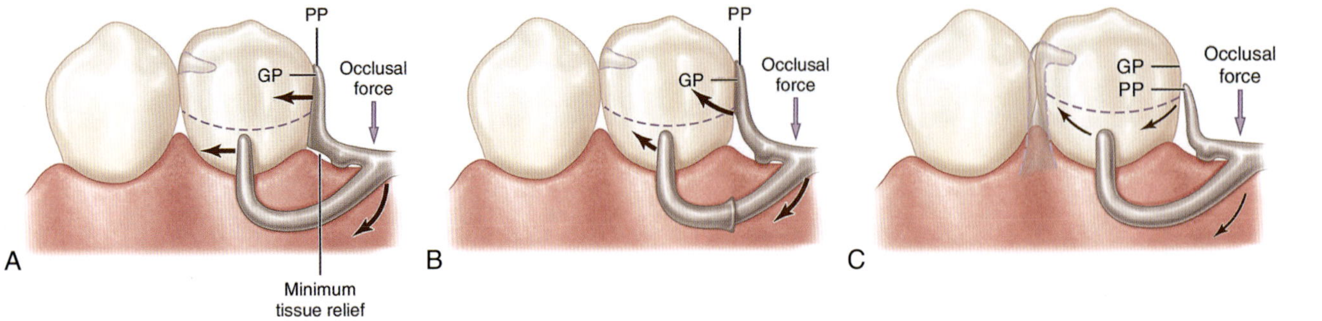

Fig. 7.26 **A,** The "Kratochvil" guide plate *(GP)* extending the entire length of the proximal tooth surface. **B,** The "Krol" proximal plate *(GP)*, contacting approximately 1–2 mm of the gingival portion of the guiding plane. **C,** The "Demer" guide plate, contacting the height of contour and bridging the slight undercut underneath with no tooth contact other than at the point of the height of contour. (*GP*) represents the proximal guide plane prepared on the proximal surface of the tooth. (*PP*) represents the proximal plate, part of the RPD framework.

adjacent to the extension base area. One approach suggested by Kratochvil[2] recommends that the guide plane and the corresponding proximal plate minor connector should extend the entire length of the proximal tooth surface. This type requires adjustment for physiologic tissue relief, eliminating impingement of the free gingival margin (Fig. 7.26, *A*). A second approach suggested by Demer[3] states that the proximal plate contacts at the height of contour only and bridges the slight undercut (see Fig. 7.26, *B*). The third approach suggested by Krol[4,5] favors a proximal plate minor connector that contacts approximately 1–2 mm of the gingival portion of the guiding plane (see Fig. 7.26, *C*).

If the abutment teeth demonstrate contraindications for a bar-type clasp (i.e., exaggerated buccal or lingual tilts, severe tissue undercut, or a shallow buccal vestibule) and the desirable undercut is located in the gingival third of the tooth away from the extension base area, the I-bar retentive clasp should be substituted for the Akers retentive clasp, hence the name "RPA" (see Fig. 7.26, *B*). The application of each approach is predicated on the distribution of load to be applied to the tooth and edentulous ridge. As circumferential clasp has become used more in place of Akers clasp, the literature has begun to replace the name of RPA with RPC.

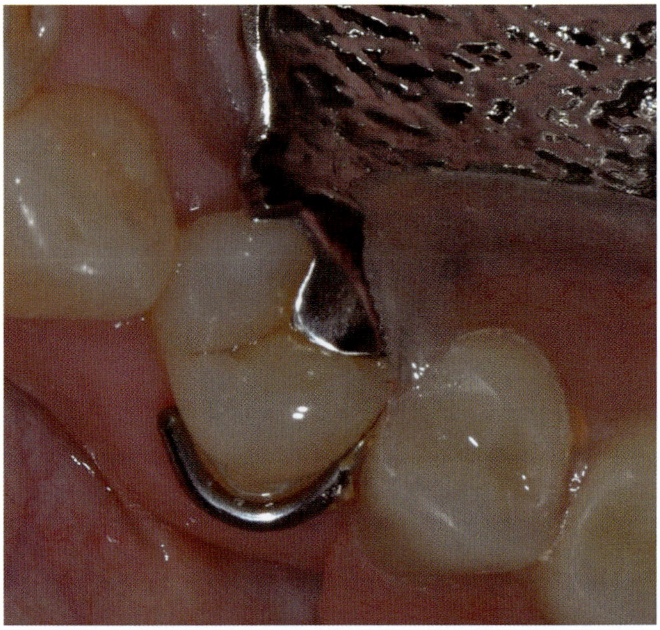

Fig. 7.27 A combination clasp assembly in a Kennedy Class II partial denture. The wrought wire engages the mesiobuccal aspect of the tooth due to rotation of the tooth; a distal rest is conveniently placed due in the open distal embrasure and the lingual plate provides reciprocation.

Combination Clasp

Another strategy that may be used to reduce the effect of the Class I lever in distal extension situations includes a flexible component in the "resistance arm"; this strategy is employed in the combination clasp (Fig. 7.27). The combination clasp consists of a wrought-wire retentive clasp arm and a cast reciprocal clasp arm (Fig. 7.28). Although the latter may be seen in the form of a bar clasp arm, it is usually a circumferential arm. The retentive arm is almost always circumferential, but it also may be used in the manner of a bar, originating gingivally from the denture base. The advantages of the combination clasp include its flexibility and adjustability and the appearance of the wrought-wire retentive arm. It is used when maximum flexibility is desirable, such as on an abutment tooth adjacent to a distal extension base or on a periodontally weak abutment tooth. It may be used for its adjustability when precise retentive requirements are unpredictable and later adjustment to increase or decrease retention may be necessary. A third justification for its use is its esthetic advantage over a cast clasp. Wrought in structure, it may be used in smaller diameters than a cast clasp, with less danger of fracture. Because it is round, light is reflected in such a manner that the display of metal is less noticeable than with the broader surfaces of a cast clasp.

The disadvantages listed previously should not prevent its use regardless of the type of alloy that is used for the cast framework. Technical problems are minimized by selecting the best wrought wire for this purpose, then casting to it, or soldering it to the cast framework. The selection of wrought wire, its attachment to the framework, and subsequent laboratory procedures to maintain its optimum physical properties are presented in Chapter 20.

The patient may be taught to avoid distortion of the wrought wire by the explanation that to remove a removable partial denture, the fingernail should always be applied to its point of origin,

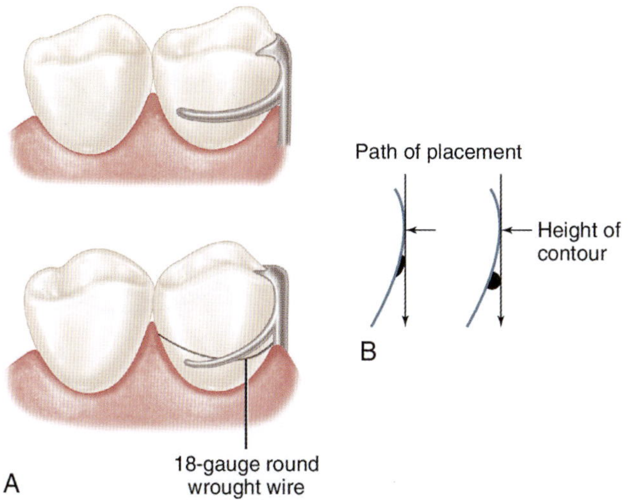

Fig. 7.28 **A,** Combination clasp consists of a cast reciprocal arm and a tapered, round wrought-wire retentive clasp arm. The latter is cast to, or soldered to, a cast framework. This design is recommended for the anterior abutment of the posterior modification space in a Kennedy Class II partially edentulous arch, where only a mesiobuccal undercut exists, to minimize the effects of a first-class lever system. **B,** In addition to the advantages of flexibility, adjustability, and appearance, a wrought-wire retentive arm makes only line contact with the abutment tooth, rather than broader contact with the cast clasp.

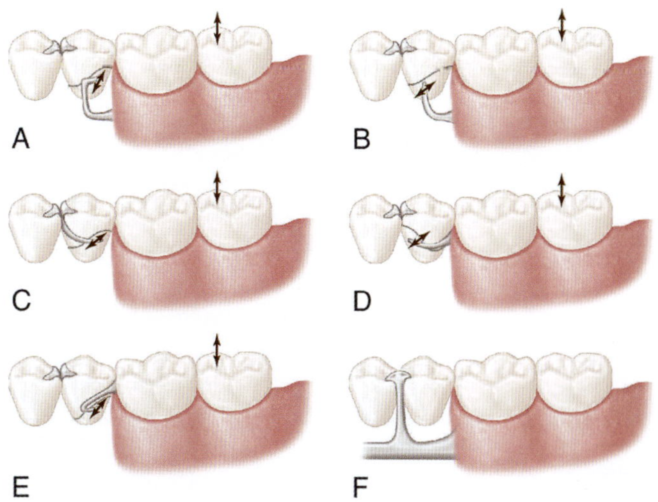

Fig. 7.29 **A,** Distobuccal undercut engaged by one-half T-type bar clasp. The portion of the clasp arm on and above the height of contour might afford some stabilization against the horizontal rotation of the denture base. **B,** I-bar placed in undercut at the middle (anteroposteriorly) of the buccal surface. This retainer contacts the tooth only at its tip. Note that the guiding plane on the distal aspect of the abutment is contacted by the metal of the denture framework and that a mesial rest is used. **C,** Interproximal ring clasp engaging the distobuccal undercut. Bar-type retainer cannot be used because tissue undercuts inferior to the buccal surface of the abutment. **D,** Round uniformly tapered wrought-wire circumferential retainer arm engaging the mesiobuccal undercut. A wrought-wire arm, instead of a cast arm, should be used in this situation because of the ability of wrought wire to flex omnidirectionally. A cast half-round retainer arm would not flex edgewise, which could result in excessive stress on the tooth when the rotation of the denture base occurs. **E,** A hairpin clasp may be used when the undercut lies cervical to the origin of the retainer arm. Both hairpin and interproximal ring clasps may be used to engage the distobuccal undercut on the terminal abutment of the distal extension removable partial denture. However, the distobuccal undercut on the terminal abutment should be engaged by a bar-type clasp as the clasp of choice in the absence of a large buccal tissue undercut cervical to the terminal abutment. Hairpin and interproximal ring clasps are the least desirable of the clasping situations illustrated here. **F,** Lingual view shows the use of an embrasure rest (double occlusal rests), connected to the lingual bar by the minor connector in illustrated designs. This design eliminates the need for a lingual clasp arm, places the fulcrum line anteriorly to make better use of the residual ridge for support, and provides stabilization against horizontal rotation of the denture base.

near the denture base, where it is held rigid by the casting, rather than to the flexible terminal end. Often, lingual retention may be used rather than buccal retention, especially on a mandibular abutment, so that the patient never touches the wrought-wire arm during denture removal. Instead, removal may be accomplished by lifting against the cast reciprocal arm located on the buccal side of the tooth. This may negate the esthetic advantage of the wrought-wire clasp arm, and esthetics should be given preference when the choice must be made between buccal and lingual retention. In most situations, however, retention must be used where it is possible, and the clasp designed accordingly.

Analysis of Tooth Contours for Retentive Clasps

Evaluation of tooth undercuts is important as it dictates the choice of clasps to be used. For example, when a distal undercut exists on a tooth with no soft tissue undercut, it may therefore be approached with a properly designed bar clasp arm. However, if there is a soft tissue undercut on that tooth, a ring clasp (despite its several disadvantages) may be the better choice into the distal undercut (Fig. 7.29). Analysis and accomplishment of tooth modification required for optimum stability and retention are necessary for the success of the prosthesis.

Critical areas of an abutment that provide for retention and stabilization (reciprocation) can be identified only with the use of a physical or digital surveyor. Surveying will be covered in detail in Chapter 11.

Physical Surveyors

The surveyor (Fig. 7.30) is a simple instrument that is essential for planning RPD. Its main working parts are the vertical arm and the adjustable table, which hold the cast in a fixed relation to the vertical arm. This relationship of the vertical arm to the cast represents the path of placement that the RPD will ultimately take when inserted or removed from the mouth (Fig. 7.31).

The adjustable table may be tilted in relation to the vertical arm of the surveyor until a path can be found that best satisfies all involved factors. A cast in a horizontal relationship to the vertical arm represents a vertical path of placement; a cast in a tilted relationship represents a path of placement toward the side of the cast that is on an upward slant. The vertical arm, when brought in contact with a tooth surface, identifies the location on the clinical crown where the greatest convexity exists. This line, called the *height of contour* or *survey line* (specific to the surveyor-defined path), is the boundary between (1) an occlusal or incisal region of the tooth that is freely accessible to a prosthesis and (2) a gingival region of the tooth that can be accessed only when a portion of the prosthesis elastically deforms and

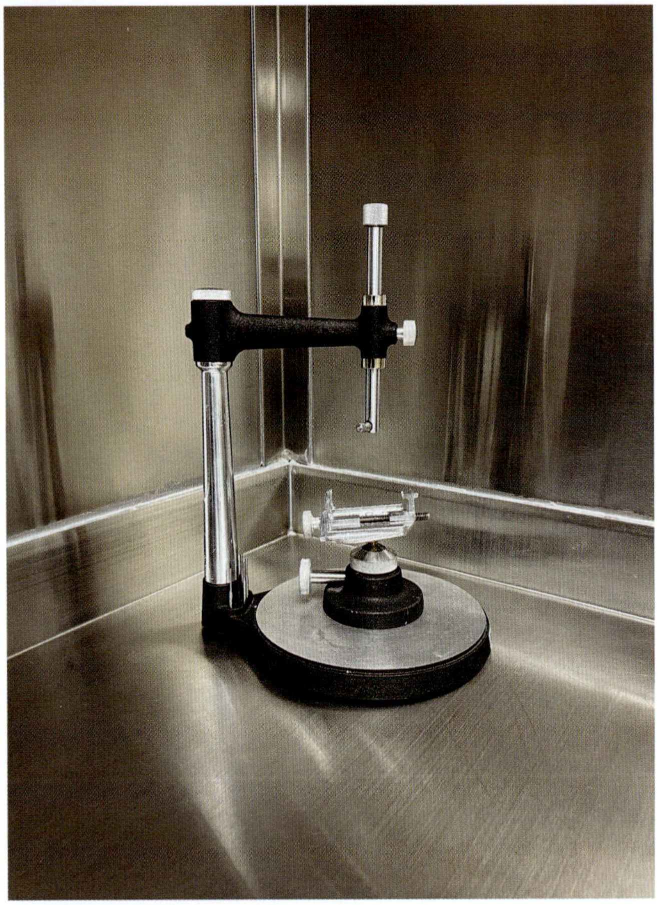

Fig. 7.30 Essential parts of a dental surveyor (Ney Parallelometer, Dentsply Ceramco, Burlington, NJ).

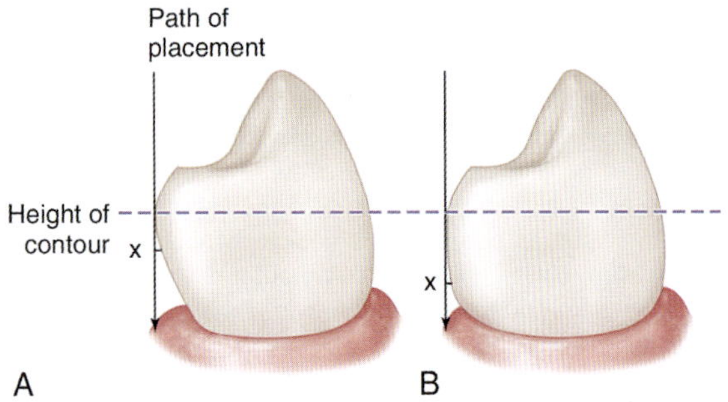

Fig. 7.31 Angle of cervical convergence on two teeth presenting dissimilar contours. A greater angle of cervical convergence on the tooth **(A)** necessitates the placement of a clasp terminus, x, nearer the height of contour than when a lesser angle exists, as in **B**. It is apparent that uniform clasp retention depends on the depth (amount) of the tooth undercut rather than on the distance below the height of the contour at which the clasp terminus is placed.

recovers to contact the tooth. This surveyor-defined path and the subsequent tooth height of contour will indicate the areas available for retention and those available for support and stabilization, as well as the existence of tooth and other tissue interference with the path of placement.

When the surveyor blade contacts a tooth on the cast at its greatest convexity, a triangle is formed. The apex of the triangle is at the point of contact of the surveyor blade with the tooth, and

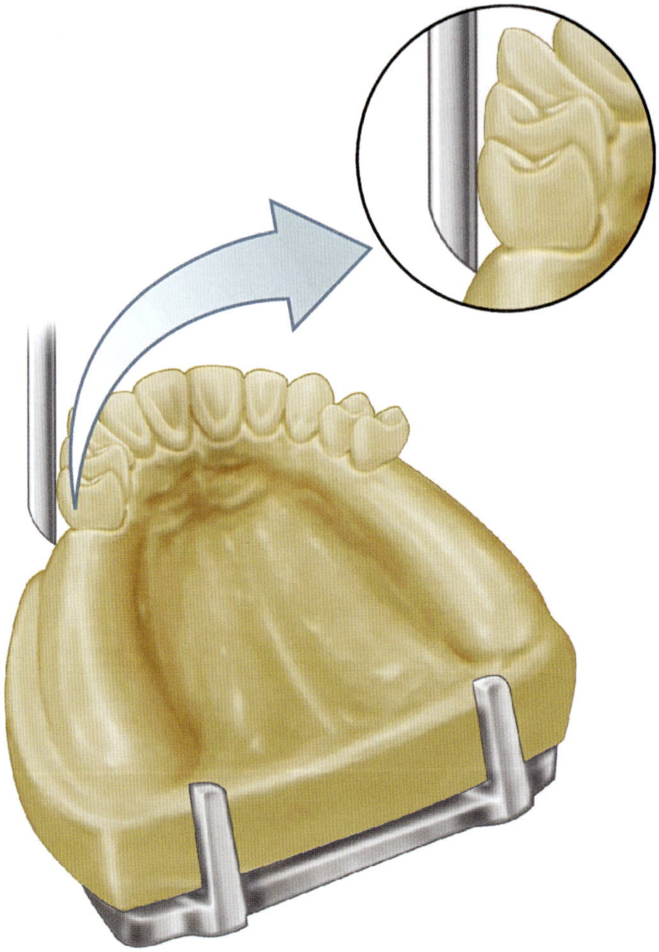

Fig. 7.32 Tooth undercut is best viewed against a good source of light passing through the triangle bounded by the surface of the abutment tooth, the surveyor blade, and the gingival tissues.

the base is the area of the cast representing the gingival tissue (Fig. 7.32). The apical angle is called the angle of cervical convergence (see Fig. 7.31). This angle may be measured as described in Chapter 11, or it may be estimated by observing the triangle of light visible between the tooth and the surveyor blade. For this reason, a wide surveyor blade rather than a small cylindrical tool is used so it is easier to see the triangle of light. The importance of this angle lies in its relationship to the amount of retention.

Digital Surveyors

Various laboratory software systems are available that allow for surveying an intraoral scan or a scanned model. Some software systems also have diagnostic surveying components (Fig. 7.33). In all instances, models or scans are loaded onto the software and oriented. After the orientation is complete, the path of insertion or draw is selected. The same criteria used for setting the path of insertion on a physical surveyor are applied when digitally surveying. In most instances, the selected path of draw is indicated by an arrow or a line that points to the direction selected. This allows the inspection of the selected path of insertion from various angles. Surveying the model or scan is the next step; digital surveyor software systems indicate the height of contour and 0.01" and 0.02" undercuts on the model using color-coded lines or areas.

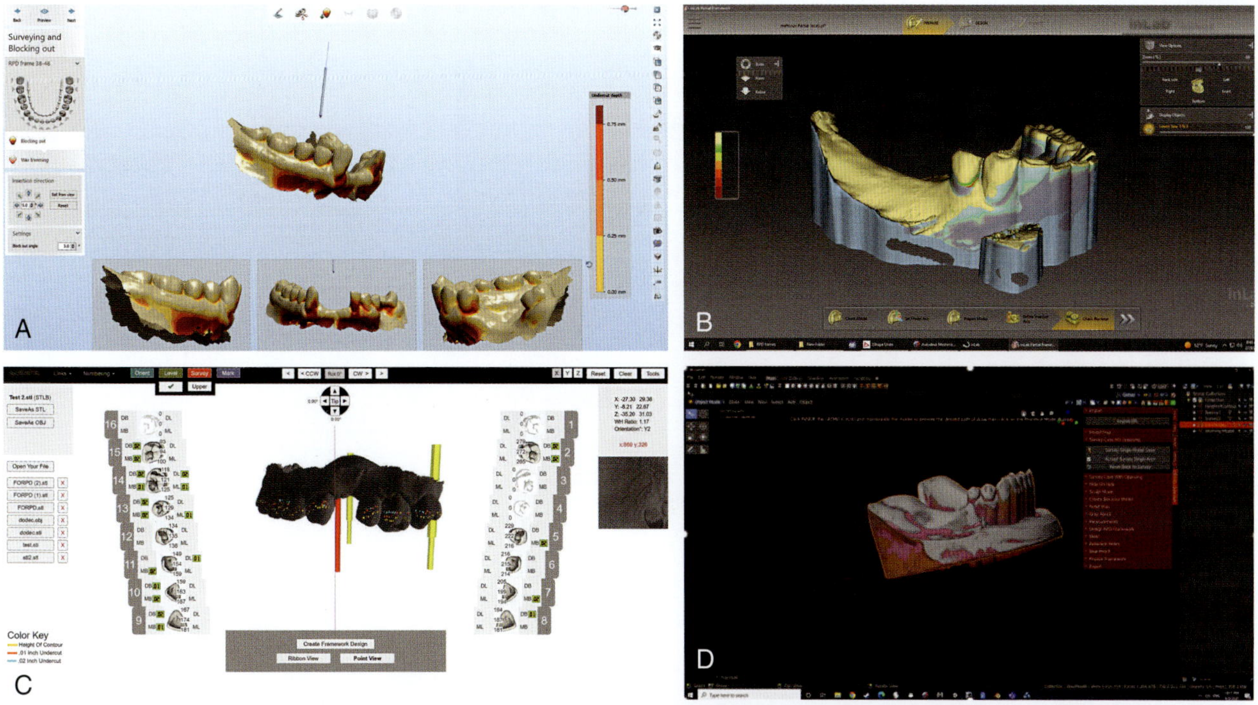

Fig. 7.33 Various virtual surveying software platforms exist: **(A and B)** license based and full laboratory design software, **(C)** diagnostic surveying and automated design software, and **(D)** free to use removable partial denture design and surveying software. All systems function similarly. A path of draw is selected, and the undercuts are depicted using different colors projected on the cast.

AMOUNT OF RETENTION

Clasp retention is based on the metal's resistance to deformation. For a clasp to be retentive, it must be placed in an undercut area of the tooth, where it is forced to deform upon application of a vertical dislodging force (Fig. 7.34). It is this resistance to deformation along an appropriately selected path that generates retention (Fig. 7.35). Such resistance to deformation is dependent on several factors and is also proportionate to the flexibility of the clasp arm.

The interaction of several factors under the clinician's control combines to produce retention. These include both tooth (planned and executed by the clinician) and prosthesis (to be planned by the dentist and executed by the laboratory technician) factors.

Tooth factors include the size of the angle of cervical convergence (depth of undercut) and how far the clasp terminal is placed into the angle of cervical convergence. Prosthesis factors include the flexibility of the clasp arm. Clasp flexibility is the product of clasp length (measured from its point of origin to its terminal end), clasp relative diameter (regardless of its cross-sectional form), clasp cross-sectional form or shape (whether it is round, half-round, or some other form), and the material used in making the clasp. The retention characteristics of gold alloy, chrome alloy, titanium, or titanium alloy depend on whether it is in cast or wrought form.

Size of and Distance Into the Angle of Cervical Convergence

To be retentive, a tooth must have an angle of convergence cervical to the height of contour. When it is surveyed, any single

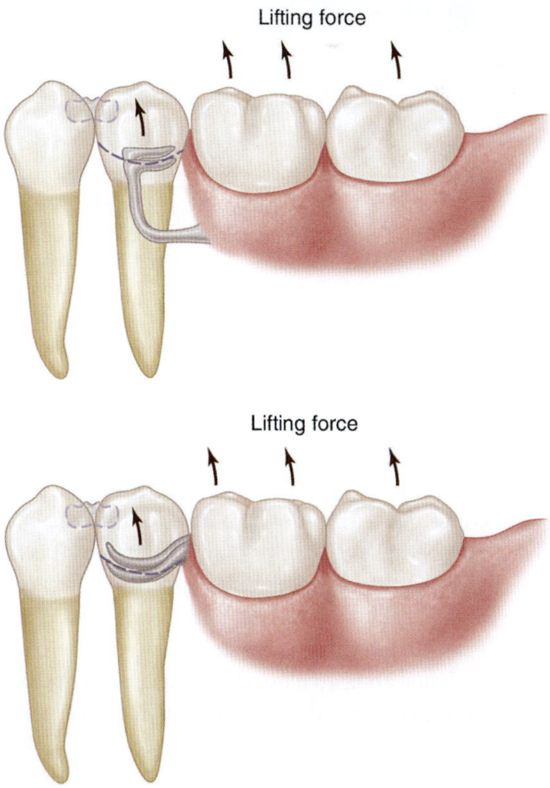

Fig. 7.34 Retention is provided primarily by the flexible portion of the clasp assembly. Retentive terminals are ideally located in measured undercuts in the gingival third of abutment crowns. When a force acts to dislodge the restoration in an occlusal direction, the retentive arm is forced to deform as it passes from the undercut location over the height of contour. The amount of retention provided by the clasp arm is determined by its length, diameter, taper, cross-sectional form, contour, type of alloy, and location and depth of undercut engaged.

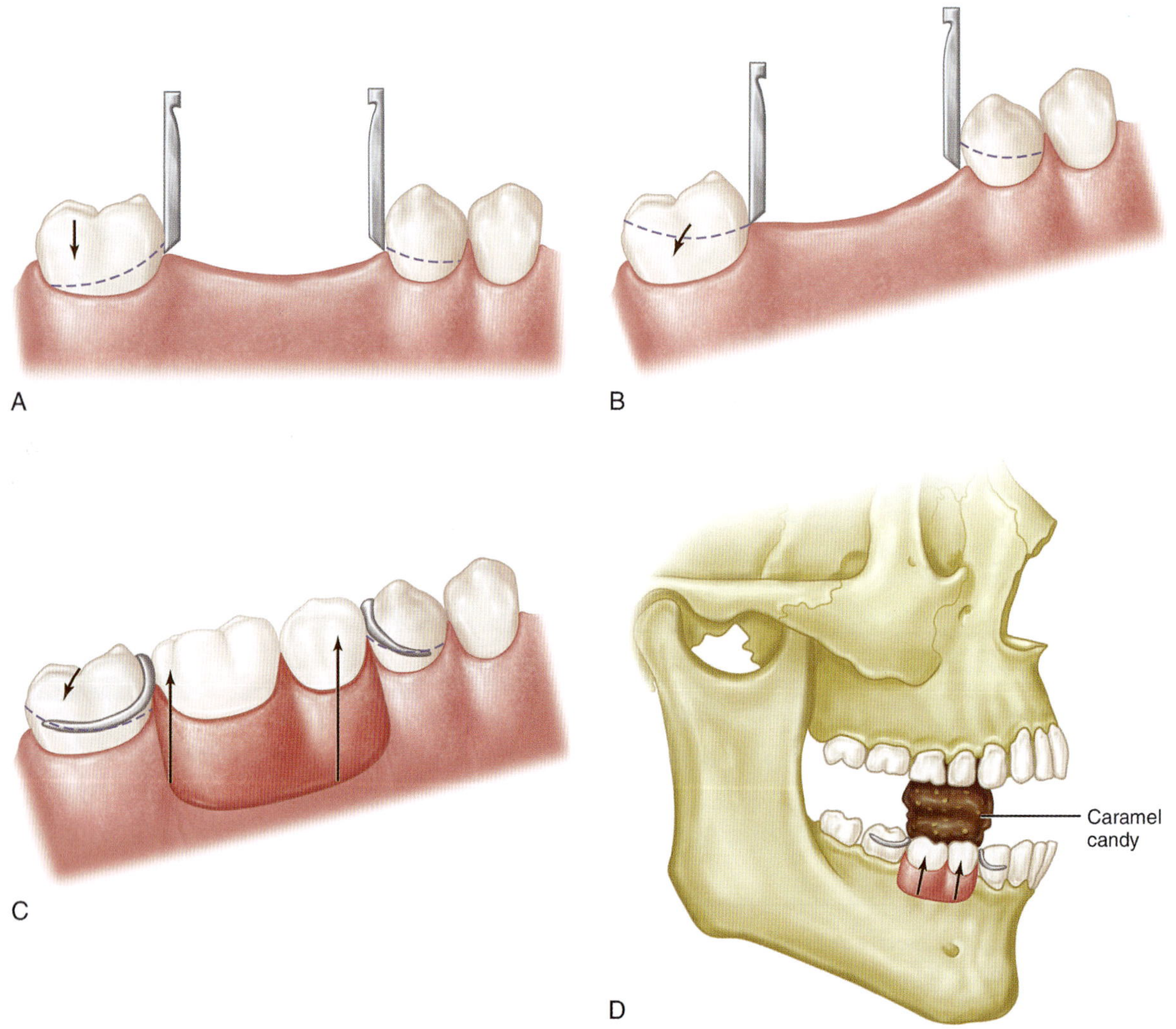

Fig. 7.35 **A,** Retentive areas are not sufficient to resist reasonable dislodging forces when a cast is surveyed at its most advantageous position (occlusal plane parallel to the surveyor table), even though guide planes could be established with minor tooth modification. **B,** Tilting cast creates functionally ineffective tooth contours, which are present only in relation to the surveying rod and do not exist when compared with the most advantageous position (position in which restoration will be subject to dislodging forces in an occlusal direction). **C** and **D,** Clasps designed at tilt are ineffective without the development of corresponding guide planes to resist displacement when the restoration is subject to dislodging forces in the occlusal direction.

tooth has a height of contour or an area of greatest convexity. Areas of cervical convergence may not exist when the tooth is viewed in relation to a given path of placement. Certain areas of cervical convergence may not be usable for the placement of retentive clasps because of their proximity to gingival tissue.

This is best illustrated by mounting a spherical object, such as an egg, on the adjustable table of a dental surveyor (Fig. 7.36). The egg now represents the cast of a dental arch or, more correctly, one tooth of a dental arch. To illustrate the height of contour, first, the egg is placed perpendicular to the base of the surveyor and is surveyed so the height of contour can be determined. The vertical arm of the surveyor represents the path of placement that a denture would take and conversely its path of removal.

With a carbon marker, a circumferential line has been drawn on the egg at its greatest circumference, as shown by the arrow in Fig. 7.36, *A*. This line, which is called the *survey line* or *height of contour*, is its greatest convexity. Cummer[6] spoke of it as the guideline because it is used as a guide in the placement of retentive and nonretentive clasps. DeVan[7] added the terms *suprabulge*, denoting the surfaces sloping superiorly, and *infrabulge*, denoting the surfaces sloping inferiorly.

Any areas cervical to the height of contour may be used for the placement of retentive clasp components, whereas areas occlusal to the height of contour may be used for the placement of nonretentive, stabilizing, or reciprocating components. Obviously, only flexible components may be placed gingival to the height of contour because rigid elements would not flex over the height of contour or contact the tooth in the undercut area.

With the original height of contour marked on the egg, the egg is now tilted from the perpendicular to an angular relation with the base of the surveyor (see Fig. 7.36, *B*). Its relation to the vertical arm of the surveyor has now been changed, just as a change in the position of a dental cast would bring about a different relationship with the surveyor. The vertical arm of the surveyor still represents the path of placement. However, its relation to the egg is totally different.

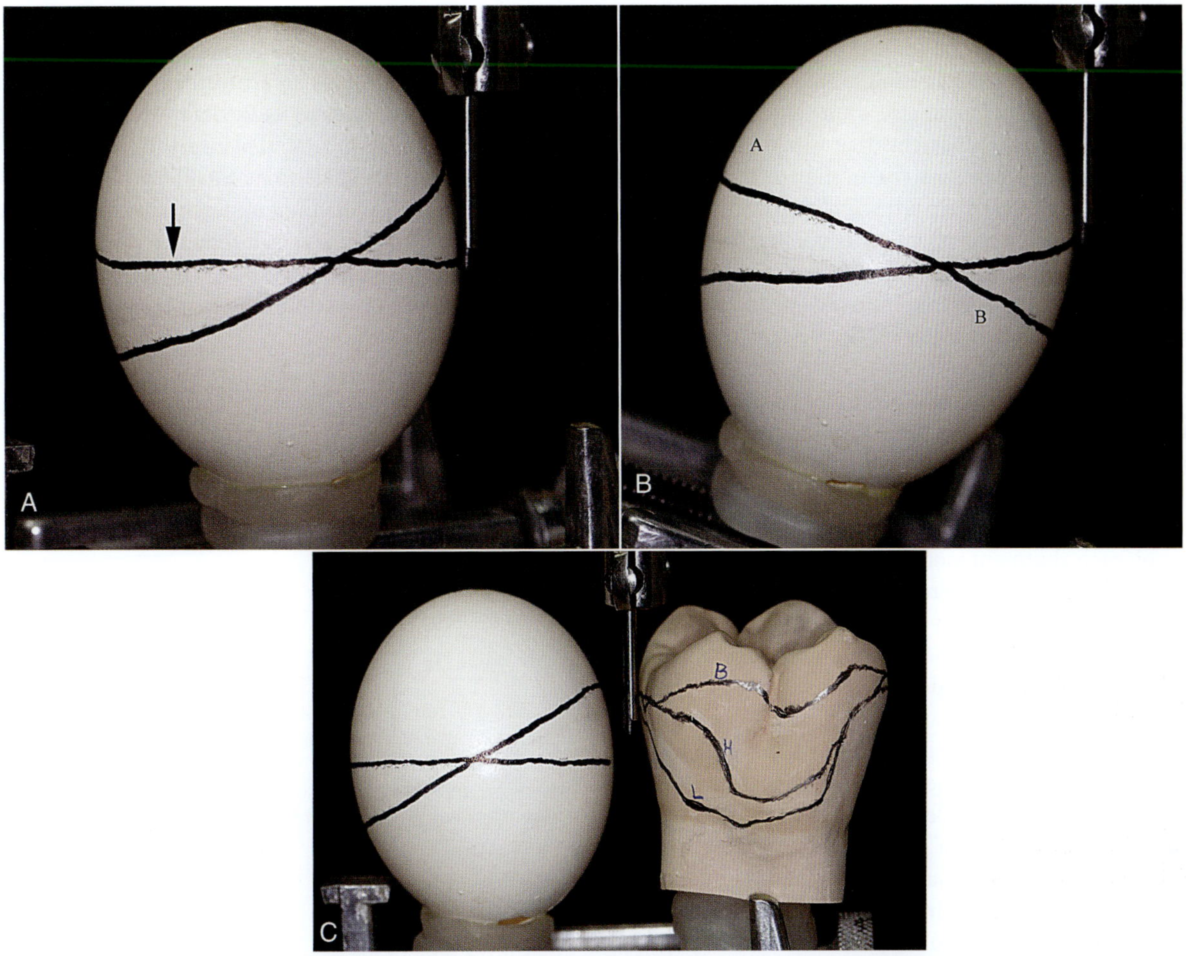

Fig. 7.36 Relationship of height of contour, suprabulge, and infrabulge. **A,** When an egg is placed with its long axis parallel to the surveying tool, the height of contour is found at its greatest circumference, here designated by the *arrow*. In this example, the second line is diagonal to the line outlining the height of contour and is either above the height of contour (right side of egg), referred to as the suprabulge region, or below the height of contour (left side of egg), referred to as the infrabulge region. **B,** If the long axis of the egg is reoriented so that the previous diagonal line is now at the greatest circumference, the original "height of contour line" no longer is at the greatest circumference. The line segment at *A* is in the suprabulge region, and the line segment *B* is in the infrabulge region. Changing the orientation alters the relationship of surfaces relative to the greatest circumference and consequently alters suprabulge and infrabulge locations. **C,** Just as the height of contour changes as orientation changes for the egg, when a tooth orientation changes, the height of contour is altered. For this molar, line *H* was produced with a horizontal orientation. When the tooth was inclined buccally, the height of contour moved to *B*, relative to the horizontal location. Alternatively, when the tooth was inclined lingually, the height of contour moved to *L*, relative to the horizontal location.

Again, the carbon marker is used to delineate the height of contour or the greatest convexity. It will be seen that areas that were formerly infrabulge are now suprabulge and vice versa. A retentive clasp arm placed below the height of contour in the original position may now be excessively retentive or totally nonretentive, whereas a nonretentive stabilizing or reciprocal arm that is located above the height of contour in the first position may now be located in an area of undercut. Fig. 7.36, *C* illustrates this principle compared with a tooth example showing that changes in tilt can significantly alter heights of contour.

The location and depth of a tooth undercut available for retention are therefore relative only to the path of placement and removal of the partial denture. At the same time, nonretentive areas on which rigid components of the clasp may be placed exist only for a given path of placement (see Fig. 7.36).

If conditions are found that are not favorable for the particular path of placement under consideration, a study should be conducted for a different path of placement. The cast is merely tilted in relation to the vertical arm until the most suitable path is found. The most suitable path of placement is generally considered to be the path of placement that requires the least amount of mouth preparation necessary to place the components of the removable partial denture in their ideal position on the tooth surfaces and in relation to the soft tissue. Then, mouth preparations are planned with a definite path of placement in mind.

It is important to remember that tooth surfaces can be recontoured through selective grinding or the placement of restorations (mouth preparations) to achieve a more suitable path of placement. In such instances, minor enameloplasty can be completed and polished after preparation to create an improved height of contour such as situation where the clasp arm should be located to avoid exposure in a smile position; this can also be accomplished using a composite resin on the smooth surface of the tooth. The path of placement also must take into consideration the presence of tissue undercuts that would interfere with the placement of major connectors, the location of vertical minor connectors, the origin of bar clasp arms, and the denture bases.

When the theory of clasp retention is applied to the abutment teeth in a dental arch during the surveying of the dental cast, each tooth may be considered individually and in relation to the other abutment teeth as far as the designs of retentive and stabilizing (reciprocating) components are concerned. This is necessary because the relationship of each tooth to the entire arch and to the design of the whole prosthesis has been considered previously when teeth were selected or modified to achieve the most suitable path of placement. Once this relationship of the cast to the surveyor has been established, the height of contour on each abutment tooth becomes fixed, and the clasp design for each must be considered separately.

A positive path of placement and removal is made possible by the contact of rigid parts of the RPD framework with parallel tooth surfaces, which act as guide planes. Because guide planes control the path of placement and removal, they can provide additional retention for the RPD by limiting the possibilities that exist for its dislodgment. The more vertical the walls (guide planes) that are prepared parallel to the path of insertion, the fewer the possibilities exist for dislodgment. If some degree of parallelism does not exist during placement and removal, trauma to the teeth and supporting structures, and strain on the RPD parts are inevitable. This ultimately results in damage to the teeth, their periodontal support or to the prosthesis itself, or both. Therefore without guide planes, clasp retention will be detrimental or practically nonexistent. If clasp retention is frictional only because of an active relationship of the clasp to the teeth, then orthodontic movement or damage to periodontal tissue, or both, will result. Instead, a clasp should bear a passive relationship to the teeth, except when a dislodging force is applied. In addition to the degree of the angle of cervical convergence and the distance a clasp is placed into the angle of cervical convergence, the amount of retention generated by a clasp depends on its flexibility. This is a function of clasp length, diameter, taper, cross-sectional form, and material.

The amount of retention also depends on the flexibility of a clasp arm. This is a function of clasp length, diameter, cross-sectional form, and material.

Length of Clasp Arm

The longer the clasp arm is, the more flexible it will be, all other factors being equal. The length of a circumferential clasp arm is measured from the point at which a uniform taper begins. Tooth modification provides increased length to a suprabulge retentive clasp by allowing the retentive tip to approach the undercut from a gingival direction optimizes clasp retention. The retentive circumferential clasp arm should be tapered uniformly from its point of origin through the full length of the clasp arm (Fig. 7.37).

The length of a bar clasp arm is also measured from the point at which a uniform taper begins. Generally, the taper of a bar clasp arm should begin at its point of origin from a metal base or at the point at which it emerges from a resin base (Fig. 7.38). Although a bar clasp arm usually will be longer than a circumferential clasp arm, its flexibility will be less because its half-round form lies in several planes; this prevents its flexibility from being proportionate to its total length. Tables 7.2 and 7.3 give an approximate depth of undercut that may be used for the cast gold and chromium-cobalt retentive clasp arms of circumferential and bar-type clasps. Based on a proportional limit of 60,000 psi and on the assumption that the clasp arm is properly

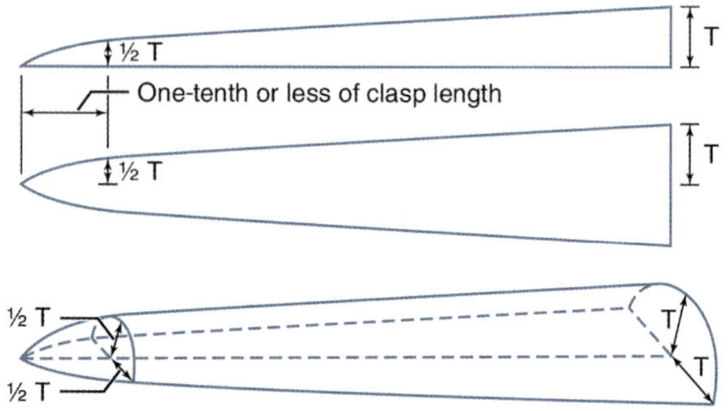

Fig. 7.37 The retentive cast clasp arm should be tapered uniformly from its point of attachment at the clasp body to its tip. Dimensions at the tip are about half those at the point of attachment. The clasp arm so tapered is approximately twice as flexible as one without any taper. *T*, Clasp thickness. (Courtesy of The Argen Corporation, New York, NY.)

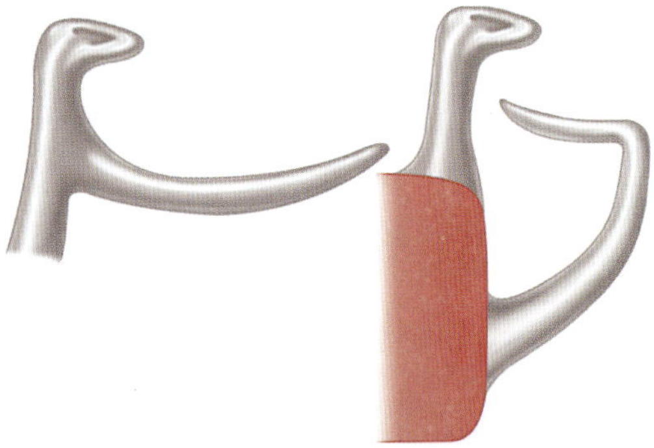

Fig. 7.38 Length of the tapered cast retentive clasp arm is measured along the center portion of the arm until it joins the clasp body (circumferential) or becomes part of the denture base or is embedded in the base (bar-type clasp).

TABLE 7.2 Permissible Flexibilities of Retentive Cast Circumferential and Bar-Type Clasp Arms of Type IV Gold Alloys[a]

Circumferential		Bar-Type	
Length (inches)	Flexibility (inches)	Length (inches)	Flexibility (inches)
0–0.3	0.01	0–0.7	0.01
0.3–0.6	0.02	0.7–0.9	0.02
0.6–0.8	0.03	0.9–1.0	0.03

[a]Based on the approximate dimensions of Jelenko preformed plastic patterns (JF Jelenko, New York, NY).

TABLE 7.3 Permissible Flexibilities of Retentive Cast Circumferential and Bar-Type Clasp Arms for Chromium-Cobalt Alloys[a]

Circumferential		Bar-Type	
Length (inches)	Flexibility (inches)	Length (inches)	Flexibility (inches)
0–0.3	0.004	0–0.7	0.004
0.3–0.6	0.008	0.7–0.9	0.008
0.6–0.8	0.012	0.9–1.0	0.012

[a]Based on the approximate dimensions of Jelenko preformed plastic patterns (JF Jelenko, New York, NY).

tapered, the clasp arm should be able to flex repeatedly within the limits stated without hardening or rupturing because of fatigue. It has been estimated that alternate stress applications of the fatigue type are placed on a retainer arm during mastication and other force-producing functions about 300,000 times a year.

Diameter of Clasp Arm

The greater the average diameter of a clasp arm is, the less flexible it will be—all other factors being equal. If its taper is uniform, the average diameter will be midway between its origin and its terminal end. If its taper is not uniform, a point of flexure—and therefore a point of weakness—will exist; this then will be the determining factor in its flexibility, regardless of the average diameter of its entire length.

Cross-Sectional Form of the Clasp Arm

Flexibility may exist in any form, but it is limited to one direction in the case of the half-round form. The only universally flexible form is the round form, which is practically impossible to obtain by casting and polishing.

Because most cast clasps are essentially half-round in form, they may flex away from the tooth, but edgewise flexing (and edgewise adjustment) is limited. For this reason, cast retentive clasp arms are more acceptable in tooth-supported partial dentures in which they are called on to flex only during placement and removal of the prosthesis. A retentive clasp arm on an abutment adjacent to a distal extension base not only must flex during placement and removal but also must be capable of flexing during functional movement of the distal extension base. It must have universal flexibility to avoid transmission of tipping stresses to the abutment tooth, or it must be capable of disengaging the undercut when vertical forces directed against the denture are toward the residual ridge. A round clasp is the only circumferential clasp form that may be safely used to engage a tooth undercut on the side of an abutment tooth away from the distal extension base. The location of the undercut is perhaps the single most important factor in the selection of a clasp for use with distal extension partial dentures.

Material Used for the Clasp Arm

Although all cast alloys used in removable partial denture construction possess flexibility, their flexibility is proportionate to their bulk. If this were not true, other components of the removable partial denture could not have the necessary rigidity. A disadvantage of a cast gold removable partial denture is that its bulk must be increased to obtain needed rigidity at the expense of added weight and increased cost. It cannot be denied that greater rigidity with less bulk is possible through the use of chromium-cobalt alloys.

Although cast gold alloys may have greater resiliency than do cast chromium-cobalt alloys, the fact remains that the structural nature of the cast clasp does not approach the flexibility and adjustable nature of the wrought-wire clasp. Because it was formed by being drawn into a wire, the wrought-wire clasp arm has toughness exceeding that of a cast clasp arm. The tensile strength of a wrought structure is at least 25% greater than that of the cast alloy from which it was made. It may therefore be used in smaller diameters to provide greater flexibility without fatigue and ultimate fracture.

Relative Uniformity of Retention

Now that the factors inherent to a determination of the amount of retention from individual clasps have been reviewed, it is important to consider the coordination of relative retention between various clasps in a single prosthesis.

The size of the angle of convergence will determine how far a given clasp arm should be placed into that angle. By disregarding—for the time being—variations in clasp flexibility, the relative uniformity of retention will depend on the location of the retentive part of the clasp arm, not in relation to the height of contour, but in relation to the angle of cervical convergence.

The retention of all principal abutments should be as equal as possible. Although esthetic placement of clasp arms is desirable, it may not be possible to place all clasp arms in the same occlusocervical relationship because of variations in tooth contours. However, retentive surfaces may be made similar by altering tooth contours or by using cast restorations with similar contours.

Measurement of the degree of undercut by mechanical means with the use of a surveyor is important. However, undercut identification is only one factor that is important to consider when one is providing appropriate retention for a RPD.

Stabilizing-Reciprocal Cast Clasp Arm or Element

When the direct retainer comes into contact with the tooth, the framework must be stabilized against horizontal movement for the required clasp deformation to occur. This stabilization is derived from cross-arch framework contacts or from a rigid reciprocal clasp or component in the same clasp assembly. To provide true reciprocation, the reciprocal clasp must be in contact during the entire period of retentive clasp deformation. This is best provided with lingual-palatal, guide plane surfaces.

A stabilizing (reciprocal) clasp arm should be rigid. Therefore it is shaped somewhat differently than the cast retentive clasp arm, which must be flexible. Its average diameter must be greater than the average diameter of the opposing retentive arm to increase the desired rigidity. A cast retentive arm is tapered in two dimensions, as illustrated in Fig. 7.37, whereas a reciprocal arm should be tapered in one dimension only, as shown in Fig. 7.39. Achieving such a form for the arm requires freehand waxing of patterns.

ATTACHMENTS

The principle of the attachment was first formulated by Dr. Herman E.S. Chayes in 1906. One such attachment manufactured commercially still carries his name. Attachments are manufactured components that are incorporated into a fixed restoration made on an RPD abutment. Almost all attachments have a matrix/patrix (male and female) component. One part resides in the removable partial denture and the other integrated into the fixed restoration on the abutment tooth. The manufactured matrix-patrix components are made to have a *precision* or *semi-precision* fit with each other. Depending on how the attachment is integrated into the fixed restoration, attachments can be classified as *intracoronal* attachments that reside mainly within the contours of the abutment teeth and *extracoronal* attachments that extend beyond the contours of the fixed restoration (Figs. 7.40 and 7.41. 7.40) (Video 7.38). Some attachments may be fabricated by the dental technician as a cast dovetail fitting into a counterpart receptacle in the abutment crown. The alloys used in manufactured attachments and the precision with which they are constructed make the ready-made cast-to attachment preferable to any type that can be fabricated in the dental laboratory.

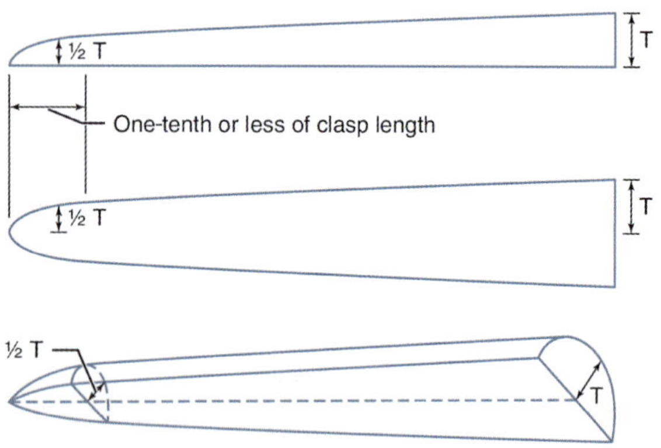

Fig. 7.39 The reciprocal arm of the direct retainer assembly should be rigid. An arm tapered both lengthwise and widthwise is more flexible than an arm of the same dimensions tapered only lengthwise. *T,* Clasp thickness.

Attachments have two major advantages over traditional clasping: (1) elimination of visible retentive and support components and (2) better vertical support through a rest seat located more favorably in relation to the horizontal axis of the abutment tooth. For these reasons, the attachment may be preferable in selected situations.

Some of the disadvantages of attachments include the following: (1) they require prepared abutments and castings; (2) they require somewhat complicated clinical and laboratory procedures; (3) they eventually wear, with progressive loss of frictional resistance to the RPD removal; (4) they are difficult to repair and replace; (5) they are effective in proportion to their length and are therefore least effective on short teeth; (6) they are difficult to place completely within the circumference of an abutment tooth because of the size of the pulp; and (7) they are considered more costly.

All the retainers that are discussed herein have merit, and much credit is due to those who have developed specific devices and techniques for the retention of RPDs. The use of patented retaining devices and other techniques falls in the same limited category as the attachment prosthesis and is for economic and

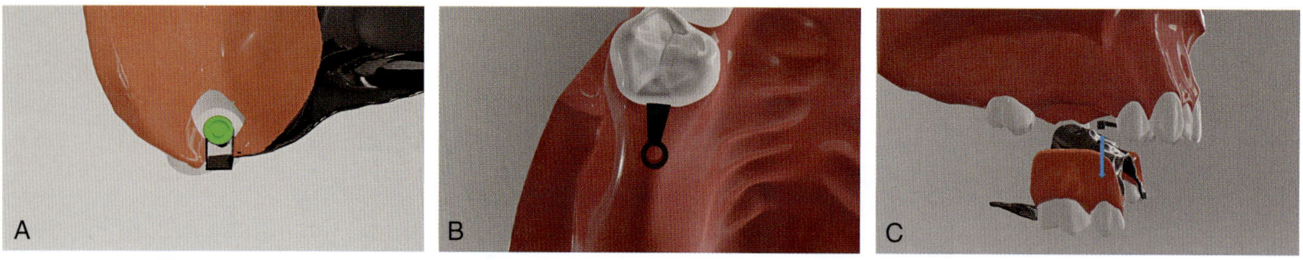

Fig. 7.40 A generic extracoronal attachment consisting of **(A)** a male component and **(B)** female components. Attachments create an esthetic alternative to clasping. **C,** Additionally, extracoronal attachments can be resilient as they are not precision milled and allow for some movement and are thus compatible with extension base situations in which movement is to be expected.

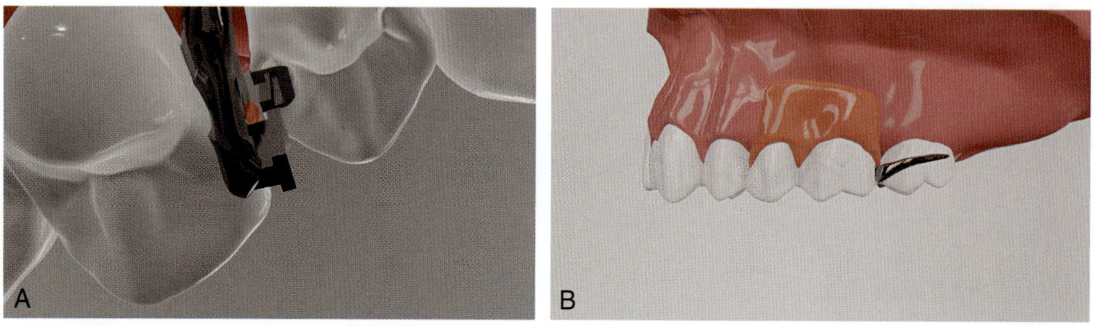

Fig. 7.41 A generic intracoronal attachment consisting of **(A)** a male (patrix) component and a female (matrix) component. **B,** Attachments create an esthetic alternative to clasping. Additionally, intracoronal attachments are precision milled and do not allow for any movement and are thus not compatible with extension base situations in which movement is to be expected.

technical reasons available to only a small percentage of those patients who need RPD service.

Attachments of the locking or dovetail type (internal attachments) unquestionably have many advantages over the clasp-type RPD in tooth-supported situations (Fig. 7.42). However, they are not indicated for distal extension RPDs because of inherent excessive leverages most often associated with these attachments.

The nonlocking type of attachments, in conjunction with sound prosthodontic principles, can be advantageously used in many distal extension base cases (Fig. 7.43). However, unless the cross-arch axis of rotation is stabilized, for the bilaterally placed attachments, torque on the abutments may be experienced. Excellent textbooks devoted to the use of manufactured intracoronal and extracoronal retainer systems are available. For this reason, this text concerns itself primarily with the extracoronal type of direct retainer assembly (clasps). Numerous well-designed attachments are available in the dental market that may be used in situations requiring special retention.

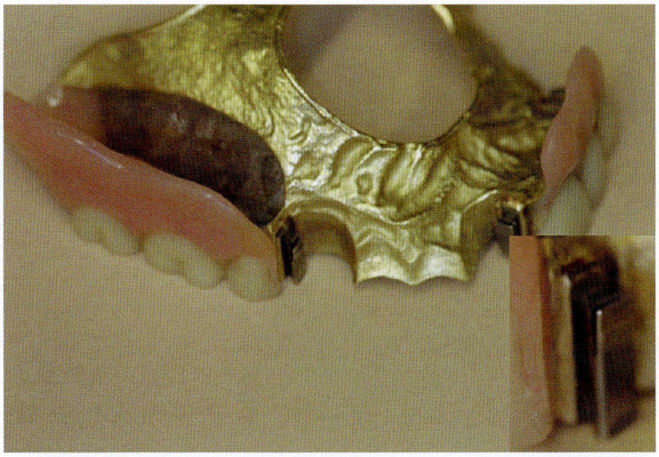

Fig. 7.42 Kennedy Classification II, modification 1, maxillary removable partial denture with three internal attachments. Gold framework with soldered attachments that gain retention through the activation of the gingival region of the male component.

Descriptive literature and technique manuals are available from the manufacturers.

Other conservative treatment of partially edentulous arches with RPDs can be accomplished in a variety of ways. Treatment is still contingent on the location and condition of the remaining teeth and the contour and quality of the residual ridges. Basic principles and concepts of design relative to support and stability must be respected even though a variety of retaining devices can be incorporated.

IMPLANTS AS DIRECT RETAINERS

In situations where additional support is needed (1) to convert a Kennedy Class I or Class II to a Kennedy Class III, (2) because the tooth anterior the edentulous area is inadequate for an abutment tooth, or (3) support requirements are adequately met by available oral tissues but there is a need to improve esthetics by eliminating visible clasps, dental implants can be used for retention. The unique aspect of implant use with RPDs is that their location can be prescribed, meaning that the clinician selects the best location. The location within the modification space must first consider anatomic characteristics of available bone. The advantage gained to a patient by placement of the implant may be minimized if extensive bone augmentation procedures were required to allow implant placement in conjunction with a RPD. In such instances, the implant-retained RPD may not be the best treatment option.

If anatomic needs are met, the location of the placement of an implant within a modification space (anterior, mid, or distal placement within the space) should be evaluated to determine which provides the best advantage with regard to retentive needs. Because retainers utilizing teeth have always been restricted to tooth locations at either end of a span, the mid-span location typically is not considered. However, the application of implants allows consideration of where the most beneficial location of retention can be provided, which forces consideration of where the most efficient resistance to movement away from the denture base can be provided. Placement at a midpoint may limit the movement of the denture base compared to the greater movement allowed at either extreme and therefore should be taken into consideration when treatment planning.

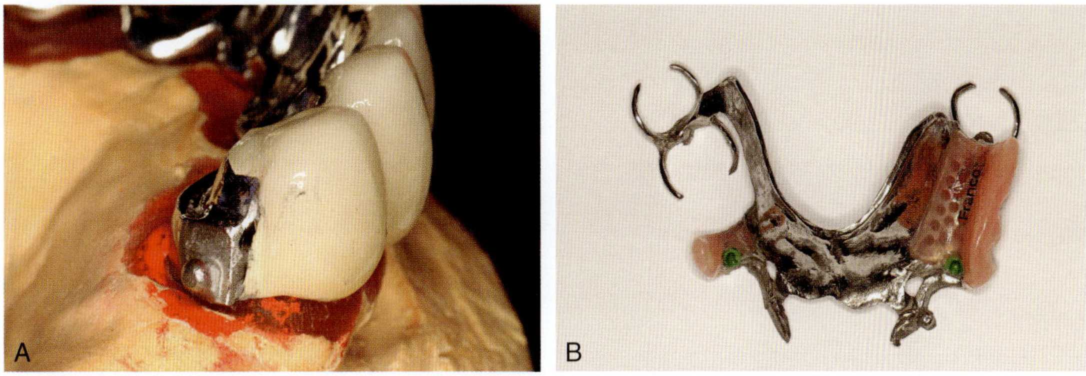

Fig. 7.43 Kennedy Classification III, modification 1 utilizing an extracoronal retainer on an anterior abutment tooth, showing a **(A)** male (patrix) component on external surface of the crown and **(B)** the female (matrix) component within the removable partial denture. Cross-arch axis of rotation is stabilized in this situation to the abutment teeth posterior to the denture bases.

REFERENCES

1. Kapur KK, et al. A randomized clinical trial of two basic removable partial denture designs. Part I: comparisons of five-year success rates and periodontal health. *J Prosthet Dent.* 1994;72:268–282. (1994).
2. Kratochvil FJ. Influence of occlusal rest position and clasp design on movement of abutment teeth. *J Prosthet Dent.* 1963;13:114–124.
3. Demer WJ. An analysis of mesial rest-I-bar clasp designs. *J Prosthet Dent.* 1976;36(3):243–253. https://doi.org/10.1016/0022-3913(76)90178-5. PMID: 784957.
4. Krol AJ. Clasp design for extension-base removable partial dentures. *J Prosthet Dent.* 1973;29(4):408–415. https://doi.org/10.1016/s0022-3913(73)80018-6. PMID: 4570914.
5. Krol AJ. RPI (rest, proximal plate, I bar) clasp retainer and its modifications. *Dent Clin North Am.* 1973;17(4):631–649. PMID: 4580355.
6. Cummer WE: Partial denture service. In: Anthony LP, editor. American Textbook of Prosthetic Dentistry, Lea & Febiger, 1942, pp. 339–452.
7. DeVan MM. Preserving natural teeth through the use of clasps. *J Prosthet Dent.* 1955;5:208–214.

8

Indirect Retainers

Lisa A. Lang, Lily T. García, and Ahmed Mahrous

CHAPTER OUTLINE

ROLE OF INDIRECT RETAINERS IN CONTROL OF PROSTHESIS MOVEMENT

As was described in Chapter 4, removable partial denture movement can exist in three planes. Tooth-supported removable partial dentures effectively use the teeth to control movement away from the tissues. Tooth-tissue–supported removable partial dentures do not have this capability because one end of the prosthesis is free to move away from the tissue (Fig. 8.1) (Video 8.1). This may occur because of the effects of gravity in the maxillary arch or adhesive foods in either arch. Indirect retainers are a component of the removable partial denture design that act to counteract this movement and increase stability during function (Fig. 8.2) (Video 8.2).

When the distal extension denture base is dislodged from its basal seat, it tends to rotate around the fulcrum lines (Fig. 8.3) (Video 8.3). Theoretically, this movement away from the tissues can be resisted by activation of the direct retainer, the stabilizing components of the clasp assembly, and the rigid components of the removable partial denture framework, which are located on definite rests at 90 degrees perpendicular to the fulcrum line, away from the distal extension base. These components are referred to as *indirect retainers* (Figs. 8.4 and 8.5). Fig. 8.5 illustrates the ideal location of the fulcrum line and indirect retainers for common Kennedy Classifications. Indirect retainer components should be placed as far as possible from the distal extension base, which provides the best leverage advantage against dislodgment (Fig. 8.6).

For the sake of clarity in the discussion of the location and functions of indirect retainers, fulcrum lines should be considered the axis about which the denture will rotate when the bases move away from the residual ridge.

An indirect retainer consists of one or more rests and the supporting minor connectors (Figs. 8.7 and 8.8). The proximal plates, adjacent to the edentulous areas, also provide indirect retention. Although it is customary to identify the entire assembly as the indirect retainer, it should be remembered that the rest is actually the indirect retainer united to the major connector by a minor connector. This is noted to avoid interpretation of any contact with tooth inclines as part of the indirect retainer. An

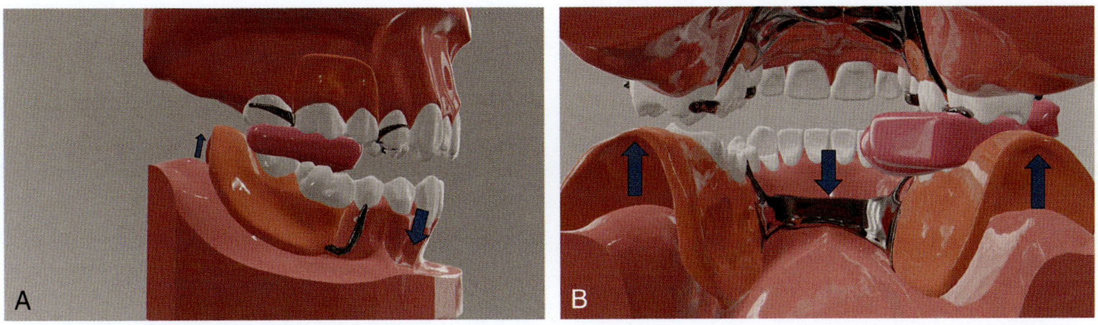

Fig. 8.1 Mandibular distal extension removable partial denture with no indirect retainers showing the distal extension base being lifted from the ridge. This can be seen from the lateral view **(A)** and posterior view **(B)**. Note how the removable partial denture movement is unhindered around the fulcrum line. This causes excessive instability and even trauma to the anterior lingual soft tissues. Courtesy of Ahmed Mahrous Copyright © 2024. All rights reserved.

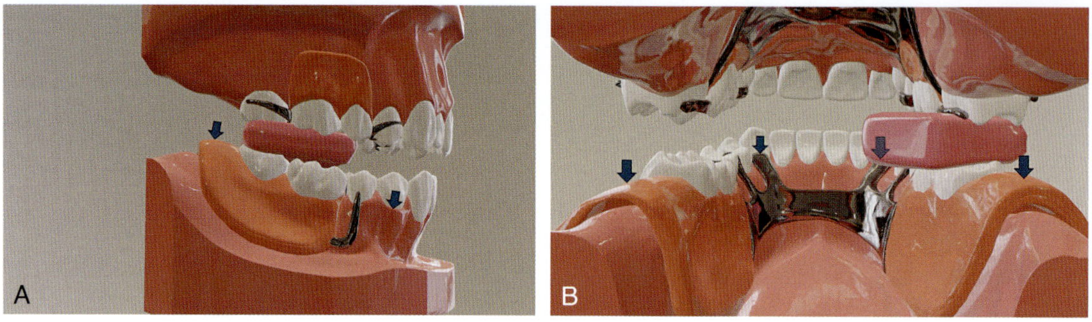

Fig. 8.2 Mandibular distal extension removable partial denture with indirect retainers showing the distal extension base being lifted from the ridge; however, the prosthesis remains relatively stationary due to the stabilizing capacity of the indirect retainers. This can be seen from the lateral view **(A)** and posterior view **(B)**. Courtesy of Ahmed Mahrous Copyright © 2024. All rights reserved.

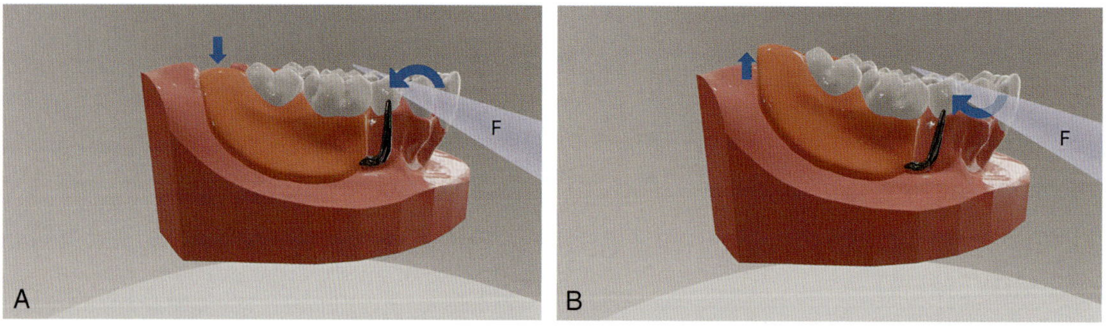

Fig. 8.3 Illustration of movement around the fulcrum line from the lateral view. The fulcrum line, an imaginary line that extends through the two terminal rests on an extension base removable partial denture (RPD) around which the removable partial denture may rotate under function, is depicted by *F* in this lateral view of an RPD. **A,** When the RPD is subjected to occlusal loads, the possible movements of the RPD extension base are counterclockwise and toward the supporting tissue. **B,** When the RPD is subjected to pulling forces, such as when eating sticky foods, the possible movements of the RPD extension base are clockwise and away from the supporting tissues. Courtesy of Ahmed Mahrous Copyright © 2024. All rights reserved.

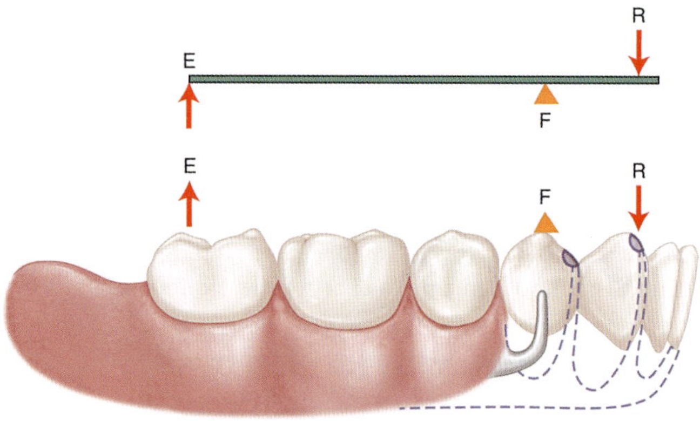

Fig. 8.4 Mandibular distal extension removable partial denture showing the distal extension base being lifted from the ridge and the clasp assembly being activated and engaged, with the indirect retainer providing stabilization against dislodgment. *E*, effort; *F*, fulcrum; *R*, resistance.

indirect retainer should be placed as far from the distal extension base as possible in a prepared rest seat on a tooth capable of supporting its function.

Although the most effective location of an indirect retainer is commonly in the vicinity of an incisor tooth, that tooth may not be strong enough to support an indirect retainer and may have steep inclines that cannot be favorably altered to support a rest. In such a situation, the nearest canine tooth or the mesio-occlusal surface of the first premolar may be the best location for the indirect retention, despite not beingas far removed from the fulcrum line. Whenever possible, two indirect retainers closer to the fulcrum line are used to compensate for the compromise in distance (see Fig. 8.8). When a distal extension is judged to be at significant risk for dislodgement away from the denture base, the use of a dental implant as a distal retainer can be considered.

FACTORS INFLUENCING EFFECTIVENESS OF INDIRECT RETAINERS

The following factors influence the effectiveness of an indirect retainer:

1. The principal occlusal rests on the primary abutment teeth must be reasonably held in their seats by the retentive arms of the direct retainers. If rests are held in their seats, rotation about an axis should occur, which subsequently would activate the indirect retainers. If total displacement of the rests occurs, no rotation about the fulcrum would occur, and the indirect retainers would not be activated.

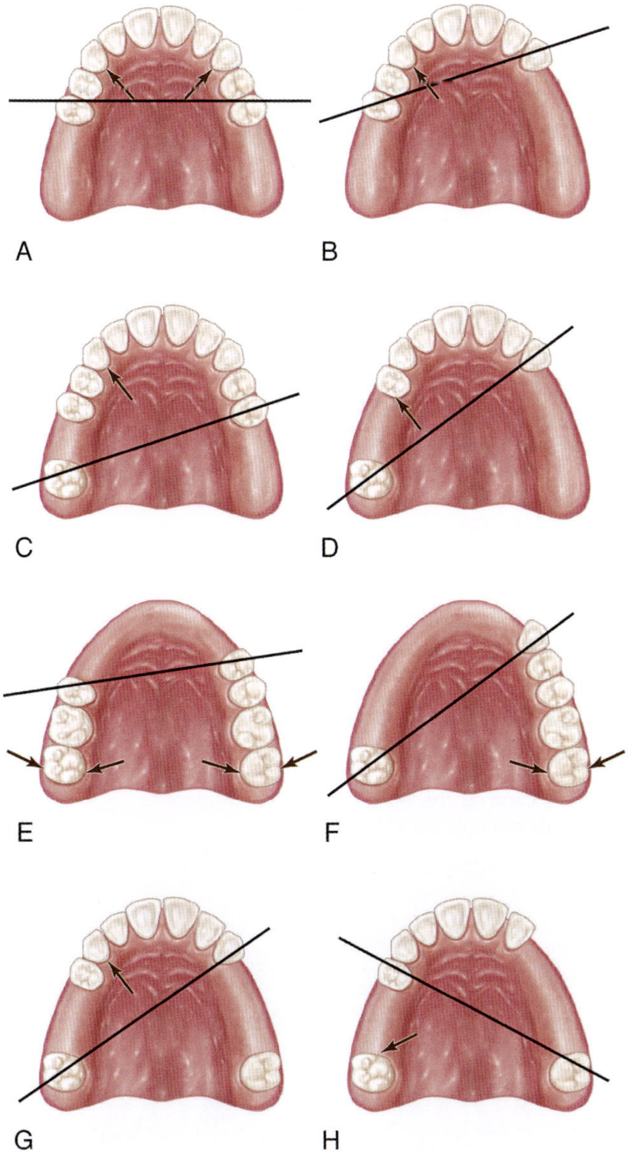

Fig. 8.5 Illustrations of the various Kennedy Classifications and partially edentulous scenarios. Fulcrum lines are outlined in several types of partially edentulous arches, around which the removable partial denture may rotate when bases are subjected to forces directed toward or away from the residual ridge. *Arrows* indicate the most advantageous position of indirect retainer(s). In a Kennedy Class I arch **(A** and **B)**, the fulcrum line passes through the most posterior abutments, provided some rigid component of the framework is occlusal to the abutment's heights of contour. **C,** In a Kennedy Class II arch, the fulcrum line is diagonal, passing through the abutment on the distal extension side and the most posterior abutment on the opposite side. **D,** If the abutment tooth anterior to the modification space lies far enough removed from the fulcrum line, it may be used effectively for support of the indirect retainer. In a Kennedy Class IV arch **(E** and **F)**, the fulcrum line passes through two abutments adjacent to the single edentulous space. **G,** In a Kennedy Class III arch, with a posterior tooth on the right side which has a poor prognosis and eventually will be lost, the fulcrum line is considered the same as though the posterior tooth was not present. Thus its future loss may not necessitate altering the original design of the removable partial denture framework. **H,** In a Kennedy Class III arch when the anterior teeth are nonsupporting, the adjacent edentulous area is the tissue-supported end; therefore the diagonal fulcrum line passes through the two principal abutments, as in a Kennedy Class II arch. The posterior abutment tooth is then used for direct and indirect retention.

2. Distance from the fulcrum line. The following three areas must be considered:
   a. Length of the distal extension base
   b. Location of the fulcrum line
   c. How far beyond the fulcrum line the indirect retainer is placed
3. Rigidity of the connectors supporting the indirect retainer. All connectors must be rigid if the indirect retainer is to function as intended.
4. Effectiveness of the supporting tooth surface. The indirect retainer must be placed on a definite rest seat on which slippage or tooth movement will not occur. Tooth inclines and weak teeth should never be used to support indirect retainers.

AUXILIARY FUNCTIONS OF INDIRECT RETAINERS

In addition to effectively activating the direct retainer to prevent movement of a distal extension base away from the tissues, an indirect retainer may serve the following auxiliary functions:

1. It tends to reduce anteroposterior tilting leverages on the principal abutments. This is particularly important when an isolated tooth is being used as an abutment—a situation that should be avoided whenever possible. Ordinarily, proximal contact with the adjacent tooth prevents such tilting of an abutment as the base lifts away from the tissues.
2. Contact of its minor connector with axial tooth surfaces aids in stabilization against horizontal movement of the denture. Such tooth surfaces, when made parallel to the path of placement, may also act as auxiliary guiding planes.
3. Anterior teeth supporting indirect retainers are stabilized against lingual movement.
4. It may act as an auxiliary rest to support a portion of the major connector, facilitating stress distribution. For example, a lingual bar may be supported against settling into the tissues by the indirect retainer acting as an auxiliary rest. One must be able to differentiate between an auxiliary rest placed for support for a major connector, one placed for indirect retention, and one serving a dual purpose. Some auxiliary rests are added solely to provide rest support to a segment of the denture and should not be confused with indirect retention.
5. It may provide the first visual indications for the need to reline an extension base removable partial denture. Deficiencies in basal seat support are manifested by the dislodgment of indirect retainers from their prepared rest seats when the denture base is depressed, and rotation occurs around the fulcrum.

These auxiliary functions derived from indirect retainers are important to consider, especially given the reported controversy as to the effectiveness of indirect retainers.

FORMS OF INDIRECT RETAINERS

The indirect retainer may take any one of several forms. All are effective in proportion to their support and distance from the fulcrum line.

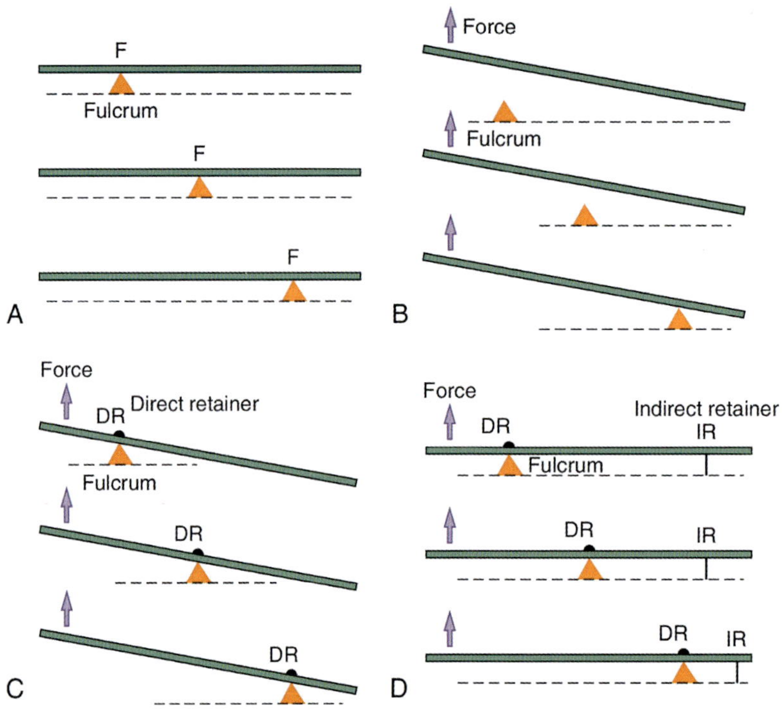

Fig. 8.6 Indirect retainer *(IR)* principle. **A,** Beams are supported at various points *(F)*. **B,** A lifting force illustrated by the lilac arrows will displace the entire beam in the absence of retainers. **C,** With direct retainers *(DRs)* at the fulcrum, the lifting force will depress one end of the beam and elevate the other end, rotating around the fulcrum point of support *(F)*. **D,** With both DRs and IRs functioning, the lifting force will not displace the beam. The farther the IR is from the fulcrum, the more efficiently it should control movement.

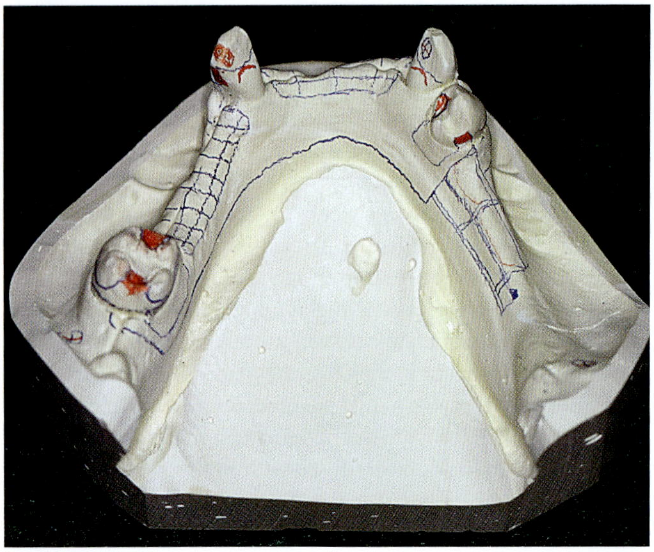

Fig. 8.7 Planning the location for an indirect retainer for a mandibular Kennedy Class II, modification 2, removable partial denture. The greatest distance from the axis of rotation around most distal rests (fulcrum line) would fall on #22. The decision to use an incisal rest or cingulum rest depends on the patient's concern for the esthetic impact of an incisal rest versus having a crown (for the cingulum rest).

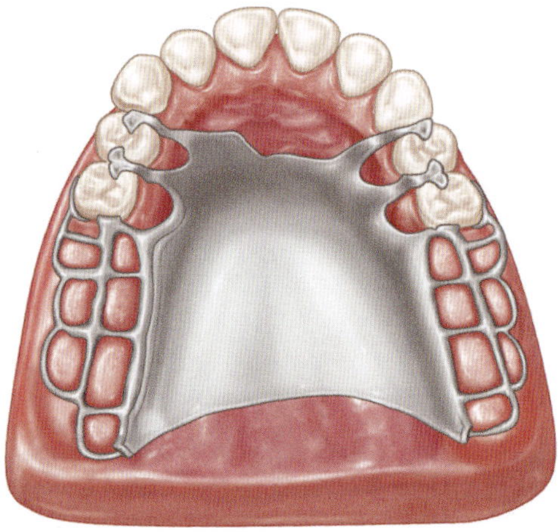

Fig. 8.8 Example of indirect retention used in conjunction with a palatal plate–type major connector. Indirect retainers are proximal plates on the second premolars and occlusal rests located on the first premolars. A secondary function of auxiliary occlusal rest assemblies is to prevent the settling of the anterior portion of the major connector and to provide stabilization against horizontal rotation.

Auxiliary Rest

The most commonly used indirect retainer is an auxiliary occlusal rest located on an occlusal surface and as far away from the distal extension base as possible. In a mandibular Kennedy Class I arch, this location is usually on the mesial marginal ridge of the first premolar on each side of the arch (Fig. 8.9). The ideal position for the indirect retainer, perpendicular to the fulcrum line, would be near the central incisors, which are often too weak, and/or have lingual surfaces that are too perpendicular to support a rest. Bilateral rests on the first premolars are quite effective, even though they are located closer to the axis of rotation. However, in certain design situations, when the distance between the primary occlusal rest of the direct retainer and the indirect retainer may result in cleansability issues, a canine rest may be more appropriate (Fig. 8.10).

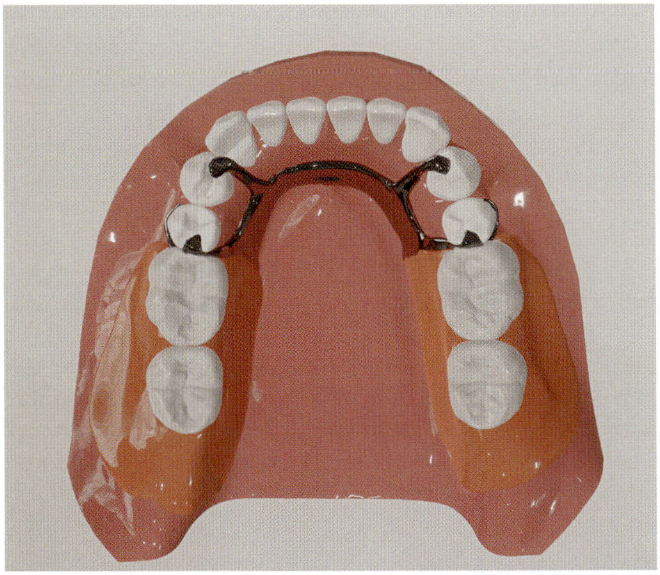

Fig. 8.9 Location of indirect retention of a mandibular Kennedy Class I removable partial denture with combination clasp assembly. The indirect retainers are on the mesial side of the first premolar. Due to anatomical considerations of mandibular incisors, cingulum rest seats may not be sufficient to support the minor connector so bilateral rests on the first premolars may be the better position for the indirect retainer. Note the indirect retainers on the mesial side of the first premolar have sufficient space to avoid food entrapment between framework components. Courtesy of Ahmed Mahrous Copyright © 2024. All rights reserved.

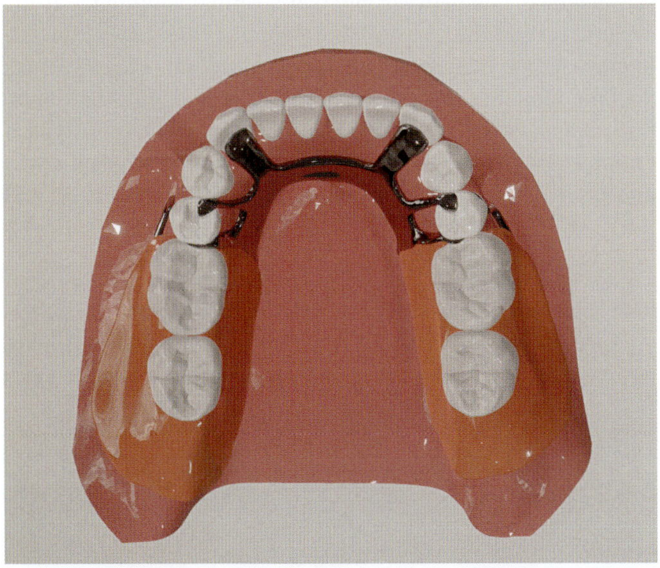

Fig. 8.10 Location of indirect retention of a mandibular Kennedy Class I removable partial denture with an RPI (rest, proximal plate, I-bar) clasp assembly. In this clasp design, the primary rest is located on the mesial of the second premolar. There is insufficient space between the second molar and the mesial of the first premolar which could result in impingement and food entrapment of the framework. Therefore the use of the canine would provide sufficient distance between the mesial primary rest and the indirect retainer. Courtesy of Ahmed Mahrous Copyright © 2024. All rights reserved.

The same principle applies to any maxillary Kennedy Class I removable partial denture when indirect retainers are used. Bilateral rest seats on the marginal ridges of the first premolars are generally preferred to rest seats on incisor teeth (see Fig. 8.8). Not only are they effective without jeopardizing the weaker single-rooted teeth, but the minor connectors cause less interference with the tongue when they can be placed in the embrasure between canine and premolar rather than anterior to the canine teeth.

Indirect retainers for Kennedy Class II removable partial dentures are usually placed on the marginal ridge of the first premolar tooth on the opposite side of the arch from the distal extension base (Fig. 8.11). Bilateral rests are seldom indicated except when an auxiliary occlusal rest is needed for support of the major connector or when the prognosis for the distal abutment is poor and provision is being considered for later conversion to a Kennedy Class I removable partial denture. Depending on the size of the arch and the number and location of missing teeth, a canine rest might be in a more favorable position for an indirect retainer (Fig. 8.12). Canine rest might also be used when the mesial marginal ridge of the first premolar is too close to the fulcrum line, or when the teeth are overlapped so that the fulcrum line is not accessible, a rest on the adjacent canine tooth may be used. Such a rest may be made more effective by placing the minor connector in the embrasure anterior to the canine, either curving back onto a prepared lingual rest seat or extending to a mesioincisal rest. The same types of canine rest as those previously outlined—lingual or incisal rests—may be used (see Chapter 6).

Occasionally, a finger extension from a premolar rest is placed on the prepared lingual slope of the adjacent canine tooth (Fig. 8.13). Such an extension is used to affect indirect retention by increasing the distance of a resisting element from the fulcrum line. This method is particularly applicable when a first premolar must serve as a primary abutment. The distance anterior to the fulcrum line is only the distance between the mesio-occlusal rest

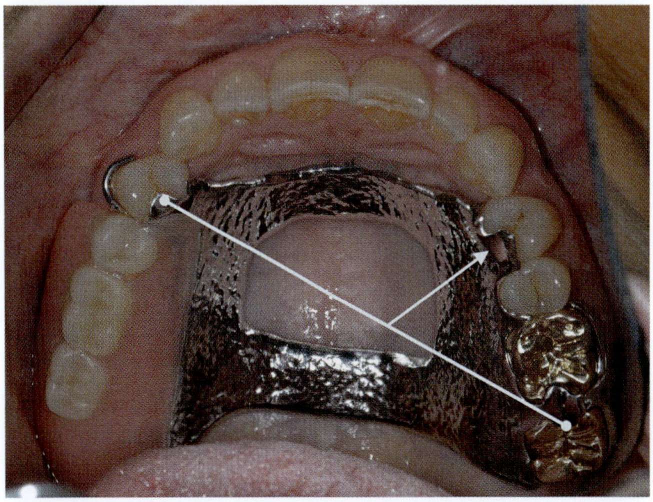

Fig. 8.11 Indirect retention for Kennedy Class II removable partial dentures is usually placed on the marginal ridge of the first premolar tooth on the opposite side of the arch from the distal extension base. If the modification space were not present, as in this unmodified maxillary Kennedy Class II arch, auxiliary occlusal rests and stabilizing components in the same position would still be essential to the design of the removable partial denture. Courtesy of Ahmed Mahrous Copyright © 2024. All rights reserved.

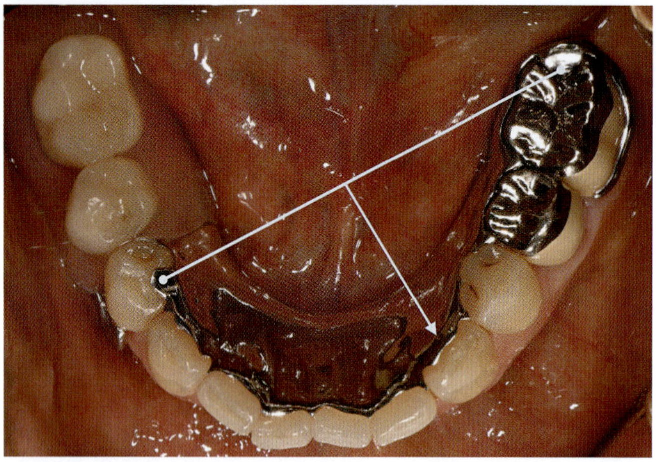

Fig. 8.12 This mandibular Kennedy Class II design shows a favorable location for the indirect retainer on the canine. This location is also at a 90-degree angle to the fulcrum line between primary rests. Courtesy of Ahmed Mahrous

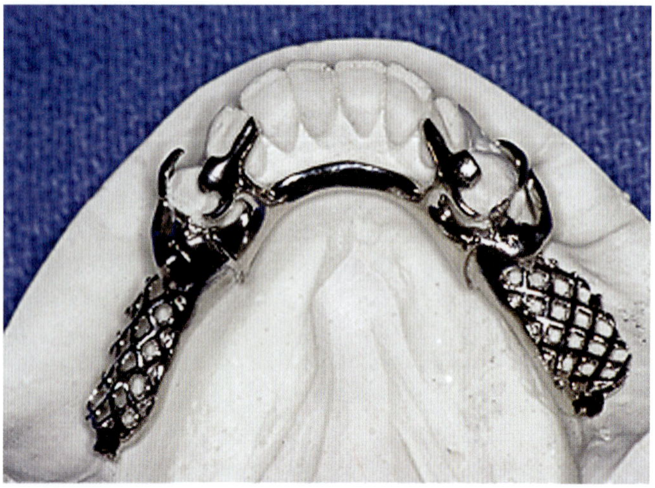

Fig. 8.13 Mandibular Kennedy Class I design using canine extensions from occlusal rests as indirect retainers. The canine extension must be placed on prepared rest seats so that resistance will be directed as nearly as possible along the long axis of the canine abutment.

and the anterior terminal of the finger extension. In this instance, although the extension rests on a prepared surface, it is used in conjunction with a terminal rest on the mesial marginal ridge of the premolar tooth. Even when they are not used as indirect retainers, canine extensions, continuous bar retainers, and lingual plates should never be used without terminal rests because of the resultant forces effective when they are placed on inclined planes alone.

Cingulum Bars (Continuous Bars) and Lingual Plates

Technically, cingulum bars (continuous bars) and lingual plates are not indirect retainers because they rest on unprepared lingual inclines of anterior teeth. The indirect retainers are the terminal rests at either end that occur in the form of auxiliary occlusal rests or canine rests (see Chapter 5).

In Kennedy Class I and Class II removable partial dentures, a cingulum bar or lingual plate may extend the effectiveness of the indirect retainer if it is used with a terminal rest at each end. In tooth-supported removable partial dentures, a cingulum bar or lingual plate is placed for other reasons but always with terminal rests (see Chapter 5).

In Kennedy Class I and Class II removable partial dentures, a continuous bar retainer or the superior border of the lingual plate should never be placed above the middle third of the teeth so that orthodontic movement during the rotation of a distal extension denture is avoided. This guideline is not so important when the six anterior teeth are almost in a straight line, but when the arch is narrow and tapering, a cingulum bar or lingual plate on the anterior teeth extends well beyond the terminal rests, and orthodontic movement of those teeth is more likely. Although these are intended primarily to stabilize weak anterior teeth, they may have the opposite effect if not used with discretion.

Modification Areas

Occasionally, the occlusal rest on an anterior abutment of a modification space in a Kennedy Class II, modification 1, removable partial denture may serve as an indirect retainer (Fig. 8.14). This use will depend on how far from the fulcrum line the secondary abutment is located. The anterior abutment on the tooth-supported side is a secondary abutment, which serves to support and retain one end of the tooth-supported segment and adds horizontal stabilization to the denture. The fulcrum line is a diagonal axis between the two terminal abutments. If the occlusal rest on the anterior abutment lies far enough from the fulcrum line, it may serve adequately as an indirect retainer. Its dual function then is tooth support for one end of the modification area and support for an indirect retainer. The most typical example is a distal occlusal rest on a first premolar when a second premolar and the first molar are missing, and the second

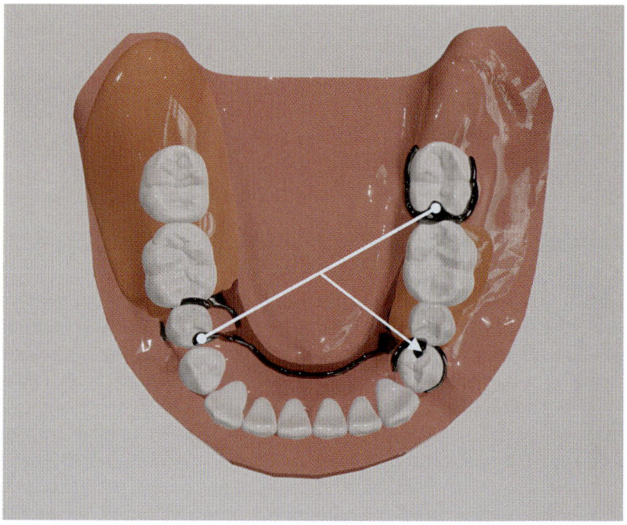

Fig. 8.14 Mandibular Kennedy Class II removable partial denture framework design. The fulcrum line runs from the patient's right second premolar to the right second molar. Forces that tend to unseat the denture from its basal seat will be resisted by supportive elements on the left first premolar as an indirect retainer. Courtesy of Ahmed Mahrous

molar serves as one of the primary abutments (see Fig. 8.14). The longest perpendicular to the fulcrum line falls near the first premolar, making the location of the indirect retainer nearly ideal.

If the modification space were not present, as in an unmodified Kennedy Class II arch, auxiliary occlusal rests and stabilizing components in the same position would still be essential to the design of the denture (Fig. 8.15).

On the other hand, if only one tooth, such as a first molar, is missing on the modification side, the occlusal rest on the second premolar abutment is too close to the fulcrum line to be effective. In such a situation, an auxiliary occlusal rest on the mesial marginal ridge of the first premolar is needed, both for indirect retention and for support for an otherwise unsupported major connector.

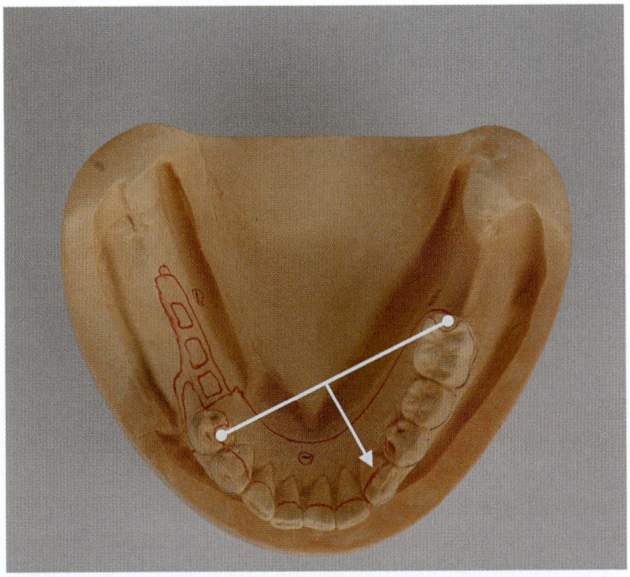

Fig. 8.15 In the surveyed cast of a mandibular Kennedy Class II arch, since there are no modification spaces present, auxiliary occlusal rests and stabilizing components are still needed as an essential component of the design of the removable partial denture. Courtesy of Ahmed Mahrous

Support for a modification area extending anteriorly to a canine abutment is obtained by any one of the accepted canine rest forms, as previously outlined in Chapter 6. In this situation, the canine tooth provides nearly ideal indirect retention and support for the major connector as well.

Rugae Support

Some clinicians consider coverage of the rugae area of the maxillary arch as a means of indirect retention because the rugae area is firm and usually well situated to provide indirect retention for a Kennedy Class I removable partial denture. Although it is true that broad coverage over the rugae area can conceivably provide some support, the facts remain that tissue support is less effective than positive tooth support and that rugae coverage is undesirable if it can be avoided.

The use of rugae support for indirect retention is usually part of a palatal horseshoe design. Because posterior retention is usually inadequate in this situation, the requirements for indirect retention are probably greater than can be satisfied by this type of tissue support alone.

In the mandibular arch, retention from the distal extension base alone is usually inadequate to prevent the base from lifting away from the tissues. In the maxillary arch, where only anterior teeth remain, full palatal coverage is usually necessary. In fact, with any Kennedy Class I maxillary removable partial denture that extends distally from the first premolar teeth, except when a maxillary torus prevents its use, palatal coverage may be used to advantage. Although complete coverage may be seen in the form of a resin base, the added retention and reduced bulk of a cast metal palate make the latter preferable (see Chapter 5). In the absence of full palatal coverage, an indirect retainer should be used with other designs of major palatal connectors for the Kennedy Class I removable partial denture.

9

Denture Base Considerations

Lisa A. Lang, Lily T. García, and Ahmed Mahrous

CHAPTER OUTLINE

The preceding chapters described removable partial denture component parts that engaged the remaining teeth (rests, direct retainers, and indirect retainers) and the cross-arch connector of all component parts, the major connector. This chapter describes the portion of the removable partial denture that contains the replacement teeth—the denture base.

FUNCTIONS OF DENTURE BASES IN CONTROL OF PROSTHESIS MOVEMENT

The denture base supports artificial teeth and consequently receives functional forces and transfers the functional forces to supporting oral structures (Fig. 9.1). This function is most critical for the distal extension prosthesis, as functional stability and comfort often relate directly to the ability to transfer forces without undue movement.

Although the primary purpose of the denture base is related to masticatory function, it may add to the cosmetic effect in prosthetic replacement, particularly when advanced techniques in tissue tinting and reproducing natural-looking contours are used. Most of the techniques for creating a natural appearance in complete denture bases are applicable to denture bases in a removable partial denture, equally well.

The denture base also provides stimulation of the supporting residual ridge tissues. Some vertical movement occurs with any denture base, even those supported entirely by the abutment teeth, because of the physiologic movement of those teeth under function. It is evident that oral tissues placed under functional stress within physiologic tolerance limits maintain form and tone better than similar tissues suffering from disuse. The term *disuse atrophy* is applicable to both periodontal tissues and the tissues of a residual ridge.

Tooth-Supported Partial Denture Base

Denture bases differ in functional purpose and may differ in terms of the material of which they are made. In a tooth-supported prosthesis, the denture base is primarily a span between two abutments supporting the artificial teeth. Thus occlusal forces are transferred directly to the natural tooth abutments along the long axis through rests. The denture base and prosthetic teeth serve to help prevent horizontal migration of remaining abutment teeth in the partially edentulous arch and vertical migration of teeth in the opposing arch.

When only posterior teeth are being replaced, esthetics is usually only a secondary consideration. However, when anterior teeth are replaced, esthetics may be of primary importance. Theoretically, the tooth-supported partial denture base that replaces anterior teeth must perform the following functions: (1) provide desirable esthetics; (2) support and retain the artificial teeth in such a way that they provide masticatory efficiency and assist in transferring occlusal forces directly to abutment teeth through rests; (3) prevent vertical and horizontal migration of remaining natural teeth; (4) eliminate undesirable food traps (oral cleanliness); and (5) stimulate the underlying tissues.

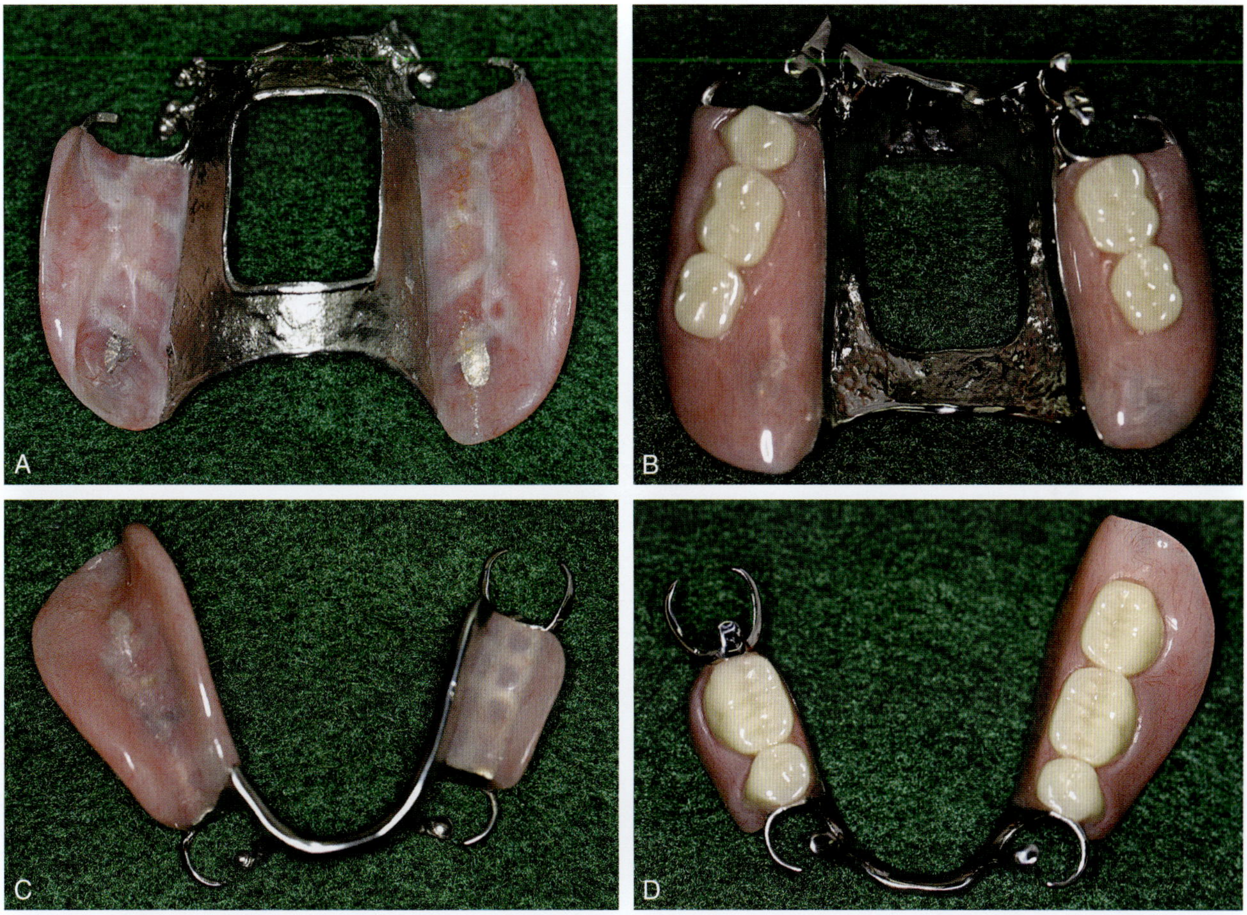

Fig. 9.1 **A,** Kennedy Class I maxillary distal extension removable partial denture showing tissue side (intaglio) of denture bases. **B,** Occlusal side of maxillary prosthesis: posterior artificial teeth are attached to the bases. **C,** Kennedy Class II, modification 1, mandibular distal extension removable partial denture shows intaglio of both extension and modification bases. **D,** Occlusal side of the mandibular prosthesis; posterior artificial teeth are attached to the bases. For both prostheses, the bases are extended within the limits of the physiologic activity of surrounding oral structures.

When an implant is placed posteriorly in a distal extension segment of a Kennedy Class I or Class II removable partial denture, the effect is to create support for the edentulous segment at both ends. In this situation, the requirements of the denture base become more like a tooth-supported base rather than a distal extension denture base.

Distal Extension Partial Denture Base

In a distal extension partial denture, denture bases that are not in tooth-supported modifications must contribute to the support of the denture. Such support is critical to the goal of minimizing functional movement and improving the stability of the prosthesis. Although the abutment teeth provide support for the distal extension base, as the distance from the abutment increases, support from the underlying ridge tissues becomes increasingly important. Maximum support from the residual ridge may be obtained by using a denture base with tissue coverage such that the occlusal load is distributed over the entire area available for such support. The space available for a denture base is determined by the hard and soft tissue and by soft tissue movement during function. Maximum support for the denture base therefore can be accomplished only by using knowledge of the limiting anatomic structures, the histologic nature of the basal seat areas, accuracy of the final impression, and accuracy of the denture base fit (Fig. 9.2). The first two of these support features relate to the gross size and cellular characteristics of the residual ridge tissues. These are highly variable between patients, and consequently, not all residual ridges can provide the same quality of support. Therefore the ability to control the functional displacement of the distal extension base is unique for individual patients.

The snowshoe principle, which suggests that broad coverage furnishes the best support with the least load per unit area, is the principle of choice for providing maximum support. Therefore hard and soft tissue support impacts the selection, design, and fabrication of a distal extension removable partial denture base. Other considerations include esthetics, stimulation of the underlying tissues, and oral hygiene maintenance. Methods used to accomplish maximum support of the restoration through design are presented in Chapters 16 and 17.

In addition to their difference in functional purposes, denture bases can be fabricated using various materials. The difference in the material selection is directly related to function since there may be a need for some denture bases to be relined. In a tooth-supported denture base segment that has an abutment

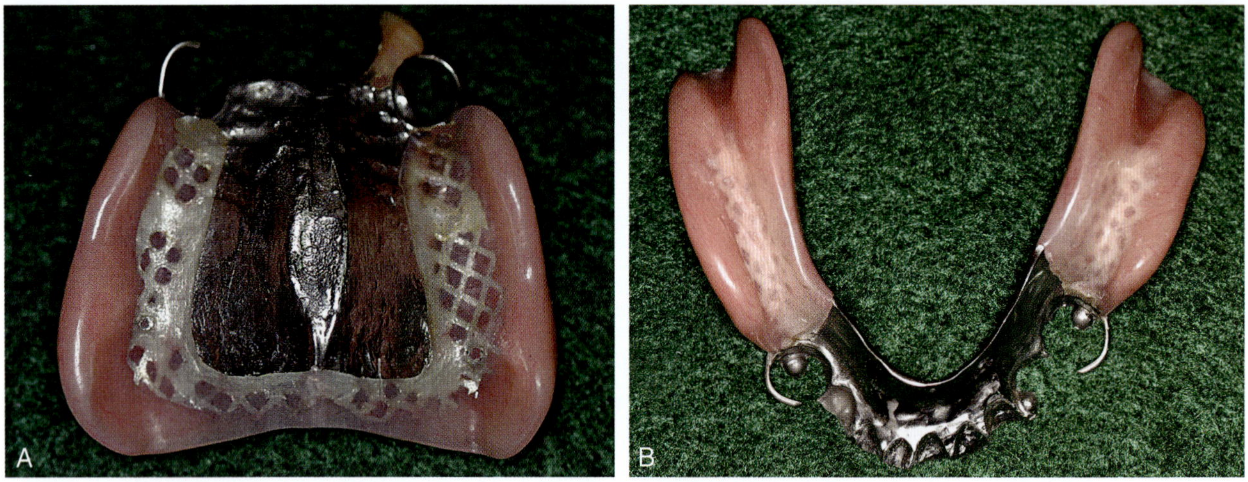

Fig. 9.2 Maxillary and mandibular distal extension removable partial dentures with resin denture bases. Bases are extended buccally within the physiologic tolerance of border structures. **A,** Maxillary denture bases cover both the maxillary tuberosities, extend into the pterygomaxillary notches and provide for adaptation along the posterior border, taking care not to extend beyond the soft palatal flexure. **B,** Mandibular bilateral distal extension removable partial denture bases cover the retromolar pads and extend into the retromylohyoid fossae. The impression procedure used established buccal shelves as primary stress-bearing areas of basal seats.

tooth at each end on which a rest has been placed, future relining or rebasing may not be necessary to reestablish support. Relining is necessary only when tissue changes have occurred beneath the tooth-supported base to the point that poor esthetics or accumulation of debris results. For these reasons alone, tooth-supported bases made soon after extractions should be of a material that permits a reline procedure at a later time. Such materials are the denture resins, the most common of which are copolymer and methyl methacrylate resins.

Primary retention for the removable partial denture is accomplished mechanically by placing retaining elements on the abutment teeth. *Secondary retention* is provided by intimate contact of denture bases and major connectors (in the instance of a maxillary major connector) with the underlying tissues. The latter is similar to the retention of complete dentures and is proportionate to the accuracy of the impression registration, the accuracy of the fit of the denture bases, and the total area of tissue contact involved.

Retention of denture bases has been described as the result of the following forces: (1) adhesion, which is the attraction of saliva to the denture and tissues; (2) cohesion, which is the attraction of the molecules of saliva to each other; (3) atmospheric pressure, which is dependent on a border seal and results in a partial vacuum beneath the denture base when a dislodging force is applied; (4) physiologic molding of the tissues around the polished surfaces of the denture; and (5) the effects of gravity on the mandibular denture.

Boucher,[1] writing on complete denture impressions, described these forces as follows:

Adhesion and cohesion are effective when there is perfect apposition of the impressioned surface of the denture base to the mucous membrane surfaces. These forces lose their effectiveness if any horizontal displacement of the denture breaks the continuity of this contact. Atmospheric pressure is effective primarily as a rescue force when extreme dislodging forces are applied to the denture. It depends on a perfect border seal to keep the pressure applied on only one side of the denture. The presence of air on the impression surface would neutralize the pressure of the air against the polished surface. Because each of these forces is directly proportional to the area covered by the denture, the dentures should be extended to the limits of the supporting structures.

The adaptation of soft tissues around the polished surfaces of denture bases helps to perfect the border seal. Also, it simulates mechanical retention at certain locations on the dentures, provided these surfaces are properly prepared. This retention is developed automatically and without effort by the patient if the impression is made with an understanding of the anatomic possibilities.

Few removable partial dentures are made without some mechanical retention. Retention made possible from the denture base can contribute significantly to the overall retention of the removable partial denture and therefore must not be discounted. Denture bases should be designed and fabricated so that they will contribute as much retention to the removable partial denture as possible. However, it is questionable whether atmospheric pressure plays as important a role in the retention of removable partial dentures because a border seal cannot be obtained as readily as it can be with complete dentures. Therefore adhesion and cohesion gained by excellent apposition of the denture base and soft tissues of the basal seat play an important retentive role.

METHODS OF ATTACHING DENTURE BASES

Acrylic-resin bases are attached to the removable partial denture framework by means of the minor connector design; to accomplish the retention of the denture base, a space is created between the framework and the underlying tissues of the residual ridge (Fig. 9.3). Relief of at least a 20-gauge thickness over the basal seat areas of the master cast is used to create the amount of space needed for the denture base material. The relief created appears as a raised platform on the investment cast on which the pattern for the retentive frame is formed (Fig. 9.4). Thus after casting, the

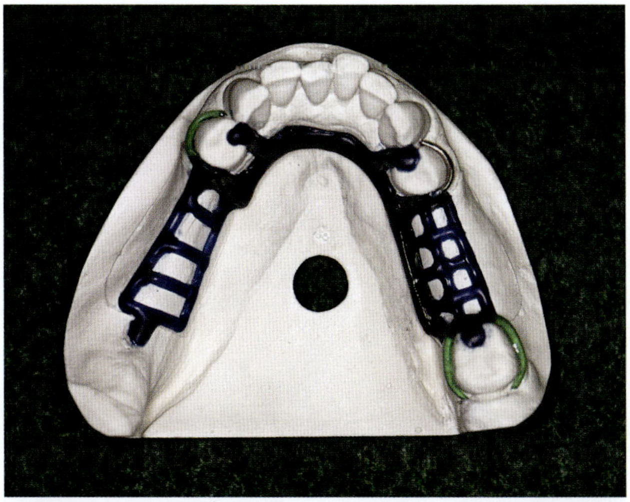

Fig. 9.3 Mandibular Kennedy Class II, modification 1, wax pattern developed on an investment cast. Adequate provision is made for attaching the resin base to the major connector on the edentulous side by way of a ladderlike minor connector and a butt-type joint. A similar minor connector design will be used for modification space. *Note*: Relief space beneath the minor connectors is established by relief wax placed on the original master cast and duplicated in this refractory cast. This allows processed resin to surround the minor connectors in creating the denture base.

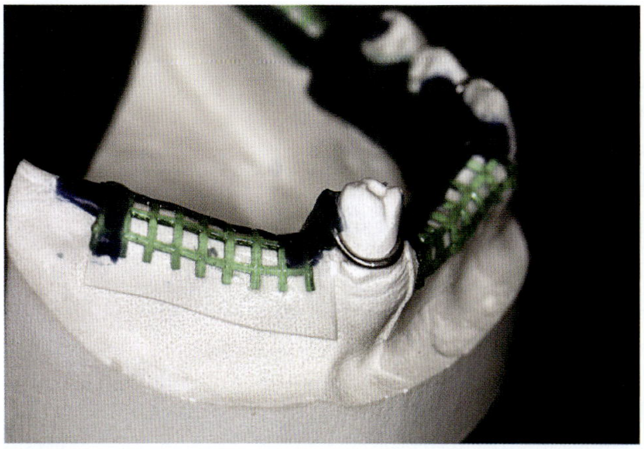

Fig. 9.4 Unlike the minor connector designs in Fig. 9.3, the designs used for this prosthesis have a plastic mesh pattern. Although such designs can be reinforced to be more rigid, the bulk of the connector itself may contribute to weakening of the resin base. A more open type of minor connector seems preferable.

portion of the retentive framework to which the acrylic-resin base will be attached will stand away from the tissue surface sufficiently to permit a flow of acrylic-resin base material beneath its surface.

The minor connector serves as retention for the denture base; the framework should be embedded or surrounded by denture base material with sufficient thickness of resin (1.5 mm) to allow for modification during an adjustment period or during relining procedures. Thickness of denture base material is also necessary to avoid weakness and subsequent fracture of the acrylic-resin base material surrounding the metal framework.

In laboratory fabrication protocol, the use of plastic mesh patterns in forming the retentive framework is generally less satisfactory than a more open framework (Fig. 9.4). Less weakening of the resin by the embedded framework results from the use of the more open form. Pieces of 12- or 14-gauge half-round wax and 18-gauge round wax are used to form a ladderlike framework rather than the finer latticework of the mesh pattern. The precise design of the retentive framework, other than that it should be located both buccally and lingually, is not as important as its effective rigidity and strength when it is embedded in the acrylic-resin base. It should also be free of interference with future adjustment, should not interfere with the arrangement of artificial teeth, and should be open enough to avoid weakening any portion of the attached acrylic resin. Designing the retentive framework for denture bases by having elements located buccal and lingual to the residual ridge not only will strengthen the acrylic-resin base but also will minimize distortion of the base created by the release of inherent strains in the acrylic-resin base during the use or storage of the restoration (Fig. 9.5).

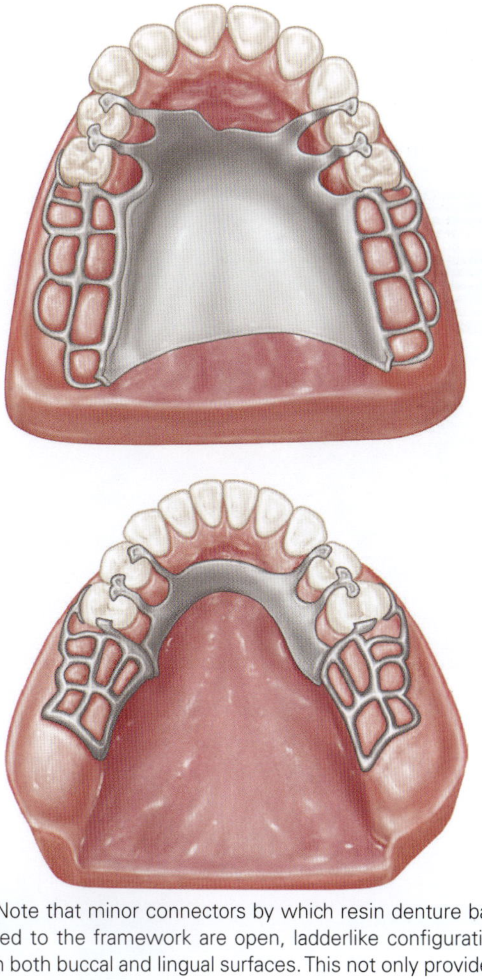

Fig. 9.5 Note that minor connectors by which resin denture bases will be attached to the framework are open, ladderlike configurations that extend on both buccal and lingual surfaces. This not only provides excellent attachment of the resin bases but minimizes the warping of bases resulting from the release of inherent strains in compression-molded resin.

Metal bases are usually cast as integral parts of the removable partial denture framework. Mandibular metal bases may be assembled and attached to the framework with acrylic resin (Fig. 9.6).

METHODS FOR INCORPORATING DENTAL IMPLANTS

When dental implants are placed, modifications can be required in the denture base, and the specific modification is dependent on how the implants will be engaged.

Implants placed anteriorly, to enhance retention by removing the need for a visible clasp, must take into account the need for adequate interocclusal clearance to have enough space to accommodate connectors within the confines of the removable partial denture, for example to have the direct connection to the metallic frame or via embedding within the acrylic-resin denture base.

Placement of the implant should take into consideration the need to minimize palatal/lingual bulk of the material, provision of adequate space for an attachment housing, acrylic resin and denture tooth, and alignment coincident with the insertion path of the prosthesis.

Modifications required for implants placed more distal, for purposes of support, typically require designing space for embedding an attachment housing within the denture base (Fig. 9.7).

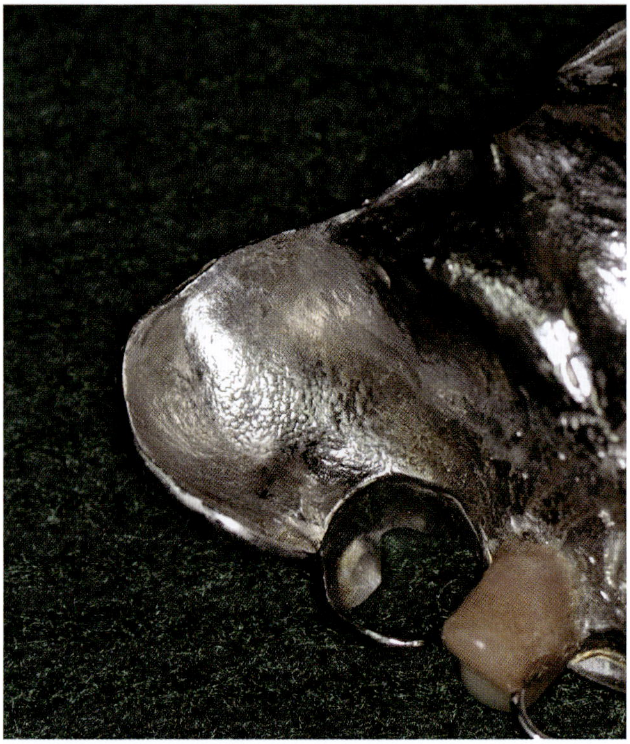

Fig. 9.6 Cast distal extension base of a maxillary removable partial denture. Cast bases are an integral part of the framework and not only provide support to the prosthetic dentition but also reinforce framework rigidity.

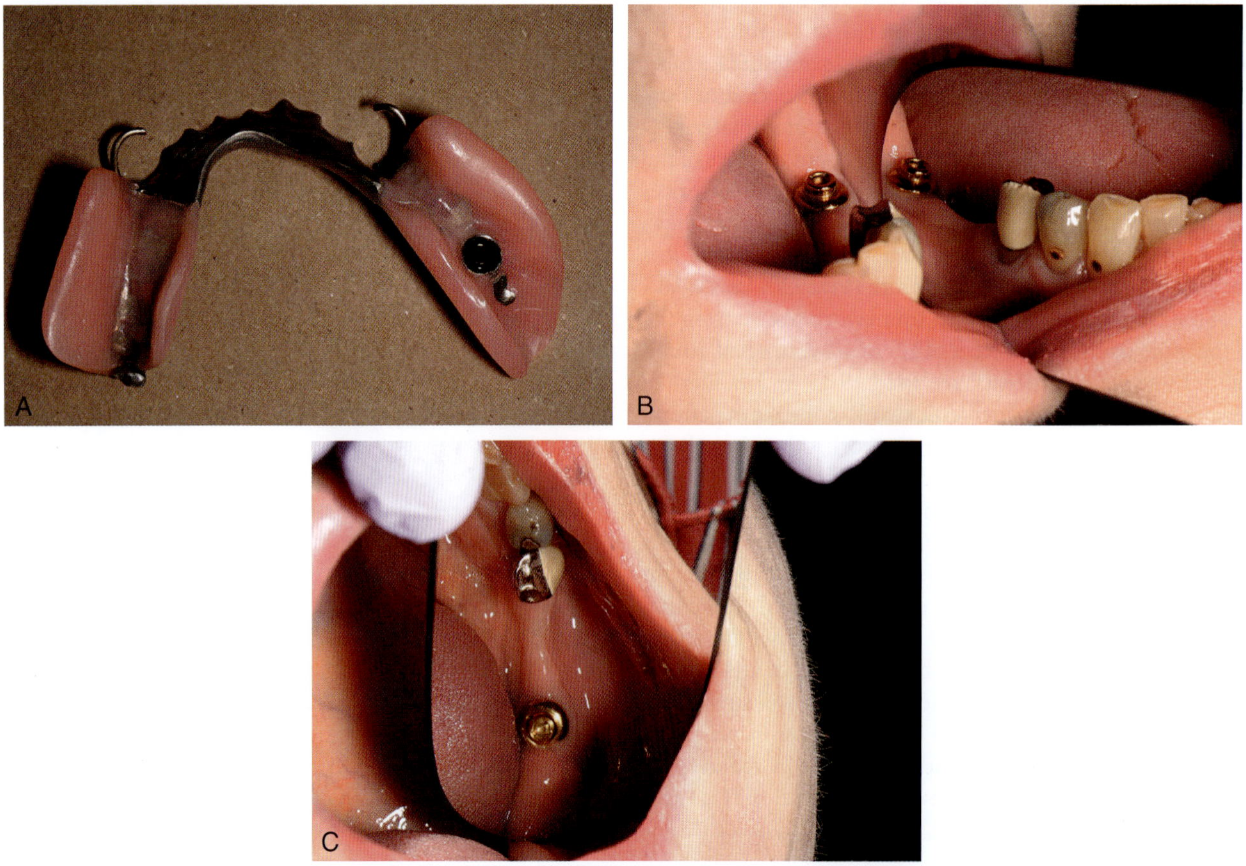

Fig. 9.7 **A,** Intaglio surface view of a locator retentive element in the posterior aspect of a distal extension base of a mandibular removable partial denture. **B,** Mirror view of the locator attachment on an implant in the distal mandible. The attachment will provide support and retention for the distal extension removable partial denture. **C,** Occlusal view of the locator attachment.

IDEAL DENTURE BASE MATERIAL

The requirements for an ideal denture base are as follows:

1. Accuracy of adaptation to the tissues, with minimal volume change
2. Dense, nonirritating surface capable of receiving and maintaining a good finish
3. Thermal conductivity
4. Low specific gravity; lightweight in the mouth
5. Sufficient strength; resistance to fracture or distortion
6. Easily kept clean
7. Esthetic acceptability
8. Potential for future relining
9. Low initial cost

Current denture base materials, whether resin or metal and regardless of the method of fabrication, come as close to this ideal as possible.

ADVANTAGES OF METAL BASES

Except for those edentulous ridges with recent extractions, metal can be used for tooth-supported bases and is thought to provide several advantages. A commonly stated advantage is that the stimulation it gives to the underlying tissues is so beneficial that it prevents some alveolar atrophy that would otherwise occur under a resin base and thereby prolongs the health of the tissues that it contacts. Some of the advantages of a metal base are discussed in the following sections. The principal disadvantage of a metal base is that metal is difficult to adjust and reline.

Accuracy and Permanence of Form

Metal bases, whether of gold, cobalt-chrome, or titanium alloy, can be cast more accurately than denture resins and can maintain accuracy of form without changes in the mouth. Internal strains that may be released later, as occurs with heat-processed acrylic bases, and cause distortion are not present. Although some resins and some processing techniques are superior to others in accuracy and permanence of form, modern cast alloys are generally superior in this respect. Evidence of this fact is that an additional posterior palatal seal may be eliminated entirely when a cast palate is used for a complete denture, as compared with the need for a definite posterior palatal seal when the palate is made of acrylic resin. Distortion of acrylic-resin base material such as in a maxillary complete denture occurs in a direction of distortion away from the palate in the midline and toward the tuberosities on the buccal flanges. The greater the palatal tissue curvature, the greater is this distortion. Similar distortions occur in a mandibular denture but are more difficult to detect. Accurate metal castings are not subject to distortion by the release of internal strains, as are most denture resins.

A metal base provides an intimacy of contact that contributes to the denture base retention. The fit is called *interfacial surface tension*, direct retention from a cast denture base is significant in proportion to the area involved. This has been mentioned previously as an important factor in both direct and direct-indirect retention of maxillary restorations. The fit of a metal base cannot be duplicated with traditional laboratory processing used in resin denture bases.

The permanence of form of the cast base is also ensured because of its resistance to abrasion from denture cleaning agents. The cleanliness of the denture base should be stressed; however, constant brushing of the tissue side of the acrylic-resin denture base inevitably causes some loss of accuracy by abrasion. The fit of the denture base to the tissue can be impacted by overzealous cleaning habits. A metal denture base can withstand repeated mechanical debridement in cleaning without significant changes in surface accuracy.

Comparative Tissue Response

Clinical observations have demonstrated that the inherent cleanliness of the cast metal base contributes to the health of oral tissues when compared with an acrylic-resin base. Perhaps, some of the reasons for this are the greater density and the bacteriostatic activity contributed by ionization and oxidation of the metal base. Acrylic-resin bases tend to accumulate mucinous deposits containing food particles, as well as calcareous deposits. Unfavorable tissue reaction to decomposing food particles and bacterial enzymes and mechanical irritation from calculus may result if the denture is not kept meticulously clean. Although calculus, which must be removed periodically, can precipitate on a cast metal base, other deposits do not accumulate as they do on an acrylic-resin base. For this reason, a metal base is naturally cleaner than an acrylic-resin base.

Thermal Conductivity

Temperature changes are transmitted through the metal base to the underlying tissues, thereby helping to maintain the health of those tissues. Freedom of interchange of temperature between the tissues covered and the surrounding external influences (temperature of liquids, solid foods, and inspired air) contributes much to the patient's acceptance of a denture and may help avoid the feeling of the presence of a foreign body. Conversely, denture acrylic resins have insulating properties that prevent interchange of temperature between the inside and the outside of the denture base.

Weight and Bulk

Metal alloy may be cast much thinner than acrylic resin and still have adequate strength and rigidity. Cast gold must be given slightly more bulk to provide the same amount of rigidity but still may be made with less thickness than acrylic-resin materials. Even less weight and bulk are possible when the denture bases are made of chrome or titanium alloys.

At times, however, both weight and thickness may be used to advantage in denture bases. In the mandibular arch, the weight of the denture may be an asset regarding retention, and for this reason, a cast gold base may be preferred. On the other hand, extreme loss of residual alveolar bone may make it necessary to add fullness to the denture base to restore normal facial contours and to fill out the buccal vestibule to prevent food from being trapped in the vestibule beneath the denture. In such situations, an acrylic-resin base may be preferred to the thinner metal base.

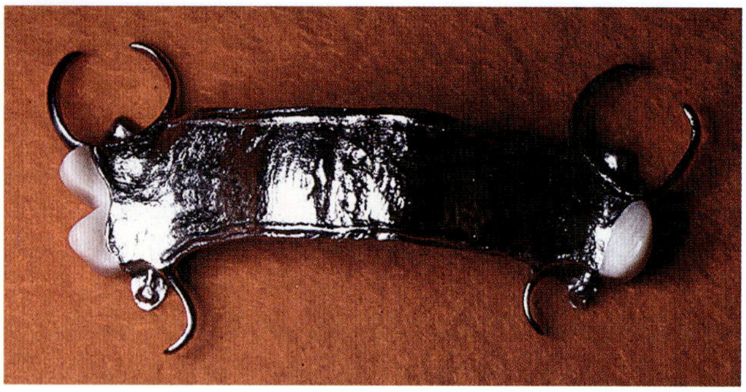

Fig. 9.8 Removable partial denture metal bases are used with a palatal strap and resin denture teeth attached directly to the cast metal bases. If needed, a buccal flange of resin could be added to such a base region; however, for these small spans, no such flange was needed.

In the maxillary arch, an acrylic-resin base may be preferred to the thinner metal base to provide fullness in the buccal flanges or to fill a maxillary buccal vestibule. Acrylic resin may also be preferred over the thinner metal base for esthetic reasons. In these instances, the thinness of the metal base may be of no advantage, but in areas where the tongue and cheek need maximum room, thinness may be desirable.

Denture base contours for functional tongue and cheek contact can best be accomplished with acrylic resin. Metal bases are usually made thin to minimize bulk and weight, whereas acrylic-resin bases may be contoured to provide ideal polished surfaces that contribute to the retention of the denture, to restore facial contours, and to avoid the accumulation of food at denture borders. Lingual surfaces usually are made concave except in the distal palatal area. Buccal surfaces are made convex at gingival margins, over root prominences, and at the border to fill the area recorded in the impression. Between the border and the gingival contours, the base can be made convex to aid in the retention and to facilitate the return of the food bolus to the occlusal table during mastication. Such contours prevent food from being entrapped in the cheek and from working under the denture. This usually cannot be accomplished with metal bases.

However, the advantages of a metal base need not be sacrificed for the sake of esthetics or desirable denture contours when the use of such a base is indicated. Denture bases may be designed to provide almost total metallic coverage, yet they have resin borders to avoid a display of metal and to add buccal fullness when needed (Fig. 9.8). The advantages of thermal conductivity are not necessarily lost by covering a portion of the metal base as long as other parts of the denture are exposed to affect temperature changes through conduction.

METHODS OF ATTACHING ARTIFICIAL TEETH

Selection of artificial teeth for form, color, and material must precede attachment to the denture. Artificial teeth may be attached to the denture bases by several means that follow: with acrylic resin, with cement, processed directly to metal, cast with the framework, and by chemical bonding. The use of acrylic resin to attach artificial teeth to a denture base is the most common method.

Porcelain or Acrylic-Resin Artificial Teeth Attached with Acrylic Resin

Artificial porcelain teeth are mechanically retained. The posterior teeth are retained by acrylic resin utilizing diatoric holes. The anterior porcelain teeth are retained by acrylic resin surrounding their lingually placed retention pins. Artificial resin teeth are retained by a chemical union with the acrylic resin of the denture base that occurs during laboratory processing procedures.

Attachment of the acrylic resin to the metal base may be accomplished by nailhead retention, retention loops, or diagonal spurs placed at random. Attachment mechanisms should be placed so that they will not interfere with the placement of the teeth on the metal base.

Any junction of the acrylic resin with metal should occur at an undercut finishing line or should be associated with some retentive undercut. Because only a mechanical attachment exists between metal and acrylic resin, every attempt should be made to avoid separation and seepage, which result in discoloration and uncleanliness. Denture odors are frequently caused by accretions at the junction of the acrylic resin with metal when only a mechanical union exists. Separation that occurs between the acrylic resin and the metal can eventually lead to loosening of the acrylic-resin base.

Porcelain or Resin Tube Teeth and Facings Cemented Directly to Metal Bases

Some disadvantages of this type of attachment are the difficulties involved in obtaining satisfactory occlusion, the lack of adequate contours for functional tongue and cheek contact, and the unesthetic display of metal at gingival margins. The latter is avoided when the tooth is butted directly to the residual ridge, but then the retention for the tooth frequently becomes inadequate.

A modification of this method is the attachment of ready-made acrylic-resin teeth to the metal base with acrylic resin of the same shade (Fig. 9.9). This is called *pressing on a resin tooth* and is not the same as using acrylic resin for cementation. It is particularly applicable to anterior tooth replacement because it is desirable to know in advance of making the casting that the shade and contours of the selected tooth will be acceptable. After a labial index of the position of the teeth is made, the lingual portion of the tooth may be cut away or a posthole prepared in the tooth for the retention on the casting. Subsequently, the tooth is attached to the denture with acrylic resin of the same shade. Because this is done under pressure, the acrylic-resin attachment is comparable with the manufactured tooth in hardness and strength.

Tube or side-groove teeth must be selected in advance of waxing the denture framework (Fig. 9.10). However, for best occlusal relationships, jaw relation records always should be made with the denture casting in the mouth. This problem may be solved by selecting tube teeth for width but with occlusal surfaces slightly higher than will be necessary. The teeth are ground to fit the ridge with sufficient clearance beneath, for a thin metal base and beveled to accommodate a boxing of metal.

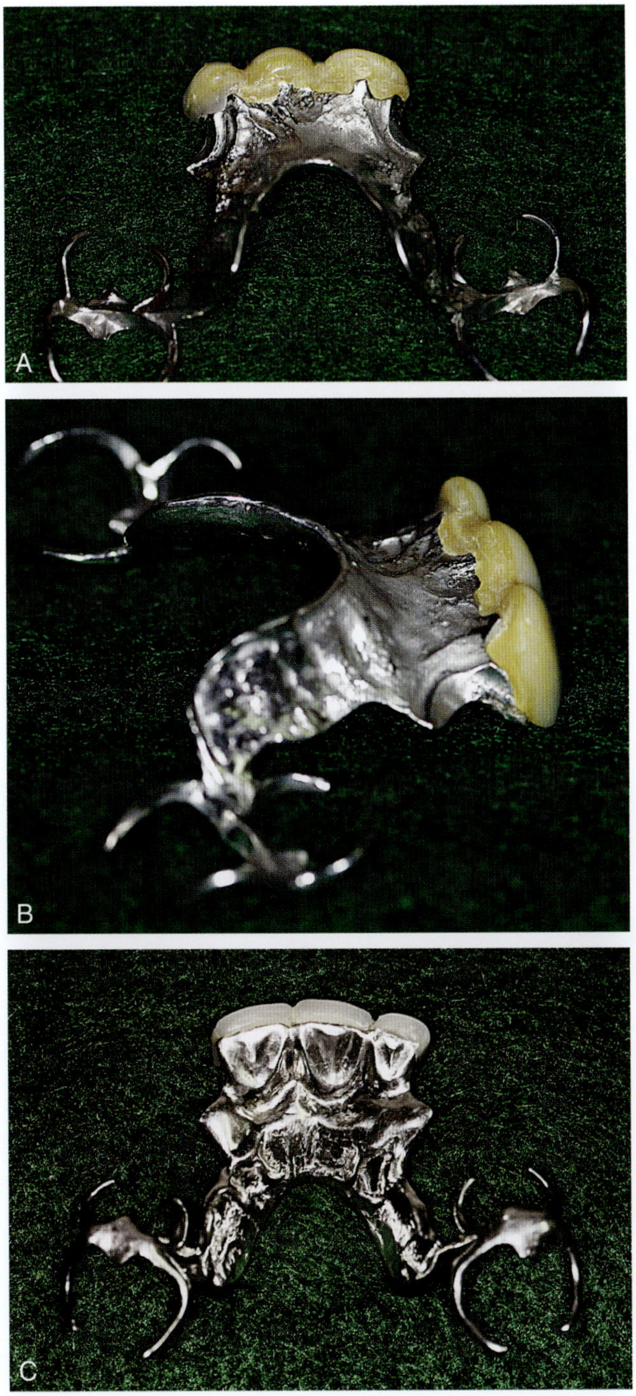

Fig. 9.9 Tissue surface of Kennedy Class IV removable partial denture in which artificial dentition was added to a metal base. **A,** Teeth were set before the completion of the framework to allow the modification space design to incorporate altered teeth. **B,** Anterior teeth were adjusted to the ridge, creating a ridge lap; then the framework was waxed to accommodate a custom tooth position. **C,** Metal reinforcement adds strength to the artificial teeth and protects against dislodgment.

If an acrylic-resin tube tooth is used, the diatoric hole should be made slightly larger than that provided. The casting is completed and tried in, occlusal relationships are recorded, and then the teeth are ground to harmonious occlusion with the opposing dentition. As is discussed in Chapter 18, artificial posterior teeth on partial dentures can hardly ever be used unaltered but rather should be considered material from which occlusal forms may be created to function harmoniously with the remaining natural occlusion.

Resin Teeth Processed Directly to Metal Bases

Modern cross-linked copolymers enable the dentist or technician to process acrylic-resin teeth that have satisfactory hardness and abrasion resistance for many situations. Thus occlusion may be created without resorting to the modification of ready-made artificial teeth (Fig. 9.11). Recesses in the denture pattern may be carved by hand or may be created around manufactured teeth that are used only to form the recess in the pattern. Occlusal relationships may be established in the mouth on the denture framework and transferred to an articulator. The teeth can then be carved and processed in acrylic resin of the proper shade to fit the opposing occlusal record. Better attachment to the metal base than by cementation is thus possible. In addition, unusually long, short, wide, or narrow teeth may be created when necessary to fill spaces not easily filled by the limited selection of commercially available teeth.

Occlusion on the acrylic-resin teeth may be reestablished to compensate for wear or settling by reprocessing new acrylic resin or using light-activated acrylic resin when this becomes necessary. A distinction always should be made between the need for relining to reestablish occlusion on a distal extension removable partial denture and the need for rebuilding occlusal surfaces on an otherwise satisfactory denture base such as on a tooth-supported or a tooth- and tissue-supported removable partial denture.

Reestablishment of occlusion may also be accomplished by placing cast gold or other suitable cast alloy restorations on existing resin teeth. Although this may be done on porcelain teeth as well, it is difficult to cut preparations in porcelain teeth unless air abrasive methods are used. Therefore if later additions to occlusal surfaces are anticipated, acrylic-resin teeth should be used, thereby facilitating the addition of new resin or cast gold surfaces. A simple technique that can be used to fabricate cast gold occlusal surfaces and attach them to resin teeth is described in Chapter 19.

Metal Teeth

Occasionally, a second molar tooth may be replaced as part of the removable partial denture casting (Fig. 9.12). This is usually done when space is too limited for the attachment of an artificial tooth and yet the addition of a second molar is desirable to prevent extrusion of an opposing second molar. Because the occlusal surface must be waxed before casting, perfect occlusion is not possible. Because metal, particularly a chrome alloy, is abrasion resistant, the area of occlusal contact should be held to a minimum to avoid damage to the periodontium of the opposing tooth and associated discomfort to the patient. Occlusal adjustment on gold occlusal surfaces is readily accomplished, whereas metal teeth made of chrome alloys are difficult to adjust and are objectionably hard for use as occlusal surfaces. Therefore they

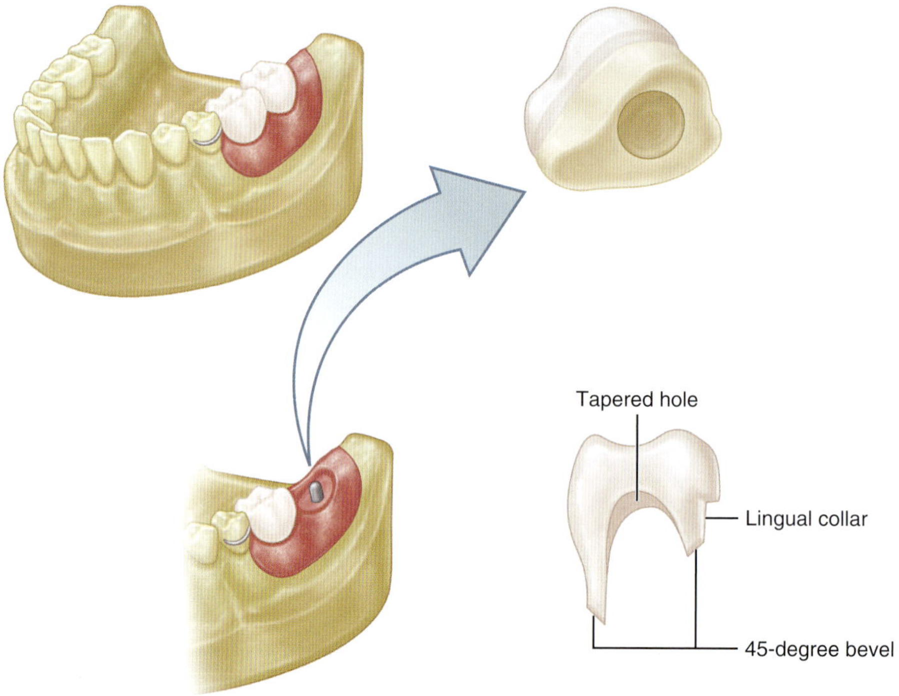

Fig. 9.10 Stock porcelain or resin tube tooth, or artificial tooth used as tube tooth, should be ground to accommodate cast coping as illustrated. A hole is drilled from the underside of the tooth, or, if a hole is already present, it is made larger. Then the tooth is ground to fit the ridge with enough clearance for minimum thickness of metal. A 45-degree bevel then is formed around the base of the tooth; finally, a collar is created on the lingual side, extending to the interproximal area. The tooth is then lubricated, and a wax pattern for the denture base is formed around it.

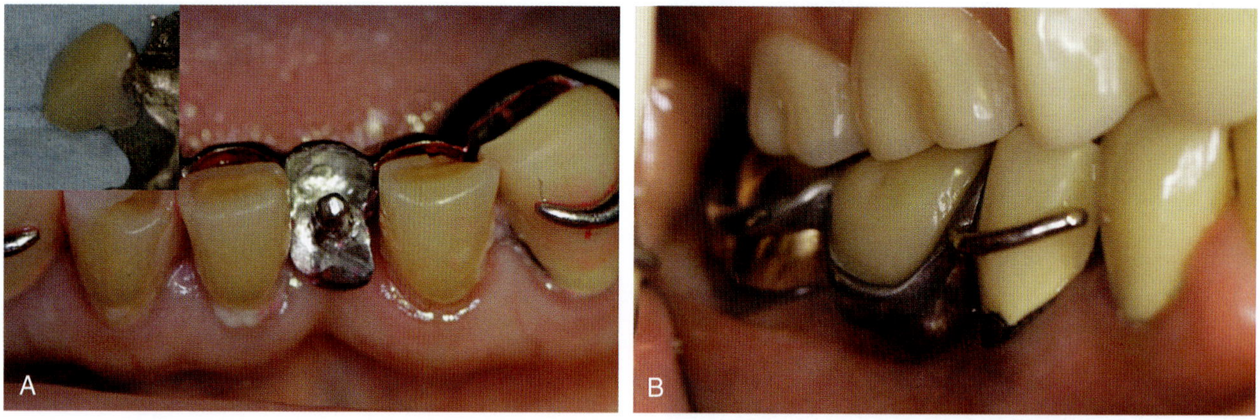

Fig. 9.11 Direct attachment of resin teeth to metal bases. **A,** Anterior modification space is prepared to receive a denture tooth, which will be reinforced with a post. **B,** Posterior molar attached to a previously waxed base to specifically receive the replacement tooth.

should be used only to fill a space and to prevent opposing natural tooth extrusion creating direct occlusal contact.

Chemical Bonding

Recent developments in resin bonding have provided a means of direct chemical bonding of acrylic resin to metal frameworks. The investing alveolar and gingival tissue replacement components can be attached without the use of loops, mesh, or surface mechanical locks. Sections of a metal framework that are used to support replacement teeth can be roughened with abrasives and then treated with a vaporized silica coating. On this surface, an acrylic-resin bonding agent is applied, followed by a thin film of acrylic resin that acts as a substrate for later attachment of replacement acrylic-resin teeth or for processing of acrylic-resin tissue replacements (Fig. 9.13).

A second method of fusing a microscopic layer of ceramic to the metal is accomplished by a process referred to as *tribochemical coating*. This system involves sandblasting the metal framework with a special silica particle material, Rocatec-Plus (3 M Espe Dental Products, Irvine, CA). Silica from these particles is attached to the framework by impact. A silane is added to this ceramic-like film to form a chemical bond between the silicate

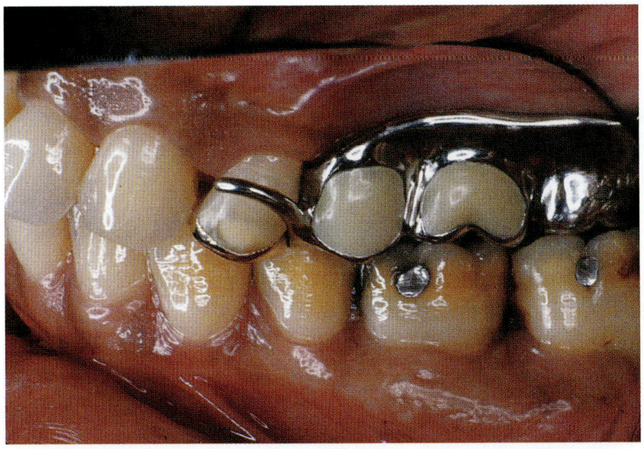

Fig. 9.12 Maxillary cast molar is designed as an integral part of the framework. Interocclusal space limitation necessitated the use of metal rather than another form of artificial posterior teeth. Note overlays on premolar and molar teeth were used to resist tooth wear. (Courtesy of Dr. C.J. Andres, Indianapolis, IN.)

layer and the denture base acrylic resin. Denture base acrylic resins formulated with 4-meta are also available and provide a mechanism for bonding acrylic resin to metal.

NEED FOR RELINING

The distal extension base differs from the tooth-supported base in several respects, one of which is that it must be made of a material that can be relined or rebased when it becomes necessary to reestablish tissue support for the distal extension base. Therefore acrylic-resin denture base materials that can be relined are generally used.

Although satisfactory techniques for making distal extension removable partial denture bases of cast metal are available, the fact that metal bases are difficult if not impossible to reline limits their use to stable ridges that will change little over a long period.

Loss of support for distal extension bases results from changes in residual ridge form over time. These changes may not be readily visible; however, manifestations of this change can be assessed. One of these is loss of occlusion between the distal extension denture base and the opposing dentition, which increases as the distance from the abutment increases (Fig. 9.14). This change is proved by having the patient close on strips of 28-gauge green casting wax, or any similar wax, and tapping in centric relation only. Indentations in a wax strip of known thickness are quantitative, whereas marks made with articulating ribbon are only qualitative. In other words, indentations in the wax may be interpreted as light, medium, or heavy, whereas it is difficult if not impossible to interpret a mark made with articulating ribbon as light or heavy. In fact, the heaviest occlusal contact may perforate paper-articulating ribbon and make a lesser mark than areas of lighter contact. Therefore the use of any articulating ribbon is of limited value in checking occlusion intraorally. In making occlusal adjustments, articulating ribbon should be used only to indicate where relief should be provided after the need for relief has been established by using wax strips

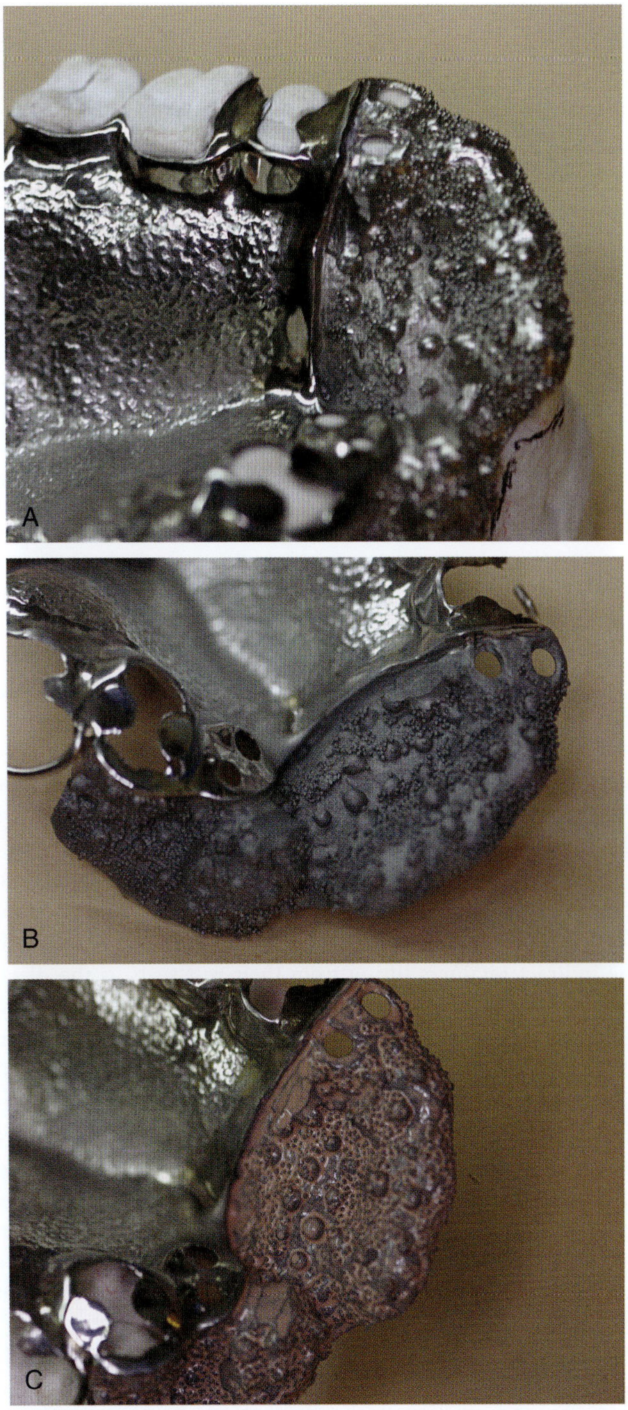

Fig. 9.13 Coating of metal framework with silica facilitates improved application and seal of resin or composite for denture base regions. Example **(A)** shows a maxillary minor with beads for added retention of the anterior denture base, **(B)** after air abrasion preparation of the surface, and **(C)** after silicoating.

of known thickness. For this purpose, 28-gauge green or blue casting wax is generally used, although the thinner 30-gauge or the thicker 26-gauge wax may be used for better evaluation of the clearance between areas not in contact.

Loss of support for a distal extension base results in loss of occlusal contact between the prosthetically supplied teeth and the opposing dentition and a return to heavy occlusal contact

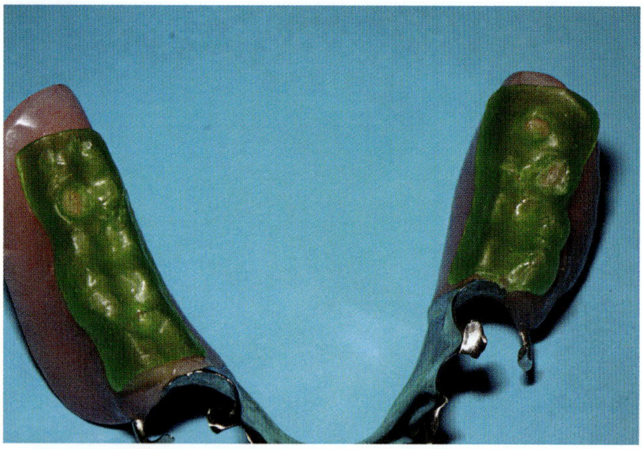

Fig. 9.14 28-Gauge soft green wax used to identify occlusal contacts between a mandibular Kennedy Class I distal extension base and an opposing complete denture.

between the remaining natural teeth. Usually, this is an indication that relining is needed to reestablish the original occlusion by reestablishing supporting contact with the residual ridge. It must be remembered, however, that occlusion on a distal extension base is sometimes maintained at the expense of extrusion of the opposing natural teeth. In such a situation, checking the occlusion alone will not show that settling of the extension base has occurred because changes in the supporting ridge may have also taken place.

A second manifestation of change also must be observable to justify relining. This second manifestation of change in the supporting ridge is evidence of rotation about the fulcrum line with the indirect retainers lifting from their rest seats as the distal extension base is pressed against the ridge tissues. Originally, if the distal extension base was made to fit the supporting form of the residual ridge, rotation about the fulcrum line is not visible. At the time the denture is initially placed, no anteroposterior rotational movement should occur when alternating finger pressure is applied to the indirect retainer and the distal end of a distal extension base or bases. After changes in the ridge form have occurred, which cause some loss of support, rotation occurs about the fulcrum line when alternating finger pressure is applied. This indicates changes in the supporting ridge that must be compensated for by relining or rebasing.

If occlusal contact has been lost and rotation about the fulcrum line is evident, relining is indicated. Conversely, if occlusal contact has been lost without any evidence of denture rotation, and if the stability of the denture base is otherwise satisfactory, reestablishing the occlusion may be needed rather than relining. For the latter, the original denture base may be used in much the same manner as the original trial base was used to record the occlusal relation. Teeth may then be reoriented to an opposing cast or to an occlusal template with the use of light-activated tooth-colored acrylic resin, tooth-colored composite, cast occlusal surfaces, or new teeth. In any event, a new occlusion should be established on the existing bases. Relining in this instance would be the wrong solution to the problem.

Loss of support may also be assessed clinically by other methods. A layer of light-bodied impression material or tissue-conditioning material can be spread on the basal seat portion of the dried denture base(s), and the restoration is returned to the patient's mouth. Care is exercised to ensure that the framework is correctly seated (rests and indirect retainers in planned positions). The restoration is removed when the material has been set. Significant thicknesses of material remaining under the bases indicate a lack of intimate contact of the bases with the residual ridges, suggesting a need for relining.

More often, however, loss of occlusion is accompanied by settling of the denture base to the extent that rotation about the fulcrum line is manifest. Because relining is the only remedy short of making completely new bases, the use of an acrylic-resin base originally facilitates later relining. For this reason, acrylic-resin bases are generally preferred for distal extension partial dentures.

The question remains as to when, if ever, metal bases with their several advantages may be used for distal extension removable partial dentures. It is debatable as to what type of ridge will most likely remain stable under functional loading without apparent change. Certainly, the age and general health of the patient will influence the ability of a residual ridge to support function. Minimum and harmonious occlusion and the accuracy with which the base fits the underlying tissues will influence the amount of trauma that will occur under function. The absence of trauma plays a big part in the ability of the ridge to maintain its original form.

The best indication for the use of metal distal extension bases is a ridge that has supported a previous partial denture without having become narrowed or flat or without consisting primarily of easily displaceable tissues. When such changes have occurred under a previous denture, further change may be anticipated because of the possibility that the oral tissues in question are not capable of supporting a denture base without further change. Despite every advantage in their favor, some individuals have ridges that respond unfavorably when called on to support any denture base.

In other instances, such as when a new removable partial denture is to be made because of the loss of additional teeth, the ridges may still be firm and healthy. Because the ridges have previously supported a denture base and have sustained occlusion, bony trabeculae will have become arranged to best support vertical and horizontal loading, cortical bone may have been formed, and tissues will have become favorable for continued support of a denture base.

If it is anticipated that there will not be a need to reline a denture base, a metal denture base can be considered. However, if the decision for a future reline is uncertain, metal bases may be used with full understanding on the part of the patient that a new denture may become necessary if unforeseen tissue changes occur. The technique shown in Fig. 9.6 permits the replacement of metal distal extension bases without the need to remake the entire denture. This method should be seriously considered any time a distal extension removable partial denture is to be made with a metal base or bases.

For reasons previously outlined, the possibility that tissues will remain healthier beneath a metal base than they will beneath an acrylic-resin base may justify wider use of metal

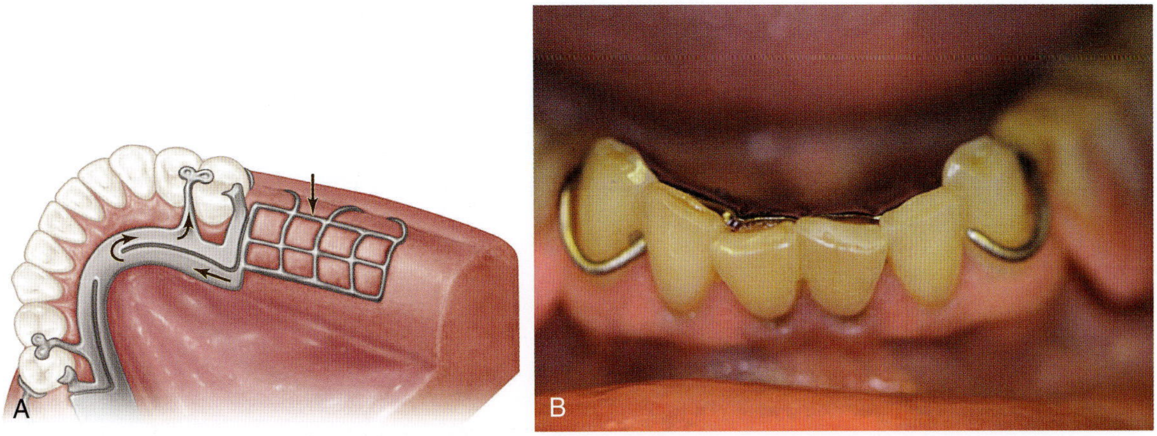

Fig. 9.15 With occlusal loading of posterior distal extensions **(A)**, the superior edge of the mandibular lingual plate major connector is displaced from the planned contact **(B)**. If appropriate contact of the major connector and teeth does not return after the release of the distal load, this suggests ridge support is poor and occlusal function is suboptimum. The denture base should be considered for a reline to reestablish occlusion contact, ensuring functional use.

bases for distal extension removable partial dentures. Through careful treatment planning, better patient education on the problems involved in making a distal extension base removable partial denture, and greater care taken in the fabrication of denture bases, metal may be used to advantage in some situations in which acrylic-resin bases are ordinarily used.

STRESS BREAKERS (STRESS EQUALIZERS)

The previous chapters describing component parts of a removable partial denture have presumed absolute rigidity of all parts of the removable partial denture framework except the retentive arm of the direct retainer. All vertical and horizontal forces applied to the artificial teeth are thus distributed throughout the supporting portions of the dental arch. A broad distribution of stress is accomplished through the rigidity of the major and minor connectors. The effects of the stabilizing components are also made possible by the rigidity of the connectors.

In distal extension situations, the use of a rigid connection between the denture base and supporting teeth must account for base movement without causing tooth or tissue damage. In such situations, stress on the abutment teeth and residual ridge is minimized through the use of functional basing, broad coverage, harmonious occlusion, and correct choice of direct retainers. Generally, two major types of clasp assemblies are used for distal extensions because of their stress-breaking design. Retentive clasp arms may be cast only if they engage undercuts on the abutment teeth in such a manner that tissue-ward movement of the extension base transmits only minimum leverage to the abutment. Otherwise, tapered wrought-wire retentive clasp arms should be used because of their greater flexibility. The tapered, round wrought-wire clasp arm acts somewhat as a stress breaker between the denture base and the abutment tooth by reducing the effects of denture base movement on the tooth through its flexibility.

Another concept of stress breaking insists on separating the actions of the retaining elements from the movement of the denture base by allowing independent movement of the denture base (or its supporting framework) and the direct retainers. This form of stress breaker, also referred to as a *stress equalizer*, has been used as a means of compensating for inappropriately designed removable partial dentures. Fig. 9.15 shows an example of a split bar major connector, which is a commonly used stress breaker.

Regardless of their design, most stress breakers effectively dissipate vertical stresses, which is the purpose for which they are used. However, this occurs at the expense of horizontal stability and the harmful effects of reduced horizontal stability (excessive ridge resorption, tissue impingement, inefficient mastication), which far outweigh the benefits of vertical stress breaking. It is the rigid nature of the more conventional removable partial denture that allows satisfaction of all requirements for support, stability, and retention without overemphasis on only one principle to the detriment of the oral tissues.

REFERENCE

1. Boucher CO. Complete denture impressions based upon the anatomy of the mouth. *J Am Dent Assoc.* 1944;31:1174–1181.

10

Principles of Removable Partial Denture Design

Ahmed Mahrous and David L. Botsko

CHAPTER OUTLINE

Before any treatment is started, it is important to consider the final design of the removable partial denture (RPD). Biomechanical considerations to control movement of the RPD under functional load are an important element in the strategy of selecting components as part of the design process. A review of the biomechanical considerations presented in Chapter 4 may be warranted. The design of the RPD may necessitate additional treatment or require modifications to existing teeth before it can be fabricated. Once a design is finalized, treatment may commence. The required tooth modifications for RPDs are as follows:

- Guide plane tooth modifications are reductions within the coronal aspect of the tooth contained in enamel surfaces only (see Fig. 10.1).
- Rest seats are prepared after the guide plane reduction and are also contained in enamel only (see Fig. 10.1).
- Heights of contour modifications are sometimes needed for both circumferential and combination clasps. The contour modification is made from the guide plane location along two-thirds of the length to the retentive clasp.

This chapter will discuss a systematic protocol for designing RPDs. Knowledge gained in previous chapters and new concepts will be utilized in designing an RPD.

DIFFERENCE IN PROSTHESIS SUPPORT AND INFLUENCE ON DESIGN

The requirements for movement control are functions of whether the prosthesis will be tooth supported or tooth-tissue supported. For a tooth-supported prosthesis, the movement potential is less because resistance to functional loading is provided by the teeth. Teeth do not vary widely in their ability to provide this support; consequently, designs for prostheses are less variable. This is the case even though the amount of supporting bone, the crown-to-root ratios, the crown and root morphologies, and the tooth number and position in the arch relative to edentulous spaces are well established and may be variable for tooth- and tooth-tissue–supported RPDs. For a tooth-tissue–supported prosthesis, the residual ridge (the remaining alveolar bone and overlying connective tissue covered with mucosa) presents with variable potential for support. Not only does the underlying alveolar bone demonstrate a highly variable form following extraction but it also continues to change with time. As the alveolar bone responds to the loss of teeth, the overlying connective tissue and mucosa undergo change that places the soft tissue at risk for pressure-induced inflammatory changes. This variable tissue support adds complexity to design considerations

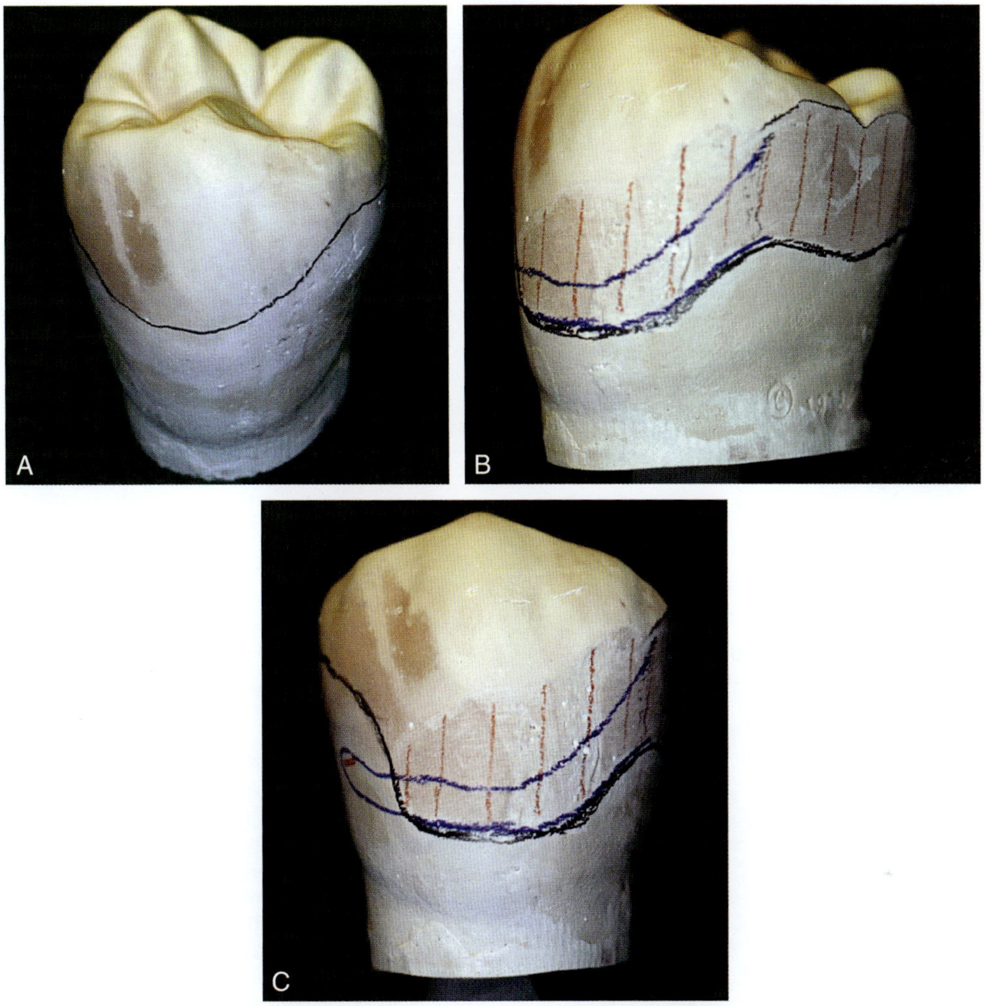

Fig. 10.1 **A,** The unmodified buccal surface of the mandibular premolar illustrates a typical height of contour location natural for this tooth (middle and occlusal thirds of the tooth). **B,** Proximal surface modification is required (hatched region) to produce a guide plane surface. **C,** Buccal surface modification is needed to position the height of contour for favorable clasp location. The tooth modification is a continuation of the proximal surface modification onto the buccal surface and generally requires less than 0.5 mm of tooth removal.

when one is dealing with tooth-tissue–supported prostheses. This occurs because unlike the efficient support provided by teeth, which results in limited prosthesis movement, the reaction of the ridge tissue to functional forces can be highly variable, leading to variable amounts of prosthesis movement. An understanding of the potential sources of functional force from the opposing arch that can affect the prosthesis's movement potential is helpful.

Factors related to the opposing arch tooth position, the existence and nature of prosthesis support in the opposing arch, and the potential for establishing a harmonious occlusion influence the RPD design. Opposing tooth positions that apply forces outside the primary support of the prosthesis can introduce leverage forces that act to dislodge the prosthesis. Such an effect is variable and is based on the nature of the opposing occlusion because the forces of occlusion differ between natural teeth, RPDs, and complete dentures. In general, RPDs opposing natural teeth require greater support and stabilization over time because of the greater functional load demands. Therefore occlusal relationships at maximum intercuspation should be broadly dissipated to the supporting units.

DIFFERENTIATION BETWEEN TWO MAIN TYPES OF REMOVABLE PARTIAL DENTURES

Based on the previous discussion, it is clear that two distinct types of RPDs exist. Certain points of difference are present between distal extension base RPDs (Kennedy Class I and Class II) and the tooth-bounded edentulous space RPDs (Kennedy Class III and Class IV).

The first consideration in designing an RPD is how each is supported. The bounded denture base type derives all its support from the abutment teeth (see Figs. 10.2, *A* and 10.3). Distal extension–type RPDs derive their primary support from tissues underlying the extension base and secondary support from the abutment teeth. The second difference between the two types, for reasons related to the manner of support, is the method of

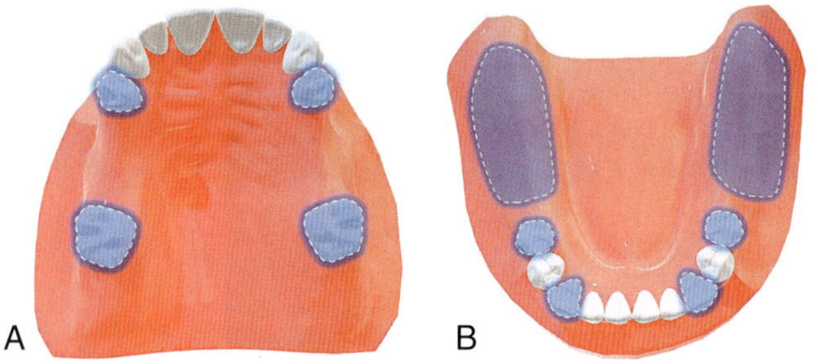

Fig. 10.2 **A,** Kennedy Class III, modification 1, partially edentulous arch provides total tooth support for the prosthesis. A removable partial denture made for this arch is totally supported by rests on properly prepared occlusal rest seats on four abutment teeth. **B,** Kennedy Class I partially edentulous arch. Major support for denture bases must come from the residual ridges, and tooth support from occlusal rests being effective only at the anterior portion of each base. (Courtesy of Ahmed Mahrous Copyright © 2024. All rights reserved.)

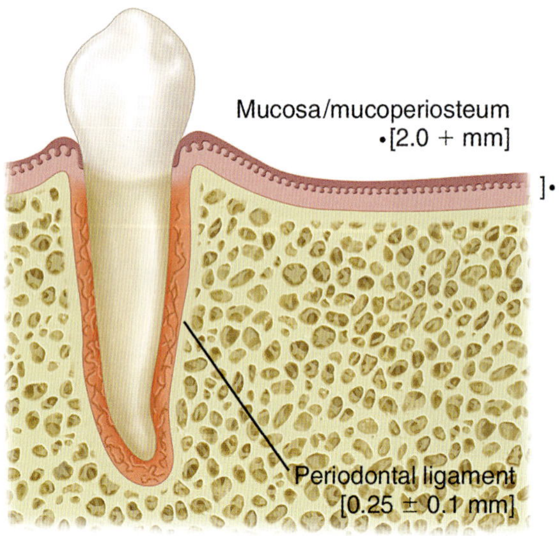

Fig. 10.3 Distortion of tissues over the edentulous ridge will be approximately 500 μm under 4 Newtons of force, whereas abutment teeth will demonstrate approximately 20 μm of intrusion under the same load.

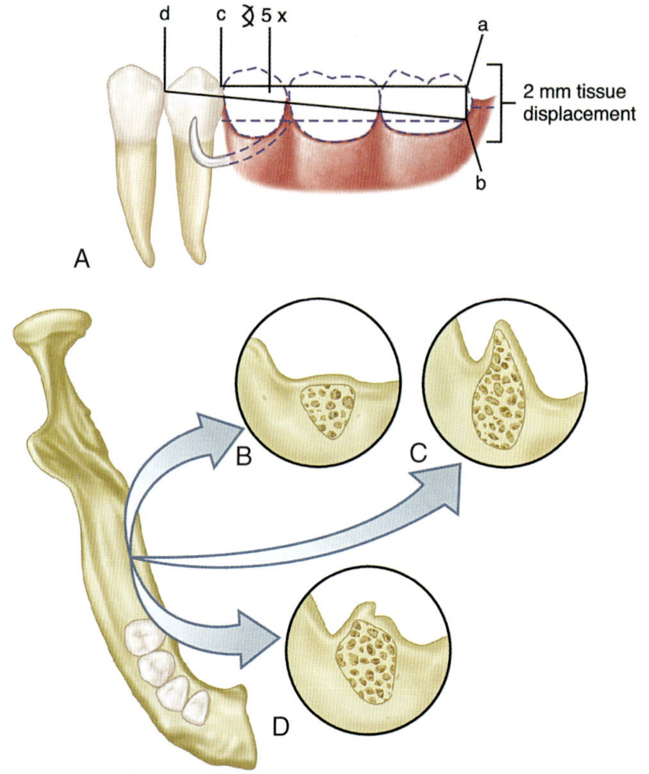

Fig. 10.4 **A,** The longer the edentulous area covered by the denture base, the greater the potential lever action on the abutment teeth. If an extension base area is 30 mm *(ac)* and tissue displacement is 2 mm *(ab)*, the amount of movement of the proximal plate on the guiding plane will be approximately 0.25 mm: [$\alpha = \sqrt{(ab)^2 + (ac)^2}$]; arc of the tangent *ab/ad* = *x/cd* (2/30 = *x*/3.75 = 0.25 mm). **B,** The flat ridge will provide good support and poor stability. **C,** The sharp spiny ridge will provide poor support and poor to fair stability. **D,** Displaceable tissue on the ridge will provide poor support and poor stability.

impression registration, and the jaw record required for each type varies.

Third, there is a need to accommodate the rotational movement of the distal extension base type of RPD around the fulcrum line. Because of the presence of an extension base that is not bounded by a retentive clasp, the RPD tends to exhibit significant rotational movement around the fulcrum line due to compressibility of the underlying soft tissue, the lifting away from the supporting tissues due to the action of sticky foods, and the movements of tissues of the mouth against the borders of the denture. In contrast, tooth-bounded RPDs have no fulcrum lines because each end of each denture base is secured by a direct retainer on an abutment tooth.

Last, because the distal extension type of RPD is supported by the residual ridge, which changes over time, it often necessitates the use of a base material that can be relined to compensate for tissue changes. Generally, acrylic resin is used as a base material for distal extension bases. The Kennedy Class III RPD, on the other hand, which is entirely tooth supported, does not require relining except when it is advisable to eliminate an unhygienic, unesthetic, or uncomfortable condition resulting from loss of tissue contact. Metal bases therefore are more frequently used in tooth-supported restorations because relining is not as likely to be necessary with them.

Differences in Support

The distal extension RPD derives its major support from the residual ridge with its fibrous connective tissue covering. The length and contour of the residual ridge significantly influence the amount of available support and stability (Fig. 10.4). Some areas of this residual ridge are firm, with limited displaceability, whereas other areas are displaceable, depending on the thickness and structural character of the tissues overlying the residual alveolar bone. The movement of the base under function determines the occlusal efficiency of the RPD and the degree to which the abutment teeth are subjected to torque and tipping stresses. The negative impact of the residual ridge character on the support provided to the occlusion in a specific arch can be addressed through the placement of a dental implant, rendering displaceable tissue with movement potential into a more resistant support for occlusion.

Impression Registration

An impression registration for the fabrication of an RPD must accurately record the anatomic form and the relationship between the remaining teeth in the dental arch and the surrounding soft tissues, so the denture will not exert pressure on those structures beyond their physiologic limits. A type of impression material that can be removed from undercut areas without permanent distortion must be used to fulfill this requirement. Elastic impression materials such as irreversible hydrocolloid, silicone impression materials (both condensation and addition reaction), and polyether impression materials are best suited for this purpose. Alternatively, an intraoral scan can be made if isolation and retraction can be accomplished adequately.

Occasionally, patients present with easily displaceable or "flabby" supporting tissues. The supporting form of the soft tissues underlying the distal extension base of the RPD should be recorded so that firm areas are used as primary stress–bearing areas and readily displaceable tissues are not overloaded. Only in this way can maximum support of the RPD base be obtained. An impression material capable of displacing tissue sufficiently to register the supporting form of the ridge should be used in those situations. A fluid mouth-temperature wax or any of the readily flowing impression materials (the silicone type or the polyethers in an individualized custom or corrected tray) may be employed for registering the supporting form. Zinc oxide–eugenol impression paste can also be used when only the extension base area is being impressed (see Chapter 16).

No single impression material can satisfactorily fulfill both previously mentioned requirements. Recording the anatomic form of both teeth and supporting tissues may result in inadequate support for the distal extension base. Because the cast may not represent the optimum coordinating form that relates the residual ridge to the teeth due to compression of the tissue overlying the residual ridge, additional impression-making techniques may need to be applied in order to obtain maximum support for the supporting tissues (see Chapter 16). This coordination of support maximizes the support capacity for the arch and minimizes movement of the RPD under function.

Differences in Clasp Design

The tooth-supported RPD, which is totally supported by the abutment teeth, is retained and stabilized by a retentive clasp at each end of each edentulous space. Because this type of prosthesis movement under function is limited to the physiologic limitations of tooth support units, the only requirement for such clasps is that they flex sufficiently over the height of contour of the teeth during placement and removal of the denture. When in its terminal position on the tooth, a retentive clasp should be passive and should not flex except when one is engaging the undercut area of the tooth for resisting a vertical dislodging force.

Cast retentive clasp arms are generally the clasp of choice for tooth-supported removable dentures. These may be occlusally approaching (suprabulge), arising from the body of the clasp and approaching the undercut from an occlusal direction like the circumferential-type retentive clasp arms, or gingivally approaching (infrabulge), arising from the base of the denture and approaching the undercut area from a gingival direction like the bar-type retentive clasps. Each of these two types of cast clasps has its advantages and disadvantages.

Distal extension base RPDs exhibit functional movement of the extension base as the RPD rotates. There are two main movements that occur during the function of an extension base RPD, each with their respective management Hyperlink to video for (Video 10.5, Fig. 10.5). The first movement is the lifting of the extension base component away from the underlying tissues as sticky foods act to pull unbound portion of the RPD toward the opposing arch. As a result, the RPD rotates around the fulcrum line causing instability and potentially tissue damage on the other side of the RPD. Indirect retainers are used to manage and counteract this type of movement (Figs. 10.6 and 10.7). A more detailed explanation may be found in Chapter 8.

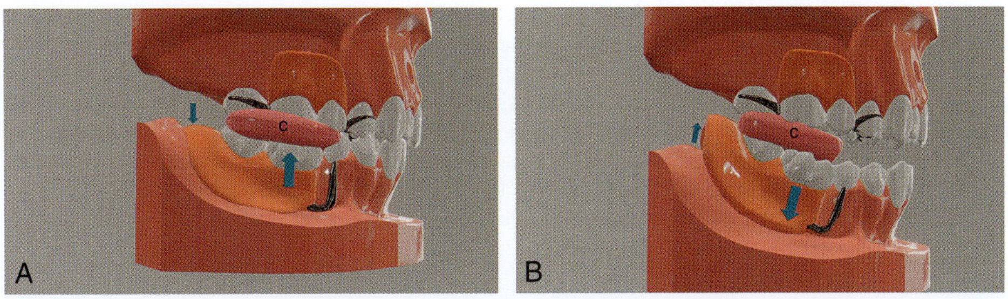

Fig. 10.5 Movement of the removable partial denture during mastication. *Large arrow* represents mandibular movement upward toward the opposing arch; *C*, bolus; *small arrow* represents movement of the prosthesis. This figure demonstrates the movement of the distal extension removable partial denture during function. The pink object *C* is a sticky food substance or bolus. **A,** During mastication as the patient bites into the object, forces are transmitted to the distal extension portion of the removable partial denture, and because of the compressible nature of the tissues in that area, the result is the downward movement of the distal extension area. **B,** As the patient continues on the chewing stroke and opens the mouth, the sticky substance acts to "pull" the distal extension area upward causing the distal extension area to lift off the tissues. It is worth noting that no such movement is seen on the maxillary tooth–supported removable partial denture as both sides of the removable partial denture are supported and retained by abutment teeth. (Courtesy of Ahmed Mahrous Copyright © 2024. All rights reserved.)

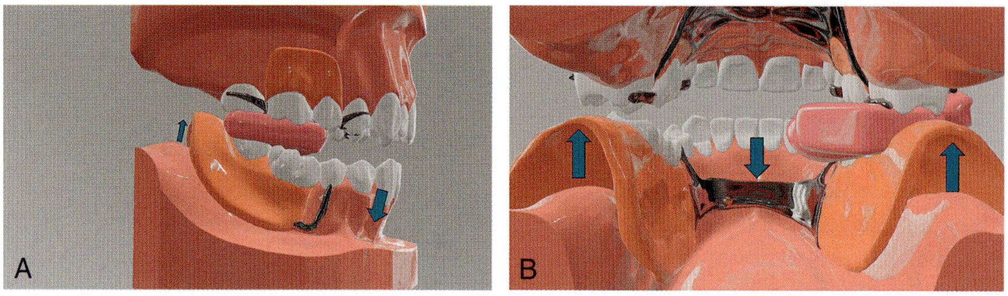

Fig. 10.6 Mandibular distal extension removable partial denture with no indirect retainers showing the distal extension base being lifted from the ridge. This can be seen from the lateral view **(A)** and posterior view **(B)**. Note how the removable partial denture movement is unhindered around the fulcrum line. This causes excessive instability and even trauma to the anterior lingual soft tissues. (Video 10.6). (Courtesy of Ahmed Mahrous Copyright © 2024. All rights reserved.)

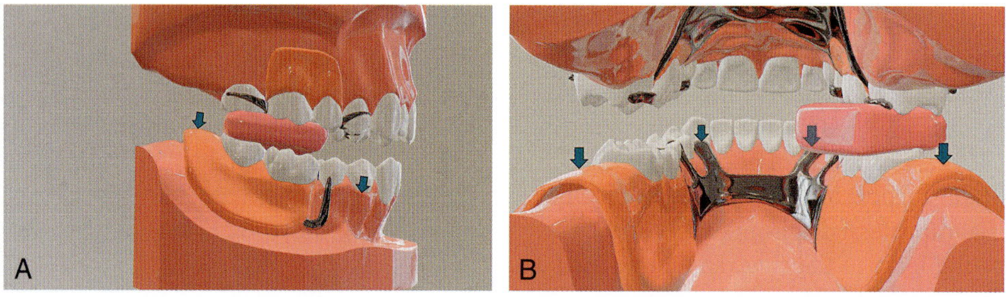

Fig. 10.7 Mandibular distal extension removable partial denture with indirect retainers showing the distal extension base being lifted from the ridge; however, the prosthesis remains relatively stationary due to the stabilizing capacity of the indirect retainers. This can be seen from the lateral view **(A)** and posterior view **(B)**. (Video 10.7) (Courtesy of Ahmed Mahrous Copyright © 2024. All rights reserved.)

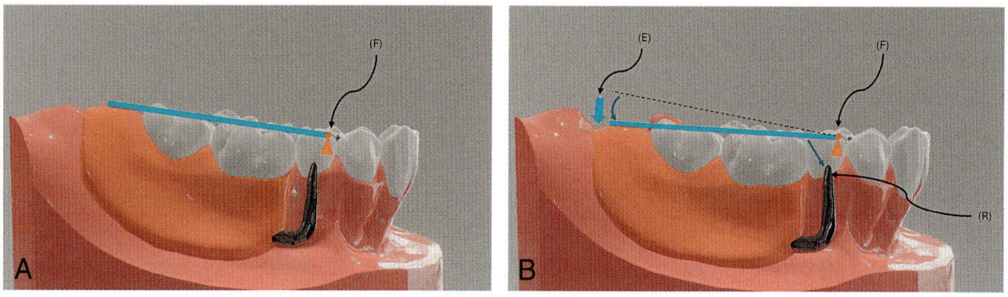

Fig. 10.8 Kennedy Class II lever removable partial denture. **A,** Stress-breaking clasp assemblies on extension base removable partial denture can reduce stress on the abutment tooth by transforming the lever system into a second-class lever. By placing the clasp tip between the fulcrum line *(F)* and the edentulous span (denture base), the lever becomes a Class II lever. This may be done by placing a rest seat on the mesial of the abutment tooth thereby making the fulcrum anterior to the clasp tip. **B,** As the removable partial denture is subjected to occlusal load, force is applied *(E)* depressing the distal denture base portion (cantilever) of the removable partial denture rotating downward toward the supporting residual ridge and the anterior portion of the clasp tip also rotates downward. Because the clasp moves in the same direction as the effort and disengages from the retentive undercut, it does not subject the tooth to excessive force. *E*, effort/force; *F*, fulcrum; *R*, load. (Courtesy of Ahmed Mahrous Copyright © 2024. All rights reserved.)

The second type of movement that occurs with distal extension base–type RPDs is the compression of the extension base into the tissues. As a result of this compression the RPD tends to rotate around the fulcrum line but in an opposite direction to that previously described. This movement is proportionate to the quality (displaceability) of the supporting soft tissues, the accuracy of the fit of the denture base, and the total occlusal load applied. Therefore the direct retainer clasp assembly adjacent to the distal extension base must perform still another function, in addition to resisting vertical displacement. The clasp assembly must also be able to dissipate stresses that otherwise would be transmitted directly to the abutment tooth as leverage. The function of the clasp assembly to reduce stress is called *stress breaking*; hence the term *stress breakers* is used to describe clasp assemblies that act to *break* the stress potentially subjected to abutment teeth they are used on (Fig. 10.8).

Stress-breaking clasp assemblies can be designed in two principal methods, (1) offsetting the retentive clasp arm tip and

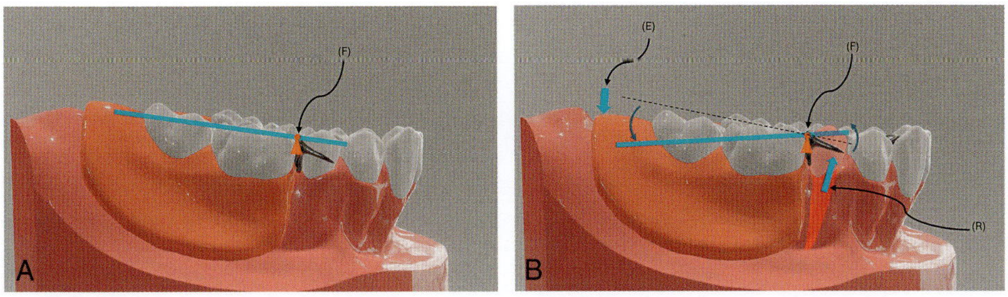

Fig. 10.9 Class I lever removable partial denture (RPD). A distal extension RPD can act as a Class I lever if the fulcrum line *(F)* connecting the terminal rests exists between the clasp and the edentulous span. The effort *(E)* represents the occlusal load being applied to the extension base. The result is a downward movement of the denture base due to the compressibility of the tissues and a corresponding opposite movement of the resistance arm *(R)* representing the clasp. As the clasp moves upward, it subjects the tooth to potentially damaging torquing forces. **A,** The fulcrum line is positioned between the clasp tip and the edentulous span, creating a cantilever (the edentulous span is distal to the fulcrum in this RPD design). **B,** As force is applied *(E)*, the distal denture base portion (cantilever) of the RPD rotates downward toward the supporting residual ridge and the anterior portion of the clasp tip rotates upward against the tooth. (Courtesy of Ahmed Mahrous Copyright © 2024. All rights reserved.)

the axis of the fulcrum line and (2) using a flexible retentive clasp arm.

Offsetting the Retentive Clasp Arm Tip and the Axis of the Fulcrum Line

As explained in Chapter 4, the movement of the RPD in a distal extension base RPD can be expected to occur as a rotational movement around the fulcrum line. Potential unwanted forces occur when the clasp exists anterior to the fulcrum line. In this arrangement the clasp acts as a Class I lever, which acts like a seesaw with the extension base on one side, the retentive clasp arm on the other, and the rest seat in the middle as the fulcrum. This arrangement could be damaging because of the potentially unwanted luxation forces subjected to the abutment tooth (Fig. 10.9). Those forces can be circumvented by changing the location of the clasp tip in relation to the rest acting as the fulcrum. To achieve this, the rest seat is moved as far away from the extension base as possible on the abutment tooth. In most Kennedy Class I and II cases, the rest is moved to the mesial side of the tooth, while the retentive clasp tip is kept as close as possible to the extension base as possible usually kept at the midbuccal region. By rearranging the clasp and the rest, the lever system is now designated as a Class II lever system where the fulcrum exists on one end of the system and both the extension base and the clasp tip exist on the other. The result is the disengagement of the clasp from the undercut as the denture base moves tissue ward breaking of the associated stress (see Fig. 10.8). Some of the most used clasp assemblies that employ such stress-breaking principles include the RPI (rest, proximal plate, and I-bar) and RPA (rest, proximal plate, and Akers) clasp assemblies described in Chapter 7.

It is important to note that such stress-breaking action gained by moving the rest away from the extension base is only effective when the rest being moved is one of the two most distal rests dictating the location of the fulcrum line. Clasps existing anterior to the fulcrum line but with rests being not part of the fulcrum line will not achieve stress breaking from moving the rest seat away from the denture base. An example of such a

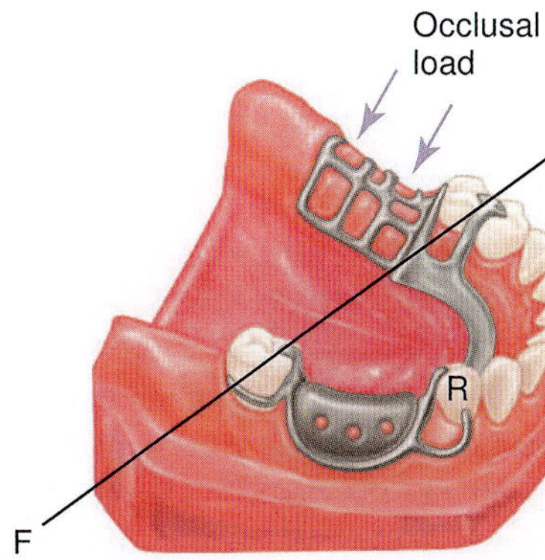

Fig. 10.10 The potential for first-class lever action can also exist in Kennedy Class II, modification 1, designs for removable partial denture frameworks. If a cast circumferential direct retainer with a mesiobuccal undercut on the right first premolar was used, force placed on the denture base could impart an upward and posteriorly moving force on the premolar, resulting in loss of contact between the premolar and canine. Tissue support from the extension base area is most important to minimize the lever action of the clasp. The retainer design could help accommodate more of an anteriorly directed force during rotation of the denture base in an attempt to maintain tooth contact. Other alternatives to the first premolar design of the direct retainer would include a tapered wrought-wire retentive arm that uses mesiobuccal undercut or that just has a buccal stabilizing arm above the height of contour. F represents the fulcrum line, while R represents the resistance arm.

situation is seen in the clasp assembly used in the anterior abutment of a modification space of a Kennedy Class II, modification 1, patient. Such clasp assemblies will need to be addressed by either removing the retentive clasp arm entirely, using a nonengaging retentive clasp arm (does not engage an undercut), or using a flexible retentive arm (Fig. 10.10).

Using a Flexible Retentive Clasp Arm

A retentive clasp arm made of wrought wire can flex more readily in all directions than can the cast half-round clasp arm. Thereby it would effectively dissipate those stresses that would otherwise be transmitted to the abutment tooth. Only the retentive arm of the circumferential clasp assembly should be made of wrought metal.

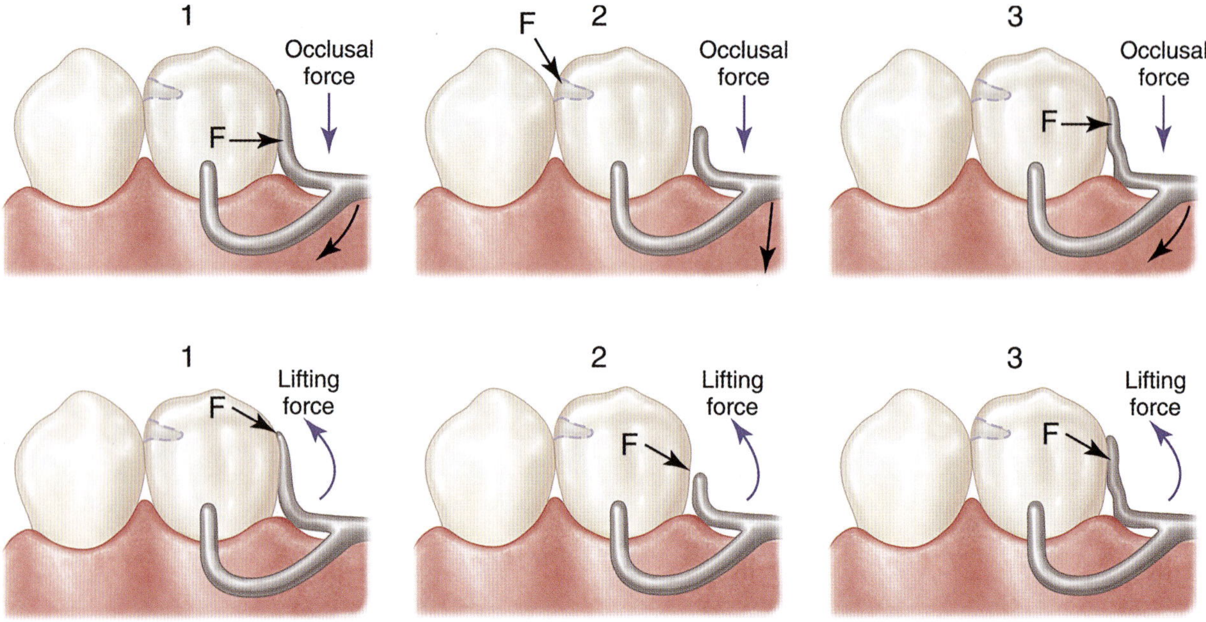

Fig. 10.11 *1*, Maximum contact of the proximal plate minor connector with the guiding plane produces a more horizontal distribution of stress to the abutment teeth. *2*, Minimum contact or disengagement of the minor connector with the guiding plane allows rotation around the fulcrum located on the mesio-occlusal rest, producing a more vertical distribution of stress to the ridge area. *3*, Minor connector contacts with the guiding plane from the marginal ridge to the junction of the middle and gingival thirds of the abutment tooth distribute load vertically to the ridge and horizontally to the abutment tooth. *F*, The location of the fulcrum of movement for the distal extension base.

Reciprocation and stabilization against lateral and torquing movements must be obtained through use of the rigid cast elements that make up the remainder of the clasp. This is called a *combination clasp assembly* because it is a combination of cast and wrought materials incorporated into one direct retainer. It is frequently used on the terminal abutment for the distal extension RPD and is indicated where a mesiobuccal, but no distobuccal undercut exists, or where a gross tissue undercut, cervical and buccal to the abutment tooth, exists. The combination clasp assembly is very useful in situations where a clasp assembly is used anterior to the fulcrum line where the rest is not associated with the fulcrum line. In those cases, the wrought wire still retains its stress-breaking ability regardless of its relationship with the fulcrum line.

It must always be remembered that the factors of length and material contribute to the flexibility of clasp arms. The shorter the arm length, the less flexible the arm will be. From a materials physical property standpoint, a short wrought-wire arm may be a destructive element because of its reduced ability to flex compared with a longer wrought-wire arm. In addition to its greater flexibility compared with the cast circumferential clasp, the combination clasp offers the advantages of adjustability, minimum tooth contact, and better esthetics, which justify its occasional use in tooth-supported designs.

The amount of stress transferred to the supporting edentulous ridge(s) and the abutment teeth will depend on: (1) the direction and magnitude of the force, (2) the length of the denture base lever arm(s), (3) the quality of resistance (support from the edentulous ridges and remaining natural teeth), and (4) the design characteristics of the RPD. As was stated in Chapter 7, the location of the rest, the design of the minor connector as it relates to its corresponding guide plane, and the location of the retentive arm are all factors that influence how a clasp system functions. The greater the surface area contact of each minor connector to its corresponding guide plane, the more horizontal the distribution of force (Fig. 10.11).

ESSENTIALS OF REMOVABLE DENTURE DESIGN

The design of the RPD framework should be systematically developed using an accurate diagnostic cast (analog or virtual) based on the following prosthesis concepts: where the prosthesis is supported, how the support is connected, how the prosthesis is retained, how the retention and support are connected, and how edentulous base support is connected.

The first step in developing the design is to determine how the RPD is to be supported. In an entirely tooth-supported RPD, the most ideal location for the support units (rests) is on prepared rest seats on the occlusal, cingulum, or incisal surface of the abutment adjacent to each edentulous space (see Fig. 10.1, *A*). The type of rest and amount of support required must be based on the interpretation of the diagnostic data collected from the patient. In evaluating the potential support that an abutment tooth can provide, consideration should be given to (1) periodontal health, (2) crown and root morphologies, (3) crown-to-root ratio, (4) bone index area (how tooth has responded to previous stress), (5) location of the tooth in the arch, (6) relationship of the tooth to other support units (length of edentulous span), and (7) the opposing dentition. For a more in-depth understanding of these considerations, review Chapters 6 and 13.

In a distal extension base RPD, the support is derived from both the teeth and the underlying tissue. In these situations, these same considerations must be given to the abutment teeth. However, equitable support must also come from the edentulous ridge areas. In evaluating the potential support available from edentulous ridge areas, consideration must be given to (1) the quality of the residual ridge, which includes contour and quality of the supporting bone (how the bone has responded to previous stress) and quality of the supporting mucosa; (2) the extent to which the residual ridge will be covered by the denture base; (3) the type and accuracy of the impression registration; (4) the accuracy of the denture base; (5) the design characteristics of the component parts of the RPD framework; and (6) the anticipated occlusal load. A full explanation of tissue support for extension base RPDs is found in Chapter 17.

Denture base areas adjacent to abutment teeth are primarily tooth supported. As one proceeds away from the abutment teeth, they become more tissue supported. Therefore it is necessary to incorporate characteristics in the RPD design that will distribute the functional load equitably between the abutment teeth and the supporting tissues of the edentulous ridge. Determining the location of tooth support and locations of rest on the principal abutment teeth and designing the minor connectors that are adjacent to the edentulous areas to contact the guide planes in such a manner that the functional load is dispersed equitably between the available tooth- and tissue-supporting units will provide designs with controlled distribution of support (see Fig. 10.11).

The second step in designing any RPD is to connect the tooth and tissue support units. This connection is facilitated by designing and locating major and minor connectors in compliance with the basic principles and concepts presented in Chapter 5.

The third step is to determine how the RPD is to be retained. The retention must be sufficient to resist reasonable dislodging forces. As was stated in Chapter 7, retention is accomplished by placement of mechanical retaining elements (clasps) on the abutment teeth and by the intimate relationship of the denture bases and major connectors (maxillary) with the underlying tissues. The key to selecting a successful clasp design for any given situation is to choose one that will (1) avoid direct transmission of tipping or torquing forces to the abutment; (2) accommodate the basic principles of clasp design by definitive location of component parts correctly positioned on abutment tooth surfaces; (3) provide retention against reasonable dislodging forces (with consideration for indirect retention); and (4) be compatible with undercut location, tissue contour, and esthetic desires of the patient. The location of the undercut is the most important single factor in the selection of a clasp. Undercut location, however, can be modified by recontouring or restoring the abutment tooth to accommodate a clasp design better suited to satisfy the criteria for clasp selection.

Avoiding direct transmission of tipping or torquing forces may be accomplished through class design philosophies such as the RPI design or stress-breaking principles such as combination clasps in distal extension base situations (Fig. 10.12).

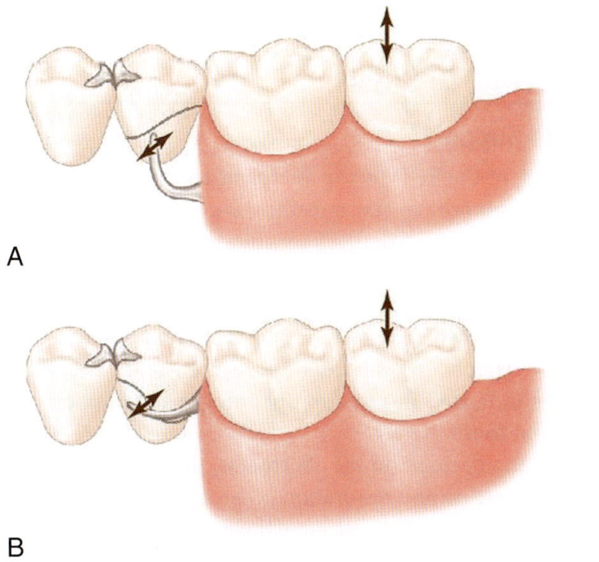

Fig. 10.12 Direct retainer assemblies that may be used on abutments adjacent to the distal extension base to avoid or minimize the effects of the cantilever design. *Arrows* indicate the general direction of movement of retentive tips of retainer arms when the denture base rotates toward and away from the edentulous ridge. **A,** Mesial rest, distal proximal plate, and I-bar placed in an undercut location at the middle (anteroposteriorly) of the buccal surface. This retainer contacts the tooth only at its tip. Note that the guide plane on the distal aspect of the abutment is contacted by the metal of the denture framework and that a mesial rest is used. **B,** Round, uniformly tapered 18-gauge wrought-wire circumferential retainer arm engaging the mesiobuccal undercut. A wrought-wire arm, instead of a cast arm, should be used in this situation because of the ability of wrought wire to flex omnidirectionally. A cast half-round retainer arm would not flex edgewise, which could result in excessive stress on the tooth when rotation of the denture base occurs. The relative importance of retention is highlighted by the results from a clinical trial investigating prosthesis design. A 5-year randomized clinical trial of two basic removable partial denture (RPD) designs—one with rest, proximal plate, and I-bar design and one with circumferential clasp design—demonstrated no discernible changes after 60 months in nine periodontal health components of the abutment teeth with either of the two designs. The overall results indicate that the two designs did not differ in terms of success rates, maintenance, or effects on abutment teeth. Therefore a well-constructed RPD supported by favorable abutments and good residual ridges that are properly prepared and maintained in a patient, who exhibits good oral hygiene, offers the best opportunity for satisfactory treatment.

The fourth step is to provide reciprocation to the retentive areas. This is provided either by rigid reciprocal clasps or any rigid metal opposing the clasp above the height of contour like the lingual plate or the minor connector and proximal plate of an RPI system (see Chapter 7).

The fifth and last step in this systematic approach to design is to ensure all components are correctly joined including retentive, support, reciprocal, and edentulous areas. This is accomplished by examining that all components are connected to the major connector. Strict attention to details of the design characteristics outlined in Chapter 9 is necessary to ensure rigidity of the base material without interfering with tooth placement.

COMPONENTS OF REMOVABLE PARTIAL DENTURE DESIGN

Tooth Support

Support of the RPD by the abutment teeth is dependent on the alveolar support of those teeth, the crown and root morphology, the rigidity of the RPD framework, and the design of the occlusal rests. Through clinical and radiographic interpretation, the dentist may evaluate the abutment teeth and decide whether they will provide adequate support. In some instances, a tooth may be deemed too weak to be used as an abutment and extraction is indicated in favor of obtaining better support from an adjacent tooth.

Having decided on the abutments, the dentist is responsible for preparation and restoration of the abutment teeth to accommodate the most ideal design of the RPD. This includes the form of the occlusal rest seats. These modifications may be prepared in sound tooth enamel or in restorative materials that will withstand the functional stress and wear of the component parts of the RPD. The dentist must sufficiently reduce the marginal ridge area of the rest seat to avoid interference from opposing teeth. If there is not an adequate reduction, then the occlusal rest will be inadequate and may fracture or the rest may result in occlusal interferences.

Ridge Support

Support for the tooth-supported RPD or the tooth-supported modification space comes entirely from the abutment teeth by means of rests. Support for the distal extension denture base comes primarily from the overlying soft tissues and the residual alveolar bone of the distal extension base area. In the latter, rest support is effective only at the abutment end of the denture base.

The effectiveness of tissue support depends on six things: (1) the quality of the residual ridge, (2) the extent to which the residual ridge will be covered by the denture base, (3) the accuracy and type of impression registration, (4) the accuracy of the denture bases, (5) the design characteristics of component parts of the RPD framework, and (6) the occlusal load applied. The quality of the residual ridge cannot be influenced, except that it can be improved by tissue conditioning.

The accuracy of the impression technique is entirely in the hands of the dentist. Maximum tissue coverage for support that encompasses the primary stress–bearing areas should be the primary objective in any RPD impression technique. The accuracy of the denture base is influenced by the choice of materials and by the exactness of the processing techniques. Inaccurate and warped denture bases adversely influence the support of the RPD. Materials and techniques that will ensure the greatest dimensional stability should be selected.

The total occlusal load applied to the residual ridge may be influenced by reducing the area of occlusal contact. This is done with the use of fewer, narrower, and more effectively shaped artificial teeth (Fig. 10.13).

The distal extension RPD is unique in that its support is derived from abutment teeth, which are comparatively unyielding, and from soft tissues overlying the bone, which may be comparatively yielding under occlusal forces. Compressible tissues, which are distorted or displaced by occlusal load, are unable to provide support for the denture base comparable with that offered by the abutment teeth.

An implant can efficiently serve to improve ridge support by replacing the tissue compression seen on functional loading with the stiff resistance offered by bone supporting an implant. The benefit for movement control is achieved as if a change was made from a tooth-tissue–borne prosthesis to a tooth-tooth–borne prosthesis. If implants are not a possibility, such compressible tissues should be recorded with the following considerations: (1) the material should record the tissues covering the primary stress–bearing areas in their supporting form, (2) tissues within the basal seat area other than primary stress–bearing areas must be recorded in their anatomic form, and (3) the total area covered by the impression should be sufficient to distribute the load over as large an area as can be tolerated by the border tissues.

A denture base processed to the functional form using a technique known as the *Altered cast* technique is typically less irregular and provides greater area coverage than does a denture base processed to the anatomic or resting form (Fig. 10.14). Moreover, and of far greater significance, a denture base made to anatomic form exhibits less stability under rotating and/or torquing forces than does a denture base processed to functional form and thus fails to maintain its occlusal relation with the opposing teeth.

Major and Minor Connectors

Major and minor connectors should be designed following the principles outlined in Chapter 5. In addition to connecting all the components of the arch, major connectors have a role to play in the support in the RPD.

The use of a lingual plate is indicated in Kennedy Class I partially edentulous arches when additional resistance to horizontal rotation of the denture is required because of excessively resorbed residual ridges. It is also used as a mechanism to splint periodontally involved teeth.

The rigidity of a palatal major connector is a major determinant in its selection. A U-shaped palatal connector is rarely justified due to its lack of rigidity, except when avoiding an inoperable palatal torus that extends to the junction of the hard and soft palates. Likewise the routine use of a narrow, single-palatal bar can rarely be justified. The combination anterior-posterior palatal strap–type major connector is mechanically and biologically sound if it is located so that it does not impinge on tissues. The broad, anatomic palatal major connector is frequently preferred because of its rigidity, better acceptance by the patient, and greater stability without tissue damage.

Direct Retention for Tooth-Supported Removable Partial Dentures

Direct retainers for tooth-supported RPDs have only two functions: (1) to retain the prosthesis against reasonable dislodging forces without damage to the abutment teeth and (2) to aid in resisting any tendency of the denture to be displaced

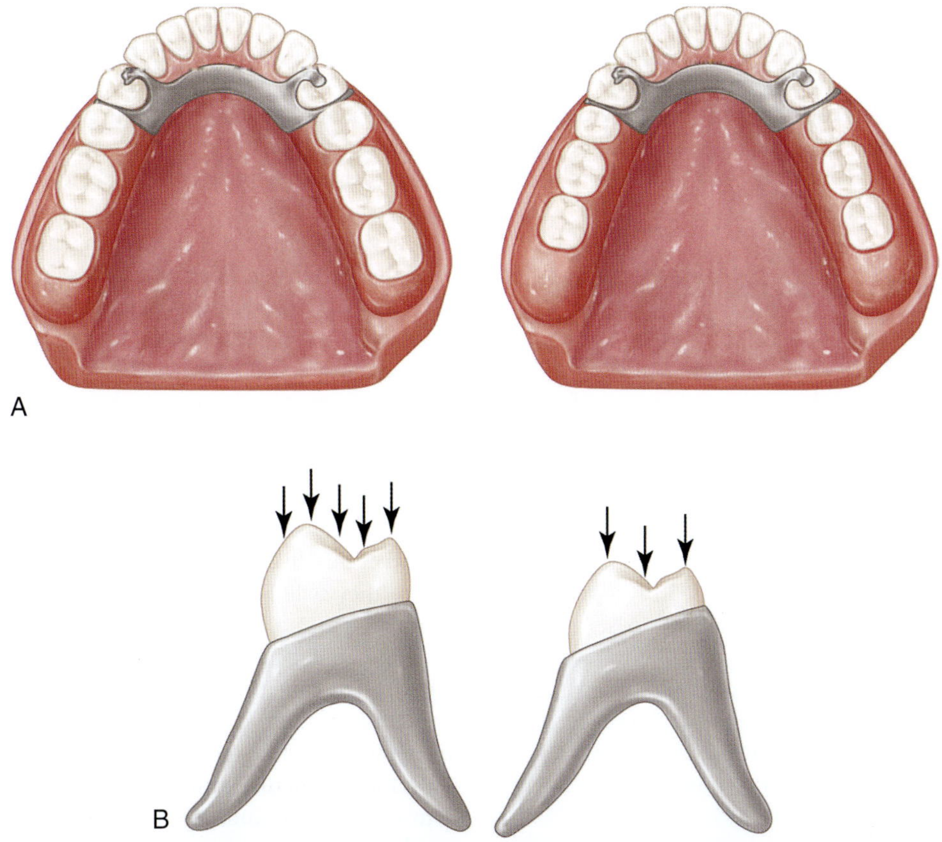

Fig. 10.13 A, The total occlusal load applied may be reduced by using comparatively smaller posterior teeth represented by the illustration on the *right*. **B,** Less muscular force will be required to penetrate a food bolus with a reduced occlusal table, thereby reducing forces to supporting oral structures.

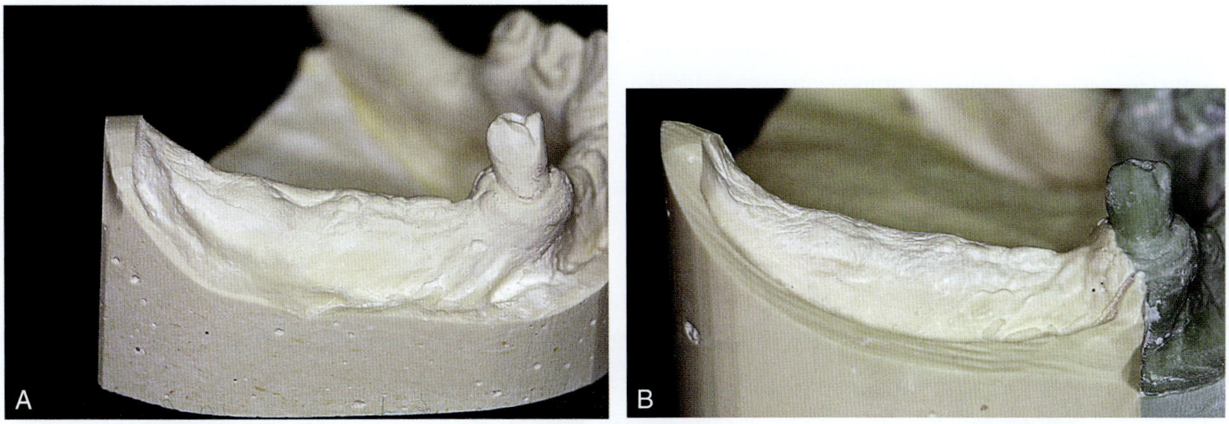

Fig. 10.14 A, Cast of the partially edentulous arch representing an anatomic form of residual ridges. An impression was made in the stock tray by using irreversible hydrocolloid. **B,** An impression recording the functional or supporting form of residual ridges was made in an individualized impression tray, permitting placement of tissues and definitive border molding.

in a horizontal plane. The prosthesis cannot move tissue ward because the retentive components of the clasp assembly are supported by the rest. No movement away from the tissues should occur, and therefore no rotation about a fulcrum, because the retentive component is secured by a direct retainer.

Any type of direct retainer is acceptable as long as the abutment tooth is not jeopardized by its presence. Circumferential and bar-type clasp retainers are mechanically effective. Therefore they are more universally used. Gingivally approaching clasps like the bar clasp should be used in the following conditions: (1) when clasp visibility is minimized due to esthetic concerns, (2) when the area for retention lies close to the gingival margin of the tooth, (3) when little tissue undercut exists relative to the abutment tooth, and (4) when sufficient vestibular depth exists relative to the abutment tooth.

Vulnerable areas on the abutment teeth must be protected by restorations with either type of retainer. The clasp retainer must not impinge on gingival tissues. The clasp must not exert excessive torque on the abutment tooth during placement and removal. It must be located the least distance into the tooth undercut for adequate retention, and it must be designed with a minimum of bulk and tooth contact.

Direct Retainers for Distal Extension Removable Partial Dentures

Direct retainers for distal extension RPDs, while retaining the prosthesis, must also be able to flex or disengage when the denture base moves tissue ward under function. Thus the retainer may act as a stress breaker. The choice for selecting an appropriate stress-breaking clasp assembly will rely on the relationship of the abutment tooth to the fulcrum line. If the abutment tooth has a rest that is part of the fulcrum line, then the options for a stress-breaking clasp assembly are an RPA, RPI, or a combination clasp assembly. However, if the abutment exists anterior to the fulcrum line and its rest is not part of the fulcrum line as is the case with anterior abutments of modification spaces of Kennedy Class I and II RPDs, then the choice becomes restricted to a combination clasp assembly or a clasp with a buccal stabilizing arm above the height of contour (see Fig. 10.10).

Stabilizing Components

The stabilizing components of the RPD framework are those that are rigid that assist in stabilizing the removable partial denture against horizontal movement. The purpose of all stabilizing components should be to distribute stresses equally to all supporting teeth without overworking any one tooth. The minor connectors that join the rests and the clasp assemblies to the major connector serve as stabilizing components.

All minor connectors that contact vertical tooth surfaces (and all reciprocal clasp arms) act as stabilizing components. It is necessary that minor connectors have sufficient bulk to be rigid and yet present as little bulk to the tongue as possible. This means that they should be confined to interdental embrasures whenever possible. When minor connectors are located on vertical tooth surfaces, it is best that these surfaces be parallel to the path of placement. When cast restorations are used, these surfaces should be made parallel.

A modification of the minor connector design has been proposed that places the minor connector in the center of the lingual surface of the abutment tooth (Fig. 10.15). Proponents of this design claim that it reduces the amount of gingival tissue coverage and provides enhanced bracing and guidance during placement. Disadvantages may include increased encroachment on the tongue space, more obvious borders, and potentially greater space between the connector and the abutment tooth. This proposed variation, however, when combined with thoughtful design principles, may provide some benefit to the periodontal health of the abutment teeth and may be acceptable to some patients.

Reciprocal clasp arms also must be rigid, and they must be placed occlusally to the height of contour of the abutment teeth, where they will be nonretentive. By their rigidity, these clasp arms reciprocate the opposing retentive clasp; they also prevent horizontal movement of the prosthesis under functional stresses. For a reciprocal clasp arm to be placed favorably, some reduction of the tooth surfaces involved may be necessary to increase the suprabulge area.

When crown restorations are used, a lingual reciprocal clasp arm may be inset into the tooth contour by providing a ledge on the crown on which the clasp arm may rest. This permits the use of a wider clasp arm and restores a more nearly normal tooth contour, while maintaining its strength and rigidity (see Chapter 15).

Guide Plane

The term *guide plane* is defined as two or more parallel, vertical surfaces of abutment teeth shaped to direct a prosthesis during placement and removal. After the most favorable path of placement has been ascertained, axial surfaces of abutment teeth are prepared parallel to the path of placement and therefore become parallel to each other. Guide planes may be contacted by various components of the RPD—the body of an extracoronal direct

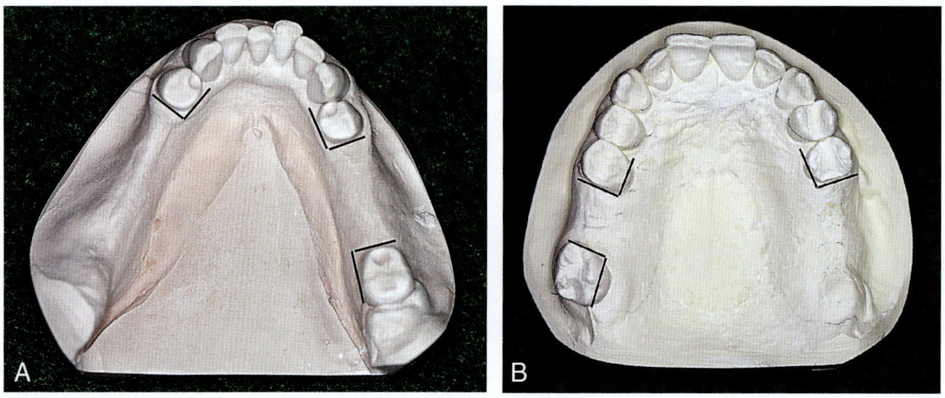

Fig. 10.15 Modifications of the abutment teeth in the form of guide planes at the height of contour of the lingual aspect of the teeth provide enhanced bracing and reduce the gingival tissue coverage. Prospective guide plane surfaces are indicated by *lines* located on the respective surfaces of abutment teeth **(A and B)**. These surfaces should be made vertically parallel to the path of placement.

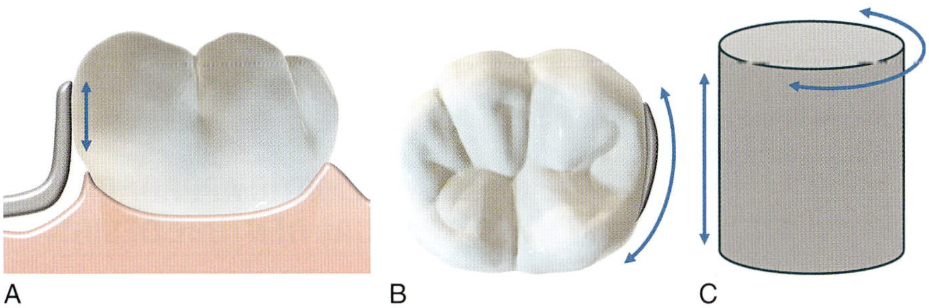

Fig. 10.16 **A,** The minor connector contacting the guiding plane surface has the same curvature as the surface. Viewed from the buccal aspect, the minor connector contacts the enamel of the tooth on its proximal surface about two-thirds its length. **B,** From an occlusal view, it tapers buccally from the thicker lingual portion, thus permitting closer contact of the abutment tooth and the prosthetically supplied tooth. **C,** The guiding plane surface should be like an area on a cylindrical object. It should be a continuous surface unbounded by *even, rounded line angles*. (Courtesy of Ahmed Mahrous Copyright © 2024. All rights reserved.)

retainer, the stabilizing arm of a direct retainer, and the minor connector portion of an indirect retainer—or by a minor connector specifically designed to contact the guide plane surface.

The functions of guide plane surfaces are as follows: (1) to provide for one path of placement and removal of the restoration (to eliminate detrimental strain to abutment teeth and framework components during placement and removal); (2) to ensure the intended actions of reciprocal, stabilizing, and retentive components (to provide retention against dislodgment of the restoration when the dislodging force is directed other than parallel to the path of removal and also to provide stabilization against horizontal rotation of the denture); and (3) to eliminate gross food traps between abutment teeth and components of the denture.

Guide plane surfaces need to be created so that they are nearly parallel to the long axes of abutment teeth as possible. Establishing guide planes on several abutment teeth (preferably more than two teeth), located at widely separated positions in the dental arch, provides for more effective use of these surfaces. The effectiveness of guide plane surfaces is enhanced if these surfaces are prepared on more than one common axial surface of the abutment teeth.

As a rule, proximal guide plane surfaces should be about one-half the width of the distance between the tips of adjacent buccal and lingual cusps or about one-third the buccal lingual width of the tooth and should extend vertically about two-thirds of the length of the enamel crown portion of the tooth from the marginal ridge cervically. In the preparation of guide plane surfaces, care must be exercised to avoid creating buccal or lingual line angles (Fig. 10.16). If it is assumed that the stabilizing or retentive arm of a direct retainer may originate in the guide plane region, a line angle preparation would weaken either or both components of the clasp assembly.

A guide plane should be located on the proximal surface of abutment adjacent to an edentulous area. However, excess torquing is inevitable if the guide planes squarely facing each other on a lone standing abutment adjacent to an extension area are used (Fig. 10.17).

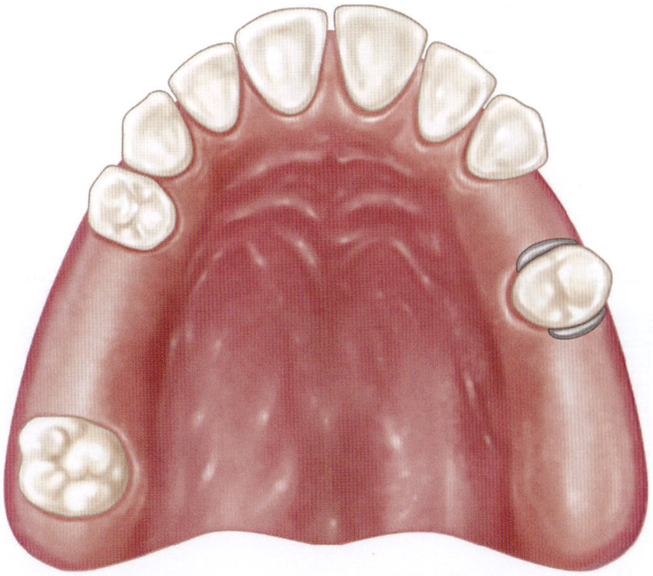

Fig. 10.17 Guiding planes squarely facing each other should not be prepared on a lone standing abutment. Minor connectors of the framework *(gray areas)* would place undue strain on the abutment when the denture is rotated vertically, either superiorly or inferiorly.

Indirect Retainers

An indirect retainer must be placed as far anterior from the fulcrum line as adequate tooth support permits if it is to function with the direct retainer to restrict movement of a distal extension base away from the basal seat tissues. The indirect retainer must be placed on a rest seat prepared in an abutment tooth that is capable of withstanding the forces placed on it. An indirect retainer cannot function effectively on an inclined tooth surface nor can a single weak incisor tooth be used for this purpose. A canine or premolar tooth should be used for the support of an indirect retainer, and the rest seat must be prepared with as much care as is given any other rest seat. An incisal rest or a lingual rest may be used on an anterior tooth, provided that a definite seat can be obtained in sound enamel or on a suitable restoration.

A second purpose that indirect retainers serve in RPD design is that of support for major connectors. A long lingual bar or an anterior palatal major connector is thereby prevented from settling into the tissues. Even without the need for indirect retention, provision for such auxiliary support is sometimes indicated.

Contrary to common use, a lingual plate does not in itself act as an indirect retainer. However, when used with a rest seat, the lingual plate acts as an indirect retainer. Because they are located on inclined tooth surfaces, without rest seats, they have the potential to serve more as orthodontic appliances than as support for RPDs. When a lingual plate or a cingulum bar is used, terminal rests should always be provided at either end to stabilize the denture and to prevent orthodontic movement of the teeth contacted. Such terminal rests may function as indirect retainers, but they would function equally well in that capacity without the continuous bar retainer or lingual plate.

SYSTEMATIC APPROACH TO REMOVABLE PARTIAL DENTURE DESIGN

The following section will cover each of the four classifications of RPDs and their recommended designs. The sequence will be as follows: Kennedy Class III, I, II, and IV.

In Table 10.1, examples are provided as a design baseline for the most common tooth loss distributions—Kennedy Class I, II, III, and IV.

TABLE 10.1 Examples of Systematic Approach to Design

	Support	Major Connector	Bracing/Stability	Retention
Class I				
Maxilla	Occlusal rest Cingulum rest Denture base palate (as needed)	AP palatal strap Full palate	Guide planes Indirect retainers Reciprocal clasp Palatal plating	RPI, RPA Combination clasp
Mandible	Occlusal rest Cingulum rest Denture base (selective pressure)	Lingual bar Lingual plate	Guide planes Indirect retainers Reciprocal clasp Lingual plating	RPI, RPA Combination clasp
Class II				
Maxilla	Occlusal rest Cingulum rest Denture base palate (uncommon)	AP palatal strap Horseshoe Full palate (uncommon)	Guide planes Indirect retainer Reciprocal clasp Palatal plating	RPI, RPA (DE side)Combination clasp (DE side) Embrasure clasp (dentate side) Circumferential clasp (dentate side)
Mandible	Occlusal rest Cingulum rest Denture base (selective pressure)	Lingual bar Lingual plate	Guide planes Indirect retainers Reciprocal clasp Lingual plating	RPI, RPA (DE side)Combination clasp (DE side) Embrasure clasp (dentate side) Circumferential clasp (dentate side)
Class III				
Maxilla	Cingulum rest Occlusal rest	Palatal strap Palatal bar	Guide planes Reciprocal clasp	Circumferential clasp I-bar clasp
Mandible	Cingulum rest Occlusal rest	Lingual bar	Guide planes Reciprocal clasp	Circumferential clasp I-bar clasp
Class IV				
Maxilla	Occlusal rest Cingulum rest Denture base palate	AP palatal strap Horseshoe Full palate	Guide planes Indirect retainer Reciprocal clasp Palatal plating	RPI, RPA (extension base type) Combination clasp (extension base type) Circumferential clasp, I-bar (bounded saddle type) Embrasure clasp, twin-flex (high esthetic requirement)
Mandible	Occlusal rest Cingulum rest Denture base	Lingual bar Lingual plate	Guide planes Indirect retainers Reciprocal clasp Lingual plating	RPI, RPA (extension base type) Combination clasp (extension base type) Circumferential clasp, I-bar (bounded saddle type) Embrasure clasp, twin-flex (high esthetic requirement)

RPA, Rest, proximal plate, Akers; *RPI*, Rest, proximal plate, and I-bar; *DE*, Distal Ex tension side.

Kennedy Class III Removable Partial Dentures

The Kennedy Class III RPD (Fig. 10.18), entirely tooth supported, may be made to fit the prepared surfaces of the anatomic form of the teeth and surrounding structures. It does not require an impression of the ridge tissues in function nor does it require indirect retention. Occlusally approaching cast circumferential clasps are the simplest and most used retentive clasp. Gingivally approaching bar-type clasps may be used in cases where esthetics are a concern if there is sufficient vestibular depth as well and no soft tissue undercuts associated with the abutment tooth. Rest seats are usually placed adjacent to the edentulous areas unless occlusal contacts or tooth angulation dictate a different position. Unless the need for later relining is anticipated, as in the situation of recently extracted teeth, the denture base may be made of metal, which offers several advantages.

Kennedy Class I Removable Partial Dentures

The Kennedy Class I, bilateral distal extension RPD differs from Kennedy Class III RPD because it lacks posterior tooth–borne support and retention. Thus this type of RPD derives most of its support from the edentulous ridge (see Fig. 10.2). The mucosa can present with varying levels of compressibility, which allows the extension base to move tissue ward upon occlusal load. Moreover, the lack of retentive clasps in the posterior region allows the extension base to move in an occlusal direction upon chewing of sticky foods or under the effects of border tissues. Both occlusal and tissue-ward movements of the extension base occur regularly during function in a rotational movement around the fulcrum line (Fig. 10.19).

Tissues that demonstrate significant compressibility may result in potential movement if a Kennedy Class I RPD is made to anatomic ridge form as it cannot provide uniform and adequate support. Thus an impression technique that will record the supporting structure in their supporting state is needed when dealing with compressible tissues.

Kennedy Class II Removable Partial Dentures

The Kennedy Class II RPD (Figs. 10.20 and 10.21) is a combination of tissue-supported and tooth-supported restorations. Due to the presence of the distal extension base, this RPD exhibits movement around the fulcrum line, which necessitates the use of indirect retention and stress-breaking clasp assemblies. In cases where the soft tissue exhibits excessive compressibility, the RPD must have adequate tissue support. Indirect retention must be provided; however, occasionally the anterior abutment on the tooth-supported side will satisfy this requirement. If additional indirect retention is needed, provisions must be made for it.

In cases, with modification spaces, on the anterior abutment of the tooth-supported side, a wrought-wire clasp design like the combination clasp assembly should be used because it may reduce the application of torque on the abutment tooth adjacent to the distal extension (see Fig. 10.10). The use of a cast circumferential clasp engaging a mesiobuccal undercut on the anterior abutment of the tooth-supported modification space may result in a Class I lever–like action if the abutment teeth have not been properly prepared and/or if tissue support from the extension base area is not adequate. Should the bar-type retainer be contraindicated because of a severe tissue undercut or the existence of only a mesiobuccal undercut on the anterior abutment, then a combination direct retainer with the retentive arm made of tapered wrought wire should be used. A thorough understanding of the advantages and disadvantages of various clasp designs is necessary in determining the type of direct retainer that is to be used for each abutment tooth.

Steps included in the fabrication of the Kennedy Class II RPD closely follow those used with the Kennedy Class I RPD, except that the distal extension base is usually made of an acrylic-resin material so that it may be relined, whereas the base for any tooth-supported area can be made of metal. This is permissible because the residual ridge beneath tooth-supported bases is not called on to provide support for the denture, and later rebasing is not as likely to be necessary.

Kennedy Class IV Removable Partial Dentures

Anterior spaces should be restored with a fixed restoration whenever possible; however, situations arise in which it is preferable to restore the space with an RPD. This can include the presence of a significant anterior defect, which requires the recreation of a significant amount of hard and soft tissue by the prosthesis. Patients might also lack the bone to support an implant restoration, or abutment teeth may not have sufficient bone support to support a fixed partial denture. Moreover, some patients might lack the manual dexterity to perform the hygiene

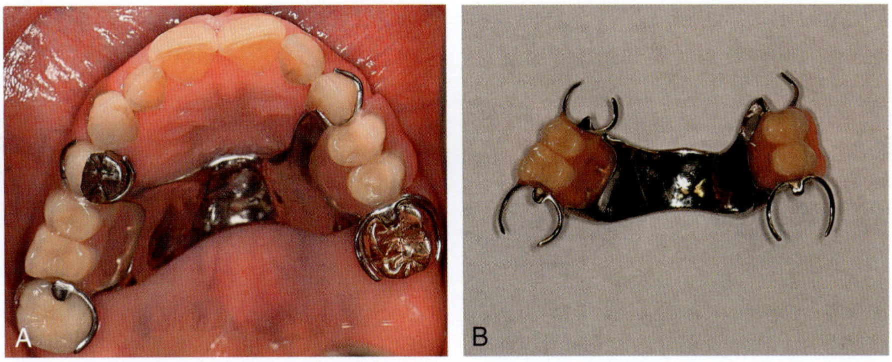

Fig. 10.18 A typical Kennedy Class III, modification I, removable partial denture with cast circumferential clasps. (Courtesy of Ahmed Mahrous Copyright © 2024. All rights reserved.)

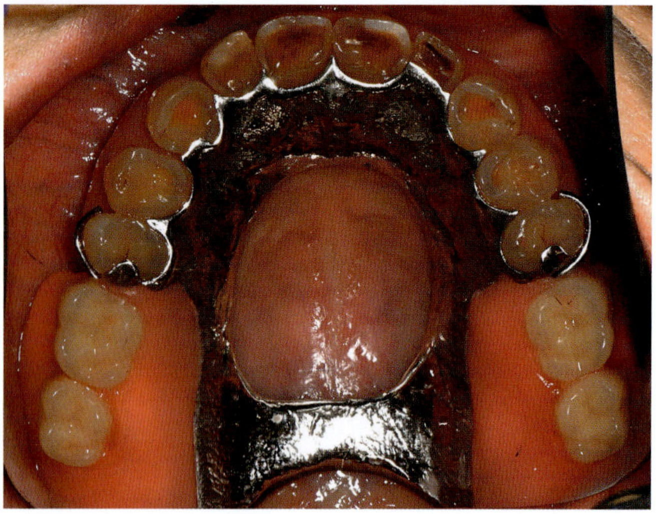

Fig. 10.19 Removable partial denture framework in a maxillary Kennedy Class I arch with wrought-wire clasps. (Courtesy of Ahmed Mahrous)

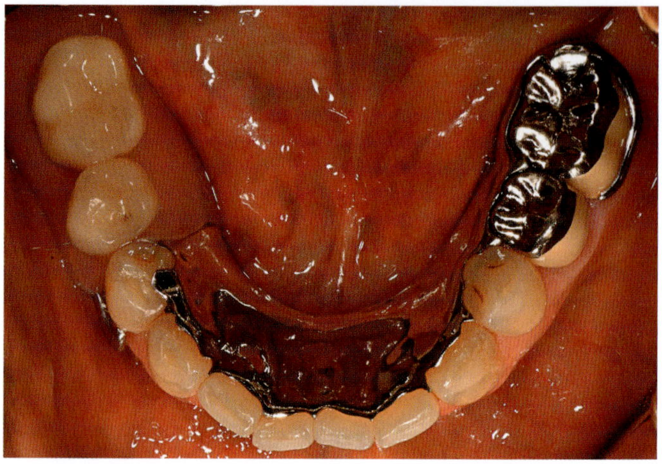

Fig. 10.21 Mandibular Class II removable partial denture. A stress-breaking rest, proximal plate, and I-bar clasp assembly is used on the mandibular right first premolar. A cast circumferential clasp was used on the mandibular left first molar. ()

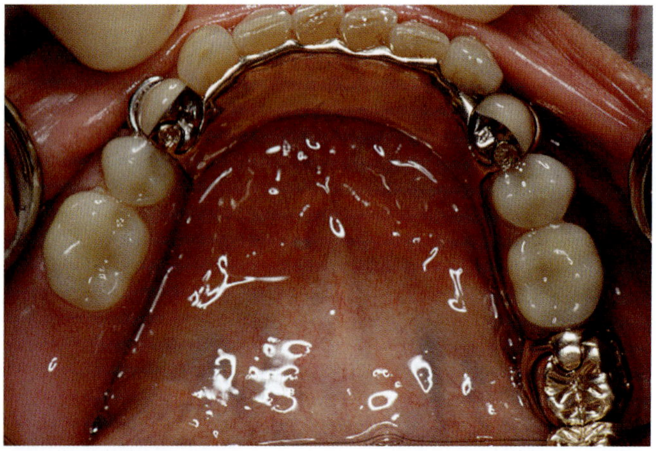

Fig. 10.20 Mandibular Class II, modification 1, removable partial denture with distal extension base. Wrought-wire clasp arms are used on both premolar abutment; this is especially important on the right first premolar to counteract as an effective stress-breaking mechanism. The rest present on the right first premolar also functions as an indirect retainer.

procedures necessary with a fixed partial denture. Last, cost may be a deterrent for some patients.

Kennedy Class IV RPDs are unique in their approach because they can behave as either a bounded type of RPD like Kennedy Class III or an extension base RPD like Kennedy Class I and II. The difference in behavior depends on the following factors:

- The curvature of the arch: Patient arches can be ovoid, tapered, or square. When missing teeth are in the anterior portion of the curvature as they are in the Kennedy Class IV partially edentulous case, the shape of the arch determines the anteroposterior position of the denture base relative to the remaining teeth. If the denture base exists anterior to the remaining teeth, it tends to create a lever arm similar to the ones seen in a distal extension base RPD. Conversely, if the denture base remains mostly at the same anteroposterior position as the existing teeth, that lever arm effect is diminished. A square arch typically allows the denture base to be in line with the remaining teeth and produces little lever arm effect. An ovoid arch would create a moderate lever arm and a tapered arch creates the most substantial lever arm (Fig. 10.22).
- Length of the span: The longer the span, the longer the extension base must be and consequently the longer the lever arm is. This effect is compounded by the shape of the arch.
- Compressibility of the ridge: Like extension base RPDs, Kennedy Class IV cases with a significantly compressible ridge will result in more tissue-ward movement upon occlusal load.
- Amount of load applied: The movement of the anterior extension base increases with an increase in applied load.

If a Kennedy Class IV RPD exhibits a minimal lever arm, the RPD case can be designed much like a tooth-bounded Kennedy Class III case. However, if the Kennedy Class IV RPD exhibits a significant lever arm, then design elements for extension base RPDs like stress breaking and indirect retention should be considered. Because the extension base in the Kennedy Class IV RPD exists anterior to the remaining teeth instead of posterior to the remaining teeth, as is the case in previously discussed extension base–type RPDs (Kennedy Class I and II cases), some adaptations will need to be made to apply extension base design concepts to the Kennedy Class IV configuration (Fig. 10.23).

The most noticeable difference is the location of the fulcrum line, in a Kennedy Class IV case with a lever arm in the location of the fulcrum line. The fulcrum line exists between the two most anterior rests instead of between the two most posterior rests in Kennedy Class I and II cases. Consequently the RPA and RPI clasps will now need to have distal rests and not mesial rests in order to provide stress-breaking action Hyperlink video 10-24. (Fig. 10.24, (Video 10.24). Last, indirect retainers will not exist posterior to the fulcrum line. In most situations, rests that are part of clasp assemblies used on posterior abutments provide indirect retention and no additional rest seats are needed (Fig. 10.25).

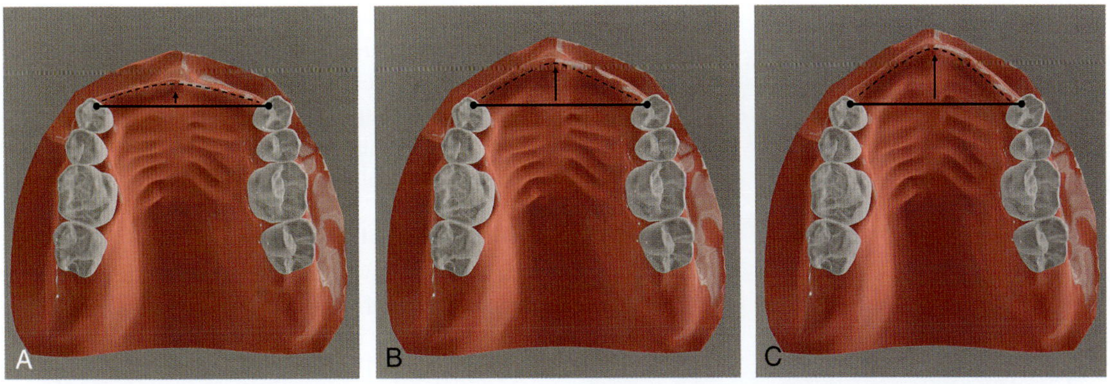

Fig. 10.22 A, The square arch typically allows the denture base to be in line with the remaining teeth and produces little lever arm effect. **B,** An ovoid arch would create a moderate lever arm. **C,** A tapered arch creates the most substantial lever arm. (Courtesy of Ahmed Mahrous Copyright © 2024. All rights reserved.)

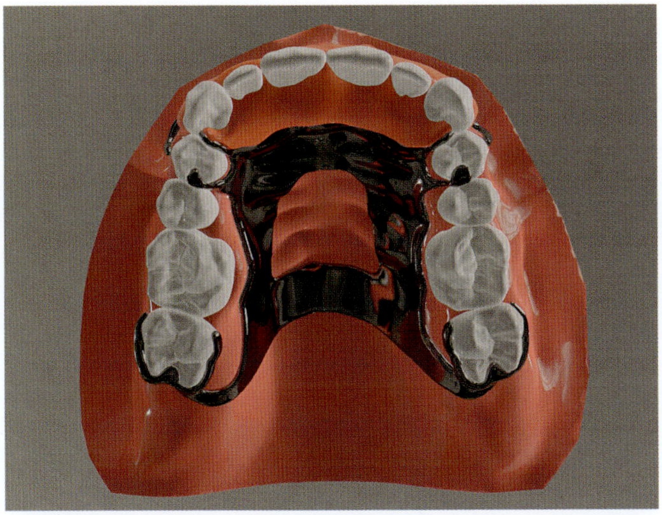

Fig. 10.23 A rest, proximal plate, and I-bar clasp used on the anterior abutments of the Kennedy Class IV configuration. In this case the rest is placed on the distal side of the first premolars instead of the mesial side as the extension base now exists on the anterior side of the arch. (Courtesy of Ahmed Mahrous Copyright © 2024. All rights reserved.)

It is important to note that most patients seeking a Kennedy Class IV RPD do so due to the esthetic compromise caused by the lack of anterior teeth. Thus greater emphasis is placed upon creating an esthetic outcome. Some of the tactics that could be employed to provide an esthetic outcome in Kennedy Class IV cases are the following:

- Using properly contoured flanges: Contouring the flanges of the denture base so that they blend with the natural anatomy of the patient could effectively camouflage the flange into the tissue (Fig. 10.26).
- Using esthetic clasp options: Gingivally approaching clasp arms generally provide better esthetics than occlusally approaching clasp arms and should be used in areas where the anterior teeth are being replaced (Fig. 10.27).
- Using alternative retentive mechanisms: The use of attachments and implants adjacent to the abutment tooth allows for the removal of the retentive clasp and provides a more esthetic outcome for the Kennedy Class IV RPD (Fig. 10.28).
- Moving clasping to distal abutment teeth: In order to provide a more esthetic outcome, embrasure clasps may be used on distally located abutments instead of on the abutments directly adjacent to the edentulous span. While biomechanically inferior in the distribution of retentive components, this configuration allows for the preservation of the retentive capacity of the direct retainers but with less esthetic compromise (see Fig. 10.27).
- Esthetic clasp options like the "twin-flex" clasp can be used (Fig. 10.29). "Twin-flex" clasps engage a 0.01-inch mesial undercut on the abutment tooth. They are soldered WW

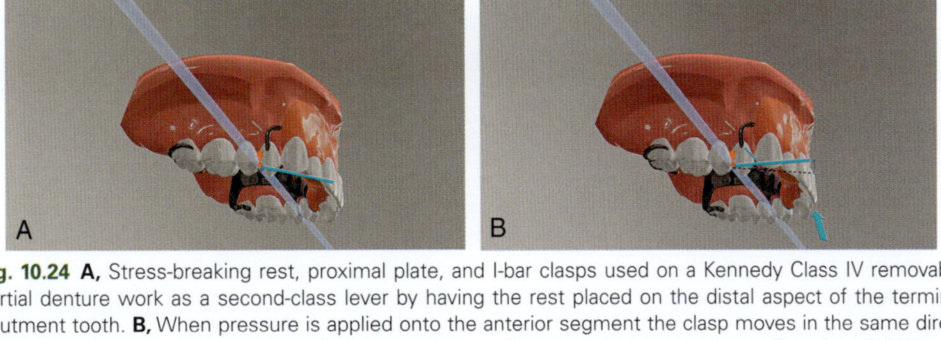

Fig. 10.24 A, Stress-breaking rest, proximal plate, and I-bar clasps used on a Kennedy Class IV removable partial denture work as a second-class lever by having the rest placed on the distal aspect of the terminal abutment tooth. **B,** When pressure is applied onto the anterior segment the clasp moves in the same direction as the effort arm and disengage from the undercut. (Courtesy of Ahmed Mahrous Copyright © 2024. All rights reserved.)

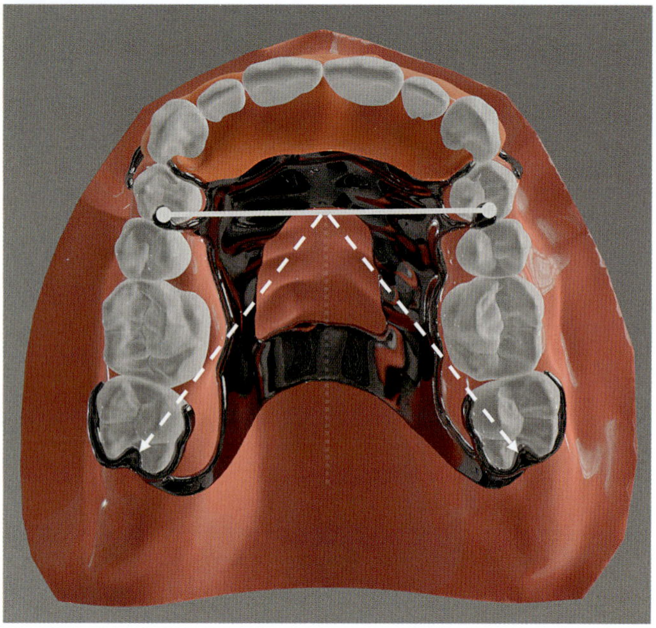

Fig. 10.25 The occlusal rests that are part of the clasp assemblies on the left and right maxillary second molars act as an indirect retainer. (Courtesy of Ahmed Mahrous Copyright © 2024. All rights reserved.)

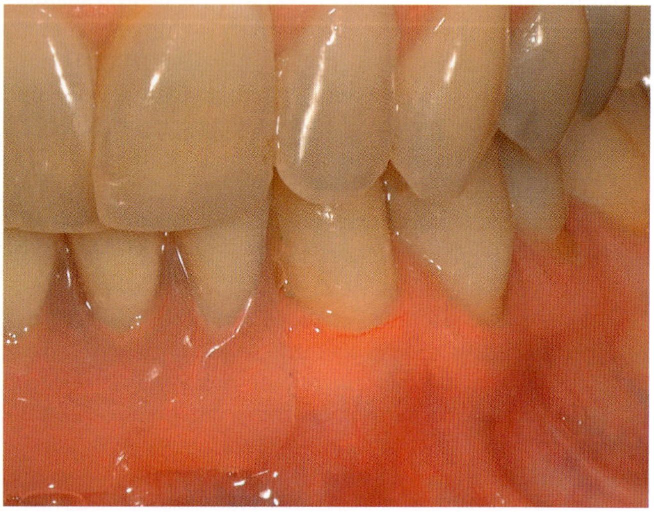

Fig. 10.26 Modifying a flange on a Kennedy Class IV or any other classification with an anterior modification so that it blends with the surrounding soft tissue. (Courtesy of Ahmed Mahrous Copyright © 2024. All rights reserved.)

under the guide planes of the framework. Twin-flex clasps derive their reciprocation from the proximal contact of the contacting tooth in the arch. When teeth are added to the RPD the clasp is occluded from view and provides a highly esthetic result. This clasp does not provide stress breaking and is difficult to manufacture, adjust, and repair.

Implant Considerations

Implants effectively reduce distal extension movement and can enhance support if placed at the distal-most tooth position. Such use of an implant changes the mechanics of a Kennedy Class I or Class II distal extension to a Kennedy Class III as both ends of the edentulous span are supported (Fig. 10.30).

If the implant is placed adjacent to the anterior tooth in an edentulous span, it can be used as a primary abutment for retention and avoiding the need of a retentive clasp in the anterior region, which provides an esthetic advantage.

ADDITIONAL CONSIDERATIONS INFLUENCING DESIGN

Every effort should be made to gain the greatest support possible for removable prostheses with the use of abutments bounding edentulous spaces. This will relieve the residual ridges of some of their obligation for support but also may allow the design of the framework to be greatly simplified. To this end, use of splint bars and overlay dentures should be considered.

Use of a Splint Bar for Denture Support

When several missing anterior teeth need to be replaced by the RPD rather than by fixed restorations and when the edentulous span is too large to ensure adequate support from the adjacent teeth, an anterior splint bar with or without a clip attachment may be considered (Fig. 10.31). An anterior splint bar may be attached to the adjacent abutment teeth in such a manner that fixed splinting of the abutment teeth results, with a smooth, contoured bar resting lightly on the gingival tissues to support the RPD. As with any fixed partial denture, the type of abutment retainers and the decision to use multiple abutments will depend on the length of the span and the available support and stability of the teeth being used as abutments. Regardless of the type of abutment retainers used, the connecting bar may be cast

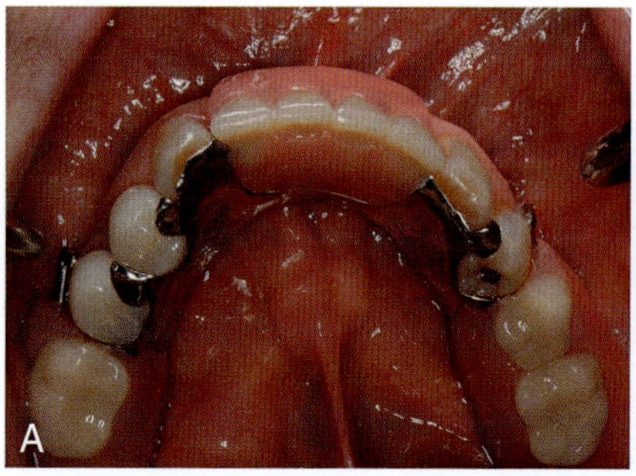

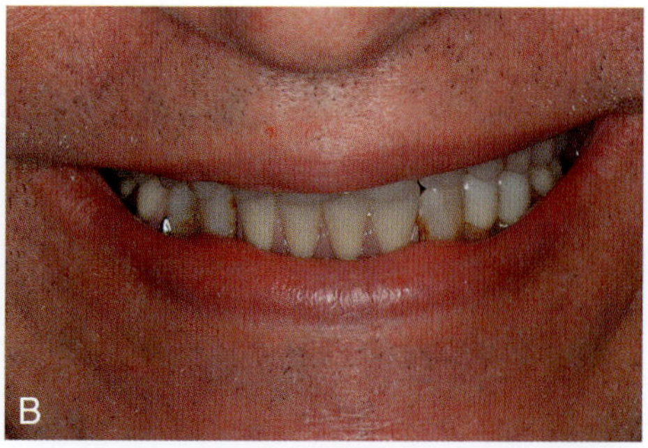

Fig. 10.27 **A,** This Kennedy Class I, modification 1, removable partial denture was designed with rest, proximal plate, and I-bar clasp assemblies on the distal abutments. No clasps were made to engage the anterior-most abutments (canines). **B,** The infrabulge I-bar clasps remain relatively hidden out of view. This is aided by placing the clasps only on the posterior abutments and avoiding the use of clasps on the anterior abutments.

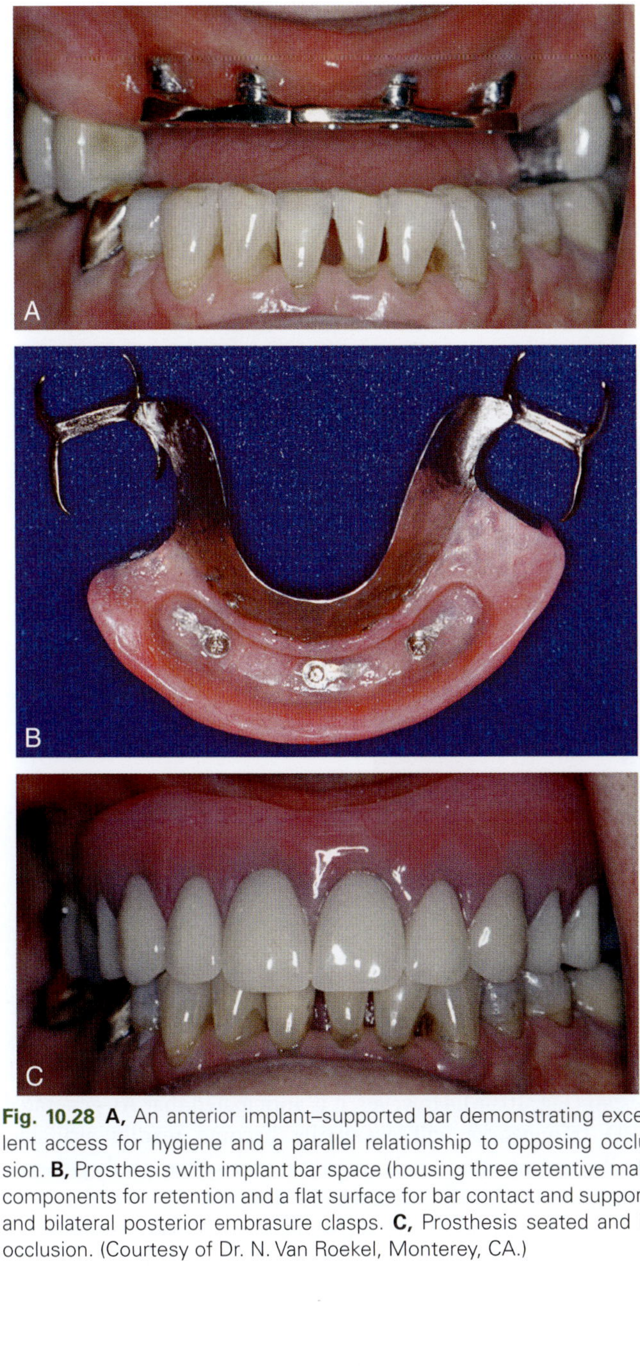

Fig. 10.28 **A,** An anterior implant–supported bar demonstrating excellent access for hygiene and a parallel relationship to opposing occlusion. **B,** Prosthesis with implant bar space (housing three retentive male components for retention and a flat surface for bar contact and support) and bilateral posterior embrasure clasps. **C,** Prosthesis seated and in occlusion. (Courtesy of Dr. N. Van Roekel, Monterey, CA.)

of a rigid alloy, or a commercially available bar may be used and cast to the abutments or attached to the abutments by soldering.

The length of the span influences the size of a splint bar. Long spans require more rigid bars (10 gauge) than short spans (13 gauge). If the bar is to be soldered, it is best that recesses be formed in the proximal surfaces of the abutments and that the connecting bar, which rests lightly on the tissues, be cast or made to fit into these recesses and then attached by soldering.

Because of the greater rigidity of chromium-cobalt alloys, the splint bar is preferably cast in one of these materials and then is attached to the abutments by soldering. The complete assembly (abutments and connecting bar) is then cemented permanently to the abutment teeth, in the same way as for a fixed partial denture. The impression for the RPD is then made, and a master cast is obtained that accurately reproduces the contours of the abutments and the splint bar. The denture framework then is made to fit the abutments and the bar by extending the major connector or minor connectors to cover and rest upon the splint bar. Retention for the attachment of a resin base, or any other acceptable means of attaching the replaced anterior teeth, is incorporated into the denture design. In those situations, wherein the RPD will be tooth supported, the splint bar may be curved to follow the crest of the residual ridge. However, in a distal extension situation, because of the vertical rotation of the denture, caution must be exercised to form the splint bar so that excessive torque will not accrue to its supporting abutments (Fig. 10.32). The proximal contours of abutments adjacent to splint bars should be parallel to the path of placement. This serves three purposes: (1) it permits a desirable arrangement of artificial teeth, (2) it aids in resisting horizontal rotation of the restoration, and (3) these components act as guide planes to direct the RPD to and from its terminal position.

The splint bar must be positioned anteroposteriorly just lingual to the residual ridge to allow an esthetic arrangement of artificial teeth. The resulting RPD offers esthetic advantages of removable anterior replacements and positive support, retention, and stability from the underlying splint bar (see Fig. 10.32).

Internal Clip Attachment

The internal clip attachment differs from the splint bar in that the internal clip attachment provides both support and retention from the connecting bar. Several preformed connecting bars are commercially available in plastic patterns. These can be customized for length and cast in the metal alloy of choice. Internal clip attachments are also commercially available in

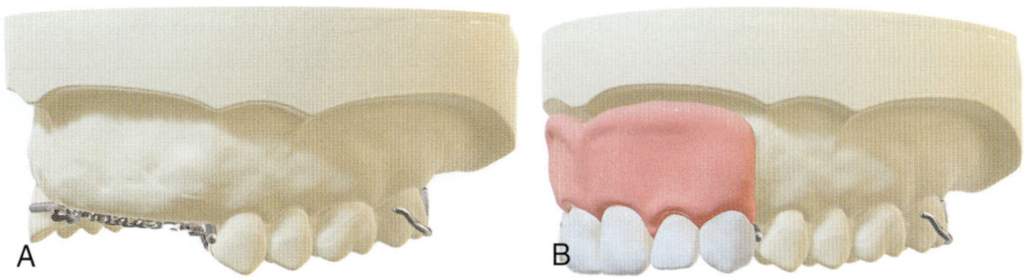

Fig. 10.29 **A,** A twin-flex clasp is a soldered piece of wrought wire that is soldered onto the framework under the proximal plate. It engages a 0.01-inch undercut on the mesial surface of the abutment tooth. **B,** When the artificial teeth are placed, the clasp is shielded from view and the esthetic result. (Courtesy of Ahmed Mahrous Copyright © 2024. All rights reserved.)

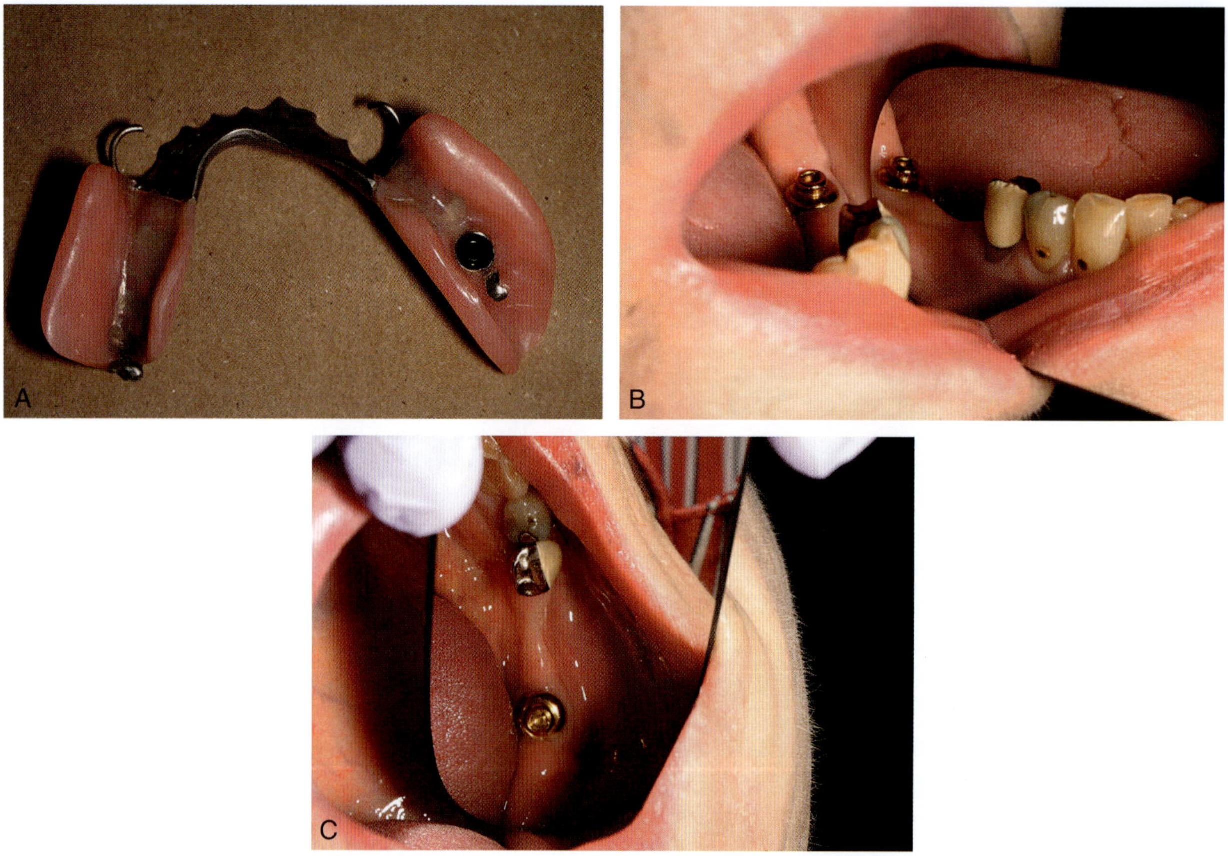

Fig. 10.30 A, Intaglio surface view of a locator retentive element in the posterior aspect of a distal extension base of a mandibular removable partial denture. **B,** Mirror view of the locator attachment on an implant in the distal mandible. The attachment will provide support and retention for the distal extension removable partial denture. **C,** Occlusal view of the locator attachment.

various metal alloys and durable nylon. When a custom-made connecting bar and clip are fabricated, the bar should be cast from 10- or 13-gauge sprue wax.

Overlay Abutment as Support for a Denture Base

Overlay RPDs are a versatile type of RPD that by definition covers parts of or the entirety of the occlusal surface of the abutment teeth (Fig. 10.33). In many instances, it is possible to salvage the roots and a portion of the crown of a badly broken-down molar through endodontic treatment. A periodontally involved molar, otherwise indicated for extraction, sometimes may be salvaged by periodontal and endodontic treatment accompanied by reduction of the clinical crown (decoronation) almost level with the gingival tissues. Overlay RPDs can also be used in cases where the absence of multiple occlusal stops leads to a loss of vertical dimension and occlusal plane discrepancies (Figs. 10.34 and 10.35). The overlay RPD can be used as a conservative alternative to more invasive treatments like complete dentures.

Automated framework design software

The use of artificial intelligence (AI) and automated design software for many aspects of dentistry has seen tremendous growth and adoption over the past decade. One area that has started to appear on the scene is automated RPD design. Currently there are only a few software systems with automated RPD framework design (Fig. 10.36). However, it is anticipated that AI-generated RPD frameworks will eventually become readily available. While current automated design software systems only generate a diagram of the RPD framework design similar to that used in a lab authorization, it is expected that software systems will eventually be able to generate 3D model design proposals ready for milling or printing with the multitude of currently available computer-aided manufacturing techniques. When considering using such automated designers, it is of utmost importance to adhere to the following guidelines.

1. Use of any automated RPD designer should only be used as an auxiliary aid to the dentist. It is impossible for any artificial algorithm to fully consider all the intricacies of RPD treatment. It is of utmost importance that the dentist makes decisions based on thorough understanding of the subject matter and considers all factors necessary to make a comprehensive treatment plan. The automated designer should only provide suggestions to RPD designs. The dentist should maintain ultimate design decision-making by allowing manual override of any design component.
2. The automated designer chosen should faithfully follow well-accepted philosophies of RPD framework design and evidence-based dentistry whenever possible.

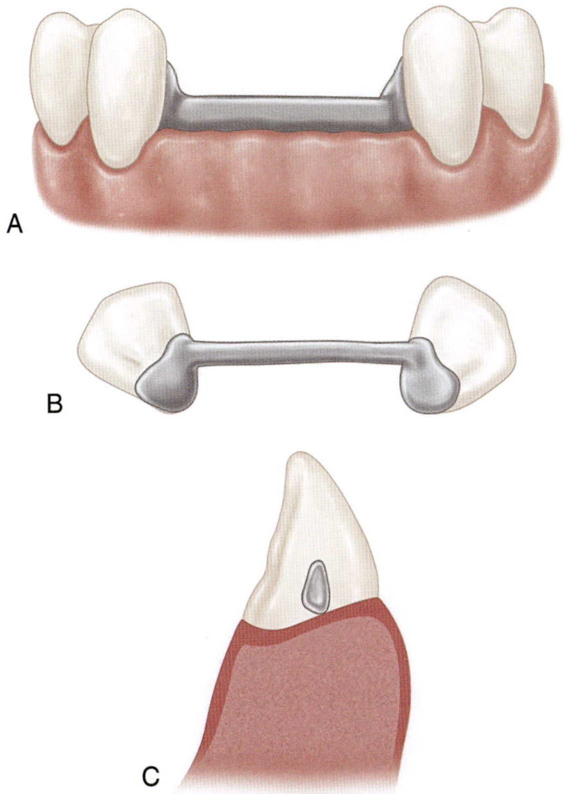

Fig. 10.31 **A,** Insofar as is possible, the splint bar should be round or ovoid. Provisions must be made in the construction and location of the bar so that dental floss may be threaded underneath the bar to allow proper cleaning by the patient. **B,** As viewed from above, the bar is in a straight line between abutments. This is especially critical for distal extension removable partial dentures (RPDs) to avoid excess torque on abutments as the denture rotates in function. **C,** Sagittal section through the bar demonstrates the rounded form of the bar making point contact with the residual ridge. The entire tissue surface of the bar is easily accessible for cleaning with dental floss. A pear-shaped bar *(in cross section)* permits rotation of the RPD without appreciable resistance or torque.

3. The automated design algorithm should consider the relevant findings that might influence the final design. Examples of such findings include the depth and location of undercuts, occlusal contacts, soft tissue undercuts, vestibular depth, and periodontal status.
4. The automated designer should provide sufficient options to address a multitude of situations and combinations of missing teeth encountered with RPD patients while maintaining the final decision to the dentist.
5. The automated designer should output clearly legible diagrams that can be interpreted by the dentist or laboratory technician.

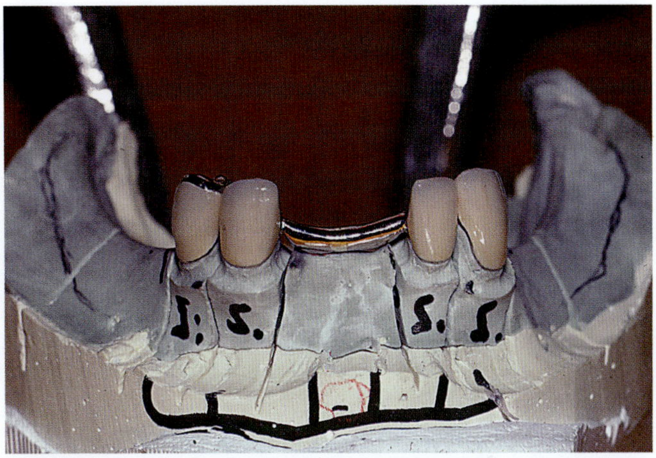

Fig. 10.32 Lower canines splinted together with a splint bar. The longevity of these teeth is greatly enhanced by splinting. Tissue surfaces are minimally contacted by the rounded form of the lower portion of the bar. The anterior and posterior slopes of the splint bar must be compatible with the path of placement of the denture. Floss will be used by the patient to clean the inferior portion of the splint bar.

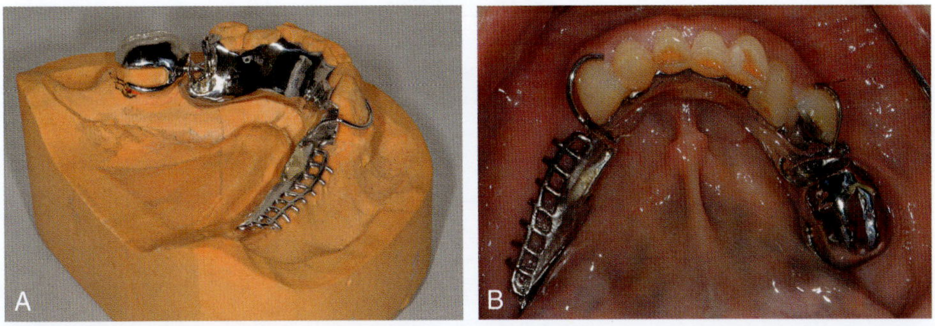

Fig. 10.33 **A,** An overlay partial denture designed to cover the gold crown on the mandibular left first molar tooth. **B,** When fully seated intraorally. wrought-wire clasps are used as stress-breaking claps on the anterior abutments. (Courtesy of Ahmed Mahrous Copyright ©. All rights reserved.)

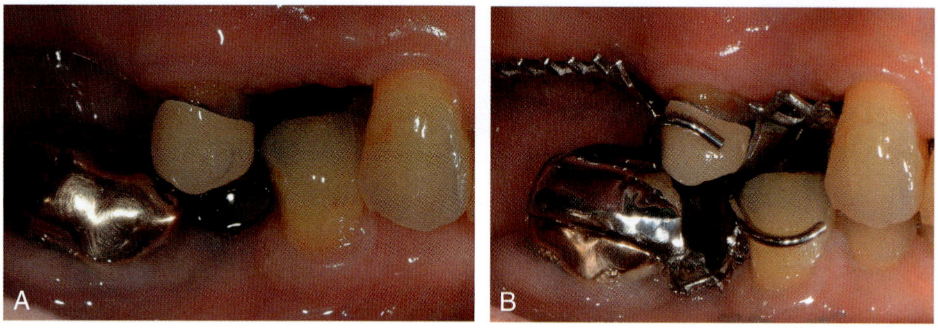

Fig. 10.34 **A,** Prolonged loss of teeth caused migration of the teeth and loss of vertical dimension. Creating insufficient space for any tooth restoration without more extensive treatment. **B,** The overlay partial denture in place increased the vertical dimension and creates adequate restorative space. (Courtesy of Mahrous Copyright © 2024. All rights reserved.)

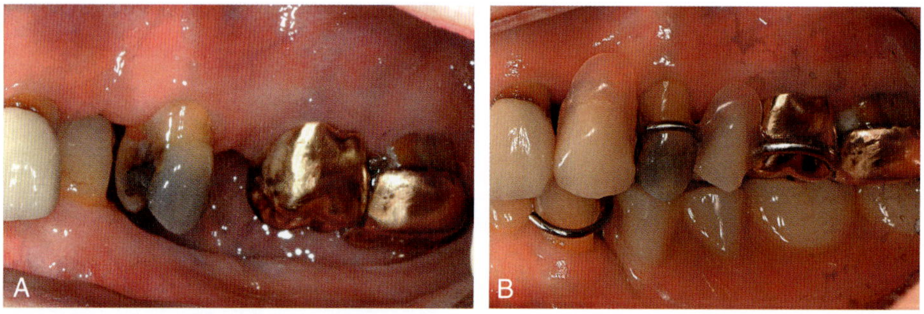

Fig. 10.35 **A,** Prolonged loss of teeth and absence of occlusal stops create a difficult restorative situation. **B,** Vertical dimension restored and the occlusal plane reestablished. (Courtesy of Ahmed Mahrous Copyright © 2024. All rights reserved.)

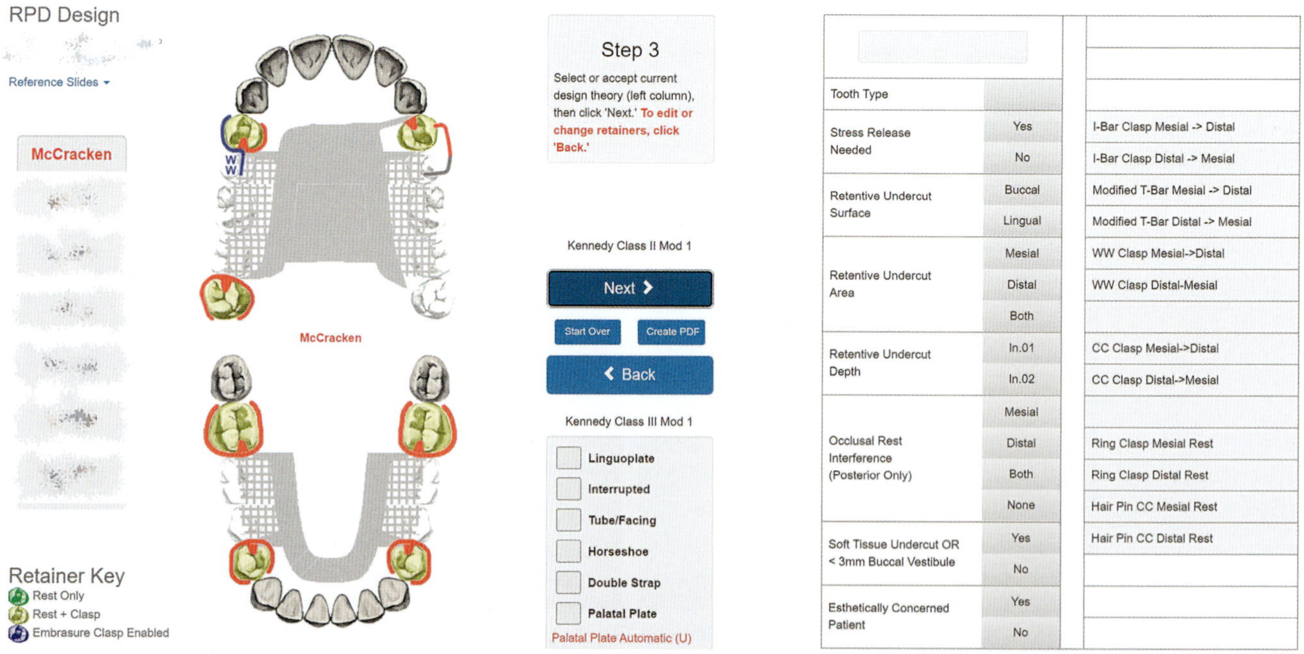

Fig. 10.36 "AiDental" is an online, algorithm-based automated removable partial denture (RPD) design software that can generate philosophy-specific RPD designs. AiDental can be used as a reference for clasp selection. Any automated clasp selector should have strict criteria and guidelines for clasp selection, and ultimate control should be left to the practicing dentist regarding clasp selection. Automated design software systems like AiDental should consider factors such as tooth type, stress breaking, location and depth of retentive undercuts, occlusal interference, soft tissue interference, and esthetic concern of patients. The algorithm provides a list of compatible clasps for each tooth and provides clear diagrams of all the RPD components with the flexibility of altering and customizing the final design. (Courtesy of Ahmed Mahrous Copyright © 2024. All rights reserved.)

11

Surveying

Ahmed Mahrous and David L. Botsko

CHAPTER OUTLINE

For a removable prosthesis, the necessity for appropriately planned and executed tooth preparation, followed by verification of a well-fitting prosthesis that engages the teeth as designed, is important. As was mentioned in Chapter 7, a dental surveyor is essential to the planning, execution, and verification of mouth modifications for a removable partial denture (RPD). Although it does not necessarily affect occlusal rest preparations on abutment teeth, the surveyor is critical for planning modifications of all tooth surfaces that will be involved in support, stabilization, and retention of the prosthesis. In this role, the use of a surveyor to determine the needed mouth preparation is vitally important in helping to provide stable and comfortable removable prostheses.

The primary purpose of surveying is to identify the location of retentive undercuts as well as modifications of oral structures that are necessary to fabricate an RPD that will have a successful prognosis. It is the modification of tooth surfaces to accommodate placement of the component parts of the partial denture in their designated ideal positions on abutment teeth that facilitates this prognosis.

A surveyor can be used to parallel internal rests and intracoronal retainers. With the addition of a handpiece holder, the surveyor can be used to machine internal rests and make the guide plane surfaces of abutment restorations parallel. Digital dentistry has also prompted the development of and ability to virtually use a digital surveyor that simulates the functions of physical surveyors.

TYPES OF SURVEYORS

Physical Surveyors

The Ney surveyor is a commonly used physical surveyor (Fig. 11.1) among others that are available and in use.

The principal parts of the Ney surveyor are as follows:

- Platform on which the base is moved.
- Vertical arm that supports the superstructure.
- Horizontal arm from which the surveying tool suspends.
- Table to which the cast is attached.
- Base on which the table swivels.
- Paralleling tool or guideline marker (this tool contacts the convex surface to be studied in a tangential manner; the relative parallelism of one surface to another may thus be determined; with substitution of a carbon marker, the height of contour may be delineated on the surfaces of the abutment teeth and on areas of interference requiring reduction on blockout).
- Mandrel for holding special tools (Fig. 11.2).

Digital Surveyors

Digital surveyors are available either as part of a dental laboratory design suite program (Fig. 11.3) or as a standalone diagnostic tool (Fig. 11.4). Digital surveyors are designed to analyze intraoral scans and scanned casts in stereolithography (.stl) format. Laboratory-based digital dental surveyors aid the dental

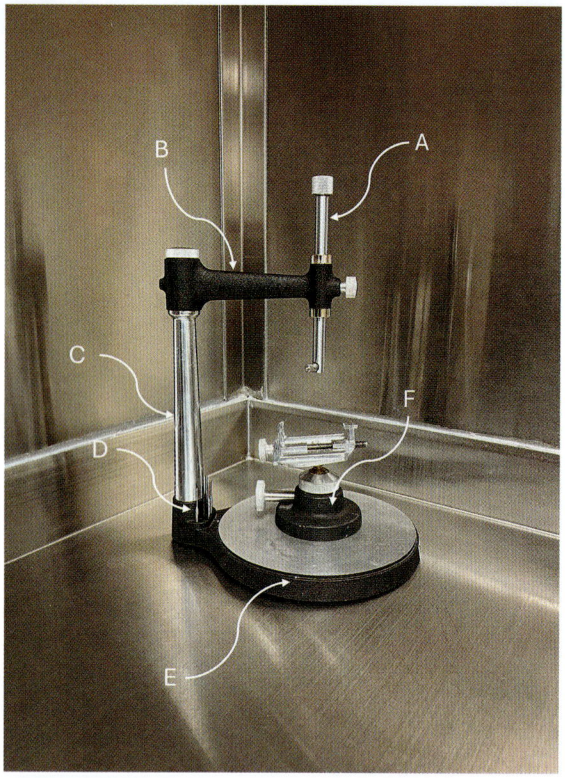

Fig. 11.1 Essential parts of a dental surveyor (Ney Parallelometer, Dentsply Ceramco, Burlington, NJ). **A,**Mandrel.**B,** Horizontal arm. **C,** Vertical arm. **D,** Tools. **E,** Base. **F,** Table and universal joint. (Courtesy of Ahmed Mahrous Copyright © 2024. All rights reserved.)

laboratory technician in fabricating an RPD metal framework following surveying, while diagnostic dental surveyors are designed to aid the dentist in planning the design of the framework. Both systems work in a similar manner by producing graphical representation of the height of contour on teeth and different depths of undercuts.

PURPOSES OF THE SURVEYOR

The surveyor is used for surveying the diagnostic cast, recontouring abutment teeth on the diagnostic cast, contouring wax patterns, measuring a specific depth of undercut, surveying ceramic veneer crowns, placing intracoronal retainers, placing internal rests, machining cast restorations, and surveying and blocking out the master cast.

Surveying the Diagnostic Cast

Surveying the diagnostic cast is essential to effective diagnosis and treatment planning. The objectives are as follows:

1. To determine the most desirable path of placement that eliminates or minimizes interference to placement and removal (Fig. 11.5): The path of placement is the direction in which a restoration moves from the point of initial contact of its rigid parts with the supporting teeth to its terminal resting position, with rests seated and the denture base in contact with the tissues. The path of removal is exactly the reverse because it is the direction of restoration movement from its terminal resting position to the last contact of its rigid parts with the supporting teeth. When the restoration is properly designed to incorporate guide planes, the patient may place and remove the restoration with ease in only one direction. This is possible only because the guide planes contact tooth surfaces appropriately, designed parallel to that path of placement.
2. To identify proximal tooth surfaces that are evaluated to determine the need to be adjusted to be parallel and serve as guide planes during placement and removal.
3. To locate and measure areas of the teeth that may be used for retention.
4. To determine whether teeth and bony areas of interference need to be eliminated surgically or by selection of a different path of placement.
5. To determine the most suitable path of placement that permits locating retainers and artificial teeth that provide the best esthetic advantage.
6. To permit accurate charting of the mouth preparations to be made: This includes the preparation of proximal tooth surfaces to provide guide planes and the reduction of excessive tooth contours to eliminate interference and to permit a more acceptable location of reciprocal and retentive clasp arms. By marking these areas on the diagnostic cast in red, using an undercut gauge to estimate the amount of tooth structure that may safely (without exposing dentin) be removed, and then trimming the marked areas on the stone cast with the surveyor blade, the angulation and extent of tooth reduction may be established before the teeth are prepared in the mouth (Fig. 11.6). With the diagnostic cast on the surveyor at the time of mouth preparation, reduction of tooth contours may be accomplished with acceptable accuracy.
7. To delineate the height of contour on abutment teeth and to locate areas of undesirable tooth undercut that are to be avoided, eliminated, or blocked out: This includes areas of the teeth to be contacted by rigid connectors, the location of nonretentive reciprocal and stabilizing arms, and the location of retentive clasp terminals.
8. To record the cast position in relation to the selected path of placement for future reference: This may be done by locating three dots or parallel lines on the cast, thus establishing the horizontal plane in relation to the vertical arm of the surveyor.

Surveying Ceramic Veneer Crowns

Ceramic veneer crowns are often used to restore abutment teeth on which extracoronal direct retainers will be placed. The surveyor is used to contour all areas of the wax pattern for the veneer crown except the buccal or labial surface. It must be remembered that one of the principal goals in using a porcelain veneer restoration is to develop an esthetic replica of a natural tooth. It is unlikely that the ceramic veneer portion can be fabricated exactly to the form required for the planned placement of retentive clasp arms without some reshaping with stones. Before the final glaze is accomplished, the abutment crowns should be returned to the surveyor on a full arch cast to ensure the correct contour of the veneered portions or

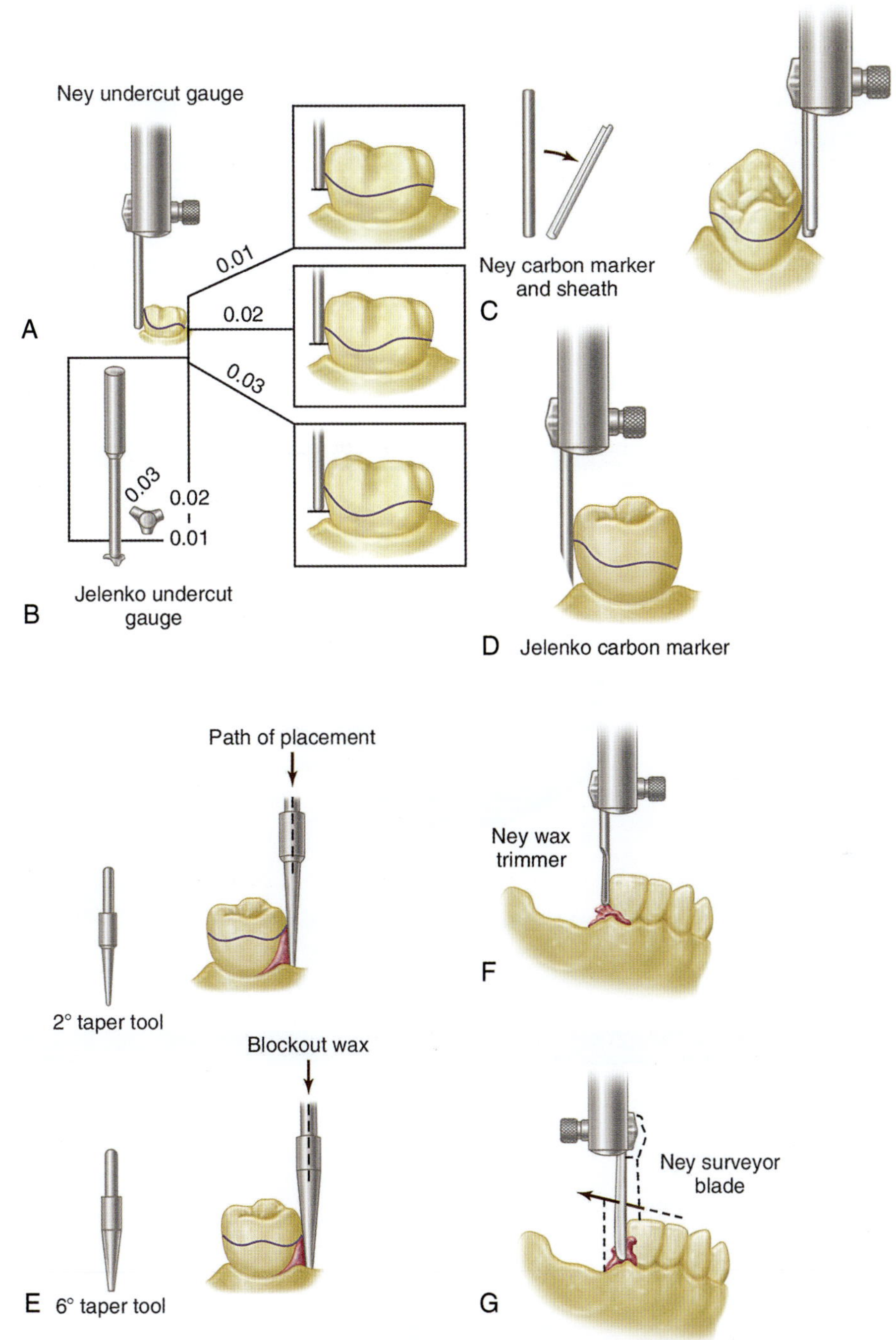

Fig. 11.2 Various tools that may be used with a dental surveyor. **A,** Ney undercut gauges. **B,** Jelenko undercut gauge. **C,** Ney carbon marker with metal reinforcement sheath. **D,** Jelenko carbon marker. **E,** 2° and 6° taper tool used to measure blockout taper. **F,** Ney wax trimmer for paralleling blockout. **G,** Surveying blade used for trimming blockout.

to locate those areas that need recontouring (Fig. 11.7). The final glaze is accomplished only after the crowns have been recontoured.

Surveying Digitally Fabricated Crowns

Milled Zirconia crowns can also be used as abutments for RPDs. However, due to the nature of their fabrication, it is often hard to assess the depth of the undercut produced or the angulation of the guide planes produced unless the crowns are associated with a printed full cast. Like ceramic veneer restorations, milled restorations should be returned to the surveyor on a full arch cast to ensure the correct contour (Fig. 11.8).

Surveying the Master Cast

The purpose of surveying the master cast begins the analysis and begins of the process of framework fabrication, which usually occurs in a dental laboratory. In most cases, the instructions provided by the surveyed diagnostic cast or scan along with a detailed laboratory authorization should be sufficient for the dental laboratory technician to create the desired framework design. However,

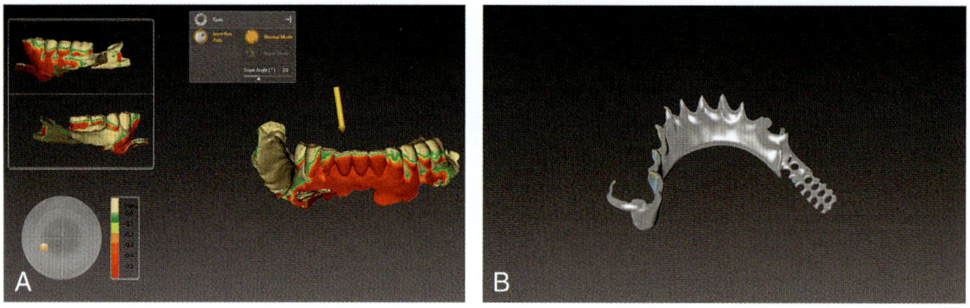

Fig. 11.3 **A,** Digital surveyors are available as part of a dental laboratory design suite. **B,** Such software systems are designed to survey models and transition to design and modeling of the framework afterwards. Such software systems are commonly seen in dental laboratories and some dental schools. (Courtesy of Ahmed Mahrous Copyright © 2024. All rights reserved.)

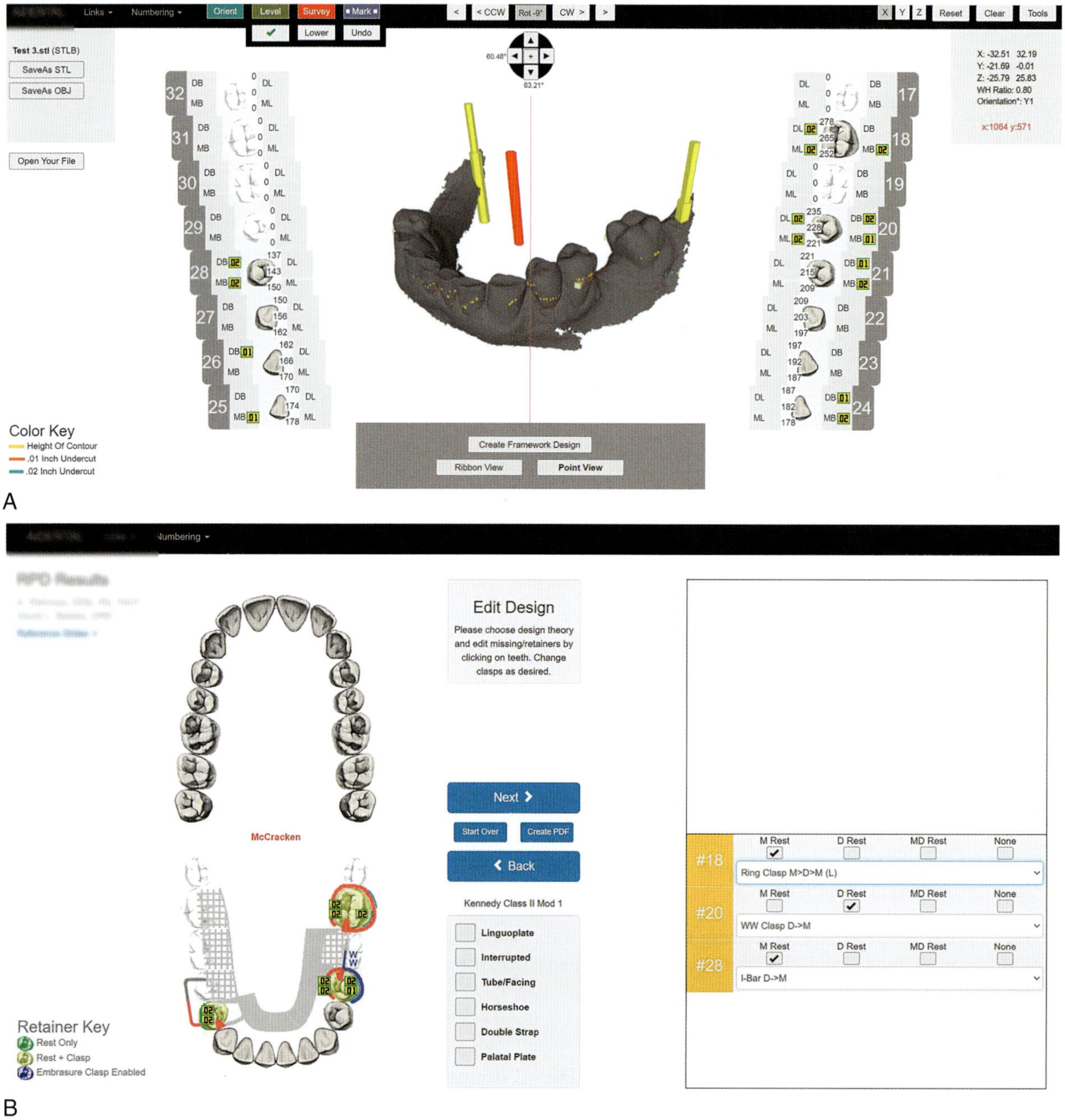

Fig. 11.4 **A,** Diagnostic surveyors available online as a standalone surveying tool. **B,** Such systems allow planning the framework design based on the available undercuts. These software systems are available online to dentists to be used during dental treatment as an alternative to physical surveyors. (Courtesy of Ahmed Mahrous Copyright © 2024. All rights reserved.)

if there is a desire to have more control over the final result, a duplicate or a printed model from a scan may be generated and surveyed and the final design may be drawn on and sent to the dental laboratory. The path of placement, the location of retentive areas, and the location of remaining interference must be known before the final design of the denture framework is completed. The objectives of surveying the master cast are as follows:

1. To select the most suitable path of placement by following mouth preparations that satisfy the requirements of guide planes, retention, noninterference, and esthetics.
2. To permit measurement of retentive areas and to identify the location of clasp terminals in proportion to the flexibility of the clasp arm being used: Flexibility depends on many of the following factors: (1) the alloy used for the clasp, (2) the design and type of clasp, (3) whether its form is round or half-round, (4) whether it is of cast or wrought material, and (5) the length of the clasp arm from its point of origin to its terminal end. Retention depends on (1) the flexibility of the clasp arm, (2) the magnitude of the tooth undercut, and (3) the depth the clasp terminal is placed into this undercut.
3. To locate undesirable undercut areas that will be crossed by rigid parts of the restoration during placement and removal and the areas marked and blocked out with a material such as a blockout wax.
4. To trim blockout material parallel to the path of placement before duplication (Fig. 11.9).

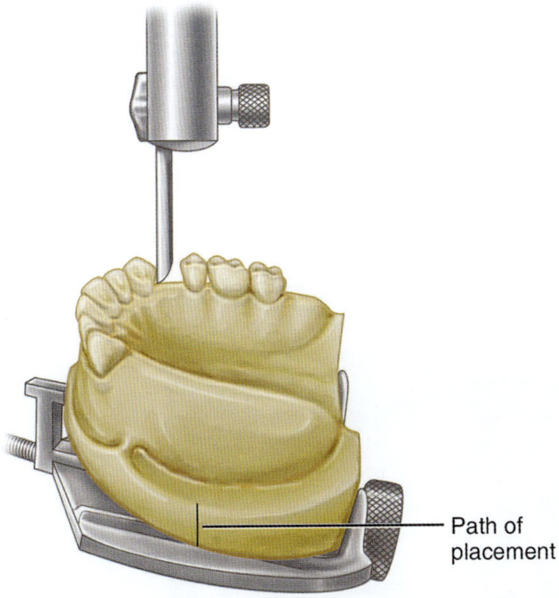

Fig. 11.5 Tilt of the cast on the adjustable table of a surveyor in relation to the vertical arm establishes the path of placement and removal that the removable partial denture will take. All mouth preparations must be made to conform to this determined path of placement, which has been recorded by scoring the base of the cast or by tripoding.

The partial denture must be designed with the following principles in mind: (1) to minimize or mitigate undue stress on abutment teeth beyond their physiologic tolerance, (2) to achieve easy placement and removal by the patient, (3) to resist against reasonable dislodging forces, and (4) to avoid creating an unfavorable appearance. Mouth preparation should therefore be planned in accordance with certain factors that will influence the path of placement and removal.

FACTORS THAT DETERMINE PATH OF PLACEMENT AND REMOVAL

The factors that determine the path of placement and removal are guide planes, retentive areas, interference, and esthetics. Additionally, if an implant is part of the design, its long axis is considered in relation to the path or placement and removal (Fig. 11.10, *B*).

Guide Planes

Proximal tooth surfaces that bear a parallel relationship to one another must be found or must be created to act as guide planes during placement and removal of the prosthesis. Guide planes are necessary to ensure the passage of rigid parts of the

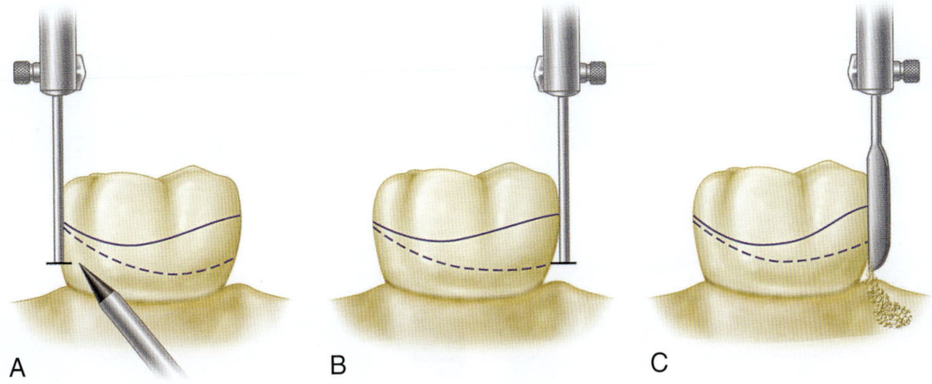

Fig. 11.6 A, *Solid line* represents the height of contour on the abutment at selected orientation of the diagnostic cast to the vertical spindle of the surveyor. *Dotted line* represents the desirable height of contour for optimally locating components of the direct retainer assembly. A 0.01-inch (0.25-mm) undercut gauge is used to mark the location of the tip of the retentive arm of the direct retainer. **B,** By reducing the axial contour of the tooth by only 0.01 inch, the optimum height of contour can be achieved without exposing the dentin. **C,** Stone tooth is trimmed with a surveyor blade to the desired height of contour. The trimmed area is marked with a red pencil and serves as a blueprint for similar recontouring in the mouth. If one can safely assume that the enamel is 1 to 1.5 mm thick in the area of contemplated reduction, only 0.25 mm of enamel is trimmed.

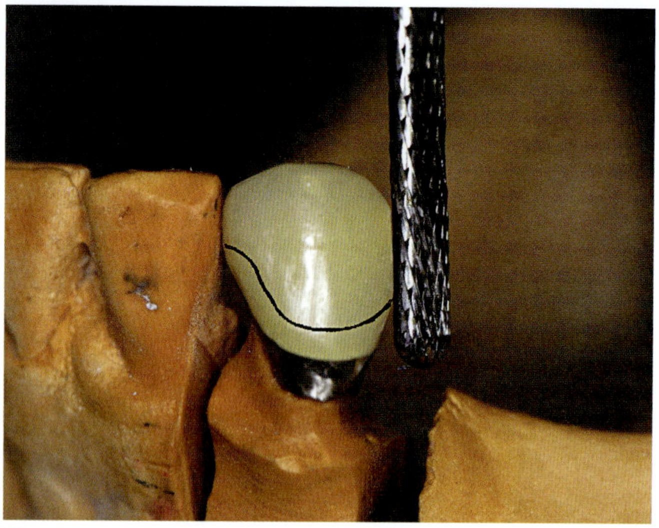

Fig. 11.7 Final glaze has not been placed on the veneer crown and required alterations of surfaces to conform to ideal placement of the retainer *(solid line)* that can be performed by machining. Final glaze is produced only after necessary recontouring is accomplished.

prosthesis past existing areas of interference. Thus the removable partial denture can be easily placed and removed by the patient without strain on the teeth contacted or on the removable partial denture itself and without damage to the underlying soft tissues.

Guide planes are also necessary to ensure predictable clasp assembly function, including retention and stabilization. For a clasp to be retentive, its retentive arm must be forced to flex. Hence, guide planes are necessary to give a positive direction to the movement of the restoration to and from its terminal position.

Retentive Areas

Retentive areas must exist for a given path of placement and must be contacted by retentive clasp arms that are forced to flex over a convex surface during placement and removal. Satisfactory clasp retention is no more than the resistance of metal to deformation. For a clasp to be retentive, its path of escapement must be other than parallel to the path of removal of the denture itself; otherwise, it would not be forced to flex and thereby generate the resistance known as retention. Clasp retention therefore depends on the existence of a definite path of placement and removal.

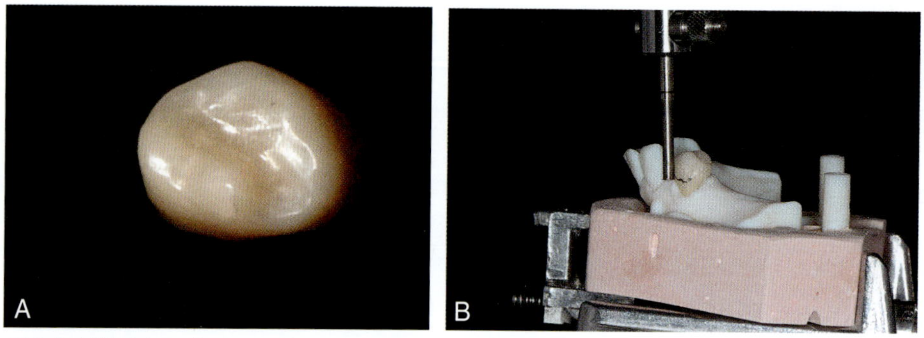

Fig. 11.8 A, Milled zirconia surveyed crown completed with guide planes, rest seats, and retentive undercut. **B,** The surveyed crown is seated onto the printed cast, and the cast is surveyed to confirm and assess the correct amount of undercut. (Courtesy of Ahmed Mahrous Copyright © 2024. All rights reserved.)

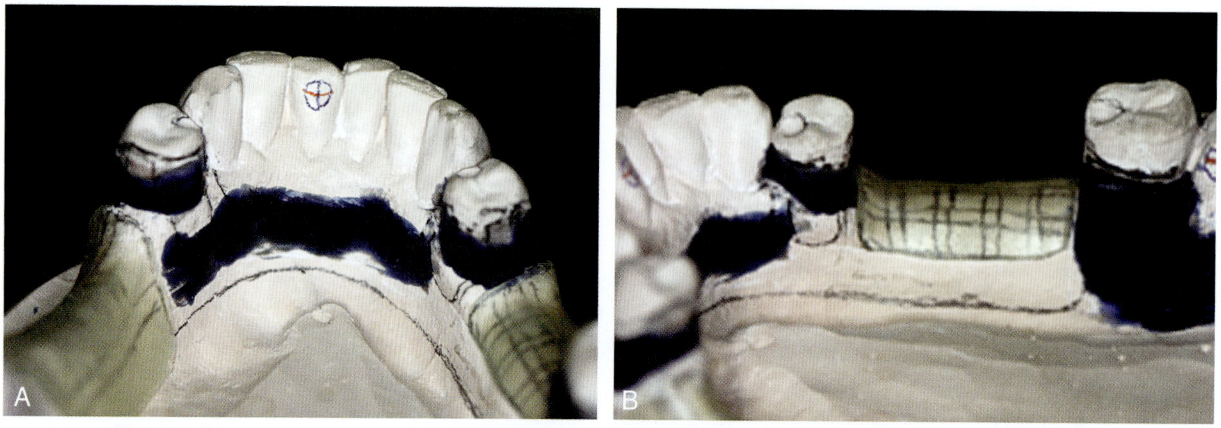

Fig. 11.9 Master casts are modified by the addition of wax relief to nonbearing regions and by placement of blockout wax parallel to the path of insertion at regions beneath the height of contour where framework contact is not planned (i.e., all areas except retentive clasp tips). **A,** Blockout wax is provided for tooth contours beneath the height of contour on teeth #21 and #28. **B,** Similar blockout was accomplished for mandibular molar #31. Blockout is carved with a straight surveyor blade to ensure parallelism with the identified path of insertion.

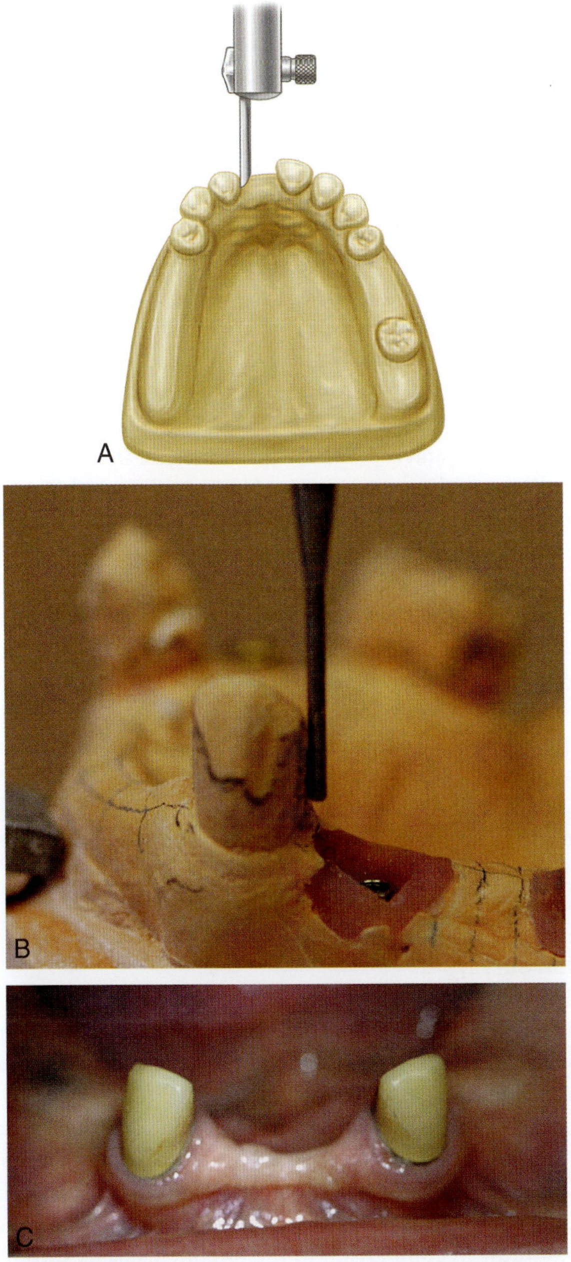

Fig. 11.10 A, When anterior teeth must be replaced with the removable partial denture, the selected vertical path should consider the junction of the natural tooth and the denture tooth. The path of insertion that requires the least amount of alteration of the natural teeth and the denture tooth (maximizing natural embrasure contours) is desirable. **B,** Distal of canine slightly altered to accommodate the path that optimizes anterior denture tooth placement. The dental implant's long axis and path of placement onto the implant abutment must be kept in mind when selecting the path of insertion/removal for the prosthesis. **C,** Canine crowns required to satisfy desired contours of the natural tooth and the denture teeth.

Although desirable, retention at each principal abutment may not be balanced in relation to the tooth on the opposite side of the arch (exactly equal and opposite in magnitude and relative location); however, positive cross-arch reciprocation to retentive elements must be present. Retention should be sufficient only to resist reasonable dislodging forces. In other words, it should be the minimum acceptable for adequate retention against reasonable dislodging forces.

Fairly even retention may be obtained by one of two means. One is to change the path of placement to increase or decrease the angle of cervical convergence of opposing retentive surfaces of abutment teeth. The other is to alter the flexibility of the clasp arm by changing its design, its size and length, or the material of which it is made.

Interference

The prosthesis must be designed so that it may be placed and removed without encountering tooth or soft tissue interference. A path of placement may be selected that encounters interference only if the interference can be eliminated during mouth preparations or on the master cast by a reasonable amount of blockout. Interference may be eliminated during mouth preparations by surgery, extraction, modification of interfering tooth surfaces, or alteration of tooth contours with restorations.

Generally, interference that cannot be eliminated for one reason or another takes precedence over the factors of retention and guide planes. Sometimes, certain areas can be made noninterfering only by selecting a different path of placement at the expense of existing retentive areas and guide planes. These must then be modified with restorations that are in harmony with the path dictated by the existing interference. However, if areas of interference can be eliminated by various reasonable means, this should be done. When this occurs, the axial contours of existing abutments may frequently be used with little alteration.

Esthetics

By one path of placement, the most esthetic location of artificial teeth is made possible, and less clasp metal and base material may be displayed.

The location of retentive areas may influence the path of placement selected; therefore retentive areas should always be selected with the most esthetic locations of clasps in mind. When restorations are to be made for other reasons, they should be contoured to permit the least display of clasp metal. Generally, less metal will be displayed if the retentive clasp is placed at a more distogingival area of tooth surface, made possible by the path of placement selected or by the contour of the restorations.

Esthetics also may dictate the choice of path selected when missing anterior teeth must be replaced with the RPD. In such situations, a more vertical path of placement is often necessary so that neither the artificial teeth nor the adjacent natural teeth will have to be modified excessively. In this instance, esthetics may take precedence over other factors. This necessitates the preparation of abutment teeth to eliminate interferences and to provide guide planes and retention in harmony with that path of placement dictated by esthetic factors.

Because the primary consideration should be the preservation of remaining oral tissues, esthetics should not be allowed to jeopardize the success of the partial denture. The replacement of missing anterior teeth, therefore, should be accomplished by means of fixed partial dentures whenever possible, especially if the mechanical and functional effectiveness of the removable partial denture will require significant tooth preparation.

STEP-BY-STEP PROCEDURES IN SURVEYING A DIAGNOSTIC CAST

Physical Surveyors

Attach the cast to the adjustable surveyor table by means of the clamp provided. Position the adjustable table so that the occlusal surfaces of the teeth are approximately parallel to the platform (Fig. 11.11). Such an orientation is a tentative but practical way to start considering the factors that influence the path of placement and removal.

Digital Surveyors

Most dental laboratory design software programs require input regarding the case information, followed by identifying the restoration type to be designed. After making the appropriate selection, a prompt will necessitate to import the .stl scan or model into the software. Diagnostic digital surveyors will start with prompting the import of the .stl.

Depending on the mechanism of scanning, the model might appear in a variety of orientations. Thus the next step in most software systems is usually to properly orient the .stl model on the screen (Fig. 11.12). The model is oriented to the horizontal axes in most cases by aligning the model to standard axes markers on the screen.

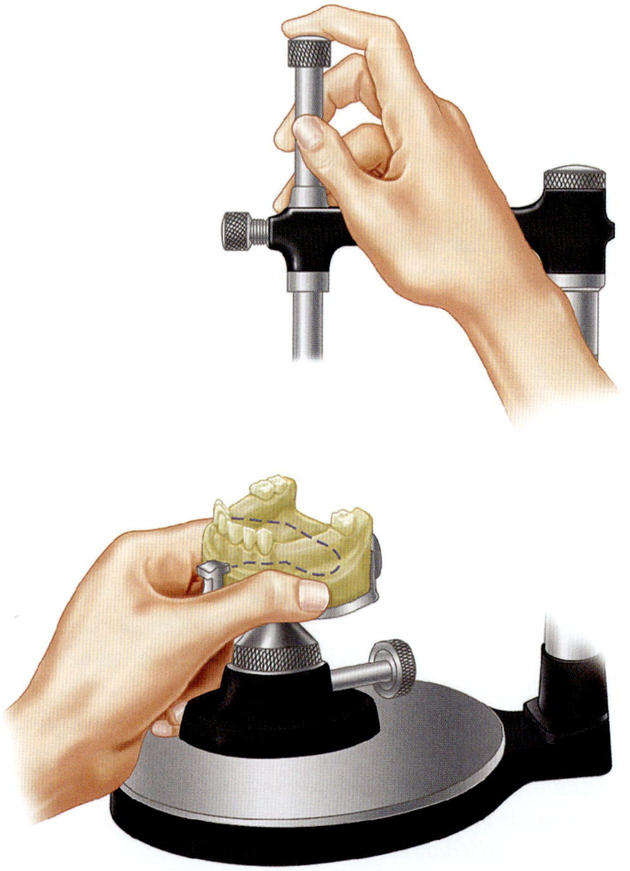

Fig. 11.11 Recommended method for manipulating the dental surveyor. The right hand is braced on the horizontal arm of the surveyor, and the fingers are used, as illustrated, to raise and lower the vertical shaft in its spindle. The left hand holding the cast on the adjustable table slides horizontally on the platform in relation to the vertical arm. The right hand must be used to loosen and tighten the tilting mechanism as a suitable anteroposterior and lateral tilt of the cast in relation to the surveyor is being determined.

Guide Planes

Physical Surveyors

Determine the relative parallelism of proximal surfaces of all of the potential abutment teeth by contacting the proximal tooth surfaces using the diagnostic stylus or straight edge with the surveyor blade. Shift the cast position anteroposteriorly until these proximal surfaces are in as close to a parallel relation to one another as possible, or near enough that they can be made parallel by recontouring. For posterior modification spaces, this determines the anteroposterior tilt of the cast in relation to the vertical arm of the surveyor (Fig. 11.13). Although the surveyor table is universally adjustable, it should be thought of as having only two axes, thus allowing only anteroposterior and lateral tilting. If an implant is to be used, the long axis of the implant should be considered in defining the guide plane reduction needs (see Fig. 11.10, *B*).

When a choice must be made between having contact with a proximal surface at the cervical area only and contact at the marginal ridge only, the latter is preferred because a plane may then be established by recontouring (Fig. 11.14). It is obvious that when only gingival contact exists, a restoration is the only means of establishing a guide plane. Therefore if a tilt that does not provide proximal contact is apparent, the proximal surface must be established with some type of restoration.

Digital Surveyors

Path of draw is usually accomplished using "line of sight." The path of draw for a prosthesis is set to the direction of the camera perspective. This is done by tilting the cast in all three axes until the most desirable path of draw is achieved (Fig. 11.15). When tilting the cast, the user should take into consideration the same factors considered when using a physical Ney surveyor. Most software systems will have a pin marking the direction of the selected path of draw. This allows the evaluation of the selected path of draw in comparison to the proximal surfaces from different angles (Fig. 11.16).

The result of selecting a suitable anteroposterior tilt should be to provide the greatest combined areas of parallel proximal surfaces that may act as guide planes. Other axial surfaces of abutment teeth may also be used as guide planes. This is realized most often by having the stabilizing component of the direct retainer assembly contacting in its entirety the axial surface of the abutment, which has been found or made parallel to the path of placement. Therefore a lateral tilt of the cast to the vertical arm of the surveyor must also be considered, as well as the anteroposterior tilt, when guide planes are used.

Retentive Areas

Physical Surveyors

Through contact of buccal and lingual surfaces of abutment teeth with the surveyor blade, the amount of retention existing below their height of convexity may be determined. This is

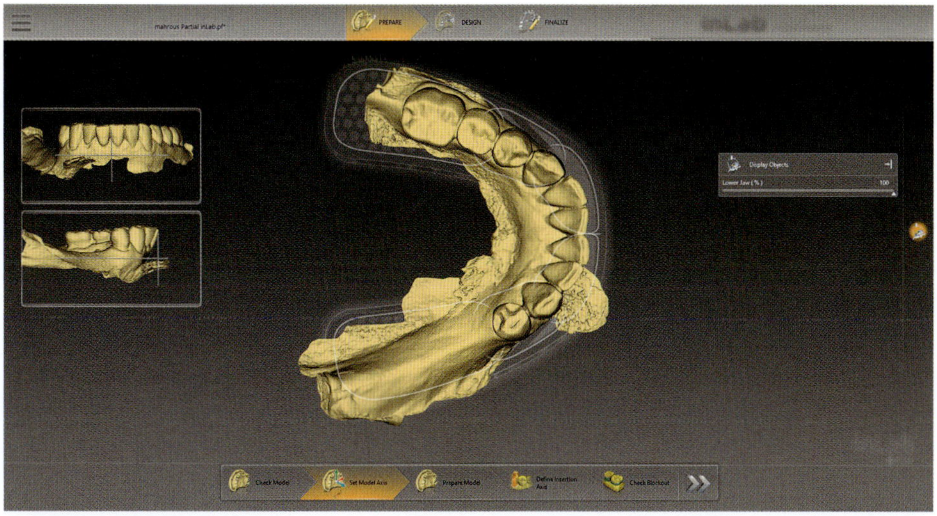

Fig. 11.12 Digital design software allows the upload of an .stl model after setting case details .stl scan. The orientation is set by aligning the model to orientation markers on the screen. (Courtesy of Ahmed Mahrous Copyright © 2024. All rights reserved.)

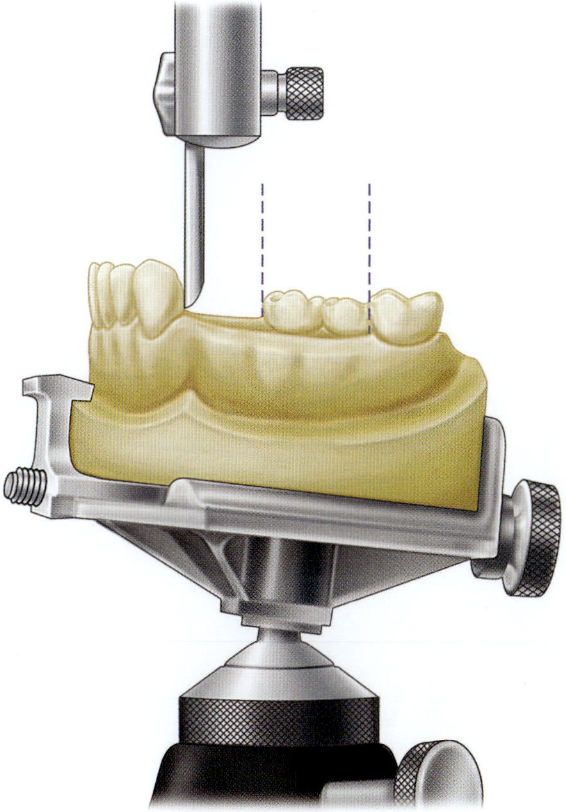

Fig. 11.13 Relative parallelism of proximal tooth surfaces determines the anteroposterior tilt of the cast in relation to the vertical arm of the surveyor.

best accomplished by directing a small source of light toward the cast from the side away from the dentist. The angle of cervical convergence is best observed as a triangle of light between the surveyor blade and the apical portion of the tooth surface being studied.

Alter the cast position by tilting it laterally until similar retentive areas exist on the principal abutment teeth. If only two

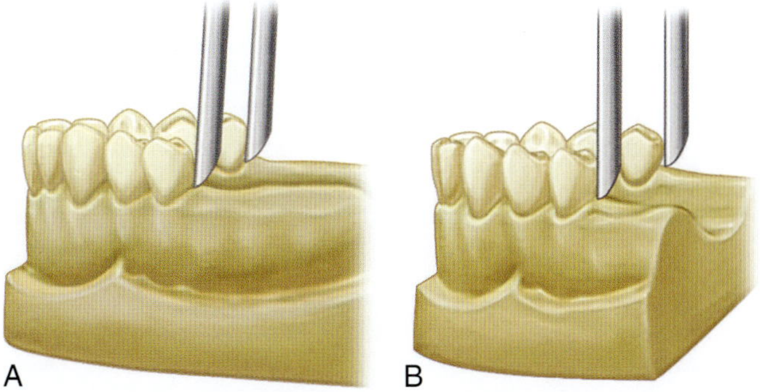

Fig. 11.14 When the most desirable anteroposterior tilt of the cast in relation to the surveyor blade is determined, a choice must be made between positions illustrated in **(A)** and **(B)**. **A,** The distal surface of the left premolar abutment would have to be extended by means of a restoration. **B,** The right premolar could be altered slightly to provide a parallel guide plane. Unless restorations are necessary for other reasons, the tilt shown in **(B)** is preferred.

abutment teeth are involved (as in a Kennedy Class I partially edentulous arch), they are both principal abutments. However, if four abutment teeth are involved (as they are in a Kennedy Class III, modification 1 arch), they are all principal abutments, and retentive areas should be located on all four. But if three abutment teeth are involved (as they are in a Kennedy Class II, modification 1 arch), the posterior abutment on the tooth-supported side and the abutment on the distal extension side are considered to be the principal abutments, and retention needs to be equalized accordingly. The third abutment may be considered secondary; less retention is expected from it than from the other two. An exception is when the posterior abutment on the tooth-supported side has a poor prognosis, and the RPD is designed to ultimately be a Kennedy Class I RPD. In such a situation, the two stronger abutments are considered the principal abutments.

When the cast is tilted laterally to establish reasonable uniformity of retention, it is necessary that the table be rotated about an imaginary longitudinal axis without disturbing the

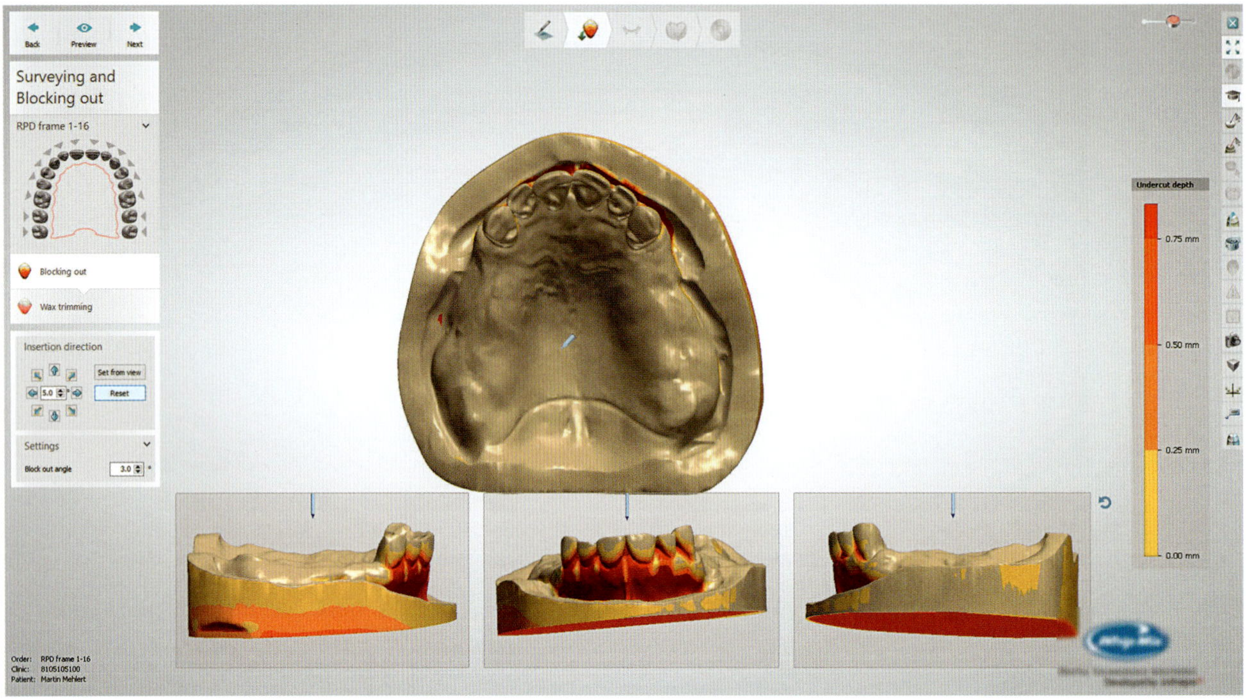

Fig. 11.15 Path of draw is set using "line of sight," which means the path is set from the angle the cast is being viewed from. (Courtesy of Ahmed Mahrous Copyright © 2024. All rights reserved.)

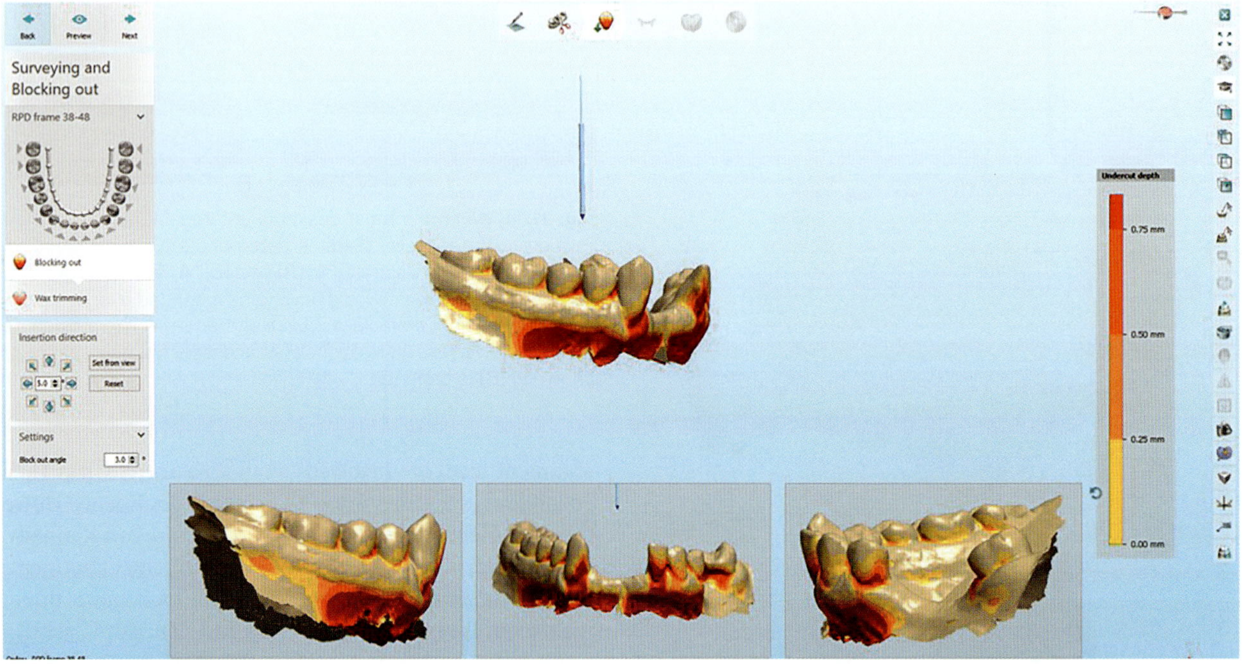

Fig. 11.16 A guide pin is seen, indicating the selected path of draw. The guide pin can be used to assess the path of draw in relation to the proximal contours of the teeth. The undercuts are identified using different colored areas on the models to indicate the different depths of the undercuts. A key usually is available on the screen to identify the depth of the undercuts. (Courtesy of Ahmed Mahrous Copyright © 2024. All rights reserved.)

anteroposterior tilt previously established. The resulting position is one that provides or makes possible parallel guide planes and provides for acceptable retention on the abutment teeth. It should be noted that this most desirable position will always require some tooth modification to be achieved. Note that possible interference to this tentative path of placement has not, as yet, been taken into consideration.

Digital Surveyors

Most digital surveyors provide a graphical representation of the height of contour as well as different colors indicating the location of different depths of undercuts underneath the height of contour. The same factors considered during evaluation of retentive areas using the Ney surveyor should be considered when evaluating undercuts using digital surveyors.

Measuring Retention

Physical Surveyors

The exact undercut that retentive clasp terminals will occupy must be measured and marked on the master cast (Fig. 11.17).

Physical surveyors like the Ney surveyor measure undercuts with an undercut gauge. The amount of undercut is measured in hundredths of an inch, with the gauges allowing measurements up to 0.03 inch. Digital surveyors will delineate the height of contour and will represent different undercut depths underneath using different colors representing the different depths.

Theoretically the amount of undercut used may vary with the clasp to be used, up to a full 0.03 inch. However, undercuts of 0.01 inch are often adequate for retention by cast retainers. Tapered wrought-wire retention may safely use up to 0.02 inch without inducing undesirable torque on the abutment tooth, provided the wire retentive arm is long enough (at least 8 mm). The use of 0.03 inch is rarely, if ever, justified with any clasp. When greater retention is required, such as when abutment teeth remain on only one side of the arch, multiple abutments should be used, rather than increased retention on any one tooth.

When a source of light is directed toward the tooth being surveyed, a triangle of light is visible. This triangle is bounded by the surface of the abutment tooth on one side and the blade of the surveyor on the other, the apex being the point of contact at the height of convexity and the base of the triangle being the gingival tissues (Fig. 11.18). Retention will be determined by (1) the magnitude of the angle of cervical convergence below the point of convexity, (2) the depth at which the clasp terminal is placed in the angle, and (3) the flexibility of the clasp arm. The intelligent application of various clasp designs with their relative flexibility is of greater importance than the ability to measure an undercut with precise accuracy.

Once an undercut is determined to be adequate for a certain clasp, the undercut is marked using a pencil mark. This mark

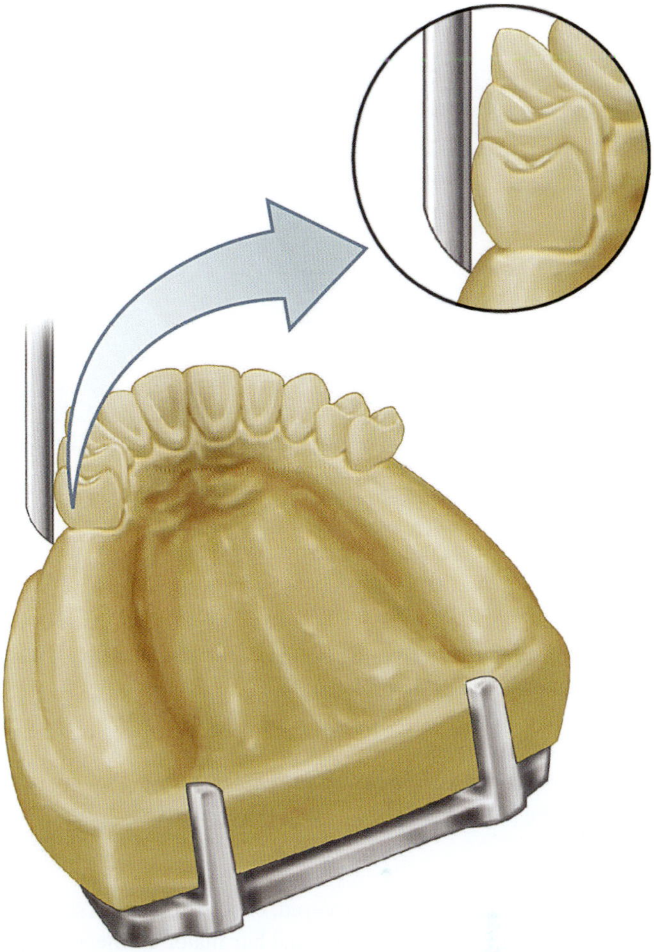

Fig. 11.18 Tooth undercut is best viewed against a good source of light passing through the triangle bounded by the surface of the abutment tooth, the surveyor blade, and the gingival tissues.

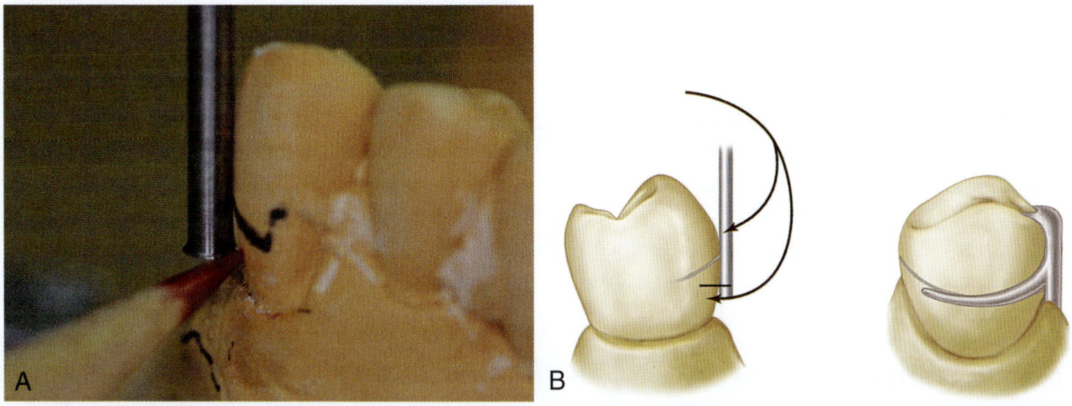

Fig. 11.17 A, Undercut gauge measures the depth of undercut below the height of contour. I-bar direct retainer will contact the tooth from the point of the undercut to the height of contour. The depth to which the retentive clasp arm can be placed depends not only on its length, taper, and diameter and the alloy from which it is made but also on the type of clasp. A circumferential clasp arm is more flexible than a bar clasp arm of the same length (see Chapter 7). **B,** Specific measurement of the undercut gingiva to the height of contour may be ascertained with the use of an undercut gauge attached to the surveyor. Simultaneous contact of the shank of the undercut gauge at the height of contour and of the lip of a specific undercut gauge on a tooth in the infrabulge area establishes definitively the degree and location of undercut. Therefore the tip of the retentive arm of the direct retainer may be placed at the planned depth of the undercut.

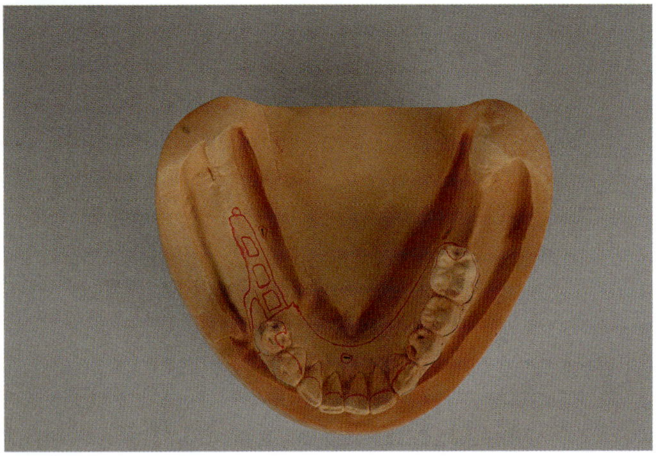

Fig. 11.19 The design is drawn onto the cast using a red pencil. The cast drawing serves as a reference for the desired size and shape of the different removable partial denture components. (Courtesy of Ahmed Mahrous Copyright © 2024. All rights reserved.)

will be used as a reference when drawing the design on the diagnostic cast. The design may be drawn on the diagnostic cast with a colored pencil (Fig. 11.19).

Digital Surveyors

Undercuts are usually displayed in real time on digital surveyors once the path of draw is selected (Fig. 11.20).

Interference

When a mandibular cast is surveyed, check the lingual surfaces that may be in contact with a lingual bar major connector during placement and removal. Bony prominences and lingually inclined premolar teeth are the most common causes of interference with a lingual bar connector.

If the interference is bilateral, surgery or recontouring of lingual tooth surfaces, or both, may be unavoidable. If the interference is only unilateral, a change in the lateral tilt may avoid an area of tooth or tissue interference. In changing the path of placement to prevent interference, previously established guide planes and an ideal location for retentive elements may be lost. Then the decision must be made whether to remove the existing interference by whatever means necessary or to resort to restorations on the abutment teeth, thereby changing the proximal and retentive areas to conform to the new path of placement.

In a like manner, bony undercuts that offer interference to the seating of denture bases must be evaluated and the decision must be made to remove them surgically, to change the path of placement at the expense of modifying or restoring teeth to achieve guide planes and retention, or to design denture bases to avoid such undercut areas. The latter may be done by shortening buccal and labial flanges and distolingual extension of the denture bases. However, it should be remembered that the maximum area available for support of the denture base should be used whenever possible.

Interference to major connectors rarely exists in the maxillary arch. Areas of interference are usually found on buccally inclined posterior teeth and those bony areas on the buccal aspect of edentulous spaces. As with the mandibular cast, the decision must be made whether to eliminate them, to change the path of placement at the expense of modifying or restoring teeth to achieve the required guide planes and retention, or to design the connectors and bases to avoid them.

Other areas of potential interference to be evaluated are those surfaces of abutment teeth that will support or be crossed by minor connectors and clasp arms. Although interference to vertical minor connectors may be blocked out, doing so may cause discomfort to the patient's tongue and may create objectionable spaces, which could result in the trapping of food. Also, it is desirable that tooth surfaces contacted by vertical minor connectors be used as auxiliary guide planes whenever possible. Excess tissue relief is preferred since insufficient relief can cause soft tissue irritation, within reason. If possible, a minor connector should pass vertically along a tooth surface that is parallel to the path of placement versus engaging into an undercut. If excessive tooth undercuts exist, they may be eliminated or minimized by slight changes in the path of placement and/or eliminated during mouth preparations. The need for such alteration should be indicated on the diagnostic cast with a red pencil after final acceptance of a path of placement.

Tooth surfaces on which reciprocal and stabilizing clasp arms will be placed should be studied to see whether sufficient areas exist above the height of convexity for the placement of these components. The addition of a clasp arm to the occlusal third of an abutment tooth adds to its occlusal dimension and therefore to the occlusal loading of that tooth. Nonretentive and stabilizing clasp arms are best located between the middle third and the gingival third of the crown rather than on the occlusal third.

Areas of interference to proper placement of clasp arms can be eliminated by reshaping tooth surfaces during mouth preparations. These areas should be indicated on the diagnostic cast. Areas of interference to the placement of clasps may necessitate minor changes in the path of placement or changes in the clasp design. For example, a bar clasp arm originating mesially from the major connector to provide reciprocation and stabilization might be substituted for a distally originating circumferential arm.

Areas of interference often overlooked are the distal line angles of premolar abutment teeth and the mesial line angles of molar abutments. These areas frequently offer interference to the origin of circumferential clasp arms. If not detected at the time of initial survey, they are not included in the plan for mouth preparations. When such an undercut exists, the following three alternatives may be considered:

1. Block out the undercut the same way as any other area of interference. This is by far the least satisfactory method because the origin of the clasp must then stand away from the tooth in proportion to the amount of blockout used. Although this is, perhaps, less objectionable than it is being placed occlusally, it may be objectionable to the tongue and the cheek and may create a food trap.
2. Circumvent the undercut by approaching the retentive area from a gingival direction with a bar clasp arm. This is often a satisfactory solution to the problem if other contraindications

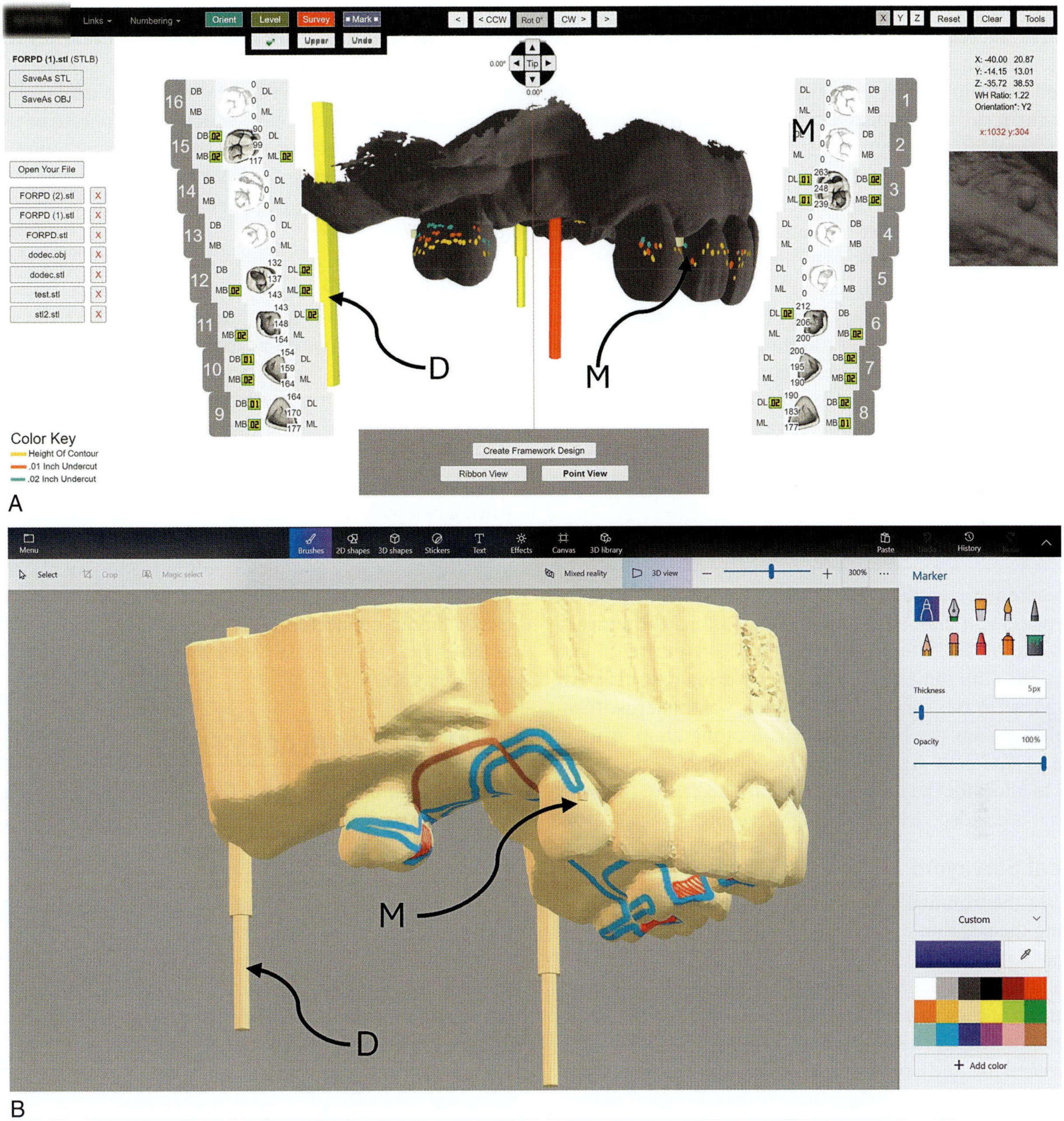

Fig. 11.20 **A,** Diagnostic surveyors are used to mark the undercuts. *(M)* The desired undercuts are marked using a square mesh. **B,** The model can then be exported, and the design can be drawn using generic 3D painting software. *(D)* The model is also exported with a Ney surveyor adaptor that can be used to reorient the printed model onto the Ney surveyor. (Courtesy of Ahmed Mahrous Copyright © 2024. All rights reserved.)

to the use of a bar clasp arm, such as a severe tissue undercut or a retentive area that is too high on the tooth, are not present.

3. Eliminate the undercut by reducing the offending tooth contour during mouth preparation. This permits the use of a circumferential clasp arm originating well below the occlusal surface in a satisfactory manner. If the tooth is to be modified during mouth preparations, it should be indicated on the diagnostic cast with a colored pencil.

When the retentive area is located objectionably high on the abutment tooth or the undercut is too severe, interference may also exist on tooth surfaces that support retentive clasps. Such areas of extreme or high convexity must be considered as areas of interference and should be reduced accordingly. These areas are likewise indicated on the diagnostic cast for reduction during mouth preparations.

Esthetics

The path of placement thus established must still be considered from the standpoint of esthetics, as to both the location of clasps and the arrangement of artificial teeth. Clasp designs that will provide satisfactory esthetics for any given path of placement usually may be selected. In some instances, gingivally placed bar clasp arms may be used to advantage; in others, circumferential clasp arms located cervically may be used. This is especially true when other abutment teeth located more posteriorly may bear the major responsibility for retention. In still other instances, a tapered wrought-wire retentive clasp arm may be placed to better esthetic advantage than a cast clasp arm. The placement of clasp arms for esthetic reasons does not ordinarily justify altering the path of placement at the expense of mechanical factors. However, it should be considered concurrently with other factors, and if a choice between two paths of insertion of equal merit permits a more esthetic placement of clasp arms by one path than the other, that path should be given preference.

When anterior replacements are involved, the choice of path is limited to a more vertical one for reasons previously stated. In this instance alone, esthetics must be given primary consideration, even at the expense of altering the path of placement and making all other factors conform. This factor should be remembered when the other three factors are considered so that compromises can be made at the time other factors are being considered.

REGISTER RELATION OF CAST TO SURVEYOR

Some method of recording the tilt of the cast in relation to the path of placement must be used so that the cast may be returned to the same tilt for future reference, especially during mouth preparations. The same applies to the need for returning any working cast to the surveyor for shaping wax patterns, trimming blackout on the master cast, or locating clasp arms in relation to undercut areas. For digital surveyors, a method is needed to allow for the mounting of a printed cast in the exact tilt as that is decided virtually during surveying.

Physical Surveyors

Obviously, the trimmed base will vary with each cast; therefore recording the position of the surveyor table is of no value. If it were, calibrations could be incorporated on the surveyor table that would allow the same position to be reestablished. Instead, the position of each cast must be established separately and any positional record applies only to that cast.

Of several methods, two seem to be the most convenient and accurate. One method is to place three widely divergent dots on the tissue surface of the cast with the tip of a carbon marker with the vertical arm of the surveyor in a locked position. Preferably these dots should not be placed on areas of the cast involved in the framework design. The dots should be encircled with a colored pencil for easy identification. When the cast is returned to the surveyor, it may be tilted until the tip of the surveyor blade or diagnostic stylus again contacts the three dots in the same plane. This approach, which will produce the original position of the cast and therefore the original path of placement, is known as *tripoding the cast* (Fig. 11.21). Some dentists prefer to make tiny pits in the cast at the location of the tripoding dots to preserve the orientation of the cast and to transfer this relationship to the refractory cast.

A second method is to score two sides and the dorsal aspect of the base of the cast with a sharp instrument held against the surveyor blade (see Fig. 11.21). When the cast is tilted until all three lines are again parallel to the surveyor blade, the original cast position can be reestablished. Fortunately, the scratch lines will be reproduced in any duplication, permitting any duplicate cast to be related to the surveyor in a similar manner. Whereas a diagnostic cast and a master cast cannot be made to be interchangeable, a refractory cast, which is a duplicate of the master cast, can be repositioned on the surveyor at any time. The technician must be cautioned not to trim the sides of the cast on the cast trimmer and thereby lose the reference marks for repositioning.

Digital Surveyors

Some virtual surveyors allow for the exporting of the surveyed model with a Ney surveyor adaptor, to allow for the mounting of the printed model on the physical surveyor to allow for the evaluation and the addition of any diagnostic markings (see Fig. 11.20).

It must be remembered that repositioning a cast on a surveyor at any time can involve a certain amount of human error. It has been estimated that an error of 0.2 mm can be anticipated when a cast with three reference points on its base is reoriented. This reorientation error can influence the placement of appropriate blockout wax and may result in ineffective placement of direct retainers into prescribed undercuts and improper contacts of minor connectors with guide planes. Therefore reorientation of the cast to the surveyor by any method must be done with great care.

FINAL PATH OF PLACEMENT

The final path of placement will be the anteroposterior and lateral position of the cast, in relation to the vertical arm of the surveyor that best satisfies all factors: guide planes, retention, interference, esthetics, and implant long axis.

All proposed mouth changes with the exception of restorations should be indicated on the diagnostic cast or model. This is done by marking the stone or printed resin cast with a red pencil or done digitally using software tools (see Fig. 11.20, *B*). Some diagnostic surveyors also allow the marking of undercut locations and incorporation of the marks in the generated .stl file. All tooth modifications may also be indicated on an accompanying chart if desired. Extractions and surgery are given priority to allow time for healing. The remaining red marks represent actual modifications of the teeth that remain to be done, which consist of the preparation of proximal surfaces, the reduction of buccal and lingual surfaces, and the preparation of rest seats. Except when they are placed in the wax pattern for a cast restoration, preparation of rest seats should always be deferred until all other mouth preparations have been completed.

The actual locations of rests will be determined by the proposed design of the removable partial denture framework. Therefore the tentative design should be marked on the diagnostic model. This is done not only to locate rest areas but also to record graphically the plan of treatment before mouth preparations. In the intervening time between patient visits, other removable partial denture restorations may have been considered. The dentist should have the plan of treatment readily available at each succeeding appointment to avoid confusion and to keep a reminder about which is to be done and the sequence that will be required.

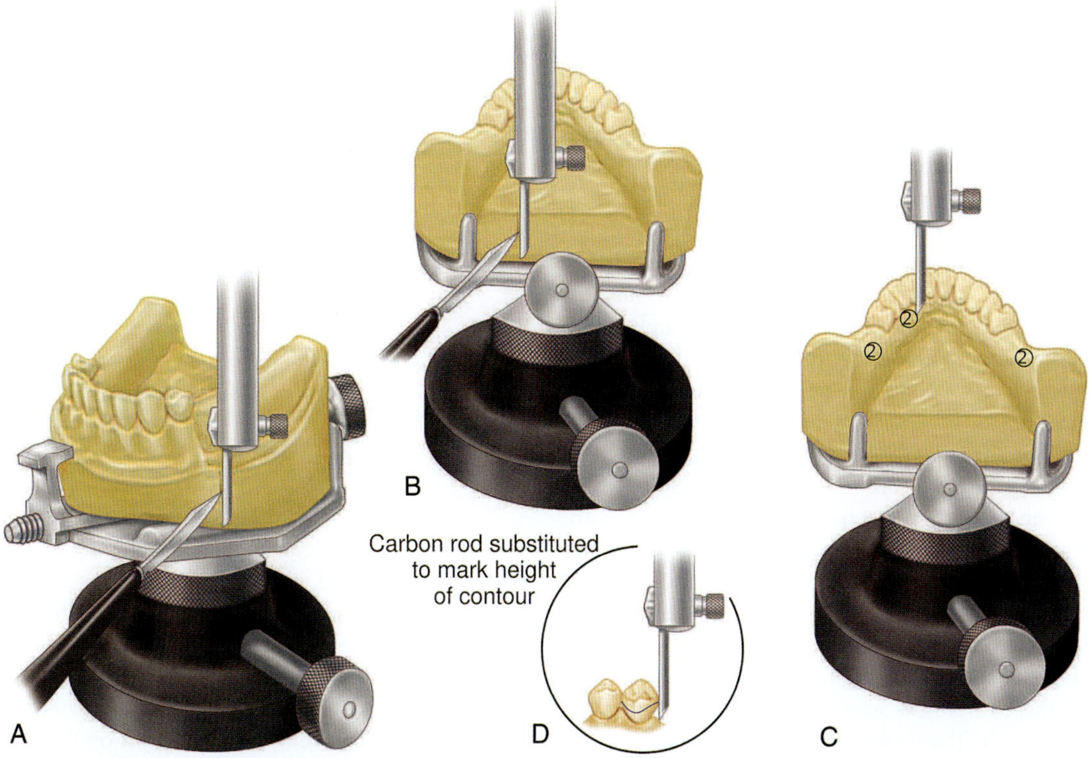

Fig. 11.21 A and **B,** The path of placement is determined, and the base of the cast is scored to record its relation to the surveyor for future repositioning. **C,** An alternate method of recording the relation of the cast to the surveyor is known as *tripoding.* A carbon marker is placed in the vertical arm of the surveyor, and the arm is adjusted to the height by which the cast can be contacted in three divergent locations. The vertical arm is locked in position, and the cast is brought into contact with the tip of the carbon marker. Three resultant marks are encircled with a colored lead pencil for ease of identification. Reorientation of the cast to the surveyor is done by tilting the surveying table that holds it until the plane created by three marks is at a right angle to the vertical arm of the surveyor. **D,** Height of contour is then delineated by a carbon marker.

The plan for treatment should include (1) the diagnostic cast with the mouth preparations and the removable partial denture design marked on it, (2) a chart showing the proposed design and the planned treatment for each abutment, (3) a working chart showing the total treatment involved that will permit a quick review and a check-off of each step as the work progresses, and (4) a record of the fee quoted for each phase of treatment that can be checked off as it is recorded on the patient's permanent record.

Red pencil marks on the diagnostic cast are used to indicate the locations of areas to be modified as well as the location of the rest seats and guide planes (see Fig. 11.17). The remaining components of the RPD framework can also be designed on the cast. The framework may be created with a red pencil or another color to discern from those areas to be modified and those that represent the framework. Although it is not necessary that rest areas be prepared on the diagnostic cast, it is advisable for the beginning student to have done this before proceeding to alter the abutment teeth. This applies equally to crown and inlay preparations on abutment teeth. It is advisable, however, for even the most experienced dentist to trim the stone teeth with the surveyor blade wherever tooth reduction is to be done. This identifies not only the amount to be removed in a given area but also the plane in which the tooth is to be prepared. For example, a proximal surface may need to be recontoured in only the upper third or the middle third to establish a guide plane that will be parallel to the path of placement. This is not usually parallel to the long axis of the tooth, and if the rotary instrument is laid against the side of the tooth, the existing surface angle will be maintained, thus avoiding the need to establish a new plane that is parallel to the path of placement.

The surveyor blade, which represents the path of placement along the straight edge, can be used to trim the surface of the abutment tooth whenever a red mark appears. The resulting surface represents the amount of tooth to be removed in the mouth and indicates the angle at which the handpiece must be held. The cut surface on the stone tooth is not marked with a red pencil again, but it is outlined with a red pencil to positively locate the area that is to be prepared.

SURVEYING THE MASTER CAST

The master cast must be surveyed in a similar manner to that used when the diagnostic cast was surveyed. Digital design software systems are usually used as the digital surveyor of choice due to their seamless transition into framework fabrication. However, in both digital and physical workflows of fabrication, the prepared proximal guide plane surfaces will indicate the correct anteroposterior tilt. Some compromises may be necessary, but the amount of guide plane surface remaining after blockout should be the maximum for each tooth. Areas above the point of contact with the surveyor blade are not considered as part of the guide plane area, and neither are gingival undercut areas, which will be blocked out.

The lateral tilt will be the position that provides equal retentive areas on all principal abutments in relation to the planned clasp design. Factors of flexibility, including the need for extraflexibility on distal extension abutments, must be considered when one is deciding what will provide equal retention on all abutment teeth. For example, cast circumferential or cast bar retention on the tooth-supported side of a Kennedy Class II design should be balanced against the 18-gauge wrought-wire retention on a distal abutment only if the more rigid cast clasp engages a lesser undercut than the wrought-wire clasp arm. Therefore the degree of undercut alone does not ensure relatively equal retention unless clasp arms of equal length, diameter, form, and material are used.

Gross interference will have been eliminated during mouth preparation. Thus for a given path of placement that is providing guide planes and balanced retention, any remaining interference must be eliminated with blockout. If mouth preparations have been adequately planned and executed, the undercuts remaining to be blocked out should be minimal.

The base of the cast is now scored, or the cast is tripoded as described previously. The surveyor blade or diagnostic stylus may then be replaced with a carbon marker, and the height of convexity of each abutment tooth and soft tissue contours may be delineated. Similarly, any areas of interference to the rigid parts of the framework during seating and removal should be indicated with the carbon marker so areas to be blocked out or relieved can be located.

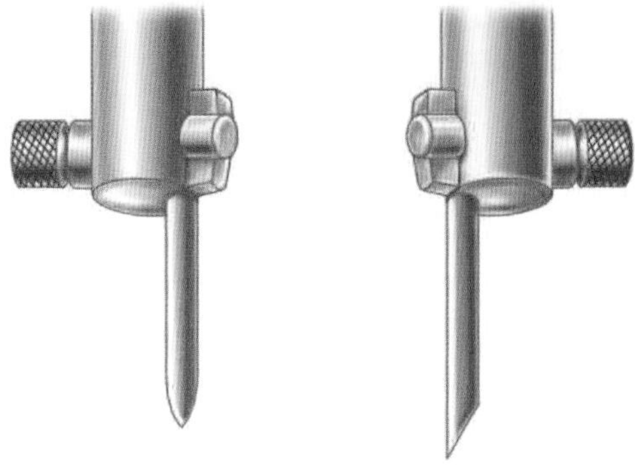

Fig. 11.22 A worn carbon marker *(left)* should be discarded because it will invariably misleadingly mark the height of contour for a given orientation of the cast to the vertical spindle of the surveyor. Unworn carbon *(right)* with an angled end is preferable for marking heights of contour on abutment teeth and performing surveys of soft tissue areas.

Carbon markers that become the slightest bit worn from use should be discarded. A worn (tapered) carbon marker will indicate heights of contour more occlusally located than those that actually exist. The carbon marker must be parallel to the vertical spindle of the surveyor (Fig. 11.22). The diagnostic stylus should always be checked to ensure that it is not bent or distorted.

The final design may now be drawn on the master cast with a fine color pencil, preferably one that will not come off during duplication. Graphite is usually lifted in duplication, but some color pencil marks will withstand duplication without smudging or transfer. Sizing or spraying the master cast to protect such pencil marks is usually not advisable unless it is done with extreme care to avoid obliterating the surface detail (see Fig. 11.19).

12

Considerations of Removable Partial Dental Materials

Ahmed Mahrous, Heba Elkassaby, and Leila Jahangiri

CHAPTER OUTLINE

Removable partial dentures (RPDs) serve as an essential treatment modality for restoring missing teeth either as an interim or a definitive treatment option for patients who either are not eligible for fixed prostheses or cannot afford them. Since its inception, RPD has had little in the way of change in both technique and material of fabrication. However, in recent years, with the advent of milling and printing technologies, there has been a rise of a multitude of novel materials and fabrication techniques for RPDs. This chapter provides a thorough review of traditional and newer materials with an appraisal of their indications, characteristics, and special considerations.

The framework material selection plays a vital role in the success of treatment, the maintenance of health, and the longevity of the remaining dentition. There are many materials used for RPD framework fabrication including, but not limited to, cobalt-chromium (Co-Cr) alloys, nickel-chromium (Ni-Cr) alloys, acetal resin, polyetheretherketone (PEEK), and titanium.

MANUFACTURING TECHNIQUES

Detailed description of the different manufacturing processes will be outlined in Chapter 20; however, a brief outline of the different fabrication techniques is discussed in the following section:

- Lost wax/resin technique: This is a traditional method which involves creating a wax/resin pattern, investing it in a refractory mold, heating the refractory to melt the wax/resin pattern, and casting with molten alloy. This technique is the most conventional and time-tested method to make the metal frameworks for RPDs.
- Milling: Digital technologies have introduced computer-aided design/computer-aided manufacturing milling, where prefabricated metal or polymer pucks are sculpted, according to the virtual framework design, using high-speed burs. In RPDs, milling is usually used to create metal or polymer-based frameworks.
- Resin printing (stereolithography [SLA]/digital light processing [DLP]): SLA and DLP printers utilize ultraviolet light to solidify layers of castable resin, enabling the creation of complex and esthetic RPD frameworks in a single step. Those resin patterns are then invested and cast similar to the conventional lost wax method.
- Metal printing (selective laser sintering [SLS]/selective laser melting [SLM]): SLS and SLM employ lasers to fuse metal powder layer by layer, producing strong and lightweight frameworks. Metal printing is used in the fabrication of RPD metal frameworks (Fig. 12.1).
- Compression molding: It is a time-tested technique of processing polymethylmethacrylate (PMMA). This technique usually uses heat-polymerized PMMA material to fabricate interim acrylic RPDs and the denture bases for framework-based RPDs. While this technique is time tested and reliable, its main drawbacks lie in polymerization shrinkage, porosities, and residual monomer.
- Injection molding: It is an evolution of the conventional compression molding; injection molding addresses the issues of polymerization shrinkage and porosity, by introducing pneumatically controlled injection under continuous pressure throughout the processing procedure.

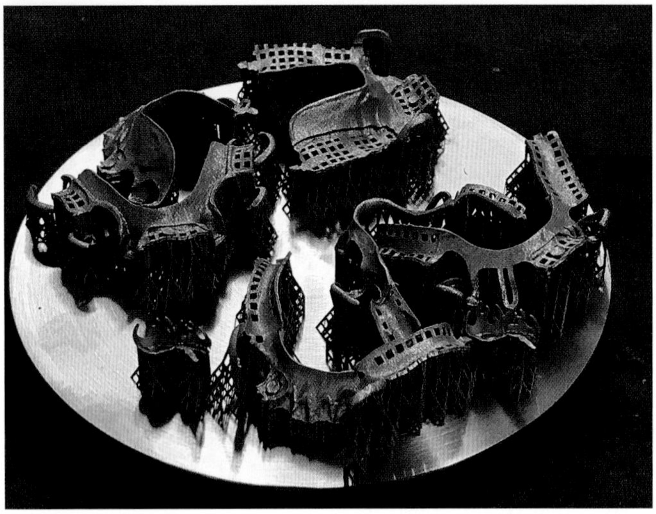

Fig. 12.1 Frameworks printed using selective laser sintering technology have metallic supports that support the framework during the printing process. All supports should be generated away from the fitting surface to avoid any possible interference and ensure optimal fit.

MATERIALS

Cobalt-Chromium and Nickel-Chromium Alloys

Metal framework RPDs offer significant advantages over all acrylic-resin RPDs. In general, the ability to predictably utilize the remaining teeth for support, stability, and retention over time is best assured when the interface between prosthesis and teeth consists of a metal structure and not a polymer. Although the utility of all acrylic-resin prostheses can be extended if wire "rests" are provided, typical polymer properties do not allow for a durable interface, which is required if one is to take advantage of the stabilizing effects of tooth contact.

Although gold alloys have been used in the past, today because of their cost, they are replaced by base-metal alloys which provides many advantages. In the 1940s, both Co-Cr and Ni-Cr revolutionized RPD frameworks, dethroning the brittle vulcanite with their superior strength and heat resistance. While both alloys offered impressive advantages, a closer look reveals the factors that led Co-Cr to ultimately ascend the throne. (1) Co-Cr is well tolerated by oral tissues; (2) Co-Cr is acceptable esthetically; (3) enamel abrasion is insignificant on vertical tooth surfaces; (4) a low-fusing Co-Cr alloy can be cast to wrought wire, and wrought-wire components may be soldered to Co-Cr alloys; (5) Co-Cr has the ability to obtain a clinically acceptable casting under strictly controlled investing and casting procedures; and (6) soldering procedures for the repair of frameworks can be performed.

The popularity of Co-Cr alloys has been attributed to the following characteristics: low density (weight), high modulus of elasticity (stiffness), low material cost, and resistance to tarnish. The term *stellite alloy* historically has referred to this class of alloy.

Co-Cr, is a blend of 60%–65% Co, 27%–30% Cr, and 5%–6% molybdenum (Mo), with the balance including silicon, manganese, iron, nitrogen (N), and carbon. The addition of controlled amounts of N (<0.5%) is reported to improve physical properties. This mixture boasts impressive properties thanks to its key ingredients:

- Co: This component is the backbone of the alloy, providing exceptional strength and hardness for long-lasting durability.
- Cr: It forms a protective oxide layer that safeguards the framework against wear and tear.
- Mo: It enhances casting properties and grain refinement, leading to smoother frameworks and improved resistance to fatigue.

This exceptional combination translates into remarkable tensile and yield strengths, exceeding 500 MPa (ASM International Handbook, 2008). Co-Cr can withstand bending, pulling, and wear and tear with unmatched resilience. Additionally, its biocompatibility and relative ease of fabrication have made it the most common material for RPDs.

Although Ni-Cr has similar strength and cost, Ni-Cr's nickel content (60%–80%) raises concerns about nickel allergies, affecting up to 15% of the population.

Traditionally, Co-Cr frameworks have been fabricated through the well-established technique of hand waxing, investing, and casting. This method delivers reliable and predictable results, supported by numerous studies.[1-4] However, advancements in additive manufacturing have introduced alternative fabrication approaches for Co-Cr frameworks, including resin printing and casting and metal printing via SLS and SLM. These newer methods offer potential advantages such as increased precision, reduced waste, and the ability to create complex geometries. Research suggests that all fabrication methods can produce clinically acceptable frameworks.[1-4] However, concerns have been raised regarding the stability of some 3D-printed castable resins during investing due to the absence of a supporting refractory cast.[5] Further research is needed to fully evaluate the long-term performance and clinical reliability of these newer fabrication techniques for Co-Cr frameworks.

Physical Properties of Cobalt-Chromium Alloys

Co-Cr alloys have high yield strength when used for RPDs. Yield strength is the resistance to plastic deformation.

The modulus of elasticity refers to the stiffness of an alloy. Greater rigidity can be obtained with the Co-Cr alloy in reduced sections in which cross-arch stabilization is required, thereby eliminating an appreciable bulk of the framework. Its greater rigidity is also an advantage when the greatest undercut that can be found on an abutment tooth is 0.005 inch. The stiffness of Co-Cr alloys can be overcome by including wrought-wire retentive elements in the framework when greater flexibility is required.

The bulk of a retentive clasp arm for a removable Co-Cr alloy is reported to work/harden, and this may lead to failure in service. When adjustments by bending are necessary, they must be executed with extreme caution and clinicians should refrain from routine and repeated adjustments to Co-Cr clasps.

Co-Cr alloys have a relatively low density (weight) which is an advantage when complete palatal coverage is indicated for the bilateral distal extension RPDs. The relative lightweight property of a cast Co-Cr maxillary complete major connector remains in position passively versus gravitational forces associated with a "heavier" material moving it out of position. Only during mastication of sticky food would the passive direct retainers be activated to maintain the prosthesis in position.

The hardness of Co-Cr alloys can be a disadvantage when a component of the framework, such as a rest, opposes a natural tooth or a restoration; the dissimilar material hardness properties could create wear of the opposing dentition or other restorations.

APPLICATIONS AND SPECIAL CONSIDERATIONS

Co-Cr is frequently chosen as the material of choice for most partial denture (Fig. 12.2). However, they are particularly indicated in cases where the patient is known to have a history of fractured prosthesis. Most commonly Co-Cr is used to make all parts of the metal framework, including major and minor connectors, rests, guiding plates, and retentive and reciprocal clasp arms. Occasionally Co-Cr can also be used to fabricate the denture base in conjunction with tube teeth (see Chapter 9). In cases where the patient might not have sufficient restorative space, mesiodistal or occlusogingival, Co-Cr can be used to fabricate the artificial teeth as well. Occasionally, Co-Cr retentive clasps can be fabricated and integrated into the denture bases of all acrylic-resin RPDs.

Titanium

Commercially pure (CP) titanium and titanium alloys containing aluminum (Al) and vanadium (V), or palladium are potential materials for RPD frameworks. In the 1970s, titanium emerged as a disruptive force in the RPD domain, offering a biocompatible and lightweight alternative to the dominant Co-Cr alloy. While exhibiting comparable tensile strength exceeding 500 MPa,[2] its initial adoption was hampered by the casting challenges of pure titanium. This obstacle was overcome through the development of dedicated titanium alloys, typically comprising 90%–94% titanium and 6%–10% Al and V.[3] These alloys retained the desired mechanical properties while facilitating fabrication.

The resultant material boasts several key advantages:

- High strength-to-weight ratio: comparable to Co-Cr, ensuring structural integrity and resistance to deformation under masticatory forces.[4]
- Superior biocompatibility: minimizing immunological reactions compared to other framework materials.[1]
- Reduced weight: nearly half that of Co-Cr, potentially minimizing patient discomfort and strain on abutment teeth.

However, titanium's adoption faces challenges. The primary hurdle is its significantly higher cost compared to Co-Cr, limiting its accessibility for some patients. Additionally, casting titanium requires specialized equipment and techniques, further increasing the cost. Fabrication limitations exist as well, with milling and printing (SLM), while offering versatility, being time consuming, and demanding a higher technical expertise.

When CP titanium is cast under dental conditions, the material properties change dramatically. During the casting procedure, the high affinity of the liquid metal for elements such as oxygen, N, and hydrogen results in their incorporation from the atmosphere. As interstitial alloying elements, their deleterious effect on mechanical properties is a problem. Additionally, reactions between molten titanium metal and the investment refractory produce gases, which cause porosity. Therefore casting

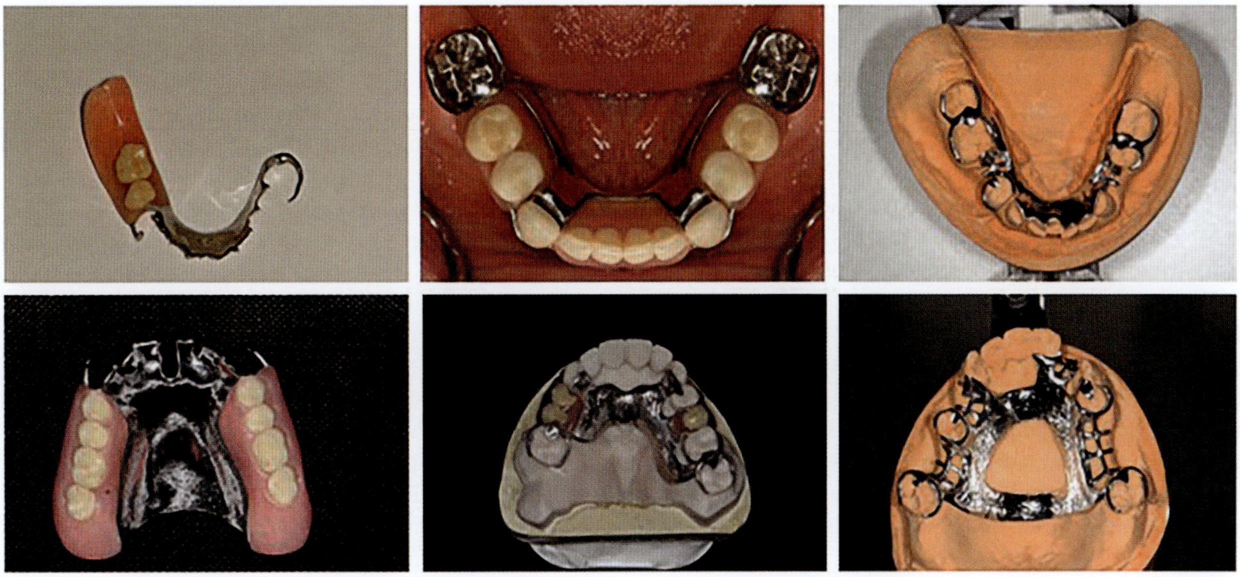

Fig. 12.2 Boasting time-tested reliability and versatility, cobalt-chromium remains the gold standard for removable partial denture framework fabrication and the benchmark for all its design principles. (Courtesy of Ahmed Mahorus Copyright © 2024. All rights reserved.)

titanium necessitates the presence of an argon gas atmosphere. With alpha-beta alloys, such as Ti-6Al-4V, a surface skin of alpha titanium can form (alpha-case zone), which has a tremendous effect on electrochemical behavior and mechanical properties. This could be important for small thin structures, such as clasp assemblies and major and minor connectors. The CP grades of titanium have yield strengths that are too low for clinical use as clasps (450 MPa minimum), although the ductility is high. The much higher yield strengths of the Ti-6Al-4V alloys are the same as that of a typical bench-cooled Co-Cr alloy but with far superior ductility. The typical Young's modulus of elasticity of titanium alloy is half that of Co-Cr and just slightly higher than that of type IV gold alloys. This would require a different approach to clasp design than is used with Co-Cr alloys and would present some advantages. Wrought titanium alloy wires are also flexible because of the same low elastic modulus. Beta alloys, which are used in orthodontics, have two-thirds the elastic modulus of CP titanium and Ti-6Al-4V. The joining of titanium by brazing is a problem, because like-casting, inert atmospheres must be used. The corrosion and fatigue behavior of brazed joints has yet to be tested for long-term corrosion resistance and clinical efficacy.

In conclusion, titanium occupies a unique niche in the RPD landscape. Its impressive combination of strength, biocompatibility, and lightweight nature positions it as a premium material. However, its higher cost and specific fabrication requirements create limitations, making it a compelling choice for patients who prioritize these qualities and have the resources to accommodate them. Continued advancements in processing technology and cost reduction may hold the key to unlocking titanium's full potential and enriching the RPD material landscape.

APPLICATIONS AND SPECIAL CONSIDERATIONS

Titanium is used in the same applications as Co-Cr.

Acetal Resin (Polyoxymethylene)

Acetal resin, formally known as polyoxymethylene (POM), holds a unique position in the world of RPD frameworks. Introduced to dentistry in the 1980s, its inherent strength and rigidity, familiar from industrial applications like gears and bearings, translated well to creating load-bearing components in RPDs. But its true claim to fame lies in its esthetic advantage—the white and pink shades blend better with natural tissues, offering a significant visual improvement over metallic frameworks (Fig. 12.3).

Composed of repeating formaldehyde units (CH2O)n, POM boasts several appealing properties:

- High strength and rigidity: This makes it suitable for clasps, retentive meshwork, and other framework components, ensuring structural stability under masticatory forces.
- Biocompatibility: While not as extensively studied as some other materials, POM generally exhibits good tolerance in most patients.

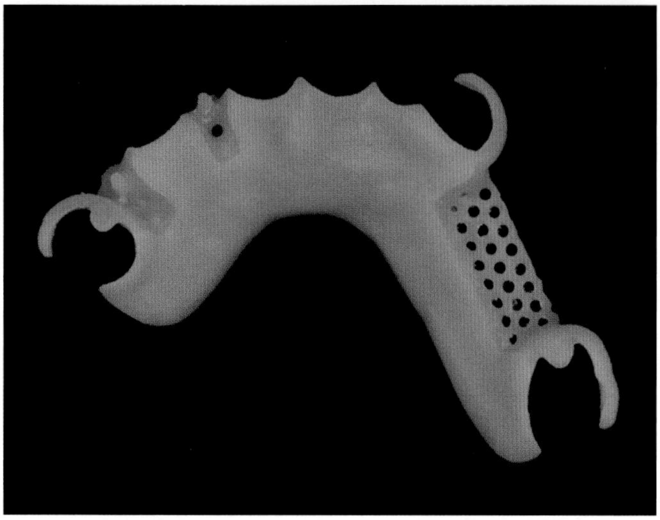

Fig. 12.3 Polyoxymethylene framework for a Kennedy Class II, modification 2. Space is provided for tube teeth on the left side of the framework, and the retentive arms are kept thicker to provide strength.

- Lightweight: Compared with metal frameworks, POM significantly reduces weight, enhancing patient comfort and potentially minimizing strain on abutment teeth.
- Ease of milling: This fabrication method allows for precise shaping of the framework, catering to individual needs and complex designs.

However, POM's limitations require careful consideration before use. Notably, its lower modulus of elasticity compared to metal alloys means clasps need to be thicker to achieve the same deflection resistance. For comparison, an acetal clasp that is 5 mm in length and 1.4 mm in cross-sectional diameter would exhibit the same modulus of elasticity as a Co-Cr clasp that is 15 mm in length and 1 mm in diameter. Studies by Turner et al.[6] and Fitton et al.[7] highlight the potential for increased plaque accumulation and gingival inflammation due to this increased coverage on the abutment teeth. Additionally, Al-Akhali et al.[8] found higher microbial colonization under POM frameworks, prompting caution for patients with compromised immune systems or those at high risk of oral infections. The material has a much higher susceptibility to discoloration, and it is contraindicated in patients with poor oral hygiene or smokers (Fig. 12.4).

Fabrication is carried out by milling POM frameworks. This typically relies on dedicated machines and prefabricated POM pucks. POM can also be injection molded, and it is fabricated by the polymerization of formaldehyde.

Despite its limitations, POM remains a valuable material in the RPD repertoire. Its esthetics, lightweight nature, and ease of milling make it a viable option for patients who prioritize these qualities and maintain diligent oral hygiene. Ultimately, the successful use of POM hinges on a thorough understanding of its properties, limitations, and appropriate milling techniques, followed by careful patient selection and ongoing oral hygiene practices.

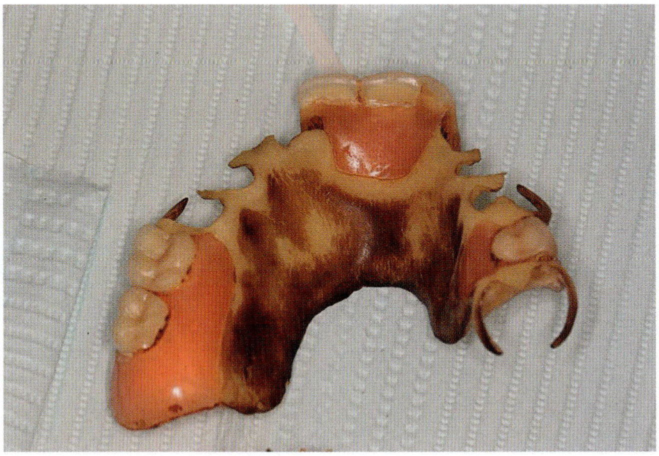

Fig. 12.4 Evident discoloration on a polyoxymethylene removable partial denture framework.

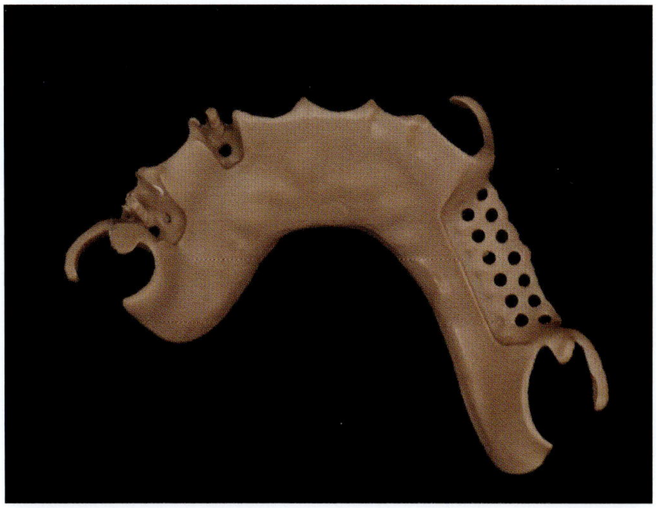

Fig. 12.5 Polyetheretherketone framework for a Kennedy Class II, modification 2. Space is provided for tube teeth on the left side of the framework, and the retentive arms are kept thicker to provide strength.

APPLICATIONS AND SPECIAL CONSIDERATIONS

Acetal resin is commonly used in the fabrication of RPD framework components, including the major and minor connectors, the retentive and reciprocal clasps as well as the rest seats. Due to its mechanical properties, all components need to be significantly thicker and thus pose more challenges to tooth modifications and patient comfort. The retentive clasps bulk can be unsightly as well as a food trap.

Polyetheretherketone

Poly(oxy-1,4-phenyleneoxy-1,4-phenylenecarbonyl-1,4-phenylene) (PEEK), a fully recyclable plastic boasting a remarkable history, emerged as a transformative force in the realm of esthetic RPDs. Introduced in the early 1980s, PEEK initially found its footing in demanding engineering applications due to its exceptional strength, rigidity, and thermal stability. This unique chemical architecture, characterized by repeating oxyphenylene and carbonyl groups, imbues PEEK with these remarkable properties, paving the way for its entry into the dental arena (Fig. 12.5). Fabrication is carried out by milling RPD frameworks from prefabricated PEEK pucks. It can also be manufactured by thermopressing of printed patterns.

PEEK's journey in dentistry began with its utilization for implant components and frameworks, capitalizing on its biocompatible nature and excellent mechanical properties. This initial success spurred further exploration, highlighting its potential for esthetic RPD frameworks. Unlike the metallic gleam of traditional frameworks, PEEK offers natural shades that better blend with oral tissues, significantly enhancing patient satisfaction and confidence. This esthetic advantage is further amplified by PEEK's superior mechanical properties.

It is PEEK's exceptional rigidity, a direct consequence of its chemical makeup, that enables the fabrication of incredibly stable yet thin-walled RPD frameworks. This translates to several benefits for patients, including minimized bulk in the oral cavity, potentially reduced stress on abutment teeth, and potentially enhanced comfort. PEEK frameworks exhibit lower stress on periodontal ligaments compared to metal alloy frameworks, suggesting a potential for improved long-term outcomes.

However, it is crucial to acknowledge that PEEK's rigidity, while advantageous in most designs, necessitates careful consideration in specific scenarios. Distal extension RPDs, for instance, may benefit more from the flexibility of materials like acetal resin (as previously discussed), as PEEK's rigidity could create high stresses on supporting tissues.[9]

In conclusion, PEEK's remarkable journey from its high-performance plastic origins to its current role as a revolutionary esthetic RPD material is a testament to its unique properties. Its biocompatible nature, remarkable strength, and esthetic advantages position it as a rising star, albeit with design considerations for specific situations.

APPLICATIONS AND SPECIAL CONSIDERATIONS

PEEK is commonly used in the fabrication of RPD framework components, including the major and minor connectors, the retentive and reciprocal clasps as well as the rest seats.

Wrought Wire

Wrought wire is used in conjunction with a variety of RPD materials specifically as a direct retainer arm which may be attached to the prosthesis by embedding a portion of the wire in a resin denture base, by soldering to the fabricated framework, or by casting the framework to a wire embedded in the wax pattern (Fig. 12.6). The physical properties of available wrought wires are the most important considerations when a

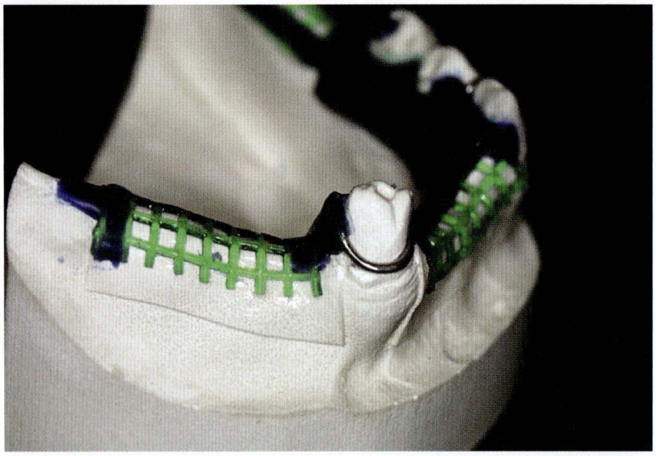

Fig. 12.6 The wrought-wire retainer arm has been contoured and incorporated into the wax pattern where it will become an integral part of the framework. The wire is contoured in two planes and will be mechanically retained in the casting.

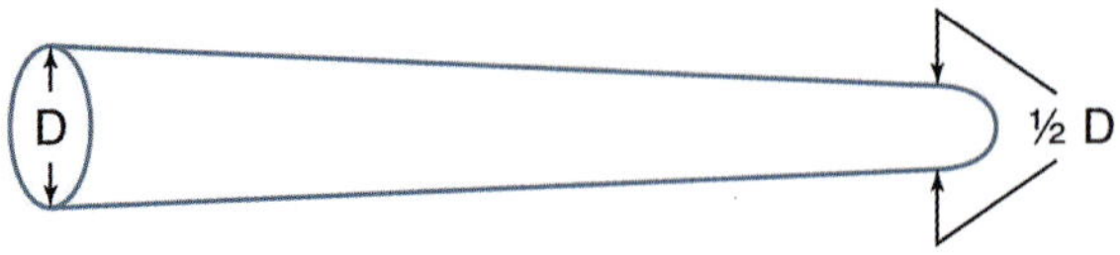

Fig. 12.7 Round, 18-gauge wrought wire for the retentive component of the direct retainer assembly (clasp) is uniformly tapered to 0.8 mm from its full diameter to its terminus. Tapering should precede contouring of the wire for the retainer arm.

proper wire for the desired method of attachment is selected. These properties include yield strength or proportional limit, percentage elongation, tensile strength, and fusion temperature. After the wire is selected, the procedures to which the wire is subjected in fabricating the prosthesis become critical. Improper laboratory procedures can diminish certain desirable physical properties of the wrought structure, rendering it relatively useless for its intended purpose. For example, when wrought wire is heated (such as in a cast-to or soldering procedure), its physical properties and microstructure may be considerably altered, depending on temperature, heating time, and cooling operation.

Regardless of the method of attaching the wrought-wire retainer that is used (i.e., embedding, soldering, or cast-to), tapering the wrought arm seems most rational. A retainer arm is in essence a cantilever that can be made more serviceable and efficient by tapering. Tapering to 0.8 mm permits more uniform distribution of service stresses throughout the length of the arm, being readily demonstrated by photoelastic stress analysis. Uniform tapering of an 18-gauge, round wire arm can be accomplished by rapidly rotating the wire in angled contact with an abrasive disk in the dental lathe. It is then polished by rotating the wire in angled contact with a mildly abrasive rubber disk in the dental lathe. The appropriate taper is shown in Fig. 12.7.

Manufacturing wrought-wire clasps involves bending and shaping the wire to conform to the desired design using specialized pliers and gauges. These preformed clasps are then soldered onto the RPD framework using a delicate technique. The solder, typically a tin-silver alloy, creates a strong yet resilient bond between the wire and the framework, allowing for the transmission of retentive forces.

While offering numerous advantages like minimal bulk, adjustability, and cost-effectiveness, wrought-wire clasps are not without drawbacks. Their flexibility can lead to unwanted movement and potential clasping forces on the teeth. Additionally, they may require more frequent adjustments and are more susceptible to breakage compared to cast clasps. However, for certain clinical scenarios, such as interim prostheses or for patients with limited financial resources, wrought-wire clasps remain a viable and valuable option in the RPD armamentarium.

APPLICATIONS AND SPECIAL CONSIDERATIONS

Wrought-wire clasps are mainly used for retentive clasp arms on cast metal RPDs as well as interim all acrylic-resin RPDs.

Polymethylmethacrylate

PMMA has established itself as the cornerstone of RPD base materials since the 1930s. This enduring dominance stems from a potent combination of desirable properties and diverse fabrication techniques.

- Biocompatible comfort: PMMA demonstrates minimal cytotoxicity and tissue irritation, making it a safe and comfortable choice for long-term oral contact.
- Desirable physical properties: PMMA boasts high flexural strength and dimensional stability, crucial for enduring masticatory stresses and maintaining optimal fit over time. Additionally, its resistance to abrasion and staining promotes longevity and esthetics. This material is easy to repair or reline.
- Esthetic versatility: PMMA's versatility allows for intrinsic tooth staining and tissue tinting, enabling integration with the existing oral tissues. This creates a natural-looking RPD. Manufacturing Techniques:
- Compression molding: This technique usually uses heat-polymerized PMMA material to fabricate interim all acrylic-resin RPDs. While this technique is time tested and reliable, its main drawbacks lie in polymerization shrinkage, porosities, and residual monomer.
- Injection molding: Molten PMMA is injected under pressure into a mold, where it cools and hardens into the desired shape. This method is relatively quick and efficient for mass production but requires specialized equipment and prefabricated molds, limiting customization.
- Milling and printing: These techniques are primarily reserved for all acrylic-resin RPDs (without metal frameworks) when clasping is not required.

Its long-lasting performance and high patient satisfaction solidify its position as the gold standard for RPD bases in most clinical scenarios.

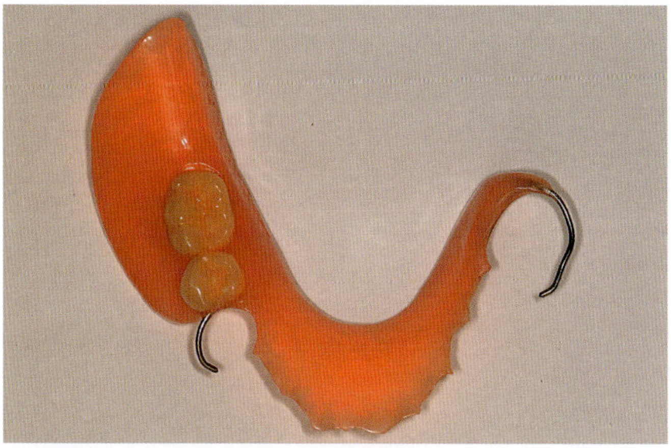

Fig. 12.8 All acrylic removable partial dentures can be very cost effective and versatile especially during transitory periods in which the patient is receiving treatment such as tooth- or implant-supported restorations. (Courtesy of Ahmed Mahorus Copyright © 2024. All rights reserved.)

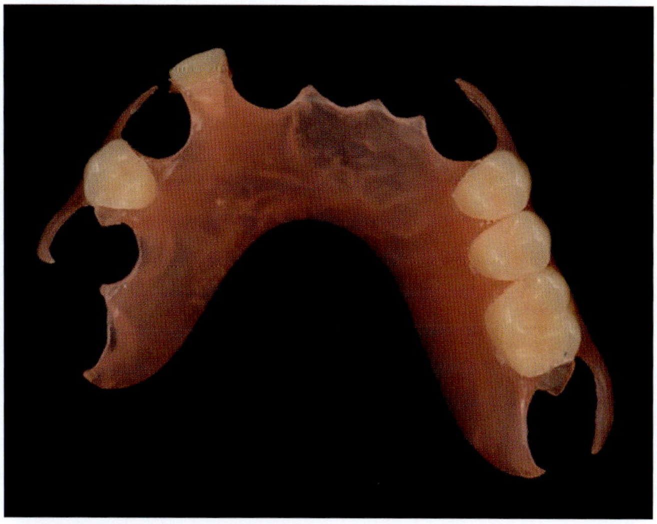

Fig. 12.9 Valplast partial denture.

APPLICATIONS AND SPECIAL CONSIDERATIONS

Denture bases for framework-based RPDs (see Fig. 12.2) as all acrylic-resin RPDs (Fig. 12.8).

Nylon-Based Materials (Thermoplastic Resins)

While PMMA reigns supreme in RPD bases, nylon-based materials such as Valplast offer unique properties and fabrication methods, appealing to specific clinical needs. Developed in the 1950s (Fig 12.9), Valplast is a nylon copolymer known for the following properties:

- Light weight and flexibility: This characteristic provides comfort for patients with sensitive tissues or difficulty tolerating clasps. Valplast's gentle flexibility reduces pressure on delicate tissues.
- Metal-free construction: For individuals with metal allergies, Valplast eliminates potential allergic reactions, making it a viable alternative to metal framework RPDs.
- Esthetics: Valplast's natural appearance provides a pleasing esthetic solution.
- Ease of fabrication: Injection molding allows for relatively quick and efficient fabrication.

However, before considering Valplast, it is crucial to understand its limitations:

- Flexural strength concerns: Studies by Takabayashi[10] and Wadachi et al.[11] report that Valplast may not meet the International Organization for Standardization (ISO) standard for Type III denture base materials, falling short of the required 65 MPa of flexural strength. This raises concerns about its long-term durability, particularly for patients with high masticatory forces.
- Increased tissue pressure: Research by Kawara et al.[12] and Vojdani and Giti[13] suggests that Valplast can exert significantly higher pressure on the supporting soft tissues compared to other resins. This could lead to discomfort or even inflammation in some patients.
- Surface softness: Compared to PMMA, Valplast exhibits a softer surface, making it more susceptible to scratches and nicks. This, together with its color instability, necessitates careful maintenance to prevent esthetic and functional compromises.
- Dimensional instability: Valplast's water absorption properties can lead to dimensional changes over time, affecting the RPD's fit and potentially compromising its function.
- Inability to repair or reline: These materials are very difficult to adjust, especially if frequent adjustments are needed such as in immediate interim RPDs where postextraction healing necessitates adjustments. Additionally, they are not suitable for reline procedures. Reline materials are generally not compatible with thermoplastic resins and result in poor bonding. Valplast clasps cannot be adjusted or repaired.

Manufacturing techniques used with nylon-based materials include injection molding. Preheated liquid Valplast is injected under pressure into a mold, where it cools and hardens into the desired shape. This method offers a relatively quick and efficient process but requires specialized equipment and prefabricated molds.

Selection Factors

While Valplast RPDs offer unique advantages, the limitations necessitate careful consideration. They are mainly suitable for a shorter-term solution. Acrylic RPDs are further expanded upon in Chapter 26.

In selecting materials, it must be remembered that fundamentals of RPDs are inviolable and do not change. It is only methods, procedures, and substances by which the dentist affects the best possible outcomes, that change. The responsibility of the decision still rests with the dentist, who must evaluate all factors in relation to the results desired. In any instance, therefore the dentist must weigh the problems involved, compare and evaluate the characteristics of different potential materials, and then make a decision that leads to delivery of the greatest possible service to the patient.

Table 12.1 summarizes current design methods, manufacturing techniques, advantages, and disadvantages of different RPD materials. Please note that materials and techniques change rapidly, and this chapter and table represent the latest information available at the time of publication of this issue.

TABLE 12.1 Summary of Current Design Methods, Manufacturing Techniques, Advantages, and Disadvantages of Different RPD Materials

RPD Material	Design Methods	Manufacturing Techniques	Advantages	Disadvantages
Cobalt-chromium	Traditional wax pattern designed Computer-aided design (CAD)	Conventional casting Conventional casting of a printed pattern Conventional casting of a milled pattern Selective laser sintering/selective laser melting (SLS/SLM) Milling Rapid prototyping	Favorable mechanical properties Easy casting Biocompatibility Longevity Durability Versatility in application Ability to have a try-in Versatility of clasp design Precision of fit and higher satisfaction with CAD/SLS/SLM	Visibility of metal components High cost Casting shrinkage Metal display Difficult milling Need for multiple appointments Fit is compromised in rapid prototyping
Clinical factors: ability to hide claps | long-term use | ability to plan for future changes | ability to handle high forces | ability to adjust clasps Patient factors: patient preference | previous experience				
Acetal resin–polyoxymethylene	CAD	Milling	Multiple shades for color matching (esthetics) High wear resistance High impact strength High elastic rebound Accuracy of fit	Require greater component thickness High microbial adhesion Increased susceptibility to discoloration Low rigidity Limited choices of clasps Increases clasp thickness
Clinical factors: medium term use | accuracy of fit Patient factors: preference for nonmetal | reduced visits | reduced cost				
Polyetheretherketone Aryl ketone polymers	CAD	Milling Thermopressing of a printed pattern	Esthetics Biocompatibility Low plaque affinity Low distortion Accuracy of fit	Transmits more forces to the underlying tissues in class I cases Thicker clasps needed for adequate strength Low rigidity Limited choices of clasps Increases clasp thickness
Clinical factors: medium-term use | accuracy of fit Patient factors: preference for nonmetal | reduced visits | more economical				
Nylons/thermoplastic resins (Valplast)	Traditional wax pattern designed	Injection molded Heat polymerized	Esthetics High strength Heat resistance Conservative tooth modification Fewer appointments Patient comfort	High surface roughness Inadequate support Low color stability Low wear resistance Low rigidity Limited choices of clasps Excessive soft tissue coverage Inability to reline/repair Inability to modify clasps
Clinical factors: short-term use Patient factors: preference for nonmetal | short fabrication time | more economical				
Polymethylmethacrylate (PMMA)	Traditional wax pattern designed CAD	Injection molded Heat polymerized Autopolymerized CAD–computer-aided manufacturing (CAM) milling CAD-CAM printing	Esthetics High strength Heat resistance Conservative tooth modification Fewer appointments Patient comfort CAD-CAM milled PMMAs Lower bacterial adherence Lower residual monomer Better color stability	Inadequate support Low wear resistance Low rigidity Excessive soft tissue coverage

TABLE 12.1 **Summary Of Current Design Methods, Manufacturing Techniques, Advantages, and Disadvantages of Different Rpd Materials—cont'd**

RPD Material	Design Methods	Manufacturing Techniques	Advantages	Disadvantages
Clinical factors: short- to medium-term use | ability to add teeth | ability to reline Patient factors: most economical | short fabrication time				
Titanium	Traditional wax pattern designed CAD	Casting Casting of a printed pattern Casting of a milled pattern SLS/SLM Milling	Favorable mechanical properties Biocompatibility Light weight For patients with known allergies to other materials	High cost Casting shrinkage Technique-sensitive casting process Difficult milling Metal display Low rigidity Difficult adjustments Few labs available for manufacturing
Clinical factors: long-term use Patient factors: light weight				

RPD, removable partial denture.

REFERENCES

1. Snosi AM, Lotfy SM, Thabet YG, Sabet ME, Rizk FN. Subtractive versus additive indirect manufacturing techniques of digitally designed partial dentures. *J Adv Prosthodontics*. 2021;13(5):327.
2. Oh KC, Yun BS, Kim JH. Accuracy of metal 3D printed frameworks for removable partial dentures evaluated by digital superimposition. *Dental Mater*. 2022;38(2):309–317.
3. Muehlemann E, Özcan M. Accuracy of removable partial denture frameworks fabricated using conventional and digital technologies. *Eur J Prosthodontics Restor Dent*. 2022;30(2):76–86.
4. Ahmed N, Abbasi MS, Haider S, et al. Fit accuracy of removable partial denture frameworks fabricated with CAD/CAM, rapid prototyping, and conventional techniques: a systematic review. *BioMed Res Int*. 2021. https://doi.org/10.1155/2021/3194433. PMID: 3194433.
5. Soltanzadeh P, Suprono MS, Kattadiyil MT, Goodacre C, Gregorius W. An in vitro investigation of accuracy and fit of conventional and CAD/CAM removable partial denture frameworks. *J Prosthodontics*. 2019;28(5):547–555.
6. Turner JW, Radford DR, Sherriff M. Flexural properties and surface finishing of acetal resin denture clasps. *J Prosthodontics*. 1999;8(3):188–195.
7. Fitton JS, Davies EH, Howlett JA, Pearson GJ. The physical properties of a polyacetal denture resin. *Clin Mater*. 1994;17(3):125–129.
8. Al-Akhali MA, El-Kerdawy MW, Ibraheim ZA, Abbas NA. Comparative study on the microbial adhesion to acetal resin and metallic removable partial denture. *Indian J Dent*. 2012;3(1):1–4.
9. Arnold C, Hey J, Schweyen R, Setz JM. Accuracy of CAD-CAM-fabricated removable partial dentures. *J Prosthet Dent*. 2018;119(4):586–592.
10. Takabayashi Y. Characteristics of denture thermoplastic resins for non-metal clasp dentures. *Dental Mater J*. 2010;29(4):353–361.
11. Wadachi J, Sato M, Igarashi Y. Evaluation of the rigidity of dentures made of injection-molded materials. *Dental Mater J*. 2013;32(3):508–511.
12. Kawara M, Iwata Y, Iwasaki M, et al. Scratch test of thermoplastic denture base resins for non-metal clasp dentures. *J Prosthodont Res*. 2014;58(1):35–40.
13. Vojdani M, Giti R. Polyamide as a denture base material: a literature review. *J Dent*. 2015;16(1 Suppl):1.

PART II

Clinical and Laboratory

13

Diagnosis and Treatment Planning

Patricia Swanson, Wendy Clark, Ramtin Sadid-Zadeh, and Ahmed Mahrous

CHAPTER OUTLINE

OBJECTIVES OF PROSTHODONTIC TREATMENT

The objectives of any prosthodontic treatment may be stated as follows: (1) the elimination of disease; (2) the preservation, restoration, and maintenance of the health of the remaining teeth and oral tissues; and (3) the selected replacement of lost teeth for the purpose of (4) restoration of function in a manner that ensures optimum stability and comfort in an esthetically pleasing manner. Preservation is a principle that utilizes all preventive and therapeutic measures to maintain oral health. It is a principle that guards decisions that place too high a premium on cosmetic concerns, underscoring the clinician's obligation to emphasize the importance of restoring the total mouth to a state of health and of preserving the remaining teeth and surrounding tissues.

Diagnosis and treatment planning for oral rehabilitation of partially edentulous mouths must take into consideration the following: control of caries and periodontal disease, restoration of individual teeth, provision of harmonious occlusal relationships, and the replacement of missing teeth by fixed (using natural teeth and/or implants) or removable prostheses. Because these procedures are integrally related, the appropriate selection and sequencing of treatment should precede all irreversible procedures.

Though the fabrication of the removable prosthesis is often the final step in a sequence of treatment, the planning (including design) should precede all but emergency treatment. This allows abutment teeth and other areas in the mouth to be properly prepared to support, stabilize, and retain the removable partial denture (RPD). This means that diagnostic casts must be made before definitive treatment is undertaken, to allow for designing and planning the removable prosthesis. After reviewing the existing condition of the remaining dentition and supporting structures, as well as the major factors that create and resist functional forces, the RPD design is drawn on the diagnostic cast and serves as the master plan for the mouth preparations and the prosthesis to follow.

Failure of RPDs can usually be attributed to factors that result in poor stability. These can result from inadequate diagnosis and failure to properly evaluate the conditions present. This results in failure to prepare the patient and the oral tissues properly before the master cast is fabricated. The importance of the examination, the consideration of favorable and unfavorable aspects relative to movement control, and the importance of planning the elimination of unfavorable influences cannot be overemphasized (see Chapter 2).

For complex treatment, two appointments are often required for obtaining diagnostic records. The first will include a preliminary oral examination (to determine the need for management of acute needs), a prophylaxis, periodontal charting, full-mouth radiographs, diagnostic casts, and mounting records if baseplates are not required. The follow-up appointment includes mounting of the diagnostic casts (when baseplates and occlusion rims are needed), a definitive oral examination, review of the radiographs to augment and correlate with clinical findings, and arrangement of additional consultations when required. Following the collection and synthesis of all patient and clinical information, including surveying of the casts, a treatment plan (often including alternative options) is presented.

The determination of each patient's treatment occurs through patient interview, clinical and radiographic examination, and diagnostic laboratory procedures. This can be divided into four distinct processes: (1) understanding the patient's desires or chief concerns/complaints regarding his or her condition (including its history) through a systematic interview process, (2) ascertaining the patient's dental needs through a diagnostic clinical examination, (3) developing a treatment plan that reflects the best management of desires and needs (with influences unique to the medical condition or oral environment), and (4) executing appropriately sequenced treatment with planned follow-up. Provision of the best care for a patient may involve no treatment, limited treatment, or extensive treatment, and the dentist must be prepared to help patients decide the best treatment option given their individual circumstances.

PATIENT INTERVIEW

A fundamental objective of the patient interview is to understand why the patient is presenting for evaluation. In addition, to information gathering, the interview is an opportunity to develop rapport with the patient. It is important to understand the patient's chief oral concerns and their motivations and apprehensions regarding care. These factors are crucial in determining the proposed treatment. Having these discussions at the outset of patient care can contribute to setting and meeting realistic patient expectations.

An initial patient interview should include the following elements, which will be reviewed in detail later in this chapter:

- Chief complaint and its history
- Medical history review
- Dental history review, especially related to previous prosthetic experience(s)
- Patient expectations

Understanding a patient's expectations is critical to determining whether an RPD will satisfy the patient. The fact that removable prostheses require a certain material thickness and often use oral soft tissues for support may be hard to comprehend for patients with no such prosthetic history. Helping the patient understand the normal phase of accommodation to such a prosthesis is an important discussion point in selection of a prosthesis. For those patients with a negative past prosthesis experience, it is necessary to determine before treatment is started whether the design, fit, occlusion, or lack of maintenance of the prosthesis can be improved to provide a more positive experience. Whenever possible, remind the patient to bring their prior prosthesis to the appointment, to allow for evaluation. This is important even if they do not currently utilize it, to determine if it was indeed the prosthesis, or instead the patient's expectations, which require adjustment.

SHARED DECISION-MAKING

The clinical practice model termed *shared decision-making* gives structure to a process where the provider and the patient identify together the best course of care. There are three main elements in shared decision-making:

- Understanding and acknowledging that the decision is shared
- Utilizing current evidence-based treatment options
- Incorporating patient values and preferences

CLINICAL EXAMINATION

ORAL EXAMINATION

A complete oral examination should precede any treatment decisions. It should include visual and digital examination of the hard and soft oral tissues to rule out pathology. Careful examination of each tooth surface is performed with a mouth mirror, explorer, and periodontal probe and supplemented by vitality tests of critical teeth. Diagnostic casts should be evaluated and surveyed. Clinical findings are augmented by and correlated with a complete intraoral radiographic survey. During the examination, the objective to be kept foremost in mind should be the consideration of possibilities for restoring and maintaining the remaining oral structures in a state of health for the longest period of time.

Sequence of Oral Examination

An oral examination should be accomplished in the following sequence: visual examination, pain relief and provisional restorations, radiographs, oral prophylaxis, evaluation of teeth and periodontium, vitality tests of individual teeth, determination of the floor of the mouth position, and impressions of each arch. An initial estimation of vertical dimension of occlusion can be evaluated, to be reviewed further with mounted casts.

- *Visual examination.* This process will reveal many of the signs of dental disease. Consideration of caries susceptibility is of primary importance, particularly as literature indicates that use of RPDs may increase caries risk. The number of restored teeth present, signs of recurrent caries, and evidence of decalcification should be noted, and caries risk assessment should be completed. Acute dental needs will be apparent and addressed next.

- *Relief of pain and discomfort by placement of temporary restorations.* If the patient is in pain, this should be addressed first so they can comfortably proceed with subsequent appointments. Treatment may include endodontic therapy or placement of protective restorations. Nonrestorable teeth and retained root tips should be extracted to prevent infection and allow time for healing of the residual ridge prior to the definitive prosthesis fabrication.
- *Oral cancer screening.* A thorough head and neck exam and an intraoral cancer screening should be performed. Evaluation of the lips, gingiva, mucosa, floor of mouth, tongue, palate, and oropharynx should be performed both visually and manually. The patient should be screened for risk factors for oral cancer, including tobacco use, alcohol use, and human papillomavirus exposure and/or vaccination status. Areas of concern should be documented with photography with a measuring device, such as a periodontal probe, to notate the size and form. Abnormalities which do not resolve within 2 weeks should be biopsied or referred to an oral pathologist for evaluation
- *A thorough and complete oral prophylaxis and periodontal evaluation.* Cursory examination may precede an oral prophylaxis, but a complete oral examination should be deferred until the teeth have been thoroughly cleansed to ensure no defects are missed. Also, accurate diagnostic casts of the dental arches can be obtained only if the teeth are clean; otherwise the teeth reproduced on the diagnostic casts are not a true representation of tooth and gingival contours. At the time of the initial examination, periodontal disease, gingival inflammation, the degree of gingival recession, and mucogingival relationships should be observed. Such an examination will not provide sufficient information to allow a definitive diagnosis and treatment plan. For this purpose, complete periodontal charting that includes pocket depths, assessment of attachment levels, furcation involvement, mucogingival problems, and tooth mobility must be performed. Bitewing radiographs are utilized to evaluate the bone level of abutment teeth most accurately. Referral to a periodontist should be completed when indicated, as periodontal health must be stabilized prior to commencing definitive treatment.
- *Complete intraoral radiographic survey* (Fig. 13.1). The objectives of a radiographic examination are (1) to locate areas of infection and other pathosis that may be present; (2) to reveal the presence of root fragments, foreign objects, bone spicules, and irregular ridge formations; (3) to reveal the presence and extent of caries and the relation of carious lesions to the pulp and periodontal attachment; (4) to permit evaluation of existing restorations; (5) to reveal the presence of endodontic treatments and posts and to permit their evaluation as to future prognosis (the design of the RPD may hinge on the decision to retain or extract an endodontically treated tooth); (6) to permit evaluation of periodontal conditions present and to establish the need and possibilities for treatment; and (7) to evaluate the alveolar support of abutment teeth, their number, the supporting length and morphology of their roots, the relative amount of alveolar bone loss suffered through pathogenic processes, and the amount of alveolar support remaining.
- *Examination of teeth, investing structures, and residual ridges.* The teeth, existing restorations, periodontium, and residual ridges can be explored by instrumentation and visual means. Recording of relevant patient history and clinical data is important to document features important to clinical presentation and must be recorded on electronic or paper charts for future reference (Figs. 13.2 and 13.3).
- *Impressions for making accurate diagnostic casts to be mounted for occlusal examination.* The casts preferably will be articulated on a suitable instrument. The importance of accurate diagnostic casts and their use will be discussed later in this chapter.
- *Caries control.* It is advisable not only to relieve discomfort arising from tooth defects but also to determine as early as possible the extent of caries. Provisional restorations can be utilized to prevent further caries activity until definitive treatment can be instituted. Additionally, caries risk evaluation should be performed and preventative treatment should be initiated as soon as possible.

The number of teeth remaining, the location of the edentulous areas, and the quality of the residual ridge will have a definite bearing on the proportionate amount of support that the RPD will receive from the teeth and edentulous ridges (Fig. 13.4). Tissue contours may appear to present a well-formed edentulous residual ridge; however, palpation often

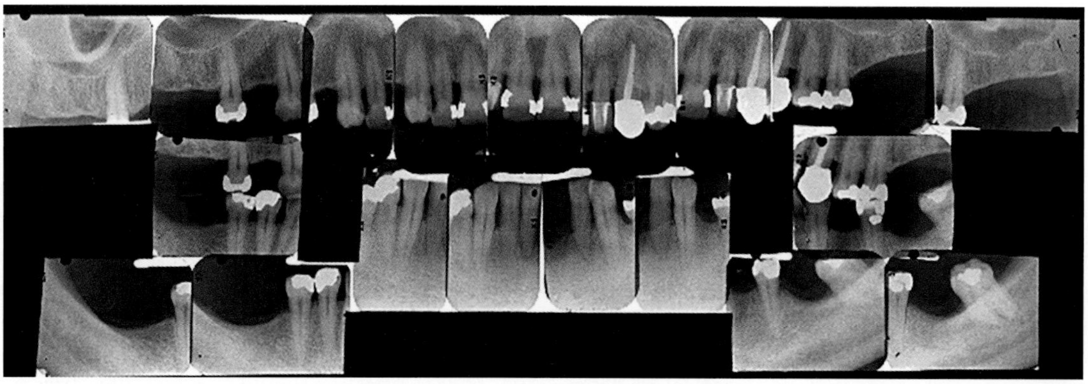

Fig. 13.1 Complete intraoral radiographic survey of remaining teeth and adjacent edentulous areas reveals much information vital to effective diagnosis and treatment planning. The response of bone to previous stress is of particular value in establishing the prognosis of teeth that are to be used as abutments.

REMOVABLE PARTIAL PROSTHODONTICS

PATIENT NAME ____________ PATIENT NUMBER ____________

☐ TREATMENT PLAN

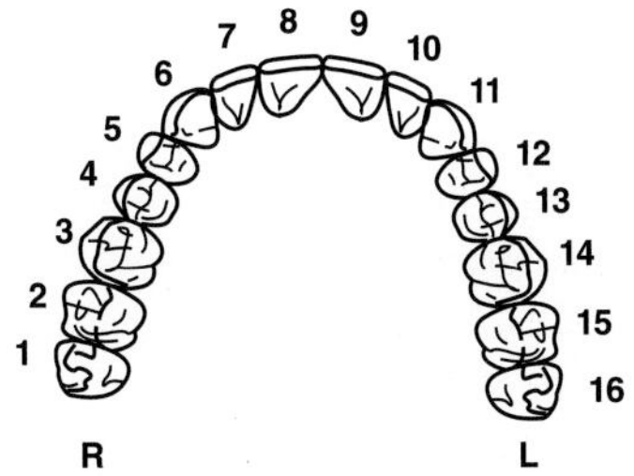

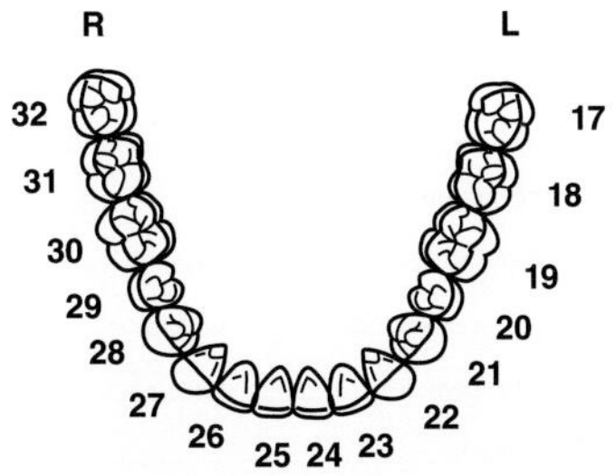

COLOR CODE:

BLUE:---- CAST METAL
RED: ----- RESIN BASE AND WROUGHT WIRE
GREEN:-- AREAS TO BE CONTOURED

INSTRUCTOR: ____________________

☐ LABORATORY INSTRUCTIONS

DESIGN SPECIFICATIONS:

1. RESTS
2. RETENTION
3. RECIPROCATION
4. MAJOR CONNECTOR
5. INDIRECT RETENTION
6. GUIDE PLANES
7. BASE RETENTION
8. AREAS TO BE MODIFIED OR CONTOURED

APPROVAL TO SEND TO LABORATORY: ______________ DATE: ________

A

Fig. 13.2 A, Diagnosis record for recording pertinent data. **B,** Treatment record chart for recording treatment plan and treatment progress.

PATIENT'S NAME John Doe CHART NO. 383838

STUDENT'S NAME Joe Smith JR. X SR. ___ STUDENT NO. 1234

STARTING DATE 1/14/99 INSTRUCTOR SIGNATURE PGreen

COMPLETION DATE ___ INSTRUCTOR SIGNATURE ___

REMOVABLE PARTIAL DENTURE

MAX RPD MAND. RPD

DIAGNOSIS

1. Are you wearing or have you worn an oral prosthesis? No___ Yes ✓. If so, what type? metal + plastic
2. If a previously worn prosthesis was not entirely satisfactory, what in your opinion were the problems with it? no retention, + teeth badly worn
3. What was the cause of loss of the natural teeth? Perio X, Caries X, Trauma___.

INTRAORAL FINDINGS

1. Oral hygiene index: Good X Fair___ 2. Caries Index: High___ Moderate___ Low X.
3. Do centric occlusion and centric relation coincide? Yes X No___.
4. Are there frenula or muscle attachments that might interfere with maximum fit and comfort? Yes___ No X.
5. Is type and quality of saliva normal? Yes X No___. Comments___
6. Examine the following areas for possible interference with optimal fit and comfort.

   Mylohyoid Ridge Normal ✓ Other:___ Alveolar Ridges Tissues Normal ✓

   Tuberosity Normal ✓ Other:___ Supporting Alveolar Bone Normal ✓

   Tori Present Yes___ No X
7. Is any surgical procedure indicated to improve the prognosis? No ✓ Note___

DIAGNOSTIC CAST ANALYSIS

On the Articulator

1. Is there adequate interridge space for the contemplated prosthesis? Yes ✓ No___
2. Is the occlusal plane retrievable? Yes ✓ Doubtful___
3. Is there adequate inter-occlusal space for contemplated rest seats and rests where they will be needed?

   Yes ✓ Note___
4. Are there anomalies which were not evident intra-orally? No ✓ Note___

On The Surveyor

1. Which teeth are the most suitable abutments? Abutment #1 20 Abutment #2 28 Abutment #3___

   Abutment #4___ Other___.
2. Do the abutments have adequate retentive undercuts in a favorable location on the tooth? Yes X No___.
3. Can suitable guiding planes be developed on the probable abutments? Yes X No___
4. Will tooth alterations be required? No___ Yes X

RADIOGRAPHIC INTERPRETATION

1. What is the crown root ratio of each abutment? Abutment #1 1:3 Abutment #2 1:3 Abutment #3___

   Abutment #4___
2. Does the supporting bone appear to be of good quality? Yes X No___.

QUALITY PRESS, INC.

B

Fig. 13.2 (Cont'd)

Name: *John Doe* Date: *July 1, 1999*

Summary Plan:

Maxillary Conventional Complete denture

Mandibular Class II mod. 1 removable partial denture

Porcelain fused to metal abutment Crowns #18, #29

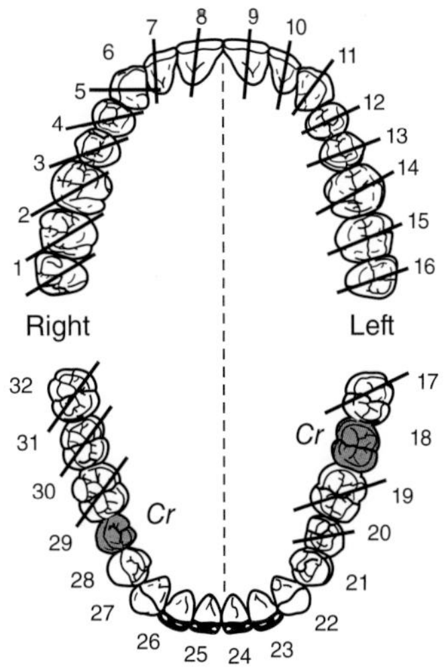

Procedures:

Tissue conditioning maxillary arch

Primary impression-both arches; make impression trays

Preparations. Contour and rest seats #21, #28. Abutment crown preparations #18, #29

Try-in abutment crowns; pick-up for cast for framework casting

Try-in abutment crowns and framework

Fluid wax functional impression: Make altered cast

Jaw relation records; shade and mold selection

Tooth arrangement

Try-in trial set-up; verify jaw relations

Placement: Mandibular crowns, partial denture, maxillary complete denture

Follow-up care

Red line each completed unit

Fig. 13.3 Simple working chart. Restorations for individual teeth, crowns, and fixed partial dentures to be made may be marked on the chart and checked off as completed during mouth preparations.

indicates that supporting bone has been resorbed and has been replaced by displaceable, fibrous connective tissue. Such a situation is common in maxillary tuberosity regions. The RPD cannot be supported adequately by tissues that are easily displaced. When the mouth is prepared, this tissue should be recontoured or removed surgically, unless otherwise contraindicated. A small but stable residual ridge is preferable to a larger unstable ridge for providing support for the denture. The presence of tori or other bony exostoses must be detected, and their presence in relation to framework design must be evaluated. Failure to palpate the tissue over the median palatal raphe to ascertain the difference in its displaceability as compared with the displaceability of the soft tissues covering the residual ridges can lead to a rocking, unstable, uncomfortable denture, and result in an unsatisfied patient. Adequate relief of the palatal major connectors must be planned, and the amount of relief required is directly proportionate to the difference in displaceability of the tissues over the midline of the palate and the tissues covering the residual ridges.

During the examination, not only each arch but also its occlusal relationship with the opposing arch must be considered separately. A situation that looks unproblematic when the teeth are apart may be complicated when the teeth are in occlusion. For example, an extreme vertical overlap may complicate the attachment of anterior teeth to a maxillary denture. Extrusion of a tooth or teeth into an opposing edentulous area may complicate the replacement of teeth in the edentulous area or may create occlusal interference, which will complicate the location and design of clasp retainers and occlusal rests. Such findings subsequently will be evaluated further by careful analysis of mounted diagnostic casts.

The fee for examination, which should include the cost of the radiographic survey and the examination of articulated diagnostic casts, should be established before the examination is performed and should not be related to the cost of treatment, but it must be understood that the examination fee is based on the time involved and the service rendered and that the material value of the radiograph and diagnostic casts is incidental to the examination's effectiveness.

DIAGNOSTIC FINDINGS

The information gathered in the patient interview and clinical examination provides the basis for establishing whether treatment is indicated, and if so, what specific treatment should be considered. More than one treatment option can be considered, and financial implications need to be considered against long-term expectations if the best decision is to be reached. Provision of an RPD does not often preclude future consideration for other treatments, a fact that is not often the case for alternative treatments. The patient interview can reveal medical considerations that influence the decision to provide any prosthesis. When it is felt that general medical health is being neglected, patients should be strongly encouraged to seek a general

Prosthodontic Diagnostic Index (PDI) Classification System

PDI Partially Edentulous Worksheet

	Class I	Class II	Class III	Class IV
Location and Extent of Edentulous Areas				
1 arch, MX ≤ 2 incisors, MD ≤ 4 incisors,≤ 2 pre-molars, ≤ one pre-molar and a molar				
Both arches and otherwise same as above, or 1/both arches and missing canine(s)				
1/both arches, posterior area > 3 teeth or two molars, antero-post area ≥ 3 teeth				
Requiring high degree of patient compliance; guarded prognosis				
Congenital or acquired maxillofacial defect				
Abutment condition				
Localized adjunctive treatment (perio, endo, ortho)				
None				
1-2 sextants				
3 sextants				
≥ 4 sextants				
Insufficient tooth structure				
None				
1-2 sextants				
3 sextants				
≥ 4 sextants				
Occlusion				
No pre-prosthetic therapy				
Localized adjunctive therapy				
Re-establish entire occlusion, no change in OVD				
Re-establish entire occlusion, with change in OVD				
Residual ridge				
Class I edentulous				
Class II edentulous				
Class III edentulous				
Class IV edentulous				
Conditions creating a guarded prognosis				
Severe oral manifestations of systemic disease				
Maxillomandibular dyskinesia and/or ataxia				
Refractory patient				
ICD-9-CM diagnostic code	525.51	525.52	525.53	525.54

Guidelines for use of the worksheet

1. Any single criterion of a more complex class places the patient into the more complex class.
2. Consideration of future treatment procedures must not influence the diagnostic level.
3. Hopeless teeth should not be considered in applying the classification.
4. Initial preprosthetic treatment and/or adjunctive therapy can change the initial classification level
5. If there is an esthetic concern/challenge, the classification is increased in complexity by one or more levels.
6. In the presence of TMD symptoms, the classification is increased in complexity in one or more levels.
7. In the situation where the patient presents with an edentulous maxilla opposing a partially edentulous mandible, each arch is diagnosed with the appropriate classification system.

Fig. 13.4 The American College of Prosthodontists created a classification for partially edentulous patients to help facilitate communication. This chart facilitates classification for clinicians. *ICD-9-CM*, International Classification of Diseases, Ninth Revision, Clinical Modification; *MX*, Maxilla; *MD*, mandible; *OVD*, occlusal vertical dimension; *TMD*, temporomandibular disorder.

medical examination. Alternatively, patients who regularly see their physician may be found to take multiple medications that can contribute to a dry mouth and, potentially, an altered oral microflora with some increased risk for plaque-induced disease. Although such a condition can influence any prosthodontic care, given the unique features of RPD service relative to the need for increased hygiene awareness and care, any factor that places an additional risk for plaque-induced disease should be emphasized with the patient and corrected if possible. Health conditions that negatively affect oral mucosal health (e.g., diabetes mellitus, Sjögren syndrome, lupus, and atrophic changes) may pose a risk for patient comfort for a tissue-supported prosthesis and factor into a treatment decision. Additional consideration should be given to a past history of cancer treatment, bisphosphonate use, or other medications related to osteonecrosis of the jaw, prior to any surgical treatments such as extractions or implant placement.

For the patient who has had previous experience with some form of prosthesis, the patient interview provides additional information that can influence treatment decisions. Identifying possible reasons (or more importantly a lack of any reason) for both positive and negative past prosthesis experiences is important for determining whether a patient can predictably be helped. Although the clinical examination will point out the oral tissue responses to such therapy, the interview will highlight the subjective patient response to therapy and provide significant information that should be pursued. It is equally important for clinicians to know when *not* to treat patients, as it is to know how to effectively treat them.

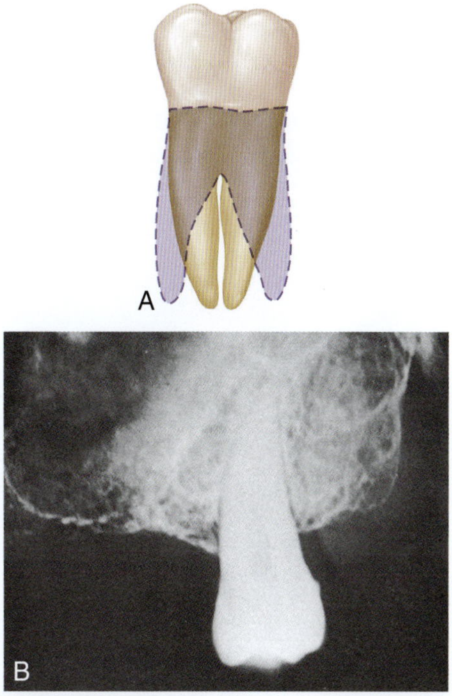

Fig. 13.5 A, The prognosis for abutment service is more favorable for a molar with divergent roots *(shaded)* than for the same tooth if its roots were fused and conical. **B,** Evidence that prospective abutment has conical and fused roots indicates the necessity for formulating a framework design that will minimize additional stresses placed on the tooth by the abutment service.

Radiographic Interpretation

An updated series of radiographs is a key piece of the diagnostic puzzle. Periapical radiographs should be taken of all remaining teeth and their apices, and bitewing radiographs should be made, when possible, of remaining posterior teeth. A panoramic radiograph can help visualize the temporomandibular joints (TMJs), as well as bony pathology and remaining bone height.

Radiographic findings should serve the dentist as an adjunct to clinical observations, and not used alone to arrive at a diagnosis. Radiographic interpretation also serves an important function when used periodically after the prosthesis has been placed, allowing for monitoring of occlusal trauma. The following may be assessed radiographically:

Disease Validation

Most commonly, radiographs are used for the diagnosis of caries location and extent, in terms of numbers of lesions and dentin/pulpal involvement, to gain insight as to the level of disease risk associated with the patient, as well as to identify what therapy is required to maintain teeth. The same is true for periodontal disease risk and severity, as such a diagnosis affects both current and future tooth prognoses for prosthesis support.

Radiographic interpretation allows diagnosis of bone lesions associated with the jaws, teeth, and adjacent structures. Surgical and postoperative management of such lesions can vary significantly with diagnosis (benign vs. malignant), and definitive prosthesis treatment is often complicated by resective procedures.

Root Morphology

The morphologic characteristics of the roots greatly determine the ability of prospective abutment teeth to resist additional rotational forces that may be placed on them. Teeth with multiple and divergent roots will resist stresses better than teeth with fused and conical roots, because the resultant forces are distributed through a greater number of periodontal fibers to a larger amount of supporting bone (Fig. 13.5).

Tooth Support

The quality of the alveolar support of an abutment tooth is of primary importance because the tooth will have to withstand greater stress loads when supporting a dental prosthesis. Bitewings will most accurately approximate the bone level, and vertically oriented bitewing radiographs can be utilized in cases of periodontal disease. Abutment teeth providing

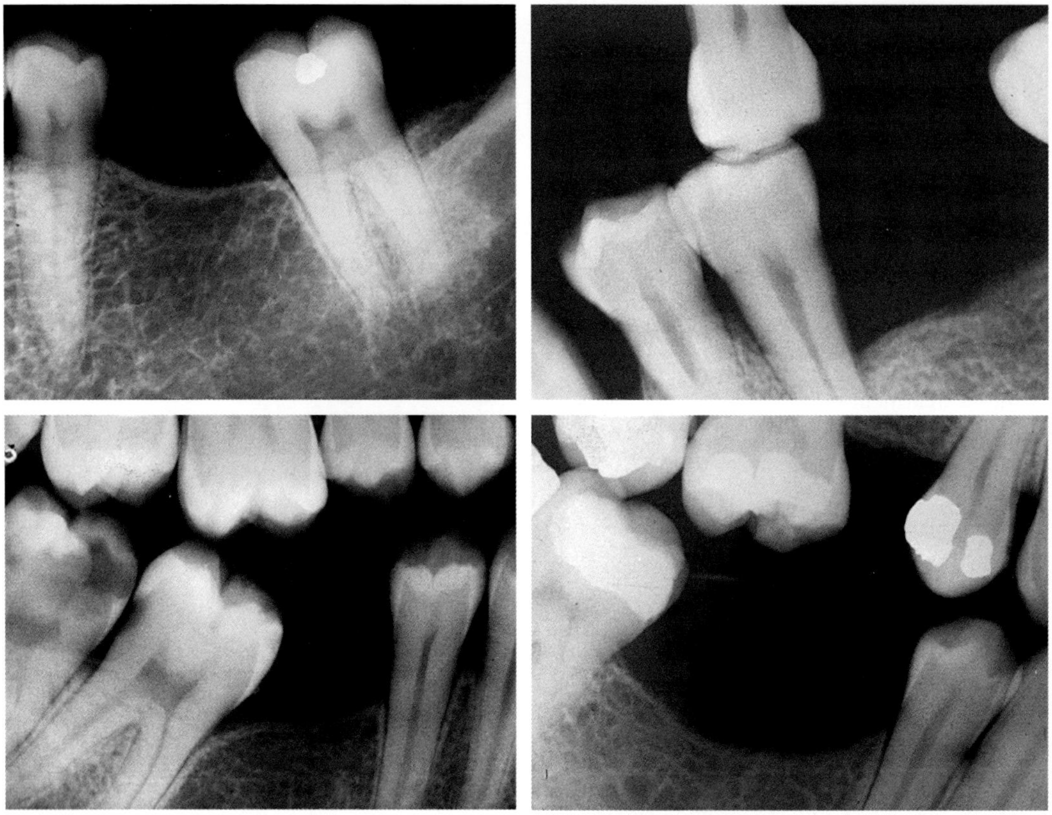

Fig. 13.6 The reaction of bone adjacent to teeth subjected to abnormal stress indicates probable reactions of that bone when such teeth are used as abutments for fixed or removable restorations. Such areas are called *index areas.*

total abutment support to the prosthesis, whether fixed or removable, will have to withstand a greater load and especially greater horizontal forces. The latter may be minimized by establishing a harmonious occlusion and by distributing the horizontal forces among several teeth through rigid connectors. Bilateral stabilization against horizontal forces is one of the attributes of a properly designed tooth-supported removable prosthesis. In many instances, abutment teeth may be aided more than weakened by the presence of a bilaterally rigid RPD (Fig. 13.6).

In contrast, abutment teeth adjacent to distal extension bases are subjected not only to vertical and horizontal forces but also to torque because of movement of the tissue-supported base. Vertical support and stabilization against horizontal movement with rigid connectors are just as important as they are with a tooth-supported prosthesis, and the RPD must be designed accordingly. It is important to judge whether the teeth and their respective periodontium can favorably respond to the demands of a prosthesis. Assessment of regions within the mouth that have been subjected to increased occlusal loads can provide some clues as to the predictability of future tooth response to increased loading by a prosthesis. An understanding of bone quality, index areas, and lamina dura response is helpful for these judgments (Fig. 13.7).

Radiographic evaluation of bone quality is hazardous but is often necessary. It is essential to emphasize that changes in bone mineralization of up to 25% often cannot be recognized by ordinary radiographic means. Optimum bone qualities are ordinarily expressed by normal-sized interdental trabecular spaces that tend to decrease slightly in size as examination of the bone proceeds from the root apex toward the coronal portion. The normal interproximal crest is ordinarily shown by a relatively thin white line crossing from the lamina dura of one tooth to the lamina dura of the adjacent tooth. Considerable variation in the size of trabecular spaces may exist within normal limits, and the radiographic appearance of crestal alveolar bone may vary considerably, depending on its shape and the direction that the ray takes as it passes through the bone.

Normal bone usually responds favorably to ordinary stresses. Abnormal stresses, however, may reduce the trabecular pattern size, particularly in that area of bone adjacent to the lamina dura of the affected tooth. This decrease in size of the trabecular pattern (i.e., so-called bone condensation) is often regarded as a favorable bone response, indicative of an improvement in bone quality. This is not necessarily an accurate interpretation. Such bone changes usually indicate stresses that should be relieved, because if the resistance of the patient decreases, the bone may exhibit a progressively less favorable response on future radiographs.

Increased width of the periodontal ligament space ordinarily suggests varying degrees of tooth mobility. This should be evaluated clinically. Radiographic evidence coupled with clinical findings may suggest to the dentist the inadvisability of using such a tooth as an abutment. Furthermore an irregular intercrestal bone surface should make the dentist suspicious of active bone deterioration.

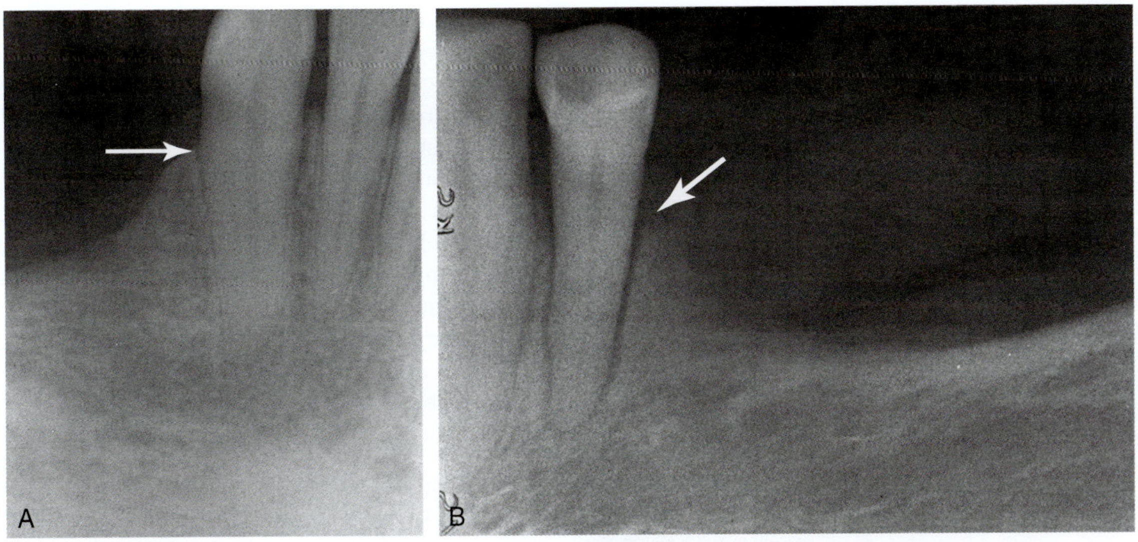

Fig. 13.7 **A,** The canine has provided support for the distal extension removable partial denture for 10 years. There has obviously been positive bone response *(arrow)* to increased stress generated by the removable partial denture. **B,** The mandibular first premolar has provided support for the distal extension denture for 3 years. Bone response *(arrow)* to past additional stress has been unfavorable.

Alveolar Lamina Dura

The alveolar lamina dura is also considered in a radiographic interpretation of abutment teeth. The lamina dura is the thin layer of hard cortical bone that normally lines the sockets of all teeth. It affords attachment for the fibers of the periodontal membrane, and as with all cortical bone, its function is to withstand mechanical strain. In a radiographic image, the lamina dura is shown as a radiopaque white line around the radiolucent dark line that represents the periodontal membrane.

When a tooth is in the process of being tipped, the center of rotation is not at the apex of the root but in the apical third. Resorption of bone occurs where there is pressure, and apposition occurs where there is tension. Therefore during the active tipping process, the lamina dura is uneven, with evidence of both pressure and tension on the same side of the root. For example, in a mesially tipping lower molar, the lamina dura will be thinner on the coronal mesial and apicodistal aspects and thicker on the apicomesial and coronal distal aspects because the axis of rotation is not at the root apex but is above it. When the tooth has been tipped into an edentulous space by some change in the occlusion and becomes set in its new position, the effects of leverage are discontinued. The lamina dura on the side to which the tooth is sloping becomes uniformly heavier, which is nature's reinforcement against abnormal stresses. The bone trabeculations are most often arranged at right angles to the heavier lamina dura.

Periodontal Considerations

An assessment of the periodontium in general and abutment teeth in particular must be made before prosthetic restoration. One must evaluate the condition of the gingiva and the degree of clinical attachment loss. The ideal periodontal condition is a disease-free periodontium with adequate keratinized mucosa in regions at or adjacent to RPD component parts that cross the gingival margins to best resist the mechanical challenges posed as the result of function and use. The condition of the supporting bone around teeth involved in the designed RPD must be evaluated, with specific attention to recession of supporting bone and mobility of teeth. If mucogingival involvements, recession of osseous tissue, or mobility patterns are recorded, the causes and potential treatment must be determined.

The oral hygiene habits of the patient must be determined, and efforts must be made to educate the patient relative to plaque control. Patients with poor oral hygiene must be motivated and educated to improve their condition prior to any definitive treatment (Fig. 13.8). Patients must be informed of the importance of continuum of care; when assessed to be high risk, periodontal maintenance with continued oral hygiene instructions should be scheduled for 3- to 4-month intervals. Referral to a periodontist for specialty care should be considered for patients with extreme clinical attachment loss, rapid progression of disease, or additional risk factors such as diabetes or smoking. In addition, the patient must be advised of the importance of regular maintenance appointments for tissue-supported prostheses to maintain occlusal relationships and soft tissue adaptation. When these ongoing observations and prophylactic requirements are described, the patient is faced with the realization that they must be willing to share responsibility for maintaining the oral health after periodontal, restorative, and prosthodontic treatment.

The remaining teeth and prosthesis require meticulous plaque control after placement of an RPD. Because of the nature of material coverage of oral tissues, the oral microflora can change with the use of a removable prosthesis. Coupled with

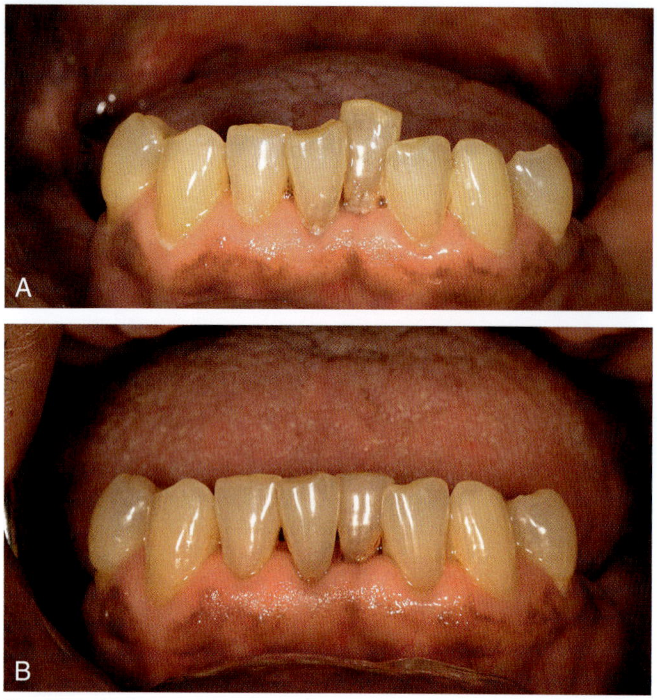

Fig. 13.8 A, Prior to initiating definitive removable prosthodontic care, this patient exhibited poor home care and a buildup of biofilm. **B,** An oral prophylaxis was completed, along with oral hygiene instructions and enameloplasty. Once excellent home care was demonstrated, the process of removable partial denture fabrication began. (Courtesy of Dr. Daniel Diaz Samayoa, Birmingham, AL.)

this microbial change is the potential for a mechanical challenge to tissue integrity if the appropriate relationship between the prosthesis and soft tissues of the residual ridge, as well as the marginal gingival, is not maintained.

Caries Risk Assessment Considerations

Caries risk should be evaluated for each patient and is of particular importance for patients receiving RPDs. Wearing a removable prosthesis increases caries risk, particularly if the prosthesis and oral cavity are not thoroughly cleaned each day (Fig. 13.9). Current evidence indicates that caries is a process that occurs on a spectrum. When the pathogenic factors (frequent exposure to carbohydrates, xerostomia, etc.) outweigh the protective factors, the bacteria that cause caries can thrive. The exam, patient interview, and treatment plan should include a discussion on the patient's current risk factors, how to mitigate them, and an appropriate recommendation to increase protective factors. If caries risk is deemed moderate or high, a caries management program should be implemented for that patient before proceeding with care, including both in office and home care regimens. The caries management by risk assessment (CAMBRA) protocol can provide guidance (Table 13.1).

Xerostomia enhances the occurrence and severity of caries, as well as contributes to irritation of the oral mucosa. Etiologies include degeneration of salivary glands (Sjögren syndrome), radiation treatment, or various medications. A viable way to alleviate xerostomia is the use of synthetic saliva, such as a supersaturated calcium phosphate solution. Another option is via a carboxymethylcellulose base, which can be enriched with fluoride to counteract caries. Frequent use provides an excellent means of maintaining high fluoride intraorally for extended periods of time, thus enhancing the remineralization of incipient caries. Although providing instructions for improvement of oral hygiene is a duty of the dental team, suspected problems of dietary deficiencies should be referred to a nutritionist.

Evaluation of the Prosthesis Foundation: Teeth and Residual Ridge

An evaluation of the prosthesis foundation is required to ensure that an appropriately stable base of sound teeth and/or residual ridge is provided to maximize prosthesis function and patient comfort.

Indications for Preprosthetic Surgery

The need for preprosthetic surgery or extractions must be evaluated. The same criteria apply to surgical intervention in the partially edentulous arch as in the completely edentulous arch. Grossly displaceable soft tissues covering basal seat areas and hyperplastic tissue should be removed to provide a firm denture foundation. Mandibular tori should be removed if they interfere with the optimum location of a lingual bar connector or a favorable path of placement. Any other areas of bone prominence, such as bilateral maxillary exostoses, that will interfere with the path of insertion should be removed also. The path of placement will be dictated primarily by the guiding plane of the abutment teeth. Clinical research in preprosthetic surgical concepts has contributed significant developments to the management of the compromised partially edentulous patient. Bone augmentation and guided bone regeneration procedures have been used with varying degrees of success as an alternative method of improving ridge support for the denture base areas. Skill and judgment must be exercised in patient selection, procedural planning, and surgical and prosthetic management to optimize clinical results. Use of osseointegrated implants can provide a foundation for developing suitable abutment support or retention for RPDs. As in any surgical procedure, results depend on careful treatment planning and cautious surgical management.

Extraction of teeth may be indicated for one of the following three reasons:

- If the tooth cannot be restored to a state of health, all reasonable avenues of treatment should be considered from both

ADA American Dental Association®
America's leading advocate for oral health

Caries Risk Assessment Form (Age >6)

Patient Name:	
Birth Date:	Date:
Age:	Initials:

		Low Risk	Moderate Risk	High Risk
	Contributing Conditions	**Check or Circle the conditions that apply**		
I.	**Fluoride Exposure** (through drinking water, supplements, professional applications, toothpaste)	☐ Yes	☐ No	
II.	**Sugary Foods or Drinks** (including juice, carbonated or non-carbonated soft drinks, energy drinks, medicinal syrups)	Primarily at mealtimes ☐		Frequent or prolonged between meal exposures/day ☐
III.	**Caries Experience of Mother, Caregiver and/or other Siblings** (for patients ages 6-14)	No carious lesions in last 24 months ☐	Carious lesions in last 7-23 months ☐	Carious lesions in last 6 months ☐
IV.	**Dental Home**: established patient of record, receiving regular dental care in a dental office	☐ Yes	☐ No	
	General Health Conditions	**Check or Circle the conditions that apply**		
I.	**Special Health Care Needs** (developmental, physical, medical or mental disabilities that prevent or limit performance of adequate oral health care by themselves or caregivers)	☐ No	Yes (over age 14) ☐	Yes (ages 6-14) ☐
II.	**Chemo/Radiation Therapy**	☐ No		☐ Yes
III.	**Eating Disorders**	☐ No	☐ Yes	
IV.	**Medications that Reduce Salivary Flow**	☐ No	☐ Yes	
V.	**Drug/Alcohol Abuse**	☐ No	☐ Yes	
	Clinical Conditions	**Check or Circle the conditions that apply**		
I.	**Cavitated or Non-Cavitated** (incipient) **Carious Lesions or Restorations** (visually or radiographically evident)	No new carious lesions or restorations in last 36 months ☐	1 or 2 new carious lesions or restorations in last 36 months ☐	3 or more carious lesions or restorations in last 36 months ☐
II.	**Teeth Missing Due to Caries in past 36 months**	☐ No		☐ Yes
III.	**Visible Plaque**	☐ No	☐ Yes	
IV.	**Unusual Tooth Morphology** that compromises oral hygiene	☐ No	☐ Yes	
V.	**Interproximal Restorations - 1 or more**	☐ No	☐ Yes	
VI.	**Exposed Root Surfaces** Present	☐ No	☐ Yes	
VII.	**Restorations with Overhangs** and/or **Open Margins; Open Contacts** with Food Impaction	☐ No	☐ Yes	
VIII.	**Dental/Orthodontic Appliances** (fixed or removable)	☐ No	☐ Yes	
IX.	**Severe Dry Mouth (Xerostomia)**	☐ No		☐ Yes

Overall assessment of dental caries risk: ☐ Low ☐ Moderate ☐ High

Patient Instructions:

Fig. 13.9 The American Dental Association (ADA) caries risk assessment form is a great tool for both diagnosis and patient education. (Permission from The American Dental Association, 2009, 2011. All rights reserved.)

TABLE 13.1 **SAFER CAMBRA Example Protocol for Patients 6–Adult**

	S		A	F		E	R	
Caries risk level	**Sealants**	**Saliva**	**Antibacterials**	**Fluoride (topical)**	**Factors favorable for remineralization (pH, Ca^{2+}, and PO^{3-}_4)**	**Effective lifestyle habits**	**Radiographs**	**Recare**
Low risk	Not indicated (optional for primary prevention of at-risk deep pits and fissures)	Saliva testing is optional or may be done for purposes of baseline records	Not indicated	OTC fluoride toothpaste used bid	Recession or sensitive roots may indicate need for supplementation	Encourage healthy dietary habits, low frequency of fermentable carbohydrates, adequate protein intake, and effective oral hygiene practices using motivational interviewing techniques. Substitute xylitol for sucrose	Every 24–36 months	Every 6 months
Moderate risk	Sealants are recommended per ICDAS code (see Table 3) for secondary prevention	Measure resting and stimulated flow and pH especially if hyposalivation is suspected	Xylitol therapy 2–3 times/ day for a total daily dose of 6–10 g. If the patient has high levels of acidogenic bacteria and then treating with the following agents, it must be understood that the evidence is very limited for antibacterials and pH neutralization, such as chlorhexidine, sodium hypochlorite, povidine iodine, and essential oils, per the manufacturer's instructions. Retest bacterial load test in 1 month, discuss and motivate patient, and repeat as needed	OTC fluoride toothpaste used bid. 0.05% NaF rinse bid. Varnish applied every 4–6 months	Low resting pH, low stimulated flow or pH may indicate need for supplementation		Every 18–24 months	Every 4–6 months

	S		A	F		E	R	
Caries risk level	**Sealants**	**Saliva**	**Antibacterials**	**Fluoride (topical)**	**Factors favorable for remineralization (pH, Ca^{2+}, and PO^{3-}_{4})**	**Effective lifestyle habits**	**Radiographs**	**Recare**
High risk		Objective measurement of acidogenic bacterial load via culturing or direct measurement of plaque ATP		5000 ppm toothpaste used od or bid. 0.05% NaF rinse bid. Varnish applied every 3–4 months	Consider supplementing if topical fluoride alone is not effective. Required if xerostomia is present		Every 6–18 months	Every 3–4 months
Extreme risk							Every 6 months until no new caries lesions	Every 3 months

Bid, Twice a day; **CAMBRA**, caries management by risk assessment; *ICDAS*, International Caries Detection and Assessment System; *od*, once daily; *OTC*, over-the-counter; *RPD*, removable partial denture. Patients with one (or more) cavitated lesion(s) are high-risk patients.

Patients with one (or more) cavitated lesion(s) and hyposalivation are extreme-risk patients. All restorative work is to be done with the minimally invasive philosophy in mind. Existing smooth surface lesions that do not significantly penetrate the DEJ and are not cavitated should be treated chemically not surgically. For extreme-risk patients with multiple cavitations, some choose to use caries control procedures with glass ionomer materials until caries progression is halted and/or reversed followed by more permanent restorative care. Patients with appliances (RPDs, orthodontics) require excellent oral hygiene together with intensive fluoride therapy (e.g., high fluoride toothpaste and fluoride varnish every 3 months). If antibacterial therapy is tried, it should be done in conjunction with fluoride therapy (and every attempt be made not to interfere with the fluoride intervention). A 1-month initial treatment evaluation may be helpful for positive reinforcement. Patients must maintain good oral hygiene (a powered toothbrush may be helpful to high- and extreme-risk patients). A diet low in frequency of fermentable carbohydrates is recommended. It is important to know the amount of xylitol in the product being recommended. Xylitol products should contain 100% xylitol (daily dosages of 6–10 g/day for antimicrobial effects) and pose extreme health risks to family pets, especially dogs.

From Young DA, Featherstone JD. Caries management by risk assessment. *Community Dent Oral Epidemiol.* 2013;41(1):e53–63.

prognostic and economic standpoints before extraction is recommended.

- A tooth may be removed if its absence permits a more serviceable and less complicated RPD design. Teeth in extreme malposition (lingually inclined mandibular teeth, buccally inclined maxillary teeth, and mesially inclined teeth posterior to an edentulous space) may be removed if an adjacent tooth is in good alignment and if good support is available for use as an abutment. Justification for extraction lies in the decision that a suitable restoration, which will provide satisfactory contour and support, cannot be fabricated or that orthodontic treatment to realign the tooth is not feasible. An exception to the arbitrary removal of a malposed tooth occurs when a distal extension RPD base would have to be made rather than using the more desirable tooth-supported base of the tooth in question. If alveolar support is adequate, a posterior abutment should be retained, if possible, in preference to a tissue-supported extension base. This is true even if the distal abutment does not have a suitable surface area for retentive clasps; even a rest on a distal abutment is preferable to a purely tissue-supported extension. Teeth deemed to have insufficient alveolar support may be extracted if their prognosis is poor and if other adjacent teeth may be used to better advantage as abutments. The decision to extract such a tooth should be based on the degree of mobility and other periodontal considerations and on the number, length, and shape of the roots contributing to its support.
- A tooth may be extracted if it is so unesthetically located as to justify its removal to improve appearance. In this situation, both orthodontics and indirect restorations should be considered in preference to removal if such treatment can satisfy the esthetic needs. If removal is advisable because of unesthetic tooth position, the biomechanical problems involved in replacing anterior teeth with an RPD must be weighed against the problems involved in making an esthetically acceptable fixed restoration.

Another consideration for preprosthetic surgery involves the decision between use of an RPD and an implant-supported prosthesis. The discussion of fixed versus removable differential treatments is discussed later in this chapter.

Endodontic Treatment

Abutments for RPDs are required to withstand various forces depending on the classification. The requirement for a distal extension abutment is different than that of a tooth-supported prosthesis in that torsional forces exist in the distal extension situation. For this reason an abutment for a distal extension that is endodontically treated carries a greater risk for complications than a similar tooth not involved in RPD function.

Because tooth support helps control prosthesis movement, teeth in the posterior part of the arch should be maintained if possible. Even if the coronal portion of the tooth must be lost, an endodontically treated root may be utilized as an overdenture abutment for RPDs. They can assist in support, and especially to control movement of distal extensions.

DIAGNOSTIC CASTS

A diagnostic cast should be an accurate reproduction of all the potential features that aid diagnosis. These include the teeth locations, contours, and occlusal plane relationship; the residual ridge contour, size, and mucosal consistency; and the oral anatomy delineating the prosthesis extensions (vestibules, retromolar pads, pterygomaxillary notch, hard/soft palatal junction, floor of the mouth, and frena). Additional information provided by appropriate cast mounting includes occlusal plane orientation and the impact on the opposing arch, tooth-to-palatal soft tissue relationship, and tooth-to-ridge relationships both vertically and horizontally.

A diagnostic cast is usually made of dental stone because of its strength and the fact that it is less easily abraded than dental plaster. The impression for the diagnostic cast is usually made with an irreversible hydrocolloid (alginate) in a stock impression tray. The size of the arch will determine the size of the tray to be used. The tray should be sufficiently oversized to ensure an optimum thickness of impression material to avoid distortion or tearing on removal from the mouth. Alternatively, digital records may be acquired. An intraoral scan can be made with any intraoral scanning system. The same requirements are necessary for digital impressions as conventional impressions, reproducing all necessary anatomical features for diagnosis. The digital casts can then be analyzed virtually or printed. The technique for making impressions is covered in more detail in Chapter 16.

Purposes of Diagnostic Casts

Diagnostic casts serve several purposes as an aid to diagnosis and treatment planning. Some of these are as follows:

- Diagnostic casts are used to supplement the oral examination by permitting a view of the occlusion from all the lingual, as well as from the buccal, aspects. Analysis of the existing occlusion is made possible when opposing casts are occluded, as is a study of the possibilities for improvement by occlusal adjustment, occlusal reconstruction, or both. The degree of overclosure, amount of interocclusal space available, and possibilities of interference with the location of rests may also be determined. As stated previously, opportunities for improvement of the occlusal scheme (by occlusal adjustment or occlusal reconstruction) are best evaluated by analysis and modification of mounted diagnostic casts. Such procedures often include diagnostic waxing to determine the possibility of enhancing the occlusion before definitive treatment is started (Fig. 13.10). In other words, diagnostic casts allow the dentist to plan ahead to avoid undesirable compromises in the patient's treatment.
- Diagnostic casts are used to permit a topographic survey of the dental arch that is to be restored by means of an RPD.

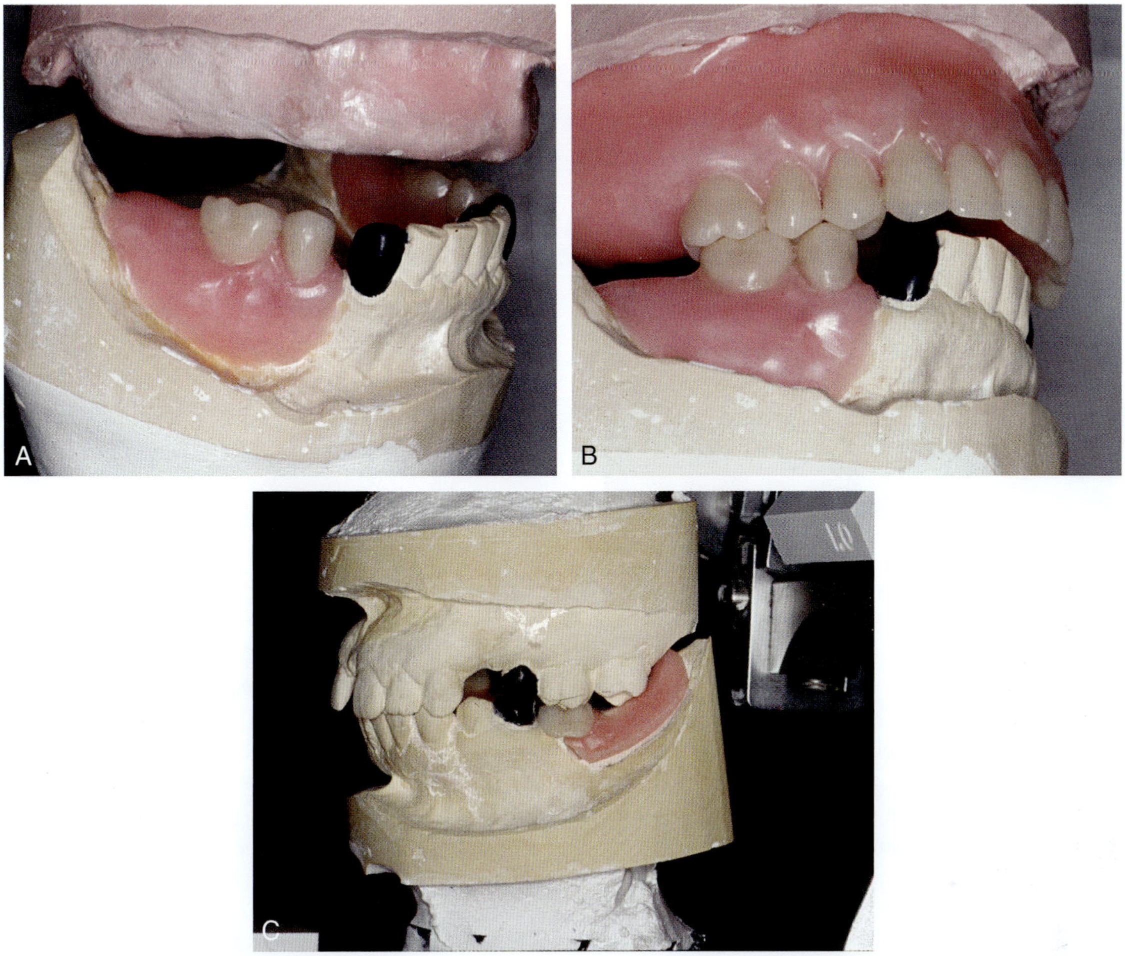

Fig. 13.10 A, Following mounting of the diagnostic casts, tooth arrangement for the mandibular occlusal plane requirements can be accomplished. **B,** Following placement of the maxillary anterior teeth in an ideal position, diagnostic arrangement of occlusion results in a space posterior to surveyed crown #27. If such a finding were objectionable, alternative arrangements could be investigated. This is not possible unless a diagnostic workup is completed. **C,** Occlusion of the mandibular removable partial denture will be enhanced by improving the maxillary posterior occlusal plane of the supererupted molars.

The cast may be surveyed to determine the parallelism of tooth surfaces involved and to establish their influence on the design of the RPD. This allows the clinician to evaluate: (1) proximal tooth surfaces, which can be made parallel to serve as guiding planes; (2) retentive areas of the abutment teeth; (3) areas of interference with placement and removal; and (4) esthetic effects of the selected path of insertion and necessary mouth preparations. From such a survey a path of placement may be selected that will satisfy requirements for parallelism and retention to the best mechanical, functional, and esthetic advantage. Then mouth preparations may be planned accordingly.

- Diagnostic casts also permit presentation to the patient of present and future restorative needs and of the hazards of future neglect. Occluded and individual diagnostic casts can be used to point out to the patient (1) evidence of tooth migration and the existing results of such migration; (2) effects of further tooth migration; (3) loss of occlusal support and its consequences; (4) hazards of traumatic occlusal contacts; and (5) cariogenic and periodontal implications of further neglect.
- Individual (custom) impression trays may be fabricated from the diagnostic casts.
- Diagnostic casts may be used as a constant reference as the work progresses. Colored marks indicating the type of restoration, the areas of tooth surfaces to be modified, the location of rests, and the design of the RPD framework, as well as the path of placement and removal, all may be recorded on the diagnostic cast for future reference (Fig. 13.11).
- Unaltered diagnostic casts should become a permanent part of the patient's record because records of conditions existing

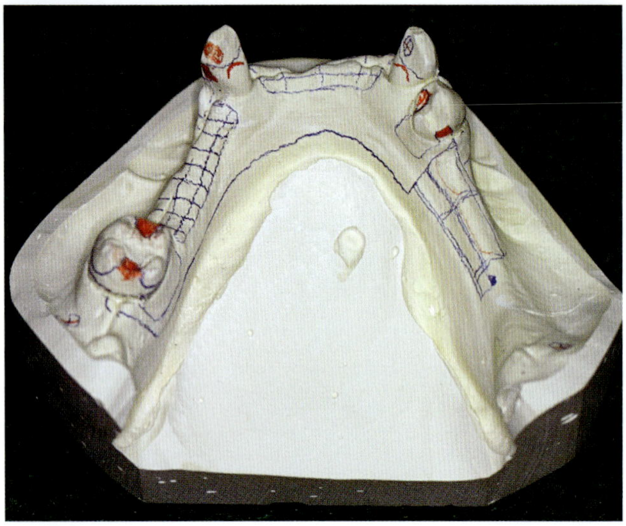

Fig. 13.11 Proposed mouth changes and design of the removable partial denture framework are indicated with a pencil on the diagnostic cast in relation to the previously determined path of placement. This serves as a means of communication with the patient and as a chair-side guide to tooth modification.

before treatment are just as important as preoperative radiographs. Therefore diagnostic casts should be duplicated, with one cast serving as a permanent record and the duplicate cast used in situations that may require alterations to it.

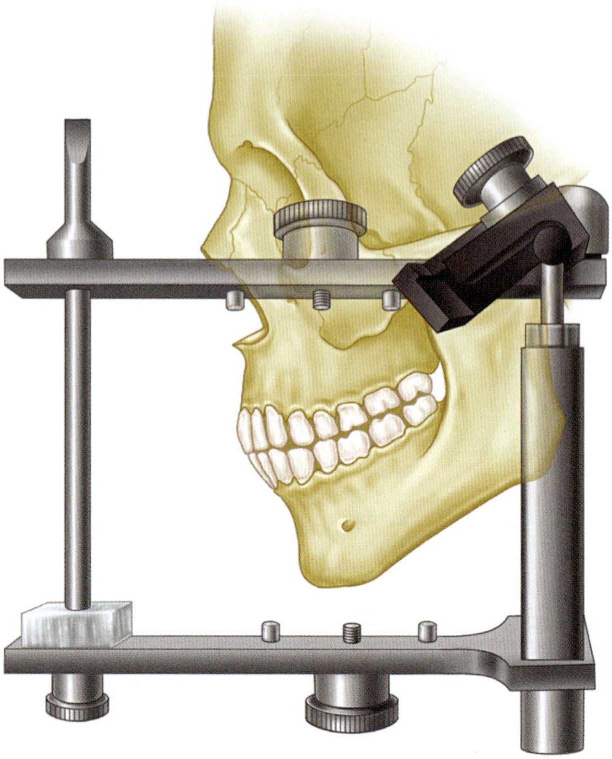

Fig. 13.12 Use of the facebow makes possible the recording of the spatial relationship of the maxilla to some anatomic reference points and transference of this relationship to an articulator.

Mounting Diagnostic Casts

For diagnostic purposes, casts should be related on an anatomically appropriate articulator to best understand the role occlusion may have in the design and functional stability of the RPD. This means placement of the maxillary cast in a position relative to the opening axis on the articulator, which is similar to the position of the maxilla in relation to the TMJ of the patient (Fig. 13.12). The mandibular cast is then mounted against the maxillary cast in maximum intercuspal position or centric relation, depending on the treatment plan.

Sequence for Mounting Maxillary Cast to Axis-Orbital Plane

The initial steps allow recording of the maxilla-TMJ relationship:

1. Identify the anterior and posterior reference points for the facebow (e.g., external auditory meatus, orbitale).
2. Prepare the bite fork and occlusion rim.
3. Place the bite fork centered to the arch, indexing it to the teeth with wax or elastomer.
4. Place the facebow over the bite fork rod anteriorly.
5. Place the bow evenly into the ears posteriorly.
6. Secure the bow anteriorly.
7. Position the bow anteriorly to the third point of reference (establishes the horizontal plane).
8. Secure the bite fork vertical rod and then the horizontal rod (holding the bow securely to prevent torque).
9. Release the bow anteriorly to allow spread and disengage from the ears.
10. Remove the fork downward and out of the mouth with the attached bow.
11. Carefully check the security of the attachments.

The next steps allow transfer of the recorded relationship to the articulator:

1. Position the posterior reference points on the articulator (usually a posterior attachment point).
2. Secure the posterior points by securing the bow anteriorly.
3. Vertically relate the secured bow to the articulator anterior reference point.
4. Seat the maxillary cast into the bite fork registration (wax or elastomer).
5. Close the articulator and check clearance for mounting plaster (modify the cast as needed).
6. Mount with low-expansion plaster.

The facebow is a relatively simple device used to obtain a transfer record for orienting a maxillary cast on an articulator. A facebow may be used to transfer a comparable radius from arbitrary reference points, or it may be designed so that the transfer can be made from hinge axis points. The latter type of transfer requires that a hinge-bow attached to the mandible should be used initially to determine the hinge axis points, to which the facebow is then adjusted for making the hinge axis transfer. An arbitrary facebow is adequate for the vast majority of cases. These facebows are not hinge axis bows and use an arbitrary point of reference. The location of that point or axis has long been the subject of controversy. Gysi[1] and others have placed it 11 to 13 mm anterior to the upper third of the tragus of the ear on a line extending from the upper margin of the external auditory meatus to the outer canthus of the eye. Others have placed it 13 mm anterior to the posterior margin of the center of the tragus of the ear on a line extending to the corner of the eye. Bergström[2] has located the arbitrary axis 10 mm anterior to the center of a spherical insert for the external auditory meatus and 7 mm below the Frankfort horizontal plane. Although most authorities agree that any of the three axes will permit transfer of the maxillary cast with reasonable accuracy, it would seem that the Bergström point compares most favorably with the kinematic axis. The lowest point on the inferior orbital margin is taken as the third point of reference for establishing the axis-orbital plane. For the sake of consistency, the right infraorbital point is generally used and the facebow is assembled in this relationship.

Commonly used with the facebow in fabrication of RPDs are semiadjustable articulators (e.g., Hanau Wide-Vue, Whip Mix 2240 [Whip Mix Corporation, Louisville, KY], and Stratos 200 [Ivoclar, Buffalo, NY]). Casts are prepared for mounting on an articulator by placing three index grooves in the base of the casts. Two V-shaped grooves are placed in the posterior section of the cast and one groove in the anterior portion (Fig. 13.13).

An occlusion rim properly oriented on a well-fitting record base should be used in facebow procedures involving the transfer of casts representative of Kennedy Class I and II partially edentulous situations (Fig. 13.14). Without occlusion rims, such casts cannot be predictably mounted due to the displaceability of the soft tissue. For illustration purposes, a facebow using the external auditory meatus as the posterior reference point, the Whip Mix Facebow technique (DB 2000, Whip Mix Corporation, Louisville, KY), will be shown. The facebow fork is covered with a paste or wax indicated for recording the interocclusal record. Polyether, polyvinyl siloxane, or a roll wax with the material is placed on the top of the facebow fork. Then the fork should be pressed lightly on the diagnostic casts with the midline of the facebow fork corresponding to the midline of the central incisors (Fig. 13.15). This will leave imprints of the occlusal and incisal surfaces of the maxillary casts and occlusion rim on the softened baseplate wax and is an aid in correctly orienting the facebow fork in the patient's mouth. The facebow fork is placed in position in the mouth, aligning with the imprints left from the rims and cast. With the facebow fork in position, the facebow toggle is slipped over the anterior

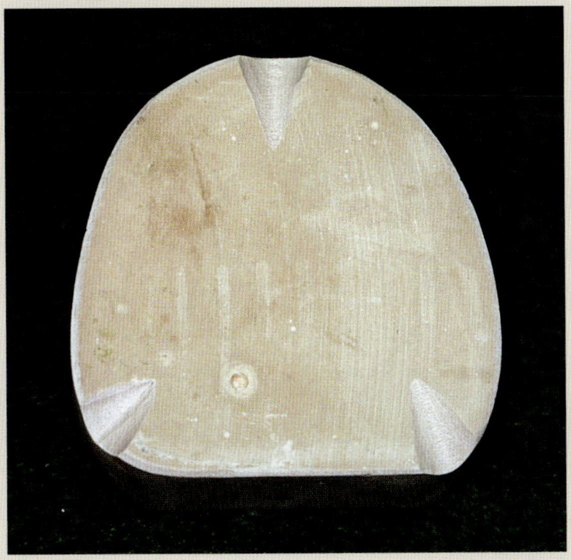

Fig. 13.13 The base of the cast has been prepared for mounting by placing three triangular grooves to allow indexing when mounted. The grooves are prepared with a 3-inch stone mounted in a laboratory lathe.

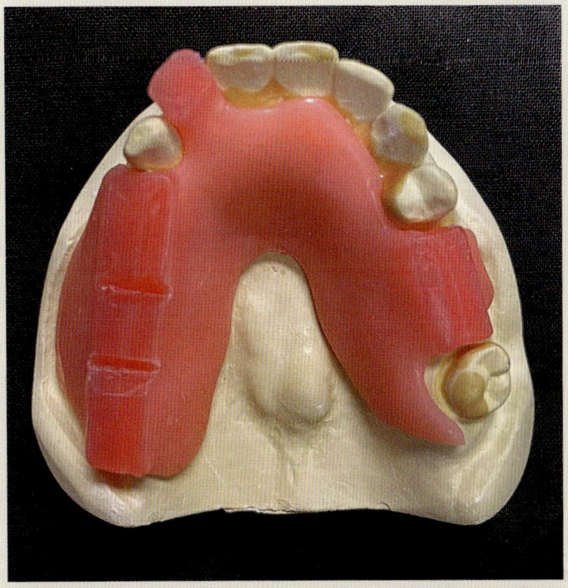

Fig. 13.14 When there is no anterior and posterior support, a record base and wax occlusion rim should be fabricated to provide stability. In this case the rim accommodates for the missing posterior support on the right side.

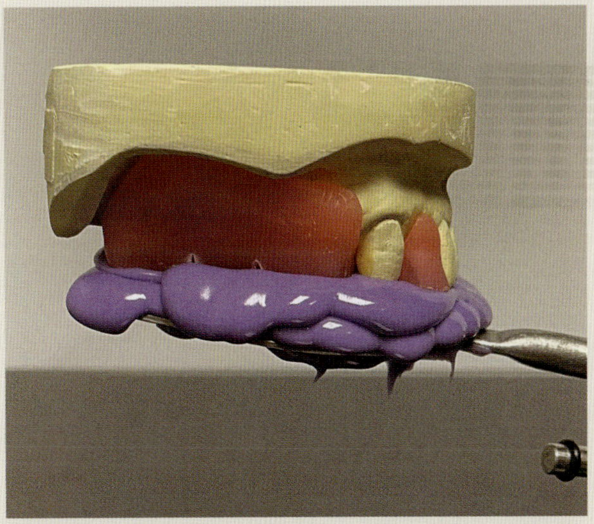

Fig. 13.15 Orienting the facebow fork to the maxillary cast and occlusion rims avoids displacing the occlusion rim in the mouth through patient closure or another uneven force. The polyvinyl siloxane material has been evenly distributed around the facebow fork, and care is exercised to position the fork to be centered at the midincisal position without any fork extension posterior to the record base, which could cause discomfort.

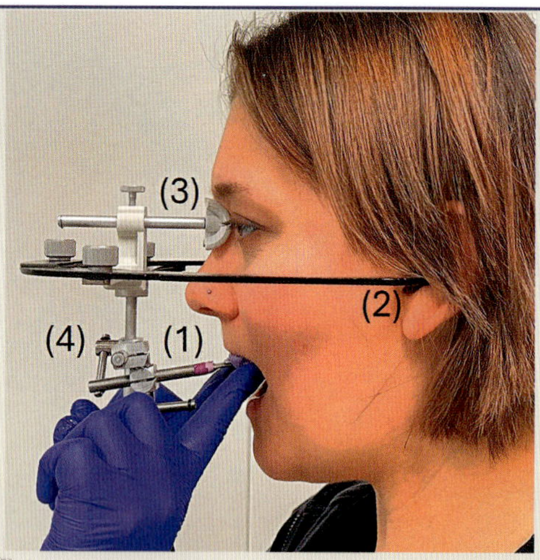

Fig. 13.16 The horizontal toggle clamp of the Whip Mix earpiece facebow *(1)* is slid onto the shaft of the facebow fork protruding from the patient's mouth. The patient then helps guide plastic earpieces into the external auditory meatus and holds them in place while the operator tightens three thumb screws *(2)* and centers the plastic nosepiece *(3)* securely on the nasion. The horizontal toggle clamp is positioned and secured near (but not touching) the lip. The T screw *(4)* on the vertical bar is tightened. Note: Extreme care should be exercised not to tilt the facebow out of position when tightening.

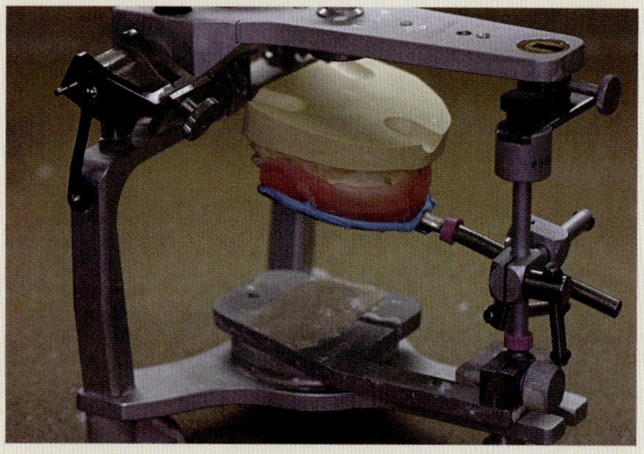

Fig. 13.17 Facebow fork support used to maintain the fork and cast in position while mounting.

projection of the facebow fork (Fig. 13.16). The patient can assist in guiding the plastic earpieces into the external auditory meatus and then hold the arms of the facebow in place with firm pressure while the operator secures the bite fork to the facebow. With all elements tightened securely, the patient is asked to open and the entire assembly is removed intact and set aside. The facebow records both the radius from the condyles to the incisal contacts of the upper central incisors and the angular relationship of the occlusal plane to the axis-orbital plane.

An auxiliary device called a *cast support* is available; it is used to support the facebow fork and the maxillary cast during the mounting operation (Fig. 13.17). With this device, the weight of the cast and the mounting stone are supported separately from the facebow, thus preventing possible downward movement resulting from their combined weight. The cast support is raised to make contact with the facebow fork after the facebow height has been adjusted to the level of the orbital plane. The keyed and lubricated maxillary cast is now attached to the upper arm of the articulator with the mounting stone, thus completing the facebow transfer (Fig. 13.18).

If a digital workflow is being utilized, a digital facebow may be utilized instead of a conventional facebow. When a full-face photo is taken, with the patient looking directly at the camera, it may be aligned in dental design software. The photo is corrected to be in parallel with the interpupillary line, which allows the facial and dental midline to be evaluated. The patient's oral scan can be aligned with the photo, so a digital smile design can be visualized. Many software programs now have accurate virtual articulators that can overlay this merged photo (Fig. 13.19). When the condylar elements of this virtual articulator are aligned with the tragus in the photograph, then a very precise virtual facebow transfer is then completed. Some programs allow input of condylar information (horizontal condylar inclination, etc.), if records are made or a condylographic tracing is completed.

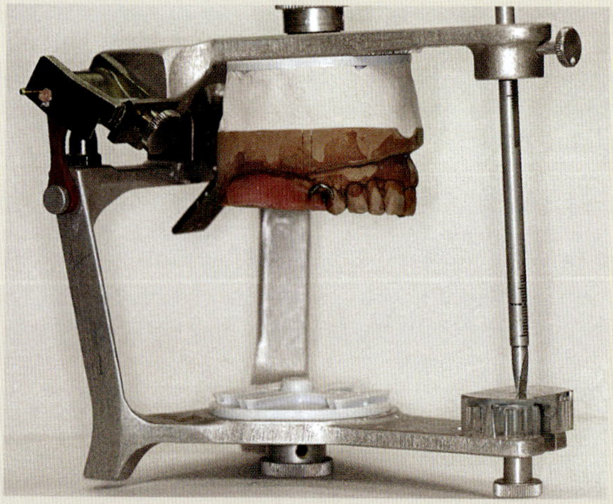

Fig. 13.18 Facebow mounting is complete. The relationship of the maxillary cast to the articulator condylar components is anatomically similar to that between the patient's maxilla and the bilateral temporomandibular joint complex. Any subsequent tooth arrangement and occlusal contact development represent the mouth more accurately than more arbitrary mountings. The benefits of the anatomic similarity are seen in more accurate occlusion for the finalized prosthesis (i.e., less intraoral adjustment required).

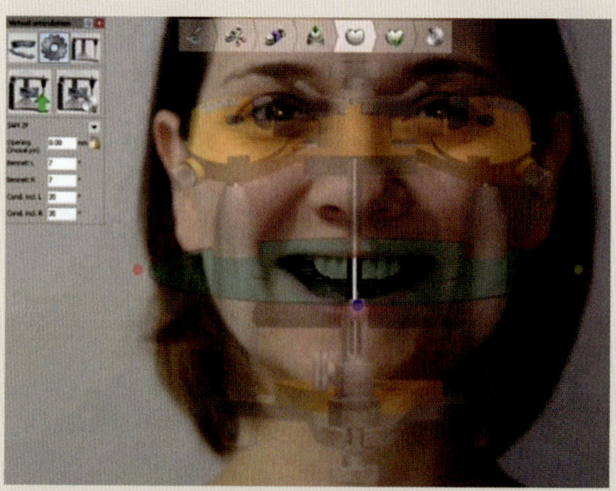

Fig. 13.19 A full-face photograph was taken for a virtual facebow transfer. The patient should be looking straight ahead. To allow for virtual articulator alignment, the ears should be visible (to locate the tragus). If the patient has long hair, it should be pulled back or tucked behind the ears.

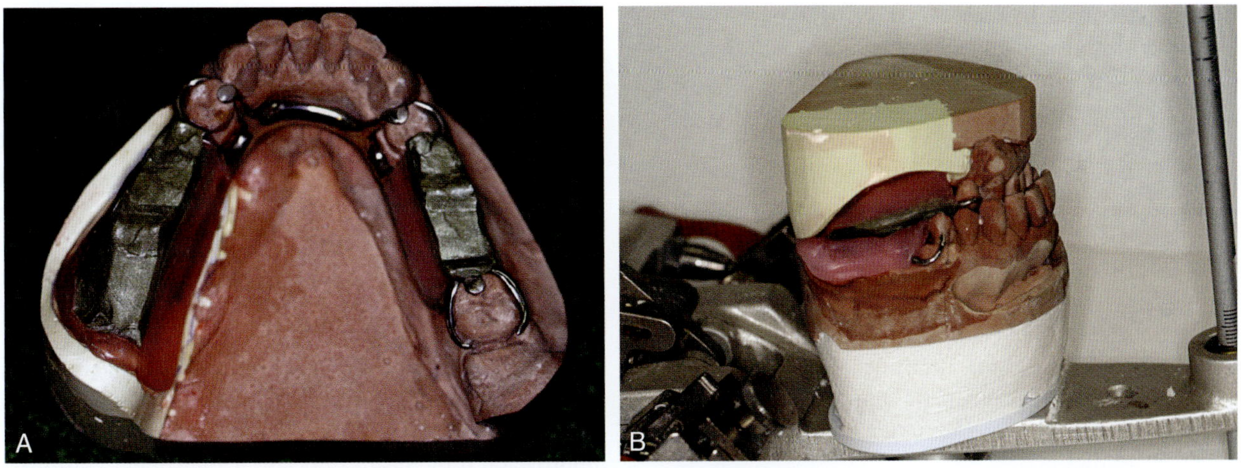

Fig. 13.20 A wax interocclusal record made on a cast framework. **A,** The modification spaces first had baseplate wax added; these were adjusted intraorally to provide space at the occlusal vertical dimension for recording wax, the wax was softened using a wax spatula and a hot water bath, the framework was placed in the mouth, and care was exercised to guide the patient to close into a previously verified (and practiced) interocclusal position deemed appropriate (in this instance, centric relation position). The record was recovered from the mouth, excess wax was removed with a warm scalpel, and the wax was chilled and replaced in the mouth to verify the record. If not verified the wax was resoftened (with additional wax added as needed) and the procedure was repeated. **B,** Immediately after verification, the framework with interocclusal registration was replaced on the mandibular cast and inverted on the maxillary cast for mounting.

Jaw Relationship Records for Diagnostic Casts

One of the first critical decisions that must be made in an RPD service involves selection of the horizontal jaw relationship to which the RPD will be fabricated (centric relation or the maximum intercuspal position). All mouth-preparation procedures depend on this analysis. Failure to make this decision correctly may result in poor prosthesis stability, discomfort, and deterioration of the residual ridges and supporting teeth.

When stable posterior contacts are not present (Kennedy Class I or II RPDs or those opposing complete dentures), the proposed prostheses should be fabricated in the horizontal jaw relationship of centric relation. When the occlusion is stable (usually Kennedy Class III and IV), the prostheses may be fabricated in the horizontal jaw relationship of maximum intercuspal position. In many instances in which edentulous spaces have not been restored, the remaining posterior teeth will have assumed malaligned positions through drifting, tipping, or extrusion. Correction of the remaining natural occlusion is indicated in such situations to improve the occlusal plane and occlusal stability.

Regardless of the selected horizontal occlusal relationship, an evaluation of the existing interocclusal relationships of the opposing natural teeth must be made and is accomplished with mounted diagnostic casts. If the casts are to be mounted in maximum intercuspal position, it is essential that at least three (preferably four) positive contacts of opposing posterior teeth are present, having widespread molar contacts on each side of the arch. If these stable contacts are not present, occlusion rims are necessary to correctly orient casts on an articulator. Scanning is advantageous in this scenario as scanners allow for capturing the relationship between opposing arches even if there is only one occlusal stop.

At times the clinician may choose to adjust the condylar settings on their semiadjustable articulator. A protrusive record can be made to adjust the horizontal condylar inclines on the articulator. Lateral eccentric records are made so that the lateral condylar inclinations can be properly adjusted. All interocclusal records should be made as near the vertical relation of occlusion as possible.

Materials and Methods for Recording Centric Relation

Materials available for recording centric relation are numerous. Commonly used materials include elastomeric materials (polyvinyl silicone or polyether materials), dimethacrylate-based materials, and wax. Of these, wax is more technique sensitive. It should be uniformly softened with a water bath before being introduced into the mouth. After removing from the mouth, it should be chilled in cold water and handled carefully to prevent distortion (Fig. 13.20).

Elastomeric materials are excellent for recording interocclusal relationships (Fig. 13.21). Some are specially formulated for this purpose and have the qualities of extremely low viscosity, minimal resistance to closure, rapid set, low rebound, lack of distortion, and stability after removal from the mouth. Prior to mounting with these materials, excess material should be trimmed to ensure that it is well adapted to the cast. Care should be exercised to ensure that no elastic rebound results when the record is used to relate the casts during the mounting procedure.

The mandibular cast should be mounted on the lower arm of the articulator, with the articulator inverted (Fig. 13.22, *A*). If the interocclusal record was made with the teeth separated, the incisal pin is adjusted so that the anterior distance between the upper and lower arms of the articulator will be increased

2 to 3 mm greater than the normal parallel relationship of the arms. This is done to compensate for the thickness of the interocclusal record so that the arms of the articulator will again be nearly parallel when the interocclusal record is removed and the opposing casts come into contact.

The base of the cast should be keyed and lightly lubricated for future removal. With the diagnostic casts accurately seated and secured in the occlusal record, the mandibular cast is affixed with stone to the lower member of the inverted articulator.

An articulator mounting thus made will have related the casts in centric relation (see Fig. 13.22, *B*). The dentist then can proceed to make an occlusal analysis by observing the influence of cusps in relation to one another after the articulator has been adjusted by using eccentric interocclusal records.

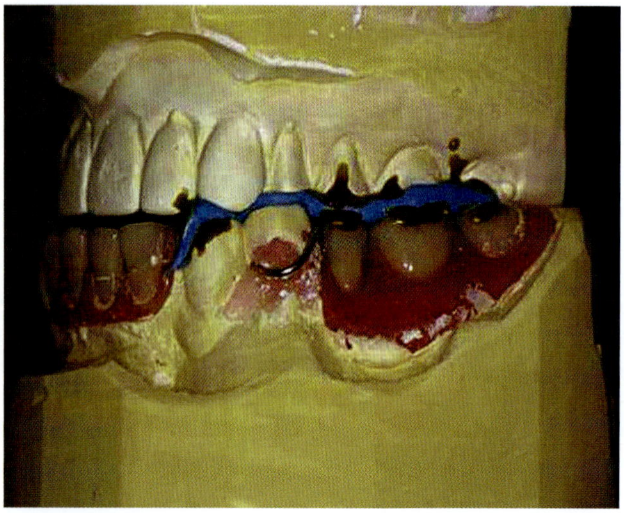

Fig. 13.21 Elastomeric interocclusal registration material used to record mandibular position.

Mounted diagnostic casts alternatively may be fabricated with the use of an intraoral scanner. The clinician may choose to scan the arches and then print the diagnostic casts. The printed casts may then be mounted on a semiadjustable articulator following the protocol described above to mount the maxillary and mandibular casts. Alternatively the casts may be mounted on a virtual articulator. After scanning, the interocclusal relationship may be scanned as well. This may be done in maximum intercuspation or in centric relation.

Analysis of Occlusal Factors

From the occlusal analysis made by evaluating the mounted diagnostic casts, the dentist must decide whether it is best to accept and maintain the existing occlusion or to attempt to improve on it by means of occlusal adjustment and/or restoration of occlusal surfaces. It must be remembered that the RPD can supplement the occlusion that exists only at the time the prosthesis is constructed. The dominant force that dictates the occlusal pattern will be the cuspal harmony or disharmony of the remaining teeth and their proprioceptive influence on mandibular movement. The goal of artificial tooth placement is to harmonize with the functional parameters of the existing occlusion providing bilateral, simultaneous functional contact.

Chapter 18 identifies schemes of occlusion recommended for partially edentulous configurations. A review of these recommendations will provide a guide for modifying the existing occlusion or developing the appropriate occlusal scheme for each partially edentulous configuration.

Improvements in the natural occlusion must be accomplished before the prosthesis is fabricated, not subsequent to its fabrication. The objective of occlusal reconstruction by any means should be occlusal harmony of the restored dentition in relation to the natural forces already present or established.

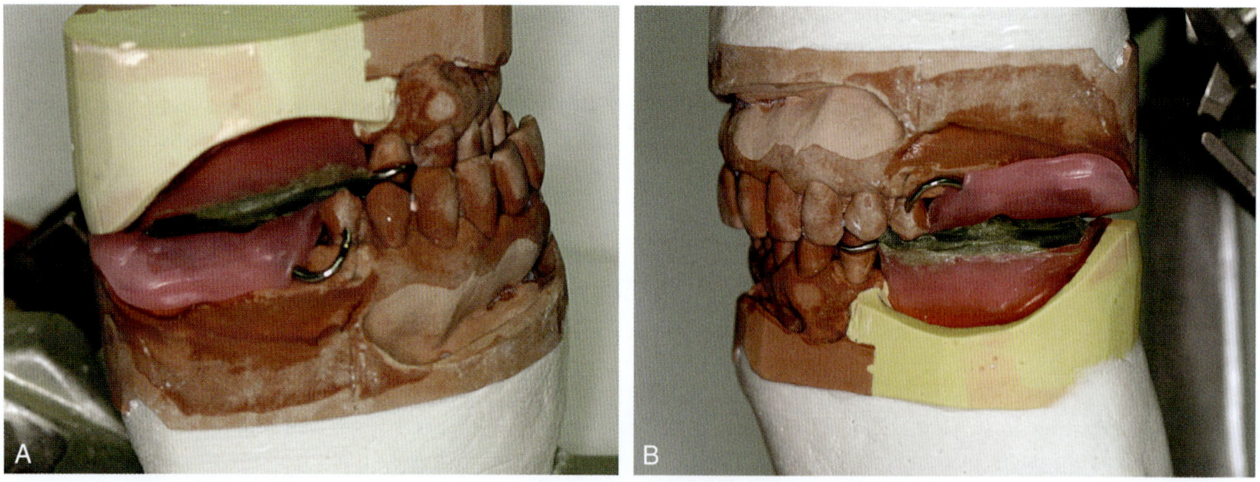

Fig. 13.22 A, Mandibular cast inverted on the mounted maxillary cast, making sure that the cast is fully seated into the interocclusal record and stabilized to the opposing cast. It is important to check the posterior occlusion rim contact to ensure that no interfering contact has altered the record. Space should be observed between the opposing record bases (or record base and opposing occlusion). **B,** Mounted casts demonstrating the occlusal plane as found in the mouth. The Frankfort horizontal plane of the patient is oriented parallel to the articulator base and the floor. Also, inspection of the posterior rims demonstrates space between the rims, which ensures that the recorded position was registered without influence from rigid contacting components, only from softened wax.

Therefore one of the earliest decisions in planning reconstructive treatment must be whether to accept or reject the existing vertical dimension of occlusion and the occlusal contact relationships in centric and eccentric positions. If occlusal adjustment is indicated, cuspal analysis always should precede any corrective procedures in the mouth by selective grinding. On the other hand, if reconstruction is to be the means of correction, the manner and sequence should be outlined as part of the overall treatment plan.

Minimum Restorative Space

Mounted diagnostic casts must be evaluated to consider the interocclusal distance and amount of restorative space for the prosthesis. Frequently, Angle Class II Division 2 patients have a severe vertical overlap, and if the maxillary anterior teeth are lost and need to be replaced with an RPD, it is difficult to do so without either increasing the vertical dimension, performing alveoloplasty, or recontouring the mandibular dentition. Similarly, supraeruption of maxillary molars which have been unopposed due to mandibular tooth loss can result in teeth which occlude with the edentulous ridge, where an RPD extension is desired to exist.

Currently available publications lack an evidence-driven determination of the minimum restorative space in RPDs specifically, but extrapolation from publications on overdentures, traditional complete dentures, and metal-acrylic fixed dental prostheses on implants can guide the practitioner in determining the space available. When minimum restorative space is not present, framework fracture or debonding of the acrylic denture tooth is a frequent complication. Based upon the thickness of relief space under latticework (0.5 mm), latticework itself (1.2–2.5 mm), minimal denture acrylic thickness (1.5–2 mm), and minimal denture tooth thickness ($\geq$2 mm), one could deduce a minimal interocclusal distance of 5.5 mm for predictable retention of a denture tooth.

When interocclusal space is limited, composite facings can be utilized to prevent debonding of denture teeth in the esthetic region (Fig. 13.23). With this technique, the RPD framework is designed to encompass the palatal and occluding surfaces of any missing teeth with limited space. A veneer of composite rather than a denture tooth replaces the facial tooth structure. In nonesthetic regions, the framework can be waxed to a full contour tooth, to entirely replace the need for a denture tooth or any composite facings which would be likely to debond due to inadequate thickness of restorative material.

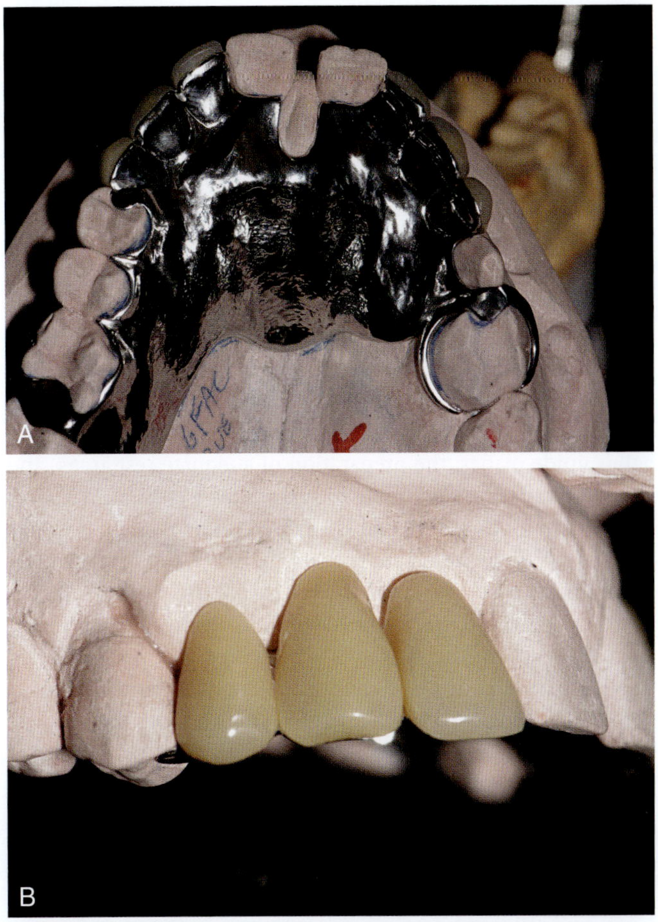

Fig. 13.23 A, Occlusal view of a framework with occlusal surfaces waxed to full contour and cast in metal, with composite facings. **B,** Facial view of composite facings on removable partial denture with limited interocclusal space. (Courtesy of Dr. Ramtin Sadid-Zadeh, Birmingham, AL.)

Fixed Restorations

The tooth position must be evaluated by a surveyor to assess contour heights, guiding plane areas, rest seats, and undercuts to accommodate the proposed RPD design. A complete coverage crown may be indicated for the abutment teeth when a significant tooth modification is required, compromising tooth health, or abutment teeth are improperly positioned in faciolingual or mesiodistal direction and cannot be rectified relative to the planned path of placement and removal of the RPD without a complete coverage crown. In addition, teeth that have been weakened by significant caries, wear, or fractures are typically unfit as abutment teeth without the placement of a complete coverage crown. Moreover, there may be a need to restore modification spaces with fixed restorations rather than include them in the RPD, especially when dealing with isolated abutment teeth. A variety of materials may be used for fixed restorations of the abutment teeth, including metal alloy, metal ceramic, and zirconia. Chapter 15 details further information on materials and techniques used to fabricate a fixed restoration for the abutment engaged in RPD abutment teeth.

Orthodontic Treatment

Occasionally, orthodontic movement of malposed teeth followed by retention through the use of fixed partial dentures makes possible a simplified RPD design, which results in a mechanically and esthetically better situation than could otherwise be accomplished. Although adequate anchorage for tooth movement can be a major limitation in partially edentulous arches, carefully placed implants that subsequently can be used for prosthesis support have been used to expand orthodontic applications for this patient group.

Need for Reshaping Remaining Teeth

The clinical crown shapes of anterior and posterior teeth are not capable of supporting an RPD framework without appropriate modification. Without the required modifications, the prosthesis does not adequately benefit from the support and stability offered by the teeth and consequently will not be comfortable for the patient. Many failures of RPDs can be attributed to the fact that the teeth were not reshaped properly to establish guiding planes or to receive clasp arms and occlusal rests before the impression for the master cast was made. Of particular importance are the paralleling of proximal tooth surfaces to act as guide planes, the preparation of adequate rest areas, and the reduction of unfavorable tooth contours (see Fig. 10.1). A malaligned tooth or one that is inclined unfavorably may make it necessary to place certain parts of the clasp so that they interfere with the opposing teeth. Unparallel proximal tooth surfaces not only will fail to provide needed guide planes during placement and removal but also will result in excessive blockout. This inevitably results in placement of the connectors so far out of contact with tooth surfaces that food traps are created. To pass lingually inclined lower teeth, clearance for a lingual bar major connector may have to be so great that a food trap will result when the restoration is fully seated. Such a lingual bar will be located so that it will interfere with tongue comfort and function. These are only some of the objectionable consequences of inadequate mouth preparations.

The amount of reduction of tooth contours should be kept to a minimum, and all modified tooth surfaces not only should be repolished after reduction but also should be subjected to fluoride treatment to lessen the incidence of caries. If it is not possible to produce the contour desired without perforating the enamel, then the teeth should be recontoured with an acceptable restorative material. The age of the patient, caries activity evidenced elsewhere in the mouth, and apparent oral hygiene habits must be taken into consideration when one is deciding between reducing the enamel and modifying tooth contours with protective restorations.

INFECTION CONTROL

The American Dental Association (ADA) follows the Centers for Disease Control (CDC) recommended infection control procedures for dentistry. The most recent recommendations were made in 2003, with a 2016 summary. Most of the updates will be familiar to practitioners and are already largely practiced routinely. They are designed to prevent or reduce the potential for disease transmission from patient to dental health care worker (DHCW), from DHCW to patient, and from patient to patient. The document emphasizes the use of Standard Precautions (which replaces the term *Universal Precautions*) for the prevention of exposure to and transmission of not only bloodborne pathogens but also other pathogens encountered in oral health care settings.

The CDC guidelines include standard precautions; work restrictions for health care personnel infected with, or occupationally exposed to, infectious diseases; management of occupational exposure to bloodborne pathogens, including postexposure prophylaxis for work exposures to hepatitis B virus (HBV), hepatitis C virus (HCV), and human immunodeficiency virus (HIV); prevention of COVID-19 transmission (SARS-CoV-2); selection and use of devices with features designed to prevent sharps injury, contact dermatitis, and latex hypersensitivity; hand hygiene; dental unit waterlines; and biofilm and water quality; special considerations include dental handpieces and other devices attached to air lines and waterlines, saliva ejectors, radiology, parenteral medications, single-use or disposable devices, preprocedural mouth rinses, oral surgical procedures, handling of biopsy specimens and extracted teeth, laser/electrosurgery plumes, *Mycobacterium tuberculosis*, Creutzfeldt-Jakob disease and other prion diseases, program evaluation, and research considerations. The recommendations provide guidance for measures to reduce the risks of disease transmission, among both DHCWs and their patients. In 2022, an additional alert was publicized by the CDC focusing on maintaining and monitoring dental waterlines, following outbreaks of nontuberculous *Mycobacteria* in dental offices in the United States. Practitioners should ensure the use of sterile saline or sterile water as coolant for all surgical procedures, and nonsurgical procedures must utilize water meeting the CDC recommendation of ≤500 CFU/mL of heterotrophic water bacteria.

Dental patients and DHCWs may be exposed to a variety of microorganisms. Exposure can occur via blood and/or oral or respiratory secretions. The microorganisms may include viruses and bacteria that infect the upper respiratory tract in general, as well as cytomegalovirus, HBV, HCV, herpes simplex virus types 1 and 2, HIV, *M. tuberculosis*, staphylococci, and streptococci. The transmission of infection in the dental operatory can occur through several routes. These include direct contact (blood, oral fluids, or other secretions), indirect contact (contaminated instruments, operatory equipment, or environmental surfaces), and contact with airborne contaminants present in droplet spatter or in aerosols of oral and respiratory fluids. For infection to occur via any of these routes, the "chain of infection" must be present. This includes a susceptible host, a pathogen with sufficient infectivity and numbers to cause infection, and a portal through which the pathogen may enter the host. For infection control procedures to be effective, one or more of these "links" in the chain must be broken.

Dental offices should adhere to CDC guidelines for environmental surface and equipment disinfection versus sterilization, with careful attention to the distinction between critical, semicritical, and noncritical items. Items that have been used in the mouth, such as impressions, bite registrations, or prostheses, must be rinsed to reduce bioburden and disinfected before they are manipulated in the laboratory (whether on site or at a remote location). Any item manipulated in the laboratory should also be cleaned and disinfected before placement in the patient's mouth. Fresh pumice with a sterile rag wheel should be used for each polishing procedure, and the pumice pan should be washed, rinsed, and dried after each procedure.

Because materials are constantly evolving, DHCWs are advised to follow manufacturers' suggested procedures for specific materials relative to disinfection procedures. As a guide, use of a chemical germicide that has at least an intermediate level of activity (i.e., "tuberculocidal hospital disinfectant") is appropriate for such disinfection. Careful communication between dental office and dental laboratory regarding the specific protocol for handling and decontamination of supplies and materials is important to prevent any cross contamination.

DIFFERENTIAL DIAGNOSIS: FIXED OR REMOVABLE PARTIAL DENTURES

Although replacement of missing teeth by means of fixed partial dentures, either tooth or implant supported, is generally the method of choice, there are many reasons why an RPD may be the better method of treatment for a specific patient. The dentist must follow the best procedure for the welfare of the patient, who is always free to seek more than one opinion. Ultimately the choice of treatment must be weighed against the patient's individual condition, economic limitations, and personal desires.

Although uncommon, unilateral tooth loss is sometimes inappropriately treated with a short-span unilateral RPD in place of a fixed partial denture. This type of prosthesis is not enhanced by cross-arch stabilization and places excessive stress on abutment teeth. Possibly more important, the risk for aspiration or ingestion is significant if such a prosthesis is dislodged during use. For these reasons, use of the unilateral RPD is strongly discouraged.

Distal Extension Spaces

Without tooth support at each end of the missing teeth, the RPD and the implant-supported prosthesis are the primary treatment considerations. When limitations to implant placement exist, the options are limited to RPD or no treatment. Current surgical options are available to correct most anatomic limitations, yet frequently implant therapy is not chosen because of patient medical factors, concerns for the risk of surgical morbidity, increased time required for treatment, and costs. It is important to note that a comparison of long-term maintenance requirements between these two options may demonstrate little cost difference over time. This is related to the effects of continued residual ridge resorption acting on the removable prosthesis and not the implant prosthesis.

Tooth-Bounded Edentulous Regions

Generally a unilateral edentulous space bounded by teeth is restored with implants if the adjacent teeth are untreated, or a fixed partial denture if the abutment teeth are already heavily restored. The length of the span and the periodontal support of the abutment teeth will determine the number of abutments required. For conventional fixed prostheses, a lack of parallelism of the abutment teeth may be counteracted with telescopic copings or precision connectors to provide parallel sectional placement. Sound abutment teeth make possible the use of more conservative retainers, such as partial-veneer crowns, or resin-bonded-to-metal restorations, rather than full crowns. The age of the patient, evidence of caries activity, oral hygiene habits, and the soundness of remaining tooth structure must be considered in any decision to use less than full coverage for abutment teeth.

Two specific contraindications for unilateral fixed restorations are known. One is a long edentulous span with abutment teeth that would not be able to withstand the trauma of nonaxial occlusal forces. The other is abutment teeth which exhibit reduced periodontal support due to periodontal disease, which would benefit from cross-arch stabilization. In either situation, a bilateral removable restoration can be used more effectively to replace the missing teeth.

Short Modification Spaces

For short spans (≤3 missing teeth), natural tooth– and implant-supported fixed prostheses and RPDs can be considered as treatment options. Implant placement requires the decision that bone volume exists or can be provided with minimal morbidity, to adequately place dental implants to support prosthetic teeth. Implant prostheses have the advantage of not requiring the use of teeth for support, stability, and retention requirements and consequently do not increase the functional burden on the natural dentition. In addition, implant-retained RPDs could be used as a transitional treatment when patients have financial limitations for an implant-supported fixed dental prosthesis. Although the predictability of contemporary implant procedures (surgery and prosthodontics) makes them a consideration for short-span prostheses, the main advantage is the opportunity to provide replacement teeth without involving adjacent teeth in the reconstruction.

Longer Modification Spaces

Longer span modification spaces (≥4 missing teeth) present a greater challenge for natural tooth–supported fixed prostheses. Consequently the RPD and the implant-supported prosthesis become preferred options. An implant prosthesis has the same bone volume requirements as stated earlier and will likely require additional implants for an increased span. Due to prosthetic and surgical needs, longer spans cause implant use to be more costly and can significantly increase the cost difference between treatment options. The increased morbidity associated with augmentation procedures can also limit universal application. Because the RPD remains largely tooth supported (unless the span includes anterior and posterior segments that may cause it to function similar to a distal extension), the functional stability requirements should be efficiently met through the tooth support.

Modification Space Position

An RPD for a Kennedy Class III arch is better supported and stabilized when a modification area on the opposite side of the arch is present. A fixed partial denture need not be used to restore such an edentulous area because its inclusion may simplify the design of the RPD. However, when a modification space is bound by a lone-standing single-rooted abutment, it is better restored by means of a fixed partial denture. This acts to stabilize the at-risk tooth, and the denture is made less complicated by not having to include other abutment teeth for the support and retention of an additional edentulous space or spaces.

When an edentulous space that is a modification of a Kennedy Class I or Class II arch exists anterior to a lone-standing abutment tooth, this tooth is subjected to trauma by the movements of a distal extension RPD far in excess of its ability to withstand such stresses. The splinting of the lone abutment to the nearest tooth could be considered. The abutment crowns should be contoured for support and retention of the RPD; in addition, a means of supporting a stabilizing component on the anterior abutment of the fixed partial denture or on the occlusal surface of the pontic usually should be provided.

Anterior Modification Spaces

While fixed tooth replacements are often the ideal treatment, sometimes a better esthetic result is obtainable when the anterior replacements are supplied by an RPD (Fig. 13.24). This is especially true when excessive tissue and bone resorption necessitate placement of the pontics in a fixed partial denture too far palatally for good esthetics or for an acceptable relation with the opposing teeth. However, in most instances, from mechanical and biological standpoints, anterior replacements are best accomplished with fixed restorations. The replacement of missing posterior teeth with an RPD is then made much less complicated and gives more satisfactory results.

Replacement of Missing Molars

For unilaterally missing molars, an implant would be the first choice to avoid involving multiple unaffected teeth with a prosthesis (Fig. 13.25). Alternatively a cantilever-fixed prosthesis on teeth could be utilized to restore only a single molar if a double abutment of the premolars with adequate periodontal support were present.

Replacing unilaterally missing molars with an RPD necessitates the use of a distal extension prosthesis. This involves the major connector joining the edentulous side to retentive and stabilizing components located on the nonedentulous side of

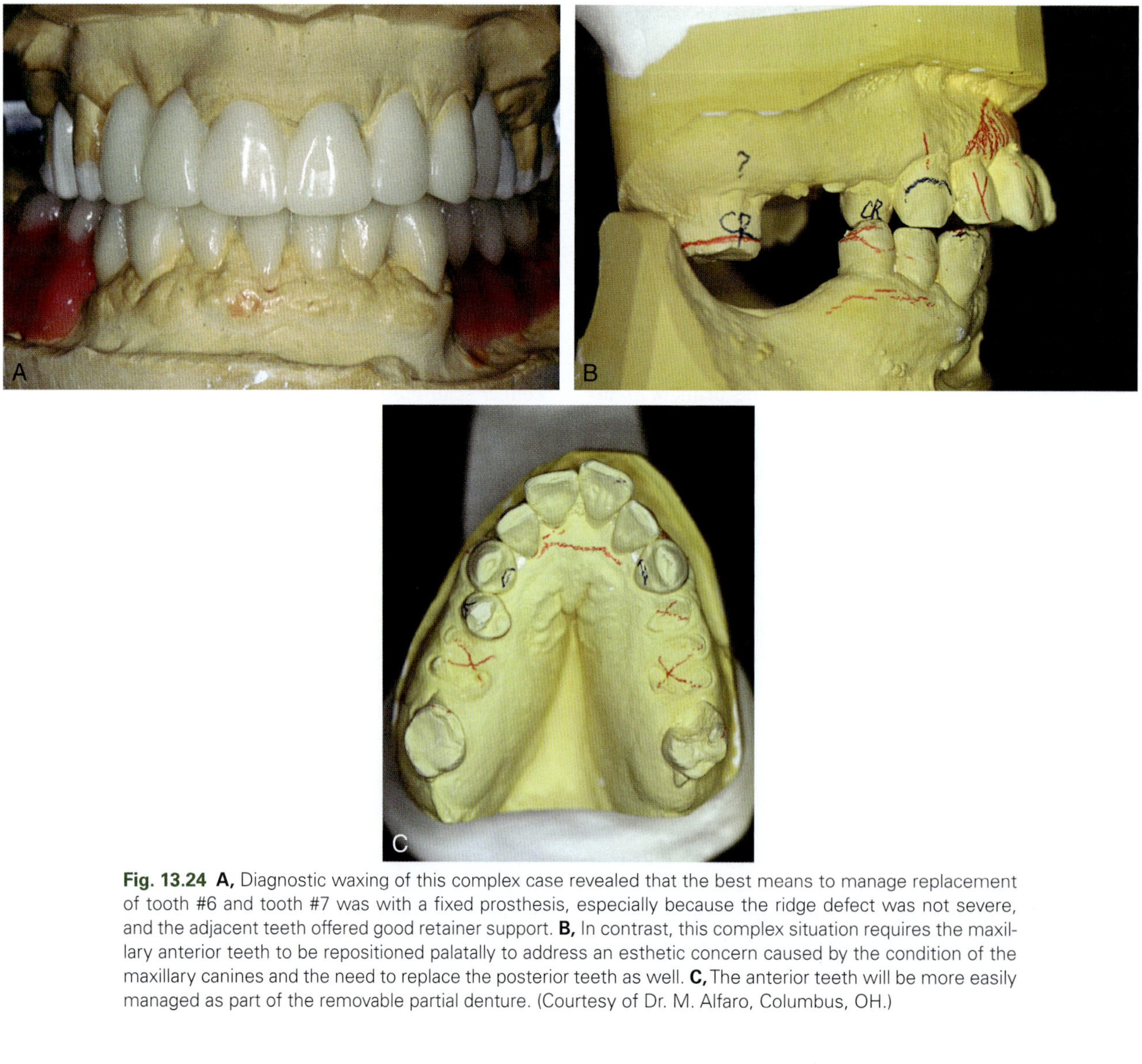

Fig. 13.24 A, Diagnostic waxing of this complex case revealed that the best means to manage replacement of tooth #6 and tooth #7 was with a fixed prosthesis, especially because the ridge defect was not severe, and the adjacent teeth offered good retainer support. **B,** In contrast, this complex situation requires the maxillary anterior teeth to be repositioned palatally to address an esthetic concern caused by the condition of the maxillary canines and the need to replace the posterior teeth as well. **C,** The anterior teeth will be more easily managed as part of the removable partial denture. (Courtesy of Dr. M. Alfaro, Columbus, OH.)

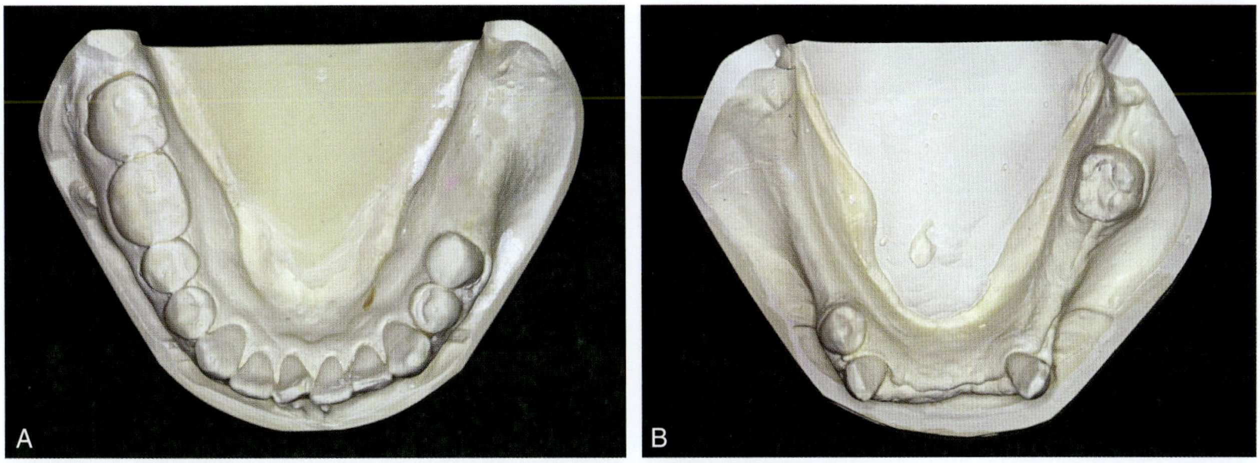

Fig. 13.25 A, Unilaterally missing molars. If the patient exhibits opposing contacts to the remaining six posterior teeth (bilateral premolars, right first and second molars), functional gain attained by replacing the left molars may be minimal. **B,** By contrast, the functional gain resulting from replacement of the posterior occlusion in this patient is likely significant.

the arch. Leverage factors are frequently unfavorable, and the retainers used on the nonedentulous side are often unsatisfactory and require preparation of otherwise uninvolved dentition. The decision to replace missing molars with either implants or an RPD is often dependent on the arch. Many patients will elect to replace maxillary molars with a prosthesis due to esthetic concern, as the edentulous sites are visible in their smile. However, patients may be more likely to elect for no replacement of missing mandibular molars, as the shortened dental arch will give them adequate function, but they should be informed of the potential for supraeruption of the opposing dentition. Two important factors to consider in making the decision to provide a unilateral, distal extension RPD include the opposing teeth and the future effect of the maxillary tuberosity.

First, the opposing teeth must be considered if it is important to prevent extrusion and migration. This influences replacement of the missing molars far more than any improvement in masticating efficiency; replacement of missing molars on one side is seldom necessary for reasons of mastication alone.

Second, the future effect of a maxillary tuberosity must be considered if concern exists for tuberosity enlargement. Often when left uncovered, the tuberosity increases in size, making future occlusal treatment difficult. However, covering the tuberosity with an RPD base, in combination with the stimulating effect of the intermittent occlusion, helps maintain tuberosity size and position. In such an instance, it may be better to make an RPD with cross-arch stabilization and retention than to leave a maxillary tuberosity uncovered.

Indications for Removable Partial Dentures

Although an RPD should be considered only when a fixed restoration is contraindicated, there are several specific indications for the use of a removable restoration.

After Recent Extractions

The replacement of teeth after recent extractions often cannot be accomplished satisfactorily with a fixed restoration. When relining will be required later or when a fixed restoration using natural teeth or implants will be constructed later, a temporary, interim RPD can be used. If an all-resin denture is used rather than a cast framework RPD, the immediate time and financial investment to the patient is much less, and the resin denture lends itself best to future temporary modifications, including those required after implant placement and before restoration.

Tissue changes are inevitable following extractions. Tooth-bounded edentulous areas (as a result of extractions) are best initially restored with RPDs. Relining of a tooth-supported resin denture base is then possible. This is usually done to improve esthetics, oral cleanliness, or patient comfort. Support for such a restoration is supplied by occlusal rests on the abutment teeth at each end of the edentulous space.

Long Span

A long-span edentulous space may be totally tooth supported if the abutments and the means of transferring the support to the denture are adequate and if the denture framework is rigid. There is little if any difference between the support afforded an RPD and that afforded a fixed restoration by the adjacent abutment teeth. However, in the absence of cross-arch stabilization, the torque and leverage on the two abutment teeth would be excessive. Instead a removable denture that derives retention, support, and stabilization from abutment teeth on the opposite side of the arch is indicated as the logical means of replacing the missing teeth.

Need for Effect of Bilateral Stabilization

In a mouth weakened by periodontal disease, a fixed restoration may jeopardize the future of the involved abutment teeth unless the splinting effect of multiple abutments is used. The RPD, on the other hand, may act as a periodontal splint through its effective cross-arch stabilizing of teeth weakened by periodontal disease. When abutment teeth throughout the arch are properly prepared and restored, the beneficial effect of an RPD can be far greater than that of a unilateral fixed partial denture.

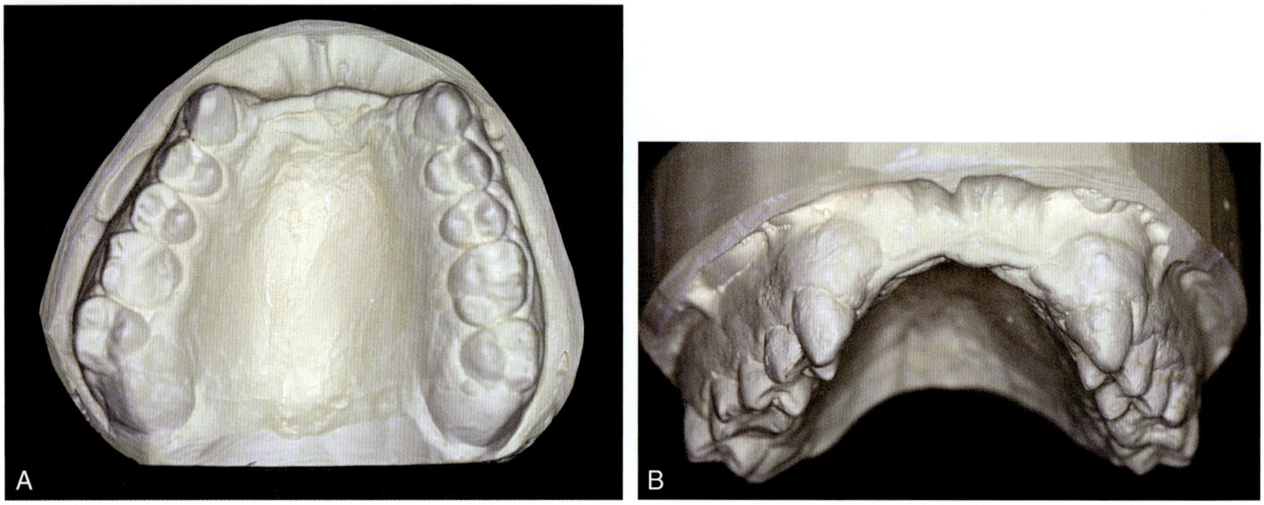

Fig. 13.26 **A,** Occlusal view of the anterior ridge defect (Kennedy Class IV) shows the palatal position of the ridge crest. The incisal edges of opposing dentition require a more labial position, which would create a difficult pontic form. **B,** Labial view of the same cast shows the significance of the vertical bone loss. Replacement of the teeth and ridge anatomy is best accomplished with a removable partial denture.

Excessive Loss of Residual Bone

The pontic of a fixed partial denture must be correctly related to the residual ridge and in such a manner that the contact with the mucosa is minimal. Whenever excessive resorption has occurred, teeth supported by a denture base may be arranged in a more acceptable buccolingual position than is possible with a fixed partial denture (Fig. 13.26).

Unlike a fixed partial denture, the artificial teeth supported by a denture base can be located without regard for the crest of the residual ridge and more nearly in the position of the natural dentition for normal tongue and cheek contacts. This is particularly true of a maxillary prosthesis.

Anteriorly, loss of residual bone occurs from the labial aspect. Often the incisive papilla lies at the crest of the residual ridge. Because the central incisors are normally located anterior to this landmark, any other location of artificial central incisors is unnatural. An anterior fixed partial denture made for such a mouth will have pontics contacting the labial aspect of this resorbed ridge and will be too far lingual to provide desirable lip support. Often the only way the incisal edges of the pontics can be made to occlude with the opposing lower anterior teeth is to use a labial inclination that is excessive and unnatural, and both esthetics and lip support suffer. Because the same condition exists with an RPD in which the anterior teeth are abutted on the residual ridge, a labial flange must be used to permit the teeth to be located closer to their natural position.

The same method of treatment applies to the replacement of missing mandibular anterior teeth. Sometimes a mandibular anterior fixed partial denture is made six or more units in length, in which the remaining space necessitates leaving out one anterior tooth or using the original number of teeth but with all of them too narrow for esthetics. In either instance the fixed partial denture is nearly in a straight line because the pontics follow the form of the resorbed ridge. An RPD will permit the location of the replaced teeth in a favorable relation to the lip and opposing dentition regardless of the shape of the residual ridge. When such a removable prosthesis is made, however, positive support must be obtained from the adjacent abutments.

Abutments with Guarded Prognoses

If the prognosis of an abutment tooth is questionable or if it becomes unfavorable while under treatment, it might be possible to compensate for its impending loss by a change in prosthesis design. The questionable or condemned tooth or teeth may then be included in the original design and, if subsequently lost, the RPD can be modified or remade (Fig. 13.27). When the tooth in question will be used as an abutment, every diagnostic aid should be used to determine its prognosis as a prospective abutment. It is usually not as difficult to add a tooth or teeth to an RPD as it is to add a retaining unit to a fixed prosthesis when the original abutment is lost, and the next adjacent tooth must be used for that purpose.

It is sometimes possible to design an RPD so that a single posterior abutment, about which there is some doubt, can be retained and used at one end of the tooth-supported base. Then if the posterior abutment is lost, it could be replaced by adding an extension base to the existing denture framework. Such an original design must include provisions for future indirect retention, flexible clasping of the future abutment, and provisions for establishing tissue support. Anterior abutments that are considered poor risks may not be so freely used because of the problems involved in adding a new abutment retainer when the original one is lost. It is rational that such questionable teeth should be condemned in favor of more suitable abutments, even though the original treatment plan must be modified accordingly.

Economic Considerations

Economics should not be the sole criterion used to arrive at a method of treatment. When, for economic reasons, definitive or

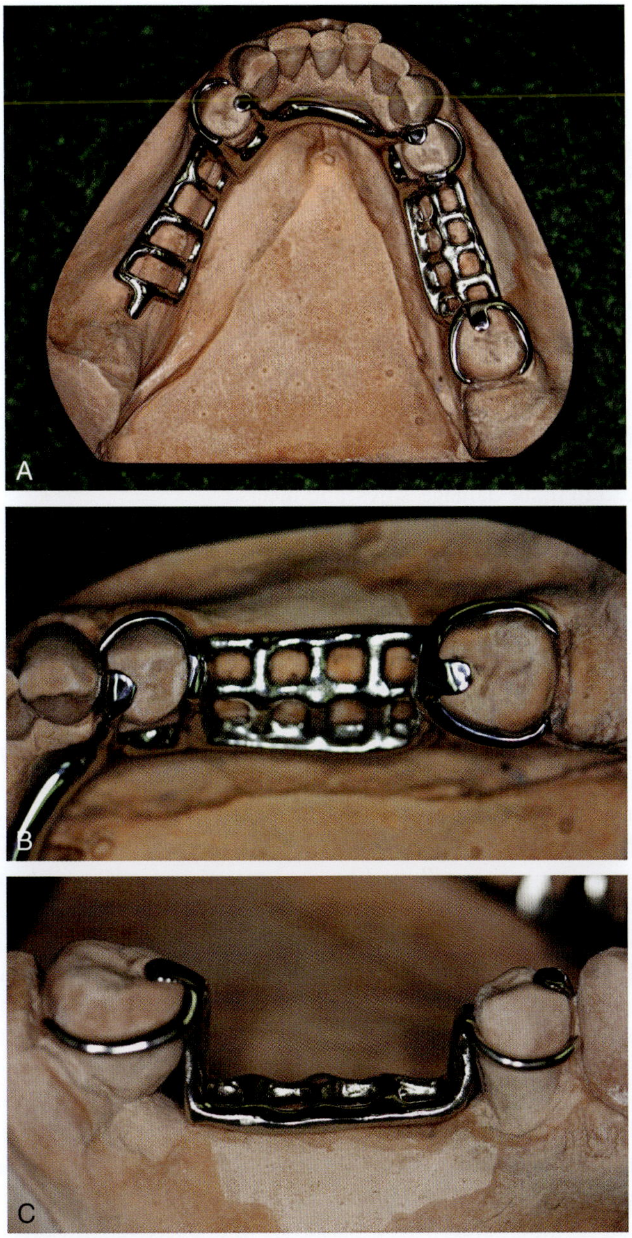

Fig. 13.27 Kennedy Class II, modification 1, where the molar abutment has a guarded prognosis. **A,** Anterior abutment of the modification space has a clasp assembly that accommodates for potential future loss of the distal molar while currently providing adequate support, stability, and retention. **B,** Premolar clasp assembly comprises a mesial rest, a distal guide plane, and a wrought-wire retainer design, which will accommodate future distal extension movement. **C,** Buccal view shows guide-plane contact and a wrought-wire location that is appropriate for a distal extension.

comprehensive treatment is out of the question and yet replacement of missing teeth is indicated, the restorative procedures dictated by these considerations must be described clearly to the patient as a compromise. A prosthesis that is made to satisfy economic considerations alone may provide only limited success and result in more costly treatment in the future.

CHOICE BETWEEN COMPLETE DENTURES AND REMOVABLE PARTIAL DENTURES

One of the more difficult decisions to make for the partially edentulous patient involves making the choice of a complete denture over an RPD. Many factors need to be considered when one is making such a decision; these generally fall under the categories of tooth-related factors, factors of comparative functional expectations between prostheses, and patient-specific factors. Because the difference between a tooth-tissue–borne prosthesis and a tissue-borne prosthesis can be significant, especially because it is difficult for the partially edentulous patient to conceptualize the tissue-borne situation, such an irreversible decision is not trivial. Providers should be careful to avoid agism in treatment planning, but careful consideration of edentulating a patient under the age of 30 should be weighed as bone resorption will only increase over time, eventually worsening the prognosis of subsequent complete dentures in a patient's lifetime.

An evaluation of the remaining teeth determines whether any caries or periodontal disease exists. The decision as to whether a tooth is useful for inclusion in a prosthetic treatment plan can be made based on an understanding that with appropriate disease management, the tooth provides a reasonable 5-year prognosis for survival. This considers the added functional demand by the prosthesis and a risk assessment for recurrent disease. Because this scenario concerns teeth with disease, the expectation is that tooth structure and/or support is compromised. The added functional burden, along with a potentially increased risk for disease, is an important concern when one is determining the long-term benefit for retaining teeth with an RPD.

If the teeth can be maintained with a reasonable prognosis, the next questions to ask are: "Do they require restoration with surveyed crowns?" and "How much improvement to the prosthesis support, stability, and retention do they provide?" If the expected prognosis for a given tooth is questionable, the costs associated with restoration are high, and the added benefit to the prosthesis is low, it is likely that the tooth should not be maintained unless the patient strongly desires to maintain all teeth. However, if the same scenario exists and the long-term impact on the support, stability, and retention of the prosthesis is great, the decision strongly favors keeping the tooth.

The question of whether retained teeth offer a significant advantage to the prosthesis from a support, stability, and retention standpoint requires comparative evaluation of potential denture-bearing foundations. If the expectation is that an edentulous arch would have unfavorable physical features (poor ridge form, poor arch configuration, displaceable mucosa, high frena attachments, minimum denture bearing area, and/or an unfavorable jaw relationship), then retention of teeth is likely to provide a more significant benefit. If retention of teeth can help prevent or delay age-related denture-bearing foundation changes seen with complete denture use, then retention of teeth can be of significant benefit.

When evaluation demonstrates that the remaining teeth have no active disease, then the often-negative impact of disease management on prognosis is not a concern. The decision to maintain teeth is again based on risk assessment, costs for use of the teeth, added benefit to prosthesis functional stability, and comparative functional expectations between a mucosal-borne denture and an RPD that uses teeth for some support, stability, and retention.

The remaining tooth location and distribution can also affect the decision to maintain teeth. It makes a difference whether the remaining teeth are located on only one side of the arch. Having bilateral teeth remaining, especially if they are in similar locations (canine-canine, canine/premolars-canine/premolars), offers advantages for prosthesis design and occlusal development compared with asymmetrical tooth locations. Some teeth may not serve well as a stabilizing component for an RPD and should not be maintained. If the remaining terminal tooth adjacent to a distal extension base is an incisor, for example, the likelihood of long-term support, stability, and retention is poor.

An additional factor for consideration when one is deciding between a complete denture and an RPD is whether there is a strong patient desire to maintain teeth. As mentioned previously, because the change to a complete denture is a significant transformation, sufficient discussion must take place before this decision is made. The dentist must be very clear that the patient understands the functional differences between a mucosal-borne prosthesis for all aspects of function (i.e., chewing, talking, etc.) and the natural dentition or an RPD.

Other patients may wish to retain their remaining teeth for an indefinite but relatively short period of time, with a planned eventual transition to complete dentures. In this instance the professional obligation may be to recommend interim RPDs without extensive mouth preparation. Such dentures will aid in mastication and provide esthetic replacements, while serving as conditioning restorations, which will make the later transition to complete dentures somewhat easier.

CLINICAL FACTORS RELATED TO REMOVABLE PARTIAL DENTURE FRAMEWORKS

The cast framework offers significant advantages over an all acrylic-resin or flexible base RPD. In general the ability to predictably utilize the remaining teeth for support, stability, and retention over time is best assured when the interface between prosthesis and teeth consists of a cast structure and not a polymer. Expectations of how the metal framework improves functional performance are related to the properties of the metal alloy, which are discussed further in Chapter 12.

Evaluation of existing prosthesis

Many times, patients present with existing RPDs, whether recently made or functioning for an extended period. A crucial step is the objective evaluation of these prostheses for inadequacies and deficiencies. Patients who have worn their dentures for a long time may not be aware of any issues, but a thorough examination can reveal problems that warrant intervention to prevent future complications.

One significant concern is the improper fit of the denture base. An overextended base, which covers more tissue than necessary, can cause immediate irritation, inflammation of the gums (gingivitis), and even ulcers. Over time, this chronic irritation can lead to permanent tissue damage and potentially contribute to the development of epulis fissuratum, a benign overgrowth of tissue. Conversely, an underextended base compromises stability and function. Patients may experience difficulty chewing and food impaction beneath the denture. Long-term consequences of an underextended base include increased tooth mobility, further tooth loss, and overloading of the remaining teeth.

Another important aspect of denture evaluation is assessing the relief provided for tender tissues. Lack of proper relief creates pressure points that cause pain and discomfort while wearing the denture. If left unaddressed, these pressure points can lead to tissue damage, sores, and ulcers.

Without proper recall and maintenance, the extension base of a Kennedy Class I RPD is subject to the loss of support caused by resorption of the underlying muco-osseous structures over a prolonged period. When combined with a maxillary complete denture, a series of interrelated pathophysiological changes may occur within the jawbone and surrounding soft tissues leading to a condition termed "combination syndrome."

While the primary etiological factor of combination syndrome is the gradual resorption of the mandibular posterior residual ridge, the sequelae of secondary factors contribute to the overall presentation. Loss of support in the mandibular RPD extension base is followed by a decrease in posterior occlusal contacts and a subsequent increase in the concentration of occlusal load on the anterior contacts. Excessive pressure on the maxillary anterior residual ridge leads to maxillary alveolar resorption, tissue mobility, and often pathological changes such as an epulis fissuratum or papillary hyperplasia (Fig. 13.28) (Video 13.30).

Anterior resorption of the maxillary ridge then triggers a discrepancy of the occlusal plane, repositioning superiorly in the anterior plane and inferiorly in the posterior plane. To maintain homeostasis, the mandibular anterior teeth extrude and compensatory hyperplasia of the posterior maxillary tuberosities develop in the absence of posterior tooth contact. In addition, anterior spatial repositioning of the mandible results from the loss of occlusal vertical dimension as well as the continued deterioration of the periodontal condition of the remaining anterior teeth. This extreme pathological response to the progressive loss of residual ridge support compromises the mechanics of both the complete denture and RPD, impacting function and comfort.

Treatment of combination syndrome, especially in the late stages, is exceptionally difficult to manage. Therefore avoiding posterior natural tooth loss in the mandible is the first line of defense. If feasible, advising the patient to invest in root canal treatment, restorations, and/or periodontal therapy to preserve a posterior stop will prevent combination syndrome. In addition, the patient should be educated regarding the risks of wearing a maxillary denture in the absence of a mandibular RPD when only mandibular anterior teeth remain. After the insertion of the mandibular RPD opposing a maxillary complete

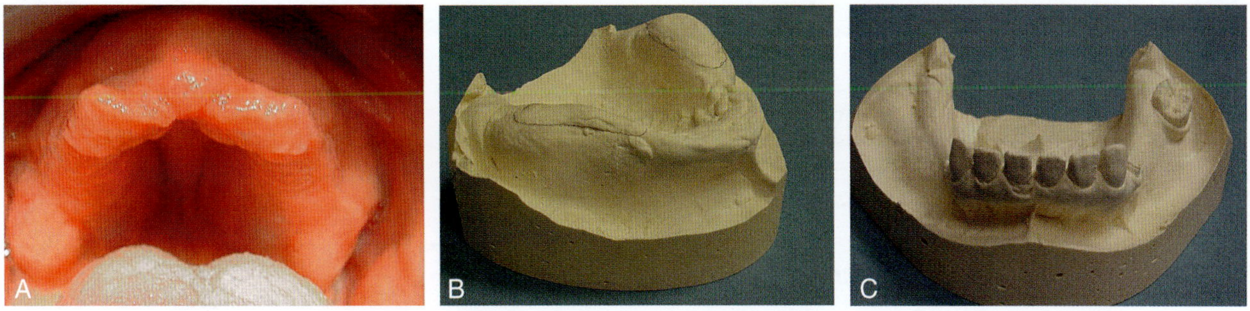

Fig. 13.28 Combination syndrome (CS) is a problem that occurs in patients who have mandibular distal extension partial dentures opposing a maxillary complete denture as seen in this patient. Clinical findings associated with CS are: loss of bone from the anterior maxillary ridge and papillary hyperplasia of the tissues of the hard palate **(A)**; down growth of the maxillary tuberosities **(B)**; and extrusion of the mandibular anterior teeth and loss of bone beneath the removable partial denture base **(C)**. Additionally the following changes may be associated with CS: loss of vertical dimension of occlusion, occlusal plane discrepancy, anterior spatial repositioning of the mandible, poor adaptation of the prosthesis, periodontal changes, and epulis fissuratum **(A)** hyperlink video CH0013_Video-Fig0013-30_Lang. (Courtesy of Dr. Lisa A. Lang.)

denture, meticulous follow-up care and maintenance protocol are paramount. Prolonging appropriate distal extension support after insertion can be achieved by a reline or rebase procedure as described in Chapter 23.

If combination syndrome is diagnosed, treatment options are available. Surgical intervention may be required to remove hyperplastic tissue or recontour the bony architecture of the residual ridge to create a more favorable foundation for denture placement. While relining the distal extension base(s) of the RPD may improve support, minimizing anterior hyperfunction requires a stable posterior occlusion and well-fitting framework. Therefore treatment of combination syndrome may require full mouth rehabilitation to include reestablishment of the vertical dimension of occlusion, recontouring or restoration of the mandibular anterior teeth into the appropriate plane of occlusion, and then remaking the maxillary complete denture and mandibular RPD. If this is not possible, a new maxillary and mandible complete denture may be the best treatment option.

Finally, extensive coverage or unhygienic designs in RPDs pose challenges with cleaning. This can lead to difficulty maintaining good oral hygiene, contributing to bad breath (halitosis) and an increased risk of fungal infections like candidiasis.

Beyond the physical consequences, deficient dentures can negatively impact a patient's self-confidence and quality of life. Difficulty speaking and eating due to poor denture fit can cause significant social and emotional distress. A thorough evaluation of existing prostheses allows for the identification of these deficiencies and the recommendation of appropriate interventions, such as adjustments, relines, or complete remakes. This proactive approach helps prevent future complications and improve patient outcomes.

RPDs require the consideration of many factors concurrently, and the importance of carefully undertaking treatment planning cannot be understated. Commitment to excellence in planning is critical to the success of the prosthesis.

REFERENCES

1. Gysi. A. The problem of articulation. *Dental Cosmos.* 1910;52:1.
2. Bergstrom G. On the production of dental articulation by means of articulators, a kinematic investigation. *Acta Odontol Scand.* 1950;9(Suppl 4).

14

Preparation of the Mouth for Removable Partial Dentures

Lisa A. Lang, Lily T. García, and Ahmed Mahrous

CHAPTER OUTLINE

The preparation of the mouth prior to fabrication of a removable partial denture is fundamental to clinical success. Mouth preparation supports the philosophy that the prescribed prosthesis not only must replace what is missing but must preserve the remaining tissues and intraoral structures. With the impact of predictable success with implants in combination with removable partial dentures, it is important to discuss dental implant treatment options when considering mouth preparation for removable prostheses.

Mouth preparation follows the preliminary diagnosis and the development of a tentative treatment plan. Final treatment planning may be deferred until the response to the preparatory procedures can be ascertained. In general, mouth preparation includes procedures that address conditions that mitigate the potential for complications and includes any tooth alterations required for proper tooth stabilization and support of the prosthesis. Key goals in mouth preparation are to create optimum health and eliminate or alter any condition that would be detrimental to the functional success of the removable partial denture.

Mouth preparations must be accomplished before impression procedures necessary to produce the master cast in fabrication of the removable partial denture. Surgical procedures should precede abutment tooth preparation and should be completed well in advance to allow the necessary healing period. A minimum of 6 weeks, preferably 3 to 6 months, should be provided between surgical procedures and restorative dentistry procedures. The time for healing depends on the extent of the surgery and potential impact on overall support, stability, and retention of the proposed prosthesis.

PREPROSTHETIC CONSIDERATIONS IN PARTIALLY EDENTULOUS MOUTHS

As a rule, all preprosthetic surgical treatment for the removable partial denture patient should be completed as early in the treatment sequence as possible. Any necessary endodontic procedures, periodontal surgery, and oral surgery should be accomplished during the same timeframe. The longer the interval between the surgical intervention and the final impression procedure, the more it allows time for complete healing and consequently the more stable the denture-bearing areas.

A variety of oral surgical techniques can prove beneficial to the clinician in preparing the patient for prosthetic replacements. However, it is not the purpose of this section to present the details of surgical correction but to review some of the more common oral conditions in which surgical intervention is indicated as an aid to removable partial denture design and fabrication, to support successful function. Other references for surgical techniques are available in text and other peer-reviewed literature. It is important to emphasize, however, that the dentist bears the responsibility for ensuring that necessary surgical intervention is accomplished in accordance with the treatment plan. Measures to control apprehension, including the use of intravenous and inhalation agents, have made the most extensive surgery acceptable to patients whether the dentist chooses to perform these procedures or elects to refer to a specialist. The important consideration is that the patient should not be deprived of any treatment that would enhance the success of the removable partial denture.

Extractions

Planned surgical procedures should occur early in the treatment regimen but not before a careful and thorough evaluation of each remaining tooth in the dental arch is completed (Fig. 14.1). Regardless of its condition, each tooth must be evaluated in terms of its strategic importance, whether it is restorable without complications to the removable partial denture design, and its potential contribution to the success of the removable partial denture.

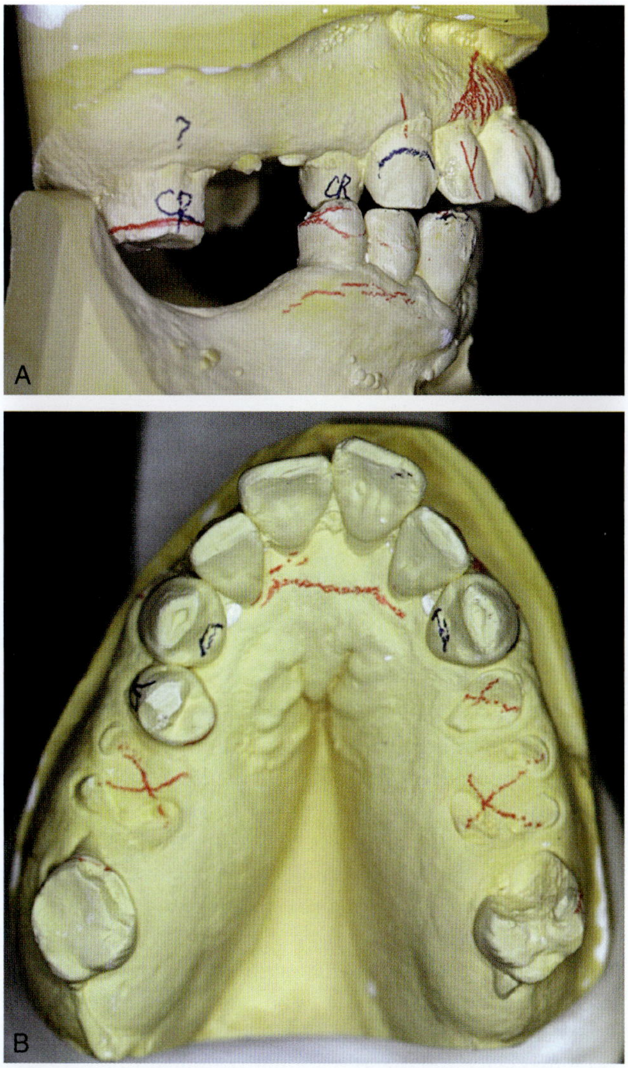

Fig. 14.1 Diagnostic mounting allows confirmation of the need for extraction after clinical examination. **A,** Anterior tooth position and chronic periodontal disease status require extraction to address the patient's concern of malpositioned and painful teeth. **B,** Root tips require immediate extraction to allow ridge healing to begin. The status of the molar (#15) requires additional workup to determine pulpal involvement of the carious lesion, and the extent of occlusal reduction required to optimize the occlusal plane. The decision to maintain this tooth, although potentially costly, must consider the stabilizing effect it will have on the posterior left functional occlusion.

Impacted Teeth

All impacted teeth, including those in edentulous areas, as well as those adjacent to abutment teeth, should be considered for removal. The periodontal implications of impacted teeth adjacent to abutments are similar to those for retained roots. These teeth are often neglected until serious periodontal implications arise. If the impacted tooth has been present for an extensive period of time in an older patient, it may not have caused nor is it likely to cause further complications.

Malposed Teeth

The loss of individual teeth or groups of teeth may lead to extrusion, drifting, or combinations of malpositioned remaining teeth (Fig. 14.2). In most instances, the alveolar bone segment moves occlusally with extruded teeth. Orthodontics may be useful in correcting many occlusal discrepancies, but for some patients, such treatment may not be practical because of lack of teeth for anchorage of the orthodontic appliances, cost, time to accomplish the treatment, or for other reasons.

Cysts and Odontogenic Tumors

Panoramic radiographs of the jaws are recommended to survey the jaws for unsuspected pathologic conditions. When a suspicious area appears on the survey film, a periapical radiograph should be taken to confirm or deny the presence of a lesion. All radiolucencies or radiopacities observed in the jaws should be

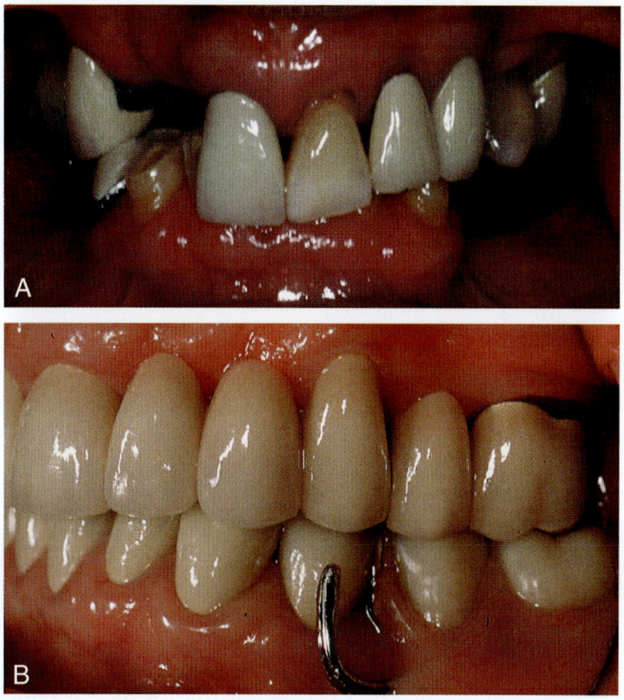

Fig. 14.2 A, Malpositioned maxillary dentition due to loss of posterior occlusion and excessive wear of opposing mandibular anterior teeth. **B,** Restored dentition made possible by a combination of endodontics, periodontics, and fixed and removable partial prosthodontics. (Courtesy of Dr. M. Alfaro, Columbus, OH.)

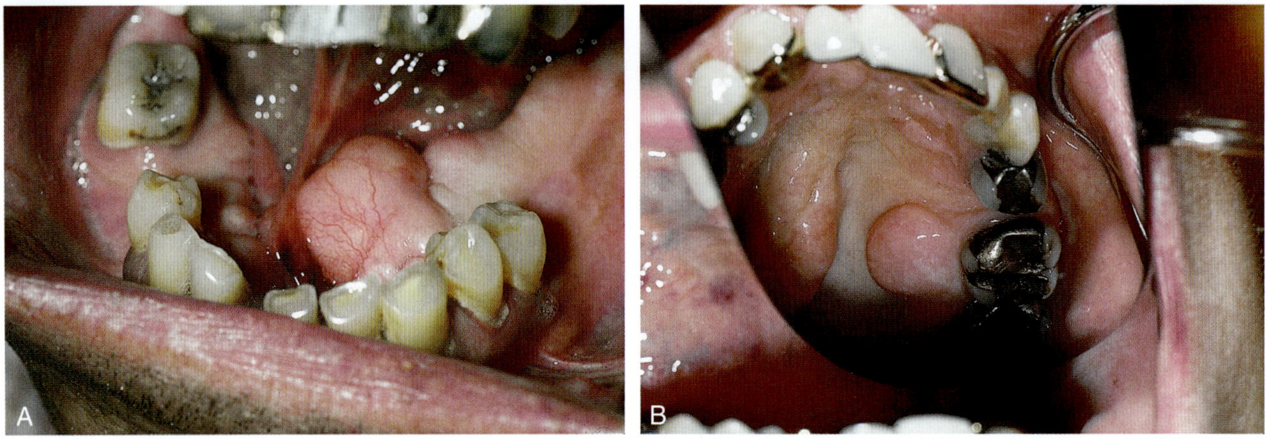

Fig. 14.3 **A,** Mandibular tori extending into the floor of the mouth, and **B,** maxillary exostoses on the palate.

investigated. Although the diagnosis may appear obvious from clinical and roentgenographic examinations, the dentist should confirm the diagnosis through appropriate consultation and, if necessary, perform a biopsy of the area and submit the specimens to a pathologist for microscopic study. The patient should be informed of the diagnosis and provided with various options for resolution of the abnormality as confirmed by the pathologist's report.

Exostoses and Tori

The existence of abnormal bony enlargements should not be allowed to compromise the design of the removable partial denture (Fig. 14.3). Although modification of removable partial denture design can, at times, accommodate for exostoses, more frequently this results in additional stress to the supporting elements and compromised function. The removal of exostoses and tori is not a complex procedure, and the advantages to be realized from such removal are great in contrast to the deleterious effects that their continued presence can create. Ordinarily, the mucosa covering bony protuberances is extremely thin and friable. Removable partial denture components in proximity to this type of tissue may cause irritation and chronic ulceration. Also, exostoses approximating gingival margins may complicate the maintenance of periodontal health and lead to the eventual loss of strategic abutment teeth.

Hyperplastic Tissue

Hyperplastic tissues are seen in the form of fibrous tuberosities, unsupported or soft flabby ridges, folds of redundant tissue in the vestibule or floor of the mouth, and palatal papillomatosis (Fig. 14.4). Consider removal of excess tissue to provide a firm base for the denture. Surgical modification of excess soft tissue produces a more stable denture, helps reduce stress and strain on the supporting teeth and tissues, and provides a favorable orientation of the occlusal plane and arch form for the arrangement of the artificial teeth in many instances. Appropriate surgical approaches should not reduce vestibular depth, making the depth shallower. Hyperplastic tissue can be removed with any preferred combination of scalpel, curette, electrosurgery, or laser. Some form of surgical stent should be considered for these patients to cover the wound sites, making healing more comfortable. An old removable partial denture that is properly modified can serve as a surgical stent.

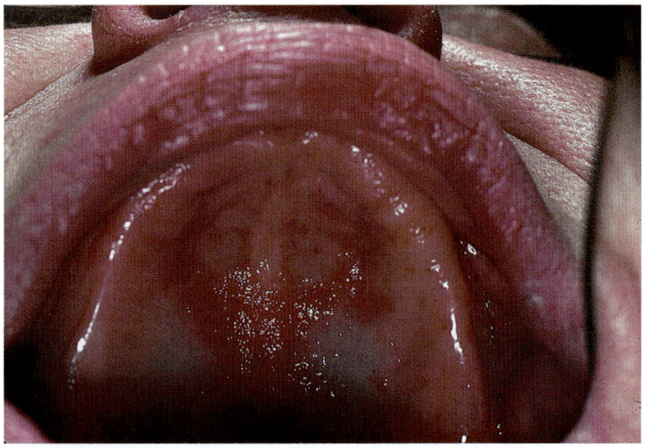

Fig. 14.4 Hyperplastic fibrous tuberosities.

Muscle Attachments and Frena

As a result of the loss of alveolar bone height, muscle attachments appear to insert on or near the residual ridge crest. The mylohyoid, buccinator, mentalis, and genioglossus muscles are most likely to introduce problems of this nature. In addition to the problem of the attachments of the muscles themselves, the mentalis and genioglossus muscles occasionally produce bony protuberances at their attachments that may also interfere with removable partial denture design. Appropriate ridge extension procedures can reposition attachments and remove bony spines, which will enhance the comfort and function of the removable partial denture.

The maxillary labial and mandibular lingual frena are common sources of interference with denture flanges. The frenum can be modified through surgical procedures to avoid compromising the fit or comfort of a removable partial denture.

Bony Spines and Knife-Edge Ridges

Sharp bony spicules should be removed and knifelike crests gently rounded. These procedures should be carried out with minimum bone loss. However, placement of a dental implant in the residual bone can effectively enhance functional comfort by creating vertical limitation of the prosthesis in occlusal function.

Polyps, Papillomas, and Traumatic Hemangiomas

All abnormal soft tissue lesions should be excised and submitted for pathologic examination before a removable partial denture is fabricated. Even though the patient may relate a history of the condition having been present for an indefinite period, its removal is indicated. New or additional stimulation to the area introduced by the prosthesis may produce discomfort or undesirable changes in the tumor.

Hyperkeratoses, Erythroplasia, and Ulcerations

All abnormal white, red, or ulcerative lesions should be investigated, regardless of their relationship to the proposed denture base or framework. A biopsy of areas larger than 5 mm should be completed; and if the lesions are large (over 2 cm in diameter), multiple biopsies should be taken. The biopsy report determines whether the margins of the tissue to be excised can be wide or narrow. The lesions should be removed and healing accomplished before the removable partial denture is fabricated. On occasion, such as after radiation treatment or procedures that create hypersensitive soft tissues, the removable partial denture design will have to be radically modified to avoid areas of possible sensitivity.

Dentofacial Deformity

Patients with a dentofacial deformity often have multiple missing teeth as part of their problem. Surgical correction of the jaw deformity can simplify the dental rehabilitation. The patient's overall problem must be evaluated thoroughly before specific problems with the dentition can be corrected. Several dental professionals (prosthodontist, oral surgeon, periodontist, orthodontist, and/or general dentist) may play a role in the patient's treatment. These individuals must be involved in producing the diagnostic database and in planning treatment for the patient. Information obtained from a general patient evaluation done to determine the patient's health status, a clinical evaluation directed toward facial esthetics and the status of the teeth and oral soft tissues, and analysis of appropriate diagnostic records create a listing of patient problems, with the most severe problem being placed at the top of the list; additional problems would follow in order of severity. It is only after this assessment that input from the team of oral health practitioners can provide a correctly sequenced final treatment plan for the patient. Surgical correction of a jaw deformity to achieve an improved appearance includes replacement of missing teeth and development of a harmonious occlusion.

Dental Implants

The use of dental implants in tooth replacement offers a significant stabilizing effect on a dental prosthesis. Brånemark and colleagues[1,2] pioneered clinical prosthodontic applications with the use of commercially pure titanium endosseous implants (Fig. 14.5). The titanium implant was designed to provide a direct titanium-to-bone interface referred to as osseointegration. Protocols developed for basic dental laboratory procedures and clinical results support the value in using dental implants as part of the treatment plan.

Implant placement using controlled surgical procedures and, in general, bone healing to the device should occur before a dental prosthesis is fabricated. Long-term clinical research has demonstrated reliable results for the treatment of complete and partially edentulous patients using dental implants. Although research on implant applications with removable partial dentures has been extremely limited, the inclusion of strategically placed implants can significantly control prosthesis movement (see Chapter 12; Figs. 14.6 through 14.8).

Augmentation of Alveolar Bone

Considerable attention has been devoted to ridge augmentation with the use of autogenous and alloplastic materials, especially in preparation for implant placement. Larger ridge volume gains necessitate consideration of autogenous grafts; however, these procedures are accompanied by concerns for surgical morbidity. Alloplastic materials have displayed short-term success; however, no randomized controlled trials have been conducted to provide evidence of long-term increases in ridge width and height for removable prostheses.

Clinical results depend on careful evaluation of the need for augmentation, the projected volume of required material, and the site and method of placement. Considerable emphasis on a thorough clinical understanding that some alloplastic materials can migrate or be displaced under occlusal loads if not appropriately supported by underlying bone and contained by buttressing soft tissues. Careful clinical judgment with sound surgical and prosthetic principles must be exercised.

PERIODONTAL PREPARATION

Periodontal preparation of the mouth usually follows any oral surgical procedure and performed simultaneously with tissue conditioning procedures. Ordinarily, tooth extraction and removal of impacted teeth, retained roots, and/or tooth or bony fragments are accomplished before definitive periodontal therapy is provided. However, it is strongly recommended that gross debridement is performed prior to surgical procedures when patients present with significant calculus accumulation. This helps limit the possibility of accidentally dislodging a piece of calculus into the extraction socket, which could lead to an infection. Elimination of exostoses, tori, hyperplastic tissue, altering muscle, and frena attachments can be incorporated with periodontal surgical techniques. In any situation, periodontal therapy should be completed before restorative dentistry procedures are begun for any dental patient. This is particularly true when a removable partial denture is contemplated because the ultimate success of this prosthesis depends directly on the health and integrity of the supporting structures. The periodontal health of the remaining teeth, especially those to be used as abutments, must be evaluated carefully by the dentist and corrective measures instituted before a removable partial denture is fabricated. It has been demonstrated that following periodontal therapy and with a good recall and oral

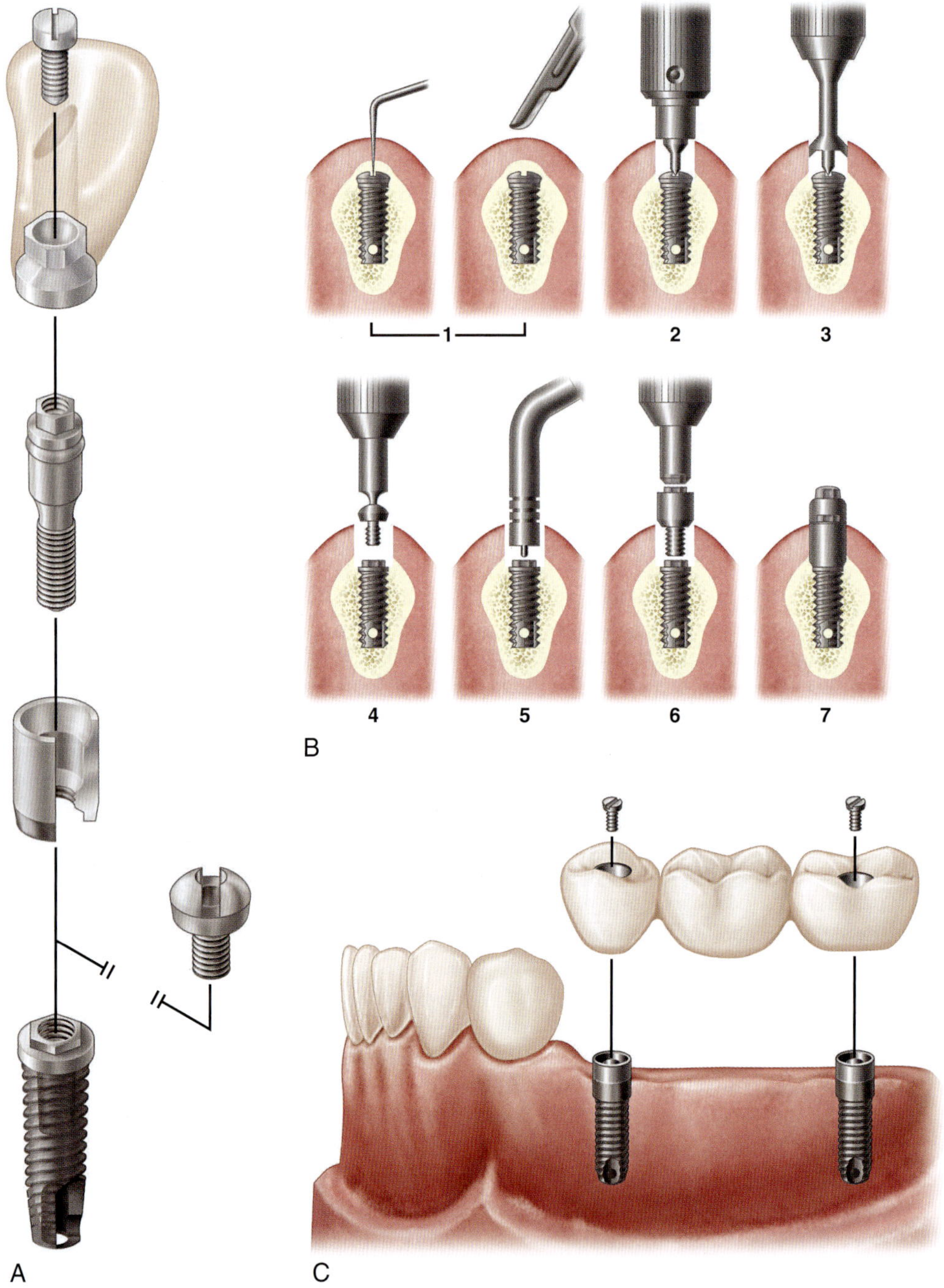

Fig. 14.5 **A,** Brånemark system components. *From lower to upper*: implant, cover screws, abutment, abutment screw, gold cylinder, and gold screw. **B,** Basic procedures in second-stage surgery: *(1)* exploration to locate cover screw; *(2)* removal of soft tissue; *(3)* removal of bony tissue; *(4)* removal of cover screw; *(5)* use of depth gauge to measure the amount of soft tissue; *(6)* abutment connection; and *(7)* placement of healing cap. **C,** Diagram of freestanding three-unit fixed partial denture supported by two osseointegrated implants that restore the extension base area, which would have been restored with a Kennedy Class II removable partial denture if implants had not been used. (A and C, Reproduced with permission from Hobo S, Ichida E, Garcia LT. *Osseointegration and Occlusal Rehabilitation*. Quintessence Publishing Company; 1989.)

hygiene program, properly designed removable partial dentures will not adversely affect the progression of periodontal disease or carious lesions.

This discussion tries to demonstrate how periodontal procedures affect diagnosis and treatment planning in a removable partial denture service rather than how the procedures are actually accomplished. For technical details, the reader is referred to any of several excellent textbooks on periodontics.

Objectives of Periodontal Therapy

The objective of periodontal therapy is the return to health of supporting structures of the teeth, creating an environment in

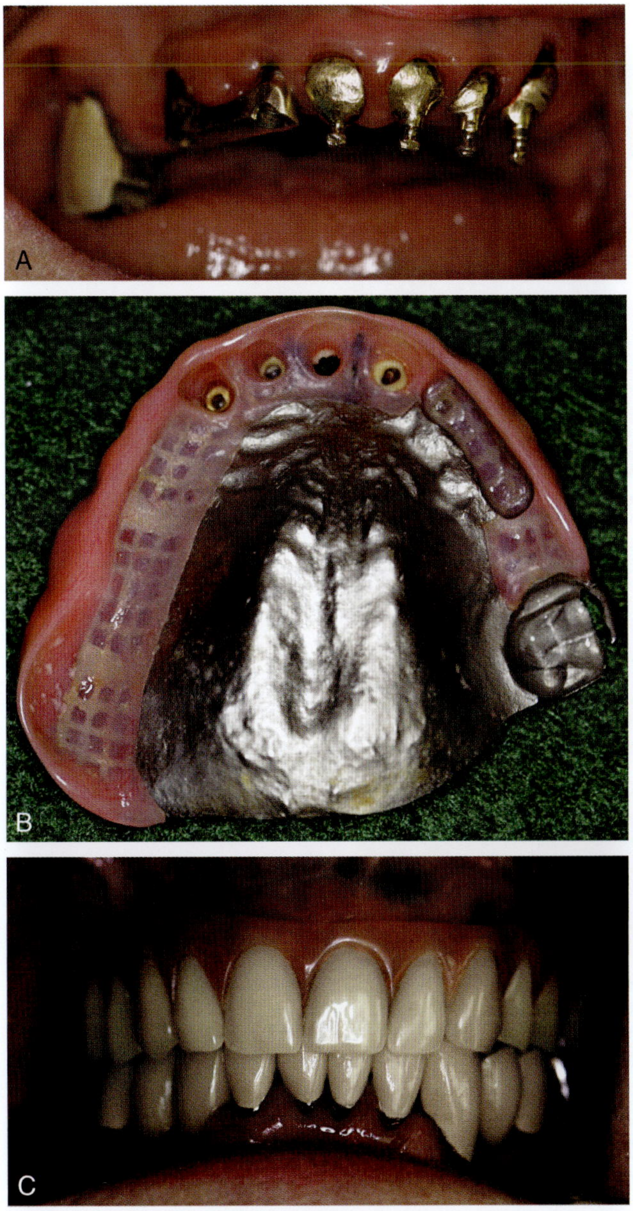

Fig. 14.6 **A,** Implant bar and natural tooth copings used to support and retain this maxillary prosthesis. **B,** Tissue side of prosthesis showing the implant bar space, which when fitted will derive both support and stability from the implants while retention is gained through resilient O-rings on the natural tooth copings. **C,** Maxillary prosthesis seated and in occlusion. (Courtesy of Dr. N. Van Roekel, Monterey, CA.)

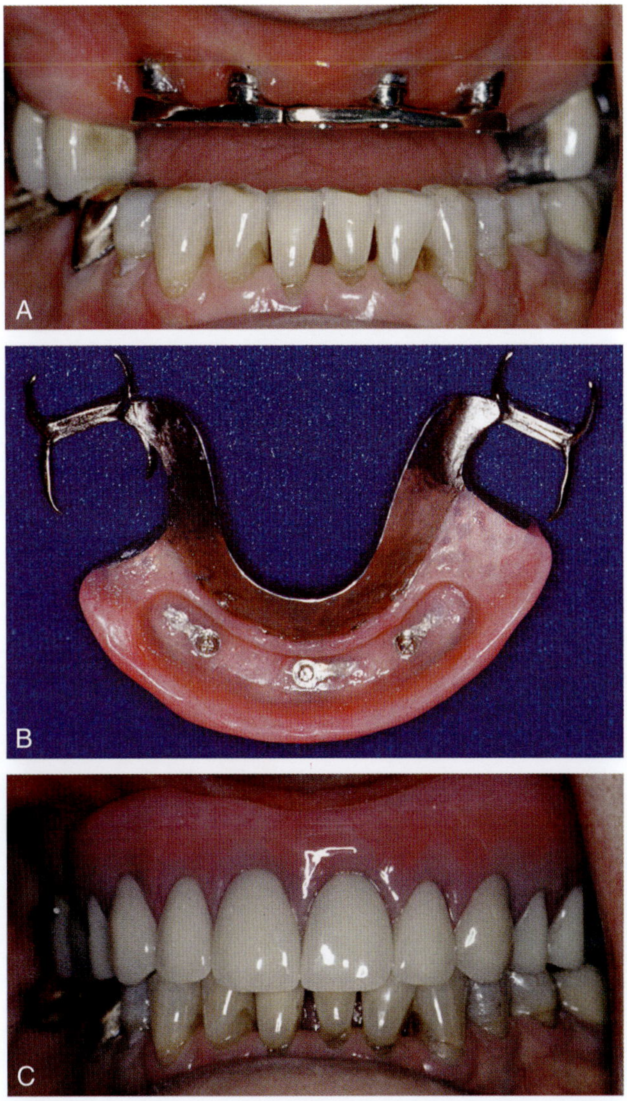

Fig. 14.7 **A,** An anterior implant-supported bar demonstrating excellent access for hygiene and a parallel relationship to opposing occlusion. **B,** Prosthesis with implant bar space (housing three retentive male components for retention and a flat surface for bar contact and support) and bilateral posterior embrasure clasps. **C,** Prosthesis seated and in occlusion. (Courtesy of Dr. N. Van Roekel, Monterey, CA.)

which the periodontium may be maintained. Criteria for satisfying this objective are as follows:

- Removal and control of all etiologic factors contributing to periodontal disease along with reduction or elimination of bleeding on probing
- Elimination of, or reduction in, the pocket depth of all pockets with the establishment of healthy gingival sulci whenever possible
- Establishment of functional atraumatic occlusal relationships and tooth stability
- Development of a personalized plaque control program and a definitive maintenance schedule

Complete periodontal charting that includes the recording of pocket depths, assessment of attachment levels, and recording of furcation involvements, mucogingival problems, and tooth mobility should be performed. Determining the severity of periodontal disease should also include the use of appropriate radiographs. The dentist who is considering removable partial denture fabrication must be certain that these criteria have been satisfied before continuing with impression procedures for the master cast.

Periodontal Diagnosis and Treatment Planning

Diagnosis

The diagnosis of periodontal diseases is based on a systematic and carefully accomplished examination of the periodontium. It follows the procurement of the health history of the patient and is performed with direct vision, palpation, a periodontal

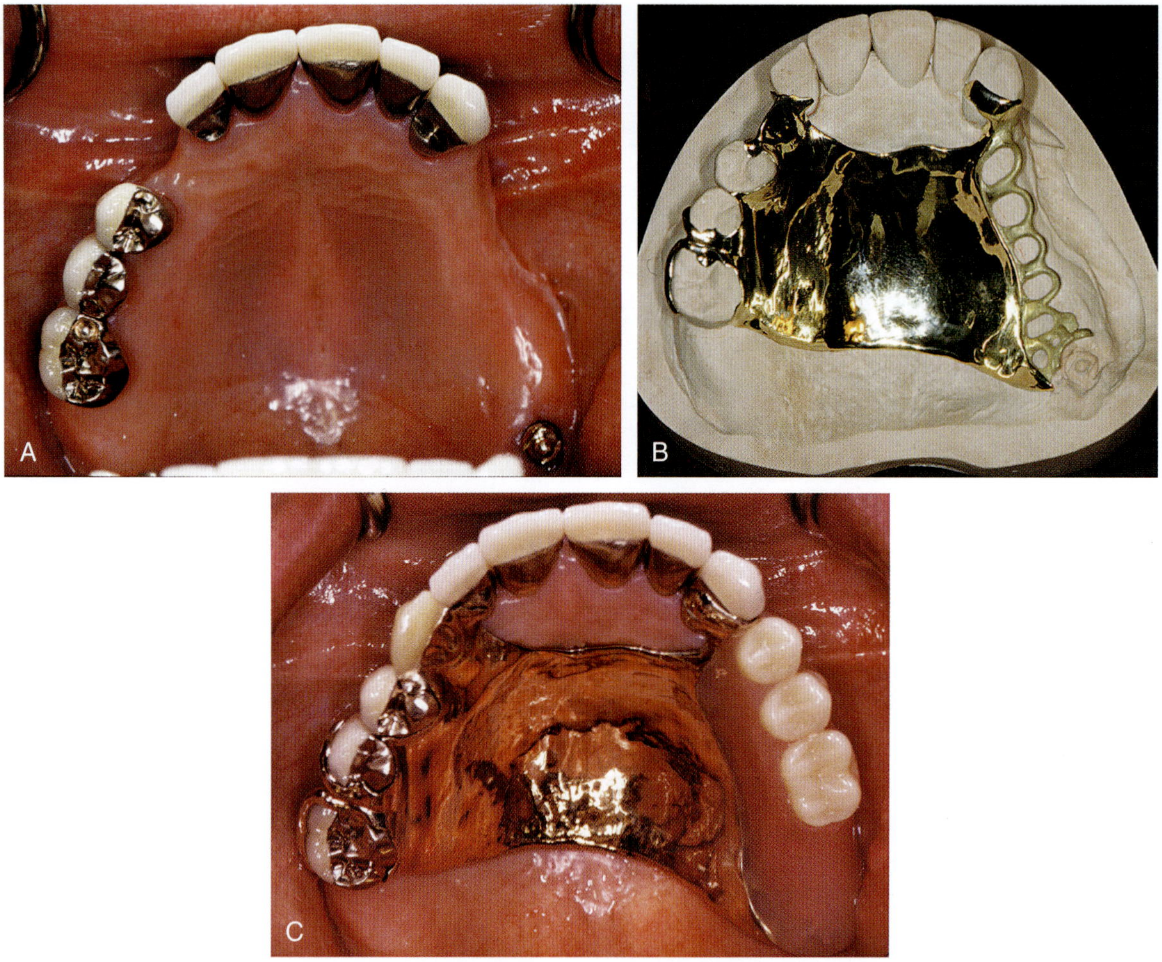

Fig. 14.8 **A,** A Kennedy Class II, modification 1, maxillary arch with a posterior implant at the distal location of the extension base. **B,** Maxillary gold framework with broad palatal coverage, maximum stabilization through palatal contacts of multiple maxillary teeth, and implant position at the distal extension base. A single implant should be protected from excessive occlusal forces; consequently, the broad palatal coverage and maximum bracing are important features of the overall design. The ball attachment abutment was used for retentive purposes. **C,** Occlusal view of the prosthesis with implant (see **A**), which provides improved retention to the distal extension base. (Courtesy of Dr. James Taylor, Ottawa, Ontario.)

probe, a mouth mirror, and other auxiliary aids, such as curved explorers, furcation probes, diagnostic casts, and appropriate radiographs.

In the examination procedure, nothing is as important as careful assessment of periodontal tissues, recording periodontal probing depths, and sites that bleed on probing, with a suitably designed periodontal probe. Under no circumstances should removable partial denture fabrication begin without an accurate diagnosis and treatment plan that includes periodontal tissue health.

Dental radiographs supplement the clinical examination and diagnosis. Clinical evaluation of the following factors should be made: (1) type, location, and severity of bone loss; (2) location, severity, and distribution of furcation involvements; (3) alterations of the periodontal ligament space; (4) alterations of the lamina dura; (5) the presence of calcified deposits; (6) the location and conformity of restorative margins; (7) evaluation of crown and root morphologies; (8) root proximity; (9) caries; and (10) evaluation of other associated anatomic features, such as the mandibular canal or sinus proximity. This information serves to substantiate clinical assessment from information obtained during the clinical examination.

In general, tooth mobility is graded according to the ease and extent of tooth movement. Normal mobility is in the order of 0.05 to 0.10 mm. Grade I mobility is present when less than 1 mm of movement occurs in a buccolingual direction; grade II is present when mobility in the buccolingual direction is between 1 and 2 mm; grade III is present when greater than 2 mm of mobility occurs in the buccolingual direction and/or the tooth is vertically depressible.

Tooth mobility is an indication of the condition of the supporting structures, namely, the periodontium, and usually caused by inflammatory changes in the periodontal ligament, traumatic occlusion, loss of attachment, or a combination of the factors. The degree of mobility present, coupled with a determination of the causative factors responsible, provides additional information that is invaluable in planning for the removable partial denture. If the causative factor can be corrected, many grade I and grade II mobile teeth can become stable and may be used successfully to help support, stabilize, and retain the removable partial denture. Mobility in itself is not an indication for extraction unless the mobile tooth cannot aid in support or stability of the removable partial denture, or mobility cannot be reduced. Grade III tooth mobility usually cannot be reversed and will not provide support or stability.

Treatment Planning

Depending on the extent and severity of the periodontal changes present, a variety of therapeutic procedures ranging from simple to relatively complex may be indicated. As was the situation with the previously discussed oral surgical procedures, it is the responsibility of the dentist rendering the removable partial denture treatment to see that the required periodontal care is accomplished for the patient. Periodontal treatment planning can usually be divided into three phases. The first phase is considered disease control or initial therapy because the objective is to eliminate or reduce local causative factors before any periodontal surgical procedures are accomplished. The procedures that are accomplished as part of the initial preparation phase include oral hygiene instruction, scaling, and root planing and polishing, as well as endodontics, occlusal adjustment, and temporary splinting, if indicated. In many instances, carefully performed scaling and root planing combined with excellent patient compliance may negate the need for periodontal surgery.

During the second, or periodontal, surgical phase, any needed periodontal surgery, such as free gingival grafts, osseous grafts, or pocket reduction, is accomplished. It is advisable to discuss the possible need for these treatment procedures with the patient at the initial examination appointment or during the initial phase of therapy because this will likely involve referral of the patient to a periodontist. The maintenance of periodontal health is accomplished in the third phase and is always ongoing. A definitive recall schedule should be established with the patient and is usually kept at 3- to 4-month intervals.

Initial Disease Control Therapy (Phase 1)

Oral Hygiene Instruction

Ordinarily, dental treatment should be introduced to the patient through instruction provided through a personalized oral hygiene home care regimen. Patient cooperation and compliance with the prescribed procedure provide the dentist perspective that reflects patient interest and help determine the long-term prognosis of treatment.

For a home care oral hygiene routine to be successful, the patient must understand the need to follow the prescribed procedure regularly. The most effective motivation techniques require a patient to understand their periodontal condition and the benefits of routine treatment. Helping a patient learn causes and consequences of managing periodontal disease, the use of aids such as a soft tissue toothbrush, and the benefits of flossing is an important component of oral hygiene instruction. At subsequent appointments, oral hygiene can be evaluated carefully, and other oral hygiene aids (such as an interdental and or sulcular brushes) can be incorporated as needed. Further treatment should be withheld until a satisfactory level of plaque control has been achieved. This is a particularly critical point for the patient who requires extensive restorative dentistry or a removable partial denture. Without good oral hygiene, any treatment intervention will have a poor prognosis. A patient's understanding and responsibility for self-care are important prior to implementation of an extensive restorative and prosthodontic treatment plan.

Occlusal Adjustment

Overhanging restoration margins and open contacts that allow food impaction should be corrected before implementing definitive prosthetic treatment. Although periodontal tissue health is essential, it may not be possible to delay all restorative procedures until complete periodontal therapy and healing have occurred. This is especially true for patients with severe carious lesions with pulpal involvement. Caries removal and restoration of defects may take precedence early in treatment. The placement of temporary or treatment fillings must not become a local causative factor.

Bacterial plaque accumulations and calculus deposits are the primary factors involved in the initiation and progression of inflammatory periodontal disease. However, poor restorative dentistry and traumatic occlusion can compromise periodontal health. Traumatic occlusal interferences should be removed by a selective grinding procedure. An attempt should be made to address deflective contacts that interfere with mandibular closure, eliminating mandibular displacement caused by occlusal interference. After which, the interocclusal relationship of the remaining teeth in various excursive mandibular movements should be observed, with special attention to cuspal contact, wear, mobility, and roentgenographic changes in the periodontium.

Accurately mounted diagnostic casts are used to determine if occlusal adjustment of the remaining natural dentition is needed. Occlusion adjustments can be coordinated yet limited to selective spot grinding. Ground tooth surfaces should be subsequently smoothed and polished. The mere presence of occlusal abnormalities, in the absence of demonstrable pathologic change associated with the occlusion, does not necessarily constitute an indication for selective grinding. The indication for occlusal adjustment is based on the presence of a pathologic condition rather than on a preconceived articulation pattern. In the natural dentition, attempts to create bilateral balance, in the prosthetic sense, have no place in the occlusal adjustment procedure. Bilateral balanced occlusion not only is difficult to obtain in a natural dentition but also is unnecessary in view of its absence in most normal healthy mouths. Occlusion on natural teeth needs to be perfected only to the point at which cuspal interference within the patient's functional range of motion is eliminated and normal physiologic function can occur.

Temporary Splinting

Teeth that are mobile at the time of the initial examination frequently present a diagnostic problem for the dentist. The cause of the mobility must be determined and then a decision made for elimination of the causative factors. The response of these teeth to temporary immobilization followed by appropriate treatment may be helpful in establishing a prognosis for them and may lead to a rational decision as to whether they should be retained or sacrificed. Secondary mobility resulting from the presence of an inflammatory lesion may be reversible if the disease process has not destroyed too much of the attachment apparatus. Primary mobility caused by occlusal interference also may disappear after selective grinding. In instances of angular types of osseous defects, one should consider guided tissue regeneration as a means of increasing attachment levels. In some situations, however, the teeth must be stabilized because of loss of supporting structure from the periodontal process.

Teeth may be immobilized during periodontal treatment by acid-etching teeth with composite resin, with fiber-reinforced resins, with cast removable splints, or with intracoronal attachments. The latter, an example of which is the A-splint, necessitates cutting tooth surfaces and embedding a ridge connector between adjacent teeth.

After periodontal treatment is performed, splinting may be accomplished with cast removable restorations or cast cemented restorations. The preferred form of permanent splinting uses two or more cast restorations soldered or cast together. They may be cemented with permanent (zinc oxyphosphate or resin) cements or temporary (zinc oxide–eugenol) cements. A properly designed removable partial denture can also stabilize mobile teeth if provision for such immobilization is planned as the denture is designed.

Use of an Occlusal Guard

The removable acrylic-resin splint, originally designed as an aid in eliminating the deleterious effects of nocturnal clenching and grinding, has been used to advantage for the removable partial denture patient. The occlusal guard may prove helpful as a form of temporary splinting if worn at night when the removable partial denture has been removed, hence referred to as nightguard. The flat occlusal surface prevents intercuspation of the teeth, which eliminates lateral occlusal forces (Fig. 14.9).

The nightguard is particularly useful before fabrication of a removable partial denture when one of the abutment teeth has been unopposed for an extended period. The periodontal ligament of a tooth without an antagonist undergoes changes characterized by loss of orientation of periodontal ligament fibers, loss of supporting bone, and narrowing of the periodontal ligament space. If such a tooth is suddenly returned to full function when it is carrying an increased burden, pain and prolonged sensitivity may result. However, if a nightguard is used to return some functional stimulation to the tooth, the periodontal ligament changes are reversed and an uneventful course can be experienced when the tooth is returned to full function.

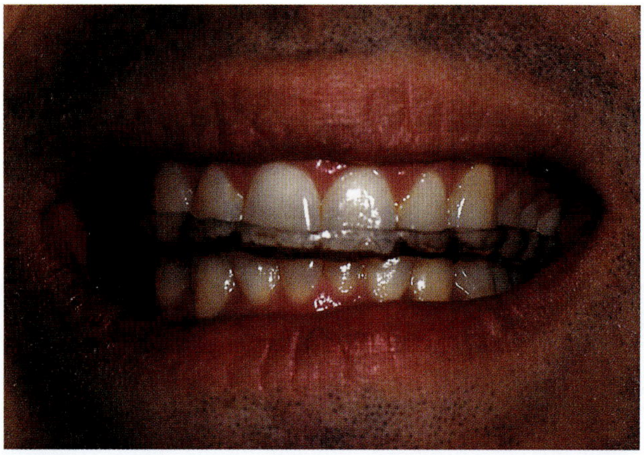

Fig. 14.9 The removable acrylic-resin splint with a flat occlusal plane can be used effectively as a form of temporary stabilization and as a means of eliminating excessive lateral forces created by clenching and grinding habits.

Minor Tooth Movement

The increased use of orthodontic procedures in conjunction with restorative and prosthetic dentistry has contributed to the success of many restorations by altering the periodontal environment in which they are placed. Malposed teeth that were once doomed to extraction should be considered now for repositioning and retention. The additional stability provided for a removable partial denture by uprighting a tilted or drifted tooth may mean much in terms of comfort to the patient. The techniques employed are not difficult to master, and the rewards in terms of a better restorative dentistry service are great.

Periodontal Treatment Intervention

One of the most important services rendered to the patient is the removal of calculus and plaque deposits from the coronal and root surfaces of the teeth. Careful scaling and root planing are fundamental to the reestablishment of periodontal health. Without meticulous removal of calculus, plaque, and toxic material in the cementum, other forms of periodontal therapy cannot be successful. Thorough scaling and root planing should precede definitive surgical periodontal procedures that may be indicated before removable partial denture fabrication.

After initial therapy is completed, the patient is reevaluated for the periodontal surgical phase. If oral hygiene is at an optimum level, yet pockets with inflammation and osseous defects are still present, a variety of periodontal surgical techniques should be considered to improve periodontal health. The procedures selected should have the potential to enhance the results obtained during initial periodontal therapy. Periodontal surgical interventions include key surgical and regenerative procedures aimed to eliminate inflammatory disease processes and restoration of the periodontal tissue attachment for sustainable long-term successful maintenance.

Advantages of Periodontal Therapy

Periodontal therapy accomplished prior to fabrication of a removable prosthesis is important to address factors of periodontal disease and improve the potential for long-term success of dental treatment. Simultaneously, restorative procedures require restorations with ideal contours to support gingival tissue health. Even in the absence of periodontal disease, certain periodontal procedures may be an invaluable aid in removable partial denture construction. Through periodontal surgical techniques, the environment of potential abutment teeth may be altered to the point of making an otherwise unacceptable tooth a most satisfactory retainer for a removable partial denture.

OPTIMIZATION OF THE FOUNDATION FOR FITTING AND FUNCTION OF THE PROSTHESIS

Conditioning of Abused and Irritated Tissues

A patient may require conditioning of supporting tissues in edentulous areas before the final impression phase of treatment begins. Patients who require conditioning treatment often demonstrate the following symptoms:

- Inflammation and irritation of the mucosa covering denture-bearing areas (Fig. 14.10)
- Distortion of normal anatomic structures, such as incisive papillae, rugae, and retromolar pads
- A burning sensation in residual ridge areas, the tongue, and the cheeks and lips

These conditions are usually associated with ill-fitting or poorly occluding removable partial dentures. However, nutritional deficiencies, endocrine imbalances, severe health problems (diabetes or blood dyscrasias), and bruxism must be considered in a differential diagnosis.

If the use of a new removable partial denture or the relining of a present denture is attempted without first correcting these conditions, the chances for successful treatment will be compromised because the same old problems will be perpetuated. The patient must be made to realize that fabrication of a new prosthesis should be delayed until the oral tissues can be returned to a healthy state. If there are unresolved systemic problems, removable partial denture treatment will usually result in failure or limited success.

The first treatment procedure should consist of immediate institution of a good home care program. A suggested home care program includes rinsing the mouth three times a day with a prescribed saline solution; massaging the residual ridge areas, palate, and tongue with a soft toothbrush; removing the prosthesis at night; and using a prescribed therapeutic multiple vitamin along with a prescribed high-protein, low-carbohydrate diet. Some inflammatory oral conditions caused by ill-fitting dentures can be resolved by removing the dentures for extended periods. However, few patients are willing to undergo such inconveniences.

Use of Tissue Conditioning Materials

The tissue conditioning materials are elastopolymers that continue to flow for an extended period, permitting distorted tissues to rebound and assume their normal form. These soft materials apparently have a massaging effect on irritated mucosa, and because they are soft, occlusal forces are probably more evenly distributed.

Maximum benefit from using tissue conditioning materials may be obtained by (1) eliminating deflective or interfering occlusal contacts of old dentures (by remounting in an articulator if necessary); (2) extending denture bases to proper form to enhance support, retention, and stability (Fig. 14.11); (3) relieving the tissue side of denture bases sufficiently (2 mm) to provide space for even thickness and distribution of conditioning material; (4) applying the material in amounts sufficient to provide support and a cushioning effect (Fig. 14.12 and (5) following the manufacturer's directions for manipulation and placement of the conditioning material.

The conditioning procedure should be repeated until the supporting tissues display an undistorted, healthy appearance. The frequency needed when changing the conditioning materials usually occurs approximately once a week or 4 to 7 days between changes. Improvement in irritated and distorted tissues is usually noted within a few visits, and in some patients a dramatic improvement will be observed. Approximately three or four tissue conditioning material changes suffice, but in some instances additional changes are required. If positive results are not seen within 3 to 4 weeks, one should consider this as indicative of a more serious health or tissue diagnosis and may require biopsy or consultation from a physician.

Abutment Restorations

Equipped with the diagnostic casts on which a tentative removable partial denture design has been drawn, the dentist is able

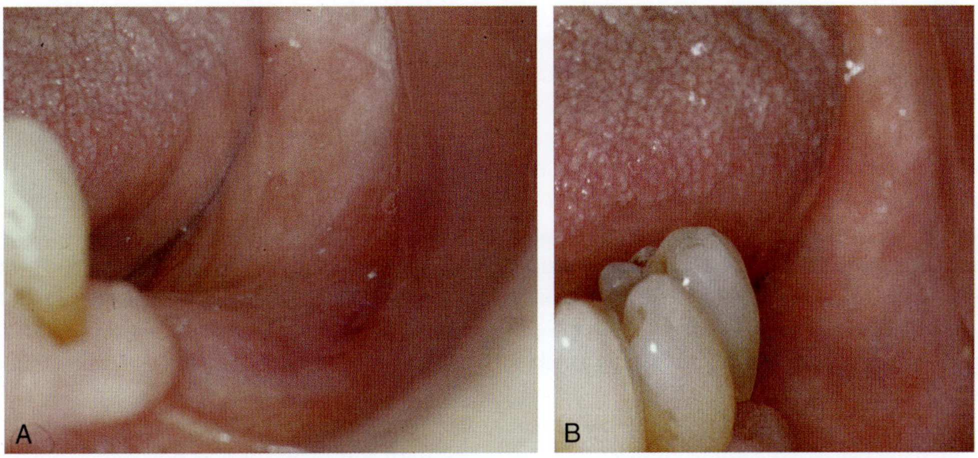

Fig. 14.10 A, Inflamed and distorted denture-bearing mucosa due to an ill-fitting prosthesis that is worn 24 hours a day. **B,** After the tissue abuse is treated via modification of the denture base with a tissue conditioning resilient liner material, the prosthesis is removed for portions of the day, and the abused tissue is massaged, the denture-bearing foundation is healthy again.

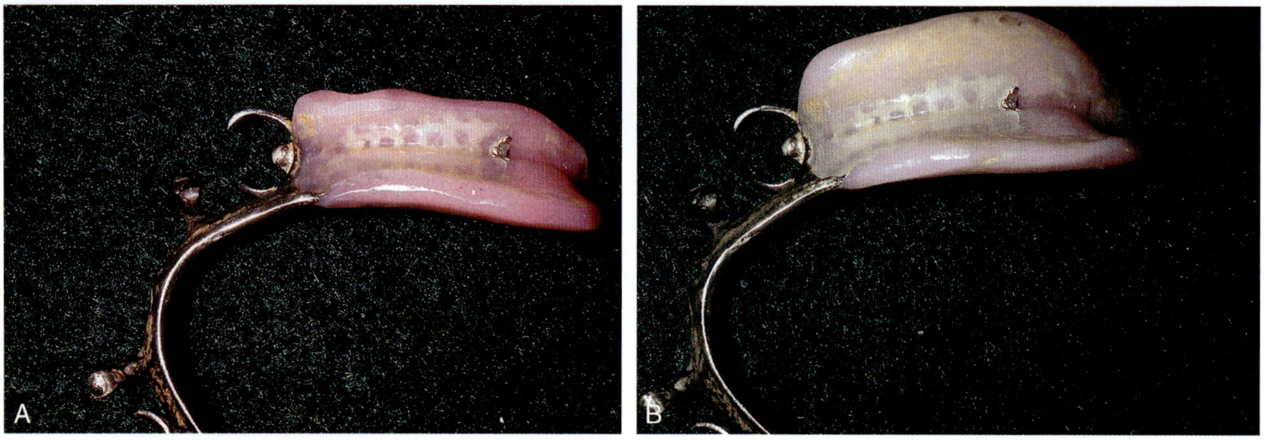

Fig. 14.11 A, Mandibular removable partial denture with underextended bases, which contributed to tissue irritation. **B,** Denture bases properly extended to enhance support, stability, and retention.

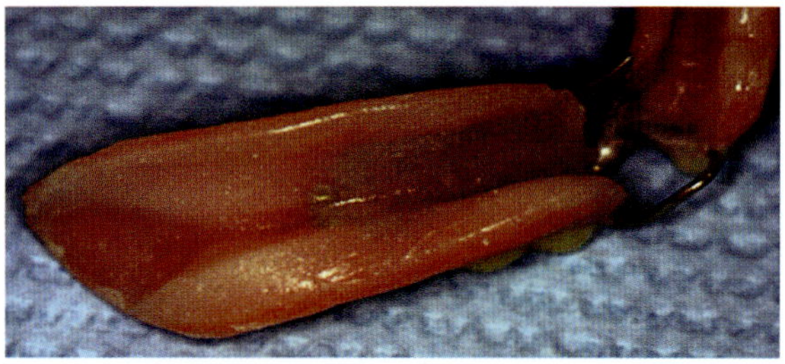

Fig. 14.12 Tissue conditioning should be of sufficient thickness to be resilient and not place undue stress on the soft tissue.

to accomplish preparation of abutment teeth with accuracy. The information at hand should include the proposed path of placement, the areas of teeth that require alteration of tooth contours, and the locations of rest seats and guiding planes.

During examination, treatment planning, and survey of diagnostic casts, each abutment tooth is considered individually as to what type of restoration is indicated. Intact abutment teeth in a patient with good oral hygiene are considered for use as removable partial denture abutments. Current oral hygiene health may not predict continued health so long-term maintenance is reinforced consistently throughout patient care for long-term success. Remember that removable partial denture clasps do not cause tooth decay; it is incumbent on the patient to maintain oral hygiene maintenance procedures to maintain oral health and keep the removable partial denture clean. At times, removable partial dentures have been condemned as cariogenic because the dentist did not instruct nor help the patient understand long-term need for oral hygiene maintenance.

Often, tooth restorations are needed; amalgam or composite restorations on teeth with proximal caries can be used although an indirect restoration (casting or milled) may be better support for occlusal rests. An amalgam restoration, properly condensed, is capable of supporting an occlusal rest without appreciable flow over a long period.

The most vulnerable area on the abutment tooth is the proximal gingival area, which lies beneath the minor connector of the removable partial denture framework and is therefore subject to accumulation of debris in an area most susceptible to caries. Even when the removable partial denture is removed, these areas are often missed by the toothbrush, which allows bacterial plaque and debris to remain for long periods. Because of this unique removable partial denture concern, special attention should be paid to these areas during patient education and follow-up. Even when a complete crown restoration is placed in this most vulnerable area, recurrent caries can occur. Caries risk is best managed through effective home care and professional follow-up procedures, rather than through the placement of restorations.

All proximal abutment surfaces that serve as guiding planes for the removable partial denture should be prepared as parallel as possible to the path of placement. Preparations may include modifying the contour of existing ceramic restorations, if necessary. This may be accomplished with abrasive stones or diamond finishing stones. A polished surface for the altered ceramic restoration may be restored by using any of several polishing kits supplied by manufacturers.

When preparing abutments that will receive surveyed crowns, it is important to plan for the tooth reduction necessary to allow placement of sufficient restorative material for durability, contour, and esthetics, as well as the contours prescribed for the desired clasp assembly (Fig. 14.13). This can be accomplished by first modifying the axial contours of the abutments to those required of the completed crown, then starting controlled tooth reduction (preparation) to accommodate the thickness of the materials for durability, contour, and esthetics. This ensures that the wax patterns and resultant crowns can be restored to the desired form.

Contouring Wax Patterns

Modern indirect techniques permit adjustment and contouring of wax patterns on the master cast with the aid of the surveyor blade. All abutment teeth to be restored with castings can be prepared at one time and an impression made that will provide an accurate stone replica of the prepared arch. Wax patterns may then be refined on separated individual dies or removable dies. All abutment surfaces adjacent to edentulous areas should be made parallel to the path of placement by the use of the surveyor blade (Fig. 14.14). This technique will provide parallel proximal surfaces eliminating the need to alter the restoration

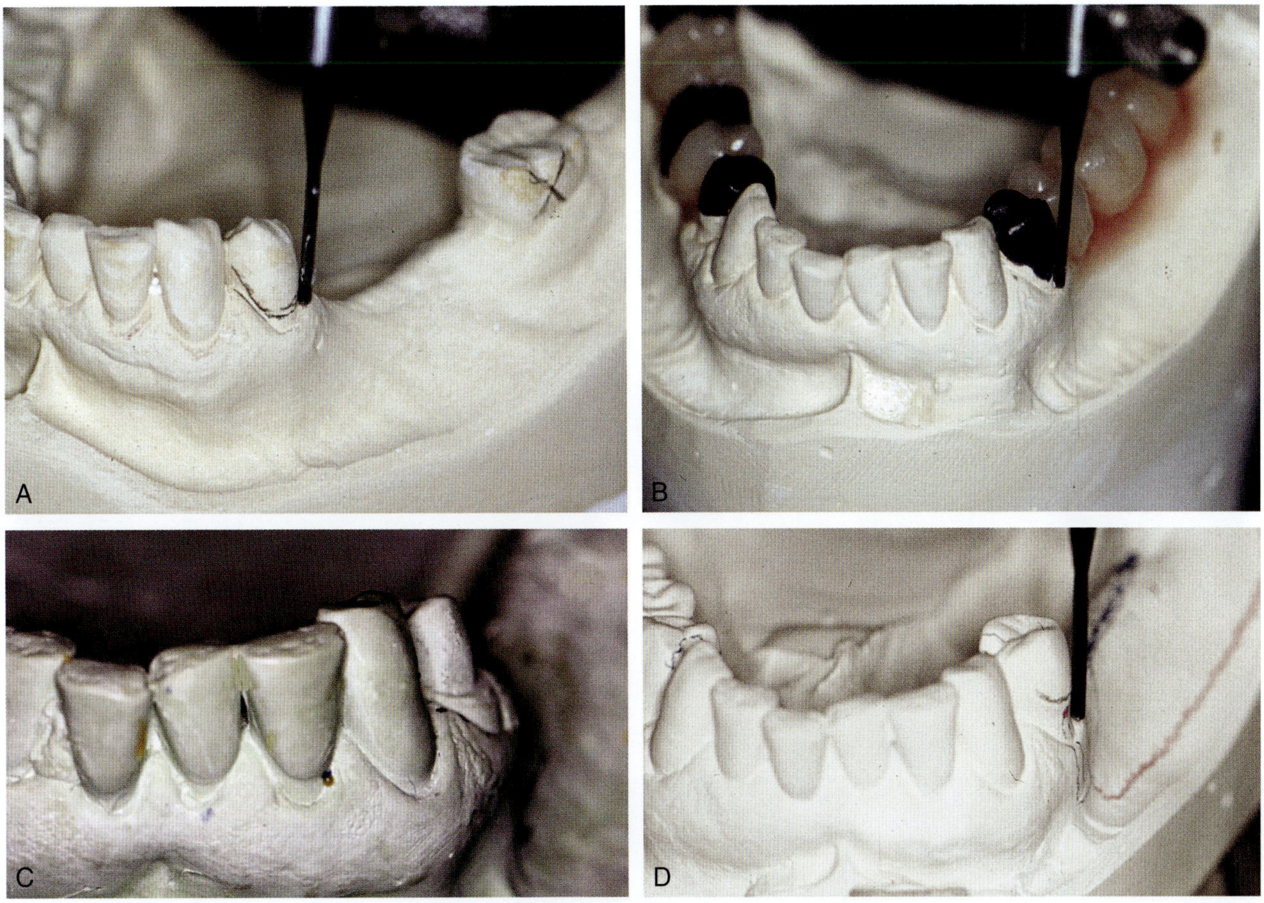

Fig. 14.13 **A,** Diagnostic cast at an orientation best for all abutments considered. The buccal survey line is too close to the marginal gingival and the distal surface does not lend itself to guide-plane preparation. A surveyed crown is indicated. **B,** Abutment contours appropriate to clasp design (distal guide plane and mid-buccal 0.01-inch undercut) are produced in wax. **C,** Cast of abutment preparation provides buccal surface reduction adequate to replace with metal ceramic material at the required contour. Without careful consideration of survey line placement needs before and during preparation, it is easy to reproduce incorrect contours in finished crowns. **D,** Cast of a seated surveyed crown demonstrates desired contours for the clasp design chosen.

intraorally, permit positive seating of the removable partial denture along the path of placement, and minimize undesirable space beneath minor connectors to avoid debris accumulation.

Rest Seats

After the proximal surfaces of the wax patterns have been made parallel, and buccal and lingual contours have been established to satisfy the requirements of stability and retention with the best possible esthetic placement of clasp arms, the occlusal rest seats should be prepared in the wax pattern rather than in the finished restoration. The placement of occlusal rests should be considered at the time the teeth are prepared to receive cast restorations so that there will be sufficient clearance beneath the floor of the occlusal rest seat and natural tooth structure. A frequent error occurs when a completed abutment crown is cemented intraorally without any provision for the occlusal rest having been made in the wax pattern. The dentist then proceeds to prepare an occlusal rest seat in the cast restoration, with the possibility of perforating the restoration to prepare a rest seat that is often too shallow.

If tooth structure has been removed to provide placement of the occlusal rest seat, it may be ideally placed in the wax pattern by using a No. 8 round bur to lower the marginal ridge and establish the outline form of the rest and then using a No. 6 round bur to slightly deepen the floor of the rest seat along the long axis of the tooth, within the confines of the marginal ridge, *not* along the marginal ridge. This approach provides an occlusal rest that best satisfies the requirements to direct occlusal force axially and avoid creating an occlusal interference with the opposing teeth.

Perhaps the most important function of a rest is the division of stress loads from the removable partial denture to provide the greatest efficiency with the least damaging effect to the supporting abutment teeth. For a distal extension removable partial denture, the rest must be able to transmit occlusal forces to the abutment teeth in a vertical direction only, thereby permitting the least possible lateral stresses to be transmitted to the abutment teeth.

For this reason, the floor of the rest seat should incline toward the center of the tooth so that the occlusal forces are

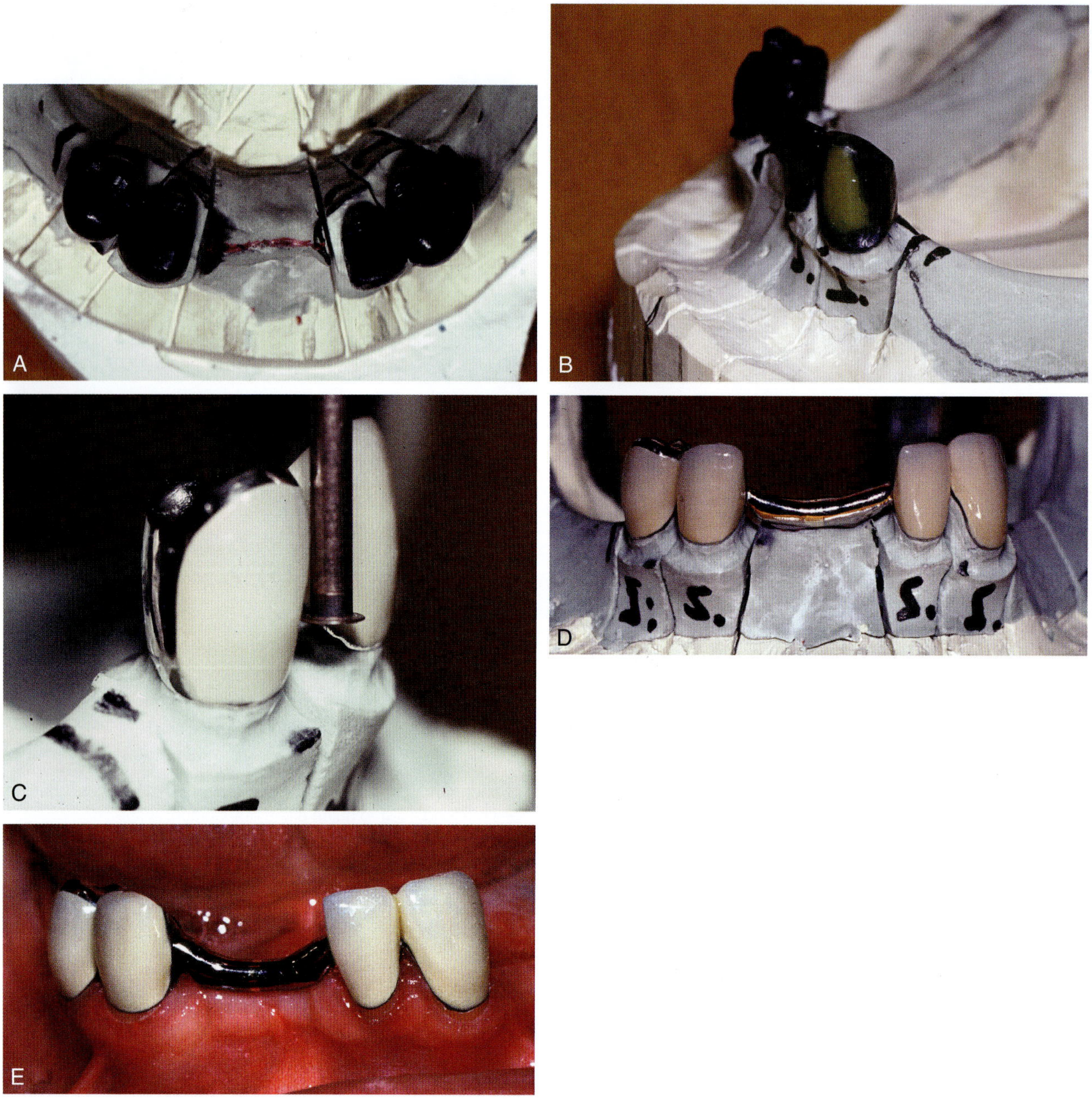

Fig. 14.14 **A,** Occlusal view of full contour wax patterns, which will be splinted between crowns and across the midline with a 13-gauge splint bar. Rests are evident on the lingual surfaces of abutment wax patterns. **B,** Wax patterns showing labial cutback for porcelain. Bilateral guide-plane surfaces will be reproduced in metal and are parallel to the path of insertion. **C,** An abutment veneered crown with an appropriate height of contour and a 0.02-inch undercut for the anticipated wrought-wire retainer. **D,** Completed prosthesis, splinted between retainer crowns and across the midline. Splint bar with added vertical support provides indirect retention. **E,** Prosthesis inserted intraorally.

directed along the long axis, centered over the root apex. Any other form but that of a spoon shape can permit locking of the occlusal rest and the transmission of tipping forces to the abutment tooth. A ball-and-socket type of relationship between occlusal rest and abutment tooth is the most desirable. At the same time, the marginal ridge must be lowered so that the angle formed by the occlusal rest, and the minor connector will stand above the occlusal surface of the abutment tooth as little as possible and avoid interference with the opposing teeth. Simultaneously, sufficient bulk must be provided to prevent weakness in the occlusal rest at the marginal ridge. The marginal ridge must be lowered and yet not be the deepest part of the rest preparation. To permit occlusal stresses to be directed toward the center of the abutment tooth, the angle formed by the floor of the occlusal rest with the minor connector should be less than 90 degrees. In other words, the floor of the occlusal rest should incline slightly from the lowered marginal ridge toward the center of the tooth.

This proper form can be readily accomplished in the wax pattern, if care is taken during crown or inlay preparation to provide the location of the rest. If direct restorations are used, sufficient bulk must be present in this area to allow proper occlusal rest seat form without weakening the restoration. There is insufficient evidence to show that direct restorations used as rest seats perform equally to enamel. When the rest seat is placed in sound enamel, this is best accomplished by the use of round carbide burs (Nos. 4, 6, and 8) that leave a smooth enamel surface.

Rest seat preparations in sound enamel (or in existing restorations that are not to be replaced) should always follow the recontouring of proximal tooth surfaces. The preparation of proximal tooth surfaces should be done first because if the occlusal portion of the rest seat is placed first and the proximal tooth surface is altered later, the outline form of the rest seat is sometimes irreparably altered.

Following proximal surface recontouring (guided plane preparation), the larger round bur is used to lower the marginal ridge 1.5 to 2.0 mm while at the same time creating the relative outline form of the rest seat. The result is a rest seat preparation with marginal ridge lowered and gross outline form established but without sufficient deepening of the rest seat preparation toward the center of the tooth. A smaller round bur (a No. 4 or 6) may then be used to deepen the floor of the rest seat to a gradual incline toward the center of the tooth. Enamel rods are then smoothed using polishing burs or abrasive rubber points to complete polishing the rest seat preparation.

The success or failure of a removable partial denture depends on how well the mouth preparations were accomplished. It is only through intelligent planning and competent execution of mouth preparations that the denture can satisfactorily restore lost dental functions and contribute to the health of the remaining oral tissues.

REFERENCES

1. Brånemark PI. Osseointegration and its experimental background. *J Prosthet Dent*. 1983;50(3):399–410. https://doi.org/10.1016/s0022-3913(83)80101-2. PMID: 6352924.
2. Brånemark P-I, Zarb GA, Albrektsson T. *Tissue-Integrated Prostheses: Osseointegration in Clinical Dentistry*. Quintessence Publishing, Co; 1985.

15

Preparation of Abutment Teeth

Lisa A. Lang, Lily T. García, Ahmed Mahrous, and Ramtin Sadid-Zadeh

CHAPTER OUTLINE

Abutment teeth may be prepared to provide support, stabilization, reciprocation, and retention for the removable partial denture after surgery, periodontal treatment, endodontic treatment, and tissue conditioning of the arch involved are completed. Rarely, if ever, is the situation encountered in which alterations of the abutment teeth are not indicated because teeth do not develop with guiding planes, rests, and contours to accommodate clasp assemblies.

A favorable clinical outcome to any deep restorations, endodontic therapy, and the results of periodontal treatment should be established before the removable partial denture is fabricated. If the prognosis of a tooth under treatment is poor and prescribed for extraction, the removable partial denture design can be modified to compensate for loss of the tooth. If teeth are lost after the removable partial denture is fabricated, then a prosthetic tooth must be added or replaced on the removable partial denture. Most removable partial denture designs are not designed for the potential postfabrication additions, sometimes making the addition of teeth or clasps difficult. Although this possibility should be considered in the original design of the framework, it typically is only when the prognosis of a tooth is fair. Every diagnostic aid should be used to determine which teeth are to be used as abutments or are potential abutments for future designs. When an original abutment is lost, it is extremely difficult to effectively modify the removable partial denture to use the next adjacent tooth to accommodate a clasp assembly, retaining unit.

It is sometimes possible to design a removable partial denture so that a single posterior abutment tooth that is questionable can be retained as an abutment and used to support one end of a tooth-supported base. Then, if that posterior abutment were lost, it could be replaced with a distal extension base. Such a design must include provision for future indirect retention, flexible clasping on the remaining terminal abutment, and provision for establishing tissue support by a secondary impression. Anterior abutments considered poor risks may not be so freely used because of the problems involved in adding a new abutment retainer when the original one is lost. Teeth with questionable prognosis should be treatment planned for extraction in favor of a better abutment in the original treatment plan.

CLASSIFICATION OF ABUTMENT TEETH

All abutment teeth must have contour modifications that are customized to the planned prosthesis design. The subject of abutment preparations may be grouped as follows: (1) abutment teeth that require only minor modifications to their coronal portions; (2) abutment teeth planned for restoration other than complete coverage crowns; and (3) abutment teeth planned for complete coverage restorations, that is, crowns.

Abutment teeth that require only minor modifications include teeth with sound enamel, those with small restorations not involved in the removable partial denture design, those with acceptable restorations that will be involved in the removable partial denture design, and those that have existing crown restorations requiring minor modification that will not jeopardize the integrity of the crown. The latter may exist as an individual crown or as the abutment of a fixed partial denture.

The use of unprotected abutments has been discussed previously. Although complete coverage of all abutments may be desirable, it is not always possible or practical. The decision to use unprotected abutments involves certain risks, of which the patient must be advised, and includes responsibility for maintaining oral hygiene and caries control. Making crown restorations fit existing denture clasps is a difficult task[1]; however, the fact that it is possible to do so may influence the decision to use uncrowned but otherwise sound teeth as abutments.

Complete coverage restorations provide the best possible support for occlusal rests (Fig. 15.1). If finances or other factors prevent the use of complete coverage restorations, then a properly condensed amalgam restoration can support an occlusal rest without appreciable flow for a long period. If an existing amalgam restoration is questionable, then the restoration should be replaced. This should be done before guide planes and occlusal rest seats are prepared, to allow the restoration to reach maximum strength and be polished.

Continued improvement in dimensional stability, strength, and wear resistance of composite resin restorations will add another option when considering preparation and modification of abutment teeth for removable partial dentures, resulting in a less invasive restoration compared to complete coverage restorations and more economical.

SEQUENCE OF ABUTMENT PREPARATIONS ON SOUND ENAMEL OR EXISTING RESTORATIONS

Abutment preparations on sound enamel or on existing restorations that have been judged as acceptable should be done in the following order:

1. Proximal surfaces parallel to the path of placement should be prepared to provide guiding planes (Fig. 15.2, *A*).
2. Tooth contours should be modified (see Fig. 15.2, *B* and *C*), lowering the height of contour so that (a) the origin of circumferential clasp arms may be placed well below the occlusal surface, preferably at the junction of the middle and gingival thirds; (b) retentive clasp terminals may be placed in the gingival third of the crown for better esthetics and better mechanical advantage; and (c) reciprocal clasp arms may be placed on and above a height of contour that is no higher than the cervical portion of the middle third of the crown of the abutment tooth.

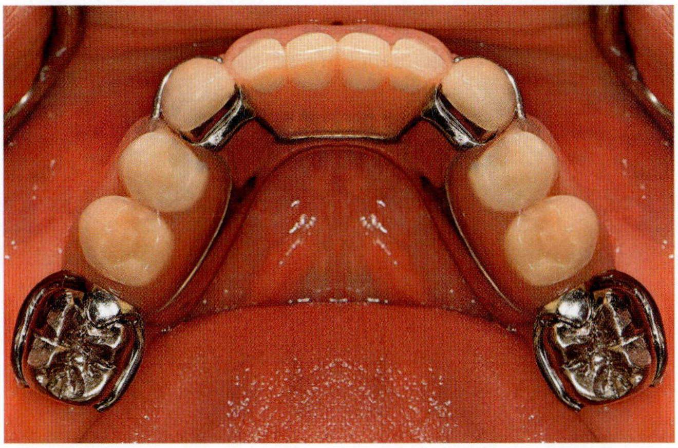

Fig. 15.1 This Kennedy Class III, modification II, partial denture is supported on all sides with cast restorations, offering exceptional fit and support. (Courtesy of Ahmed Mahrous Copyright © 2024. All rights reserved.)

3. After alterations of axial contours are accomplished and before rest seat preparations are instituted, an impression of the arch should be made in irreversible hydrocolloid and a cast formed in a fast-setting stone. This cast can be returned to the surveyor to determine the adequacy of axial alterations before proceeding with rest seat preparations. If axial surfaces require additional axial recontouring, this can be performed during the same appointment and without compromise.
4. Occlusal rest areas should be prepared that will direct occlusal forces along the long axis of the abutment tooth (see Fig. 15.2, *D*). Mouth preparation should follow the removable partial denture design that was outlined on the diagnostic cast at the time the cast was surveyed and the treatment plan confirmed. Proposed changes to abutment teeth should be made on the diagnostic cast and outlined in colored pencil to indicate the area, amount, and angulation of the modification to be done (see Chapter 13). Although occlusal rest seats may also be prepared on the diagnostic cast, indication of their location in colored pencil is usually sufficient for the experienced dentist because rest preparations follow a definite pattern (see Chapter 6).

ABUTMENT PREPARATIONS USING CONSERVATIVE RESTORATIONS

Conventional inlay preparations are permissible on the proximal surface of a tooth not to be contacted by a minor connector of the removable partial denture. However, proximal and occlusal surfaces that support minor connectors and occlusal rests require somewhat different treatment. The extent of occlusal coverage (i.e., whether cusps are covered) will be governed by the usual factors, such as the extent of caries, the presence of unsupported enamel walls, and the extent of occlusal abrasion and attrition.

When an inlay is the restoration of choice for an abutment tooth, certain modifications of the outline form are necessary. To prevent the buccal and lingual proximal margins from lying at or near the minor connector or the occlusal rest, these margins must be extended well beyond the line angles of the tooth. This additional extension may be accomplished by widening the conventional box preparation. However, the margin of a cast restoration produced for such a preparation may be quite thin and may be damaged by the clasp during placement or removal of the removable partial denture. This hazard may be avoided by extending the outline of the box beyond the line angle, thus producing a strong restoration-to-tooth junction.

In this type of preparation, the pulp is particularly vulnerable unless the axial wall is curved to conform to the external proximal curvature of the tooth. When caries is of minimal depth, the gingival seat should have an axial depth at all points about the width of a No. 559 fissure bur. It is of utmost importance that the gingival seat be placed where it can be easily accessed to maintain good oral hygiene. The proximal contour necessary to produce the proper guide plane surface and the close proximity of the minor connector render this area particularly vulnerable to future caries. Every effort should be made to provide the

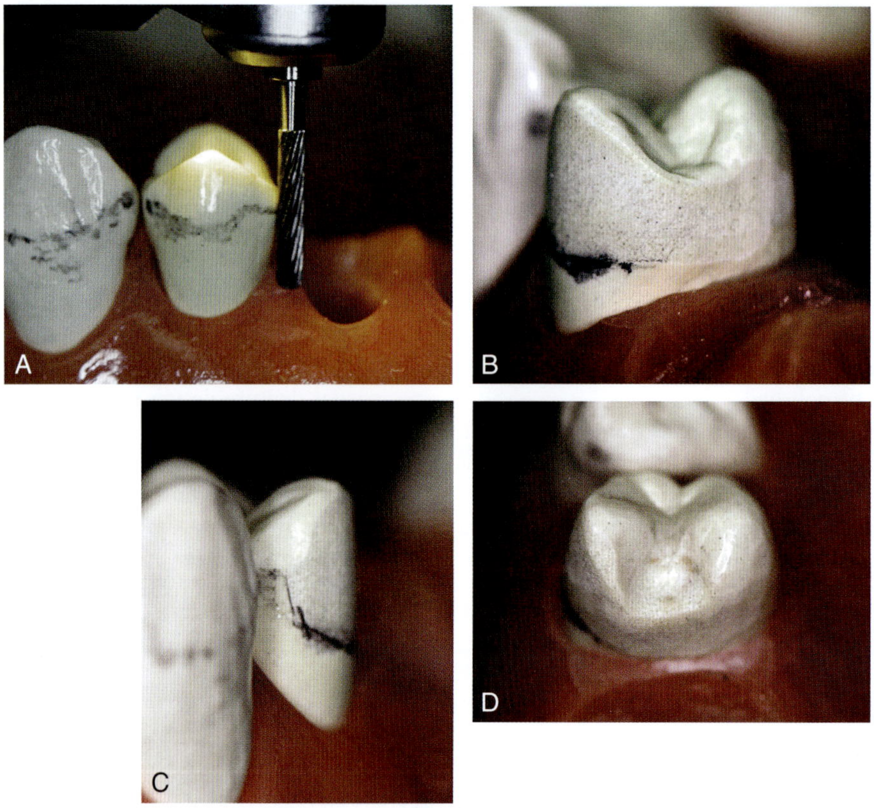

Fig. 15.2 Abutment contours should be altered during mouth preparations in the following sequence. **A,** The proximal surface is prepared parallel to the path of placement to create a guide plane. **B,** Height of contour on the buccal and lingual surfaces is lowered when necessary to permit the retentive clasp terminus to be located within the gingival third of the crown, bracing part of the retentive arm at the junction of the middle and gingival thirds of the crown, and the reciprocal clasp arm on the opposite side of the tooth to be placed no higher than the cervical portion of the middle third of the crown. **C,** The area of the tooth at which the retentive clasp arm originates should be altered if necessary to permit a more direct approach to the gingival third of the tooth: (1) incorrect position of retentive clasp arm, (2) area of tooth modified to accommodate better position of retentive clasp arm, and (3) more ideal position of retentive clasp arm. **D,** Occlusal rest preparation that will direct occlusal forces along the long axis of the tooth should be the final step in mouth preparations.

restoration with maximum resistance and retention as well as clinically imperceptible margins. The first requisite can be satisfied by preparing the opposing cavity walls 5 degrees or less from parallel and producing flat floors and sharp, clean line angles.

It is sometimes necessary to use an inlay on a mandibular first premolar for the support of an indirect retainer. The narrow occlusal width buccolingually and the lingual inclination of the occlusal surface of such a tooth often complicate the two-surface inlay preparation. Even the most exacting occlusal cavity preparation often leaves a thin and weak lingual cusp remaining.

ABUTMENT PREPARATIONS USING CROWNS

When multiple crowns are to be restored as removable partial denture abutments, it is best that all wax patterns be made at the same time. A cast of the arch with removable dies may be used if they are stable and sufficiently keyed for accuracy. If preferred, contouring wax patterns and making them parallel may be done on a solid cast of the arch (Fig. 15.3), with individual dies used to refine margins. Modern impression materials and indirect techniques make either method equally satisfactory.

The same sequence for preparing teeth in the mouth applies to the contouring of wax patterns. After the cast has been placed on the surveyor to conform to the selected path of placement and after the wax patterns have been preliminarily carved for occlusion and contact, proximal surfaces that are to act as guide planes are carved parallel to the path of placement with a surveyor blade. Guide planes are extended from the marginal ridge to the junction of the middle and gingival thirds of the tooth surface involved. One must be careful not to extend the guide plane to the gingival margin because the minor connector must be relieved when it crosses the gingivae. A guide plane that includes the occlusal two-thirds or even one-third of the proximal area is usually adequate without endangering gingival tissues.

After the guide planes are parallel and any other contouring to accommodate the removable partial denture design is accomplished, occlusal rest seats are carved in the wax pattern. This method has been outlined in Chapter 6.

It should be emphasized that critical areas prepared in wax should not be destroyed by poor sprue position or overpolishing the final restoration. The wax pattern should be sprued to

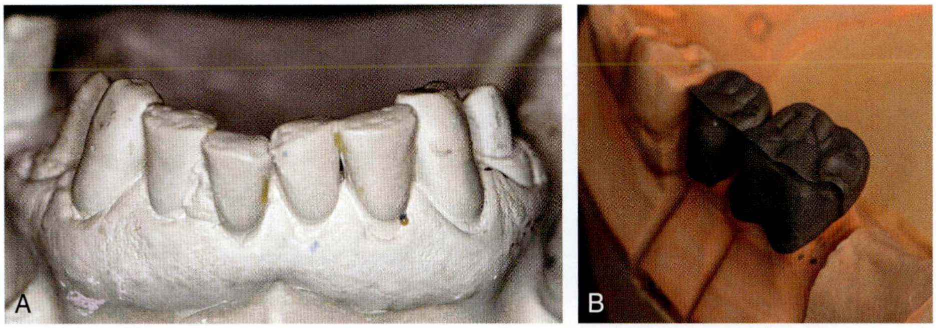

Fig. 15.3 **A,** Solid cast of multiple abutment crowns for a removable partial denture. Wax patterns for crown #21, #28, #30, and #31 can be completed at the same time using the identical cast orientation. This allows control of the path of insertion features on all fitting surfaces of the removable prostheses. **B,** Metal frameworks for metal-ceramic crowns tried in on individual dies after fabrication.

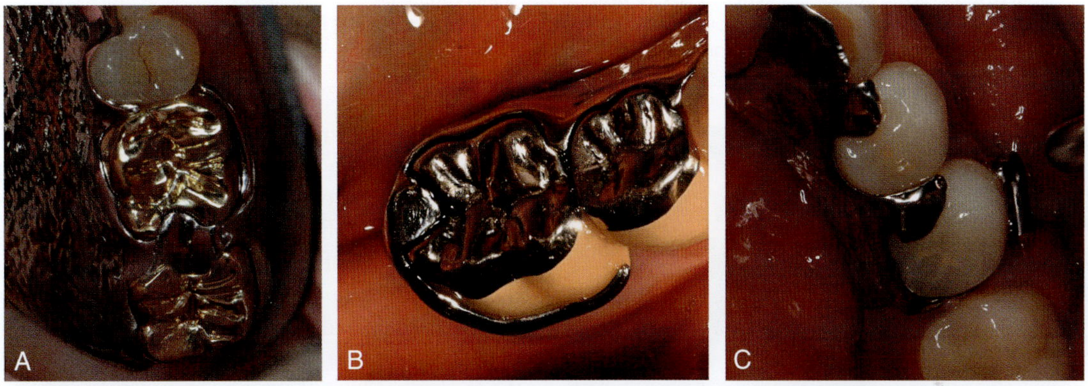

Fig. 15.4 Full coverage crowns used as surveyed crowns designed with rest seats and the appropriate retentive undercut. Those restorations can be made as complete cast **(A),** metal-ceramic **(B),** or zirconia crowns **(C)**. (Courtesy of Ahmed Mahrous Copyright © 2024. All rights reserved.)

preserve paralleled surfaces and rest areas. Polishing should consist of little more than burnishing. Rest seat areas should need only refining with round finishing burs. If some interference by spruing is unavoidable, the casting must be returned to the surveyor for proximal surface refinement. This can be done accurately with the aid of a handpiece holder attached to the vertical spindle of the surveyor or some similar machining device.

One of the advantages of making cast restorations for abutment teeth is that mouth preparations that would otherwise have to be done in the mouth may be done on the surveyor with far greater accuracy. It is generally impossible to make several proximal surfaces parallel to one another when preparing them intraorally. The opportunity for contouring wax patterns and making them parallel on the surveyor in relation to a path of placement should be used to its full advantage whenever cast restorations are being made.

The ideal crown restoration for a removable partial denture abutment is the complete coverage crown, which can be carved, cast, and finished to ideally satisfy all requirements for support, stabilization, and retention without compromise for cosmetic reasons (Fig. 15.4). Porcelain veneer crowns can be made equally satisfactory[2] but only by the added step of contouring the veneered surface on the surveyor before the final glaze. If this is not done, retentive contours may be excessive or inadequate. Digitally fabricated crowns allow the practitioner to confirm the presence of sufficient clearance during the preparation appointment (Fig. 15.5).

The three-quarter crown does not permit creation of retentive areas as does the complete coverage crown. However, if buccal or labial surfaces are sound and retentive areas are acceptable or can be made so by slight modification of tooth surfaces, the three-quarter crown is a conservative restoration of merit. The same criteria apply in the decision to leave a portion of an abutment unprotected, as in the decision to leave any tooth unprotected that is to serve as a removable partial denture abutment.

Regardless of the type of crown used, preparation should be made to provide the appropriate depth for the occlusal rest seat. This is best accomplished by altering the axial contours of the tooth to the ideal before preparing the tooth and creating a depression in the prepared tooth at the occlusal rest area (Fig. 15.6).

Since the location of occlusal rests is established early in the treatment planning phase, rest seat positions will be known in advance of any tooth preparations. If, for example, double occlusal rests are to be used, this will be known so that the tooth can be prepared to accommodate the depth of both rests. It is inexcusable when waxing a pattern to find that a rest seat has to be made shallower than is desirable because of posttreatment planning. It can also create serious problems when a rest seat must be made shallow in an existing crown or inlay because its thickness is unknown. The opportunity for creating an ideal

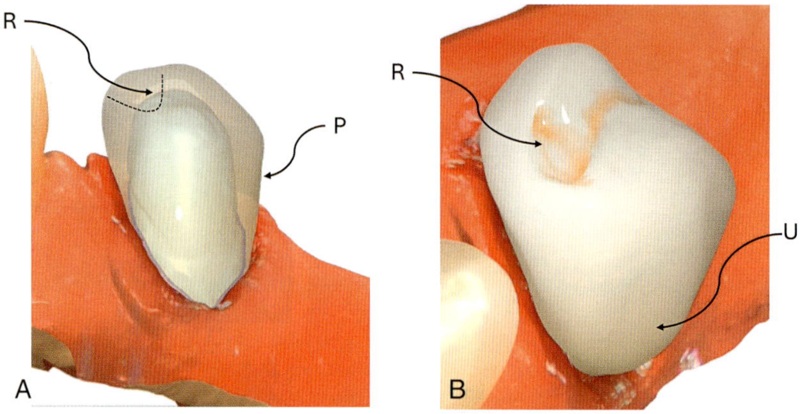

Fig. 15.5 A surveyed crown being digitally designed. **A,** Most software systems allow the user to turn the crown transparent in order to assess the clearance and reduction. This is especially important in the case of surveyed crowns because it is necessary to provide additional reduction in the area of the rest seat *(R)* and proximal plate *(P)*. **B,** The crown should be designed with a retentive undercut *(U)*, proximal plate *(P)*, and rest seat *(R)*. (Courtesy of Ahmed Mahrous Copyright © 2024. All rights reserved.)

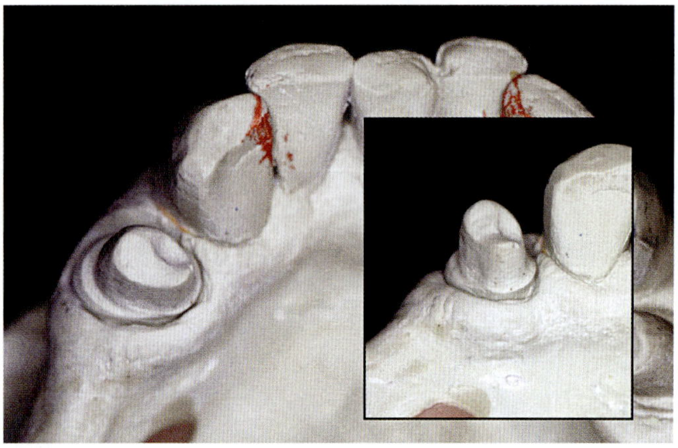

Fig. 15.6 Metal-ceramic crown preparation on tooth #21 shows mesial-occlusal rest space provided in the crown preparation at the mesial. The *inset picture* gives a perspective of the vertical height this provides for the rest to be prepared in the wax pattern.

rest seat is realized with proper treatment planning to create the space necessary to accommodate the rest.

Ledges can be incorporated into a surveyed crown in order to provide reciprocation during the entire path of placement and removal (Fig. 15.7). Ledges also contribute to support and indirect retention and can be designed so that the reciprocal clasp can seamlessly blend into the contours of the tooth.

The crown ledge may be used on any complete or three-quarter crown restored surface that is opposite the retentive side of an abutment tooth. It is used most frequently on premolars and molars but also may be used on canine restorations. It is not ordinarily used on buccal surfaces for reciprocation against lingual retention because of the excessive display of metal, but it may be used just as effectively on posterior abutments when esthetics is not a factor.

That a crown ledge is to be used should be known before crown preparation to ensure sufficient removal of tooth structure in this area. Though a shoulder or ledge is not included in the preparation itself, adequate space must be provided so that the ledge may be made sufficiently wide and the surface above it made parallel to the path of placement. The ledge should be placed at the junction of the gingival and middle thirds of the tooth, curving slightly to follow the curvature of the gingival tissues. On the side of the tooth where the clasp arm will originate, the ledge must be kept low enough to allow the origin of the clasp arm to be wide enough for sufficient strength and rigidity.

In forming the crown ledge, which is usually located on the lingual surface, the wax pattern of the crown is completed except for refinement of the margins before the ledge is carved. After the proximal guide planes and the occlusal rests and retentive contours are formed, the ledge is carved with the surveyor blade so that the surface above is parallel to the path of placement. Thus a continuous guide plane surface will exist from the proximal surface around the lingual surface.

The parallelism of proximal guide planes needs to be perfected after casting and polishing. Although it is possible to approximate parallelism and, at the same time, form the crown ledge on the wax pattern with a surveyor blade, some of its accuracy is lost in casting and polishing. The use of suitable burs such as No. 557, 558, and 559 fissure burs and true cylindrical carborundum stones in the handpiece holder permits the paralleling of all guiding planes on the finished casting with the accuracy necessary for the effectiveness of those guide plane surfaces.

Porcelain and Zirconia Crowns

For cosmetic reasons, zirconia and porcelain veneer crowns are used on abutment teeth that would otherwise display an objectionable amount of metal (Fig. 15.8). Veneer crowns must be contoured to provide suitable retention. This means that the veneer must be slightly overcontoured and then shaped to provide the desired undercut for the location of the retentive clasp arm (Fig. 15.9). Similarly, when digital zirconia crowns are fabricated, a full arch scan is completed in tandem. The completed crown should be seated onto the printed full arch model and then mounted onto a dental surveyor to confirm that the designed guide planes and the retentive undercuts are adequately contoured (Fig. 15.10).

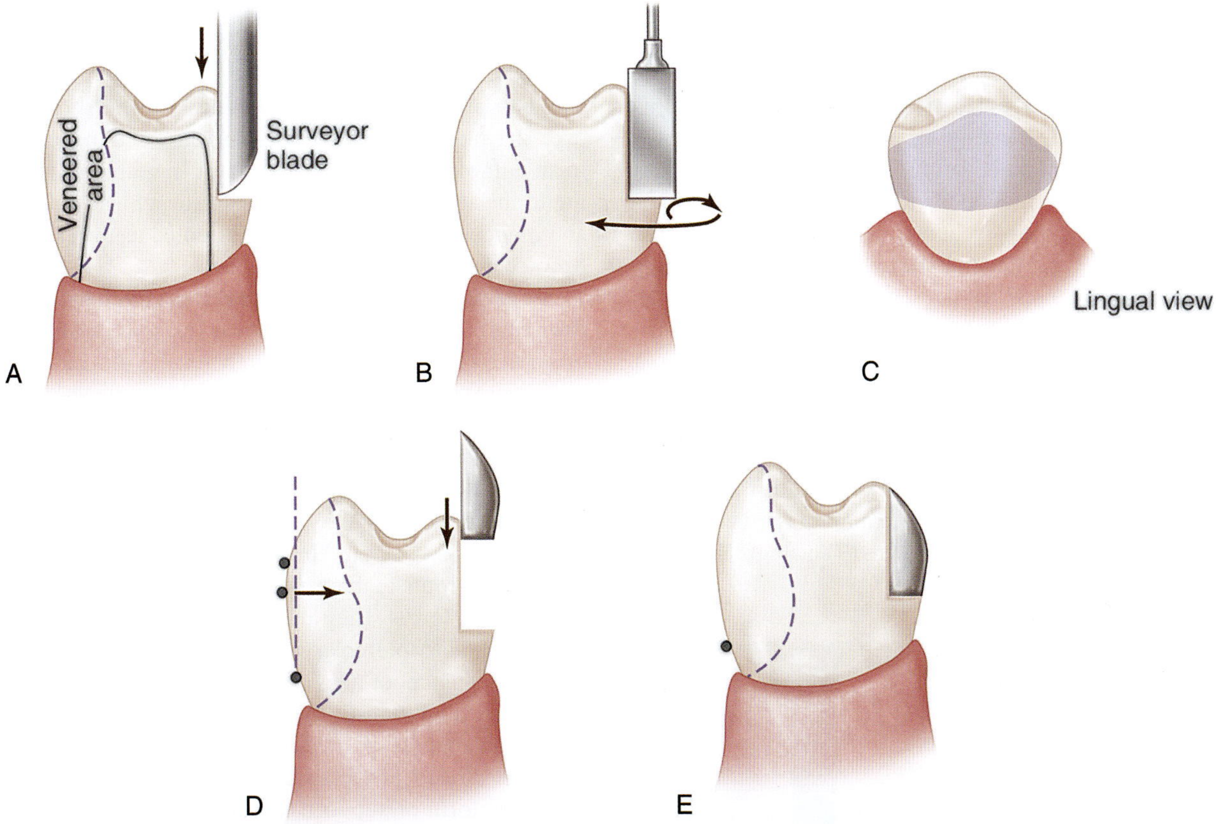

Fig. 15.7 **A,** Preparation of the ledge in a wax pattern with a surveyor blade parallel to the path of placement. **B,** Refinement of the ledge on casting, using a suitable stone or milling device in a handpiece attached to the dental surveyor or a specialized drill press for the same purpose. **C,** Approximate width and depth of the ledge formed on the abutment crown, which will permit the reciprocal clasp arm to be inlaid within the normal contours of the tooth. **D,** True reciprocation throughout the full path of placement and removal is possible when the reciprocal clasp arm is inlaid onto the ledge on the abutment crown. **E,** Direct retainer assembly is fully seated. The reciprocal arm restores the lingual contour of the abutment.

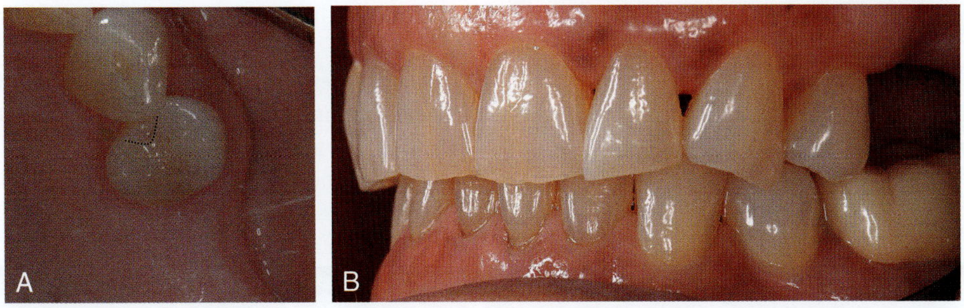

Fig. 15.8 Zirconia surveyed crown made on the maxillary left first premolar. **A,** The rest seat is prepared on the mesial aspect of the tooth. **B,** The buccal view of the same crown shows the esthetic advantage of zirconia surveyed crowns. (Courtesy of Ahmed Mahrous Copyright © 2024. All rights reserved.)

If the veneer is of porcelain, this procedure must precede glazing. If this important step in making veneered abutments is neglected or omitted, excessive or inadequate retentive contours may result.

In limited clinical trials,[3,4] porcelain laminates demonstrated resistance to wear of 5-year equivalence. The porcelain, however, resulted in slight wear on the clasps.

The flat underside of the cast clasp makes sufficient contact with the surface of the veneer so that abrasion of a resin veneer may result. Although the underside of the clasp may be polished (with some loss in accuracy of fit), abrasion results from the trapping and holding of food debris against the tooth surface as the clasp moves during function. Therefore unless the retentive clasp terminal rests on metal, glazed porcelain[5] should be used to ensure the future retentiveness of the veneered surface. Present-day acrylic resins, which are cross-linked copolymers, will withstand abrasion for considerable time, but not nearly to the same degree as porcelain. Therefore acrylic-resin veneers are best used in conjunction with a metal that supports the half-round clasp terminal.

Despite the lack of clinical trials, zirconia crowns are being used on abutment teeth for esthetic reasons. Zirconia is a non-metal that is chemically inert and corrosion resistant. However, clinicians need to be aware of various zirconia available in dentistry, ranging from 3% mol. to 5% mol. yttria-stabilized zirconia polycrystalline. Three percent mol. yttria-stabilized zirconia polycrystalline has high flexural strength, fracture toughness, hardness, and elastic modulus.

Zirconia was found to have comparable strength to a complete cast crown and a digital file of the final restoration. Zirconia was also found to have comparable retention of cobalt-chromium clasps when compared with complete cast crowns. The outcome of this in vitro study showed a comparable retention force of 11.4 and 11.5 N, respectively. However, further studies are needed to assess the long-term retention of removable partial dentures when using zirconia crowns as an abutment.

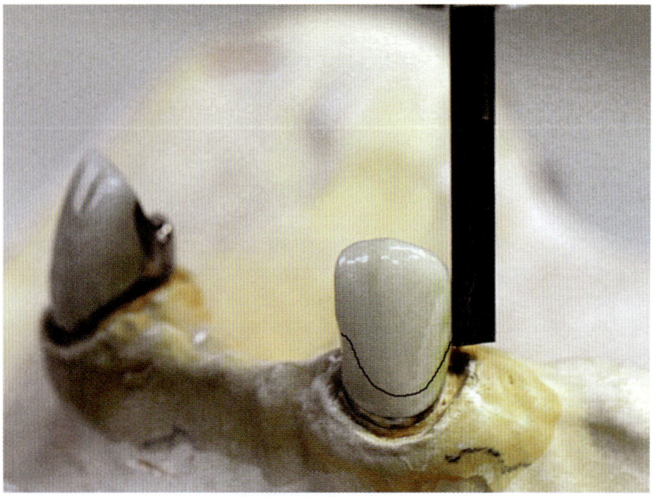

Fig. 15.9 A porcelain veneer crown is resurveyed following adjustment, glazing, and polishing. It is important to survey crowns returned from the laboratory before cementation. The best time to ensure control of all abutment contours for a removable partial denture is when surveyed crowns are used and they are resurveyed before permanent placement.

SPLINTING OF ABUTMENT TEETH

Often, a tooth is considered too weak to use alone as a removable partial denture abutment because of the short length or excessive taper of a single root, or because of bone loss resulting in an unfavorable crown-to-root ratio. In such instances, splinting to the adjacent tooth or teeth can be a means of improving abutment support. Thus two single-rooted teeth serve as a multirooted abutment.

Splinting should not be used to retain a tooth that would otherwise be condemned for periodontal reasons. When the length of service of a restoration depends on the serviceability of an abutment, any periodontally questionable tooth should be condemned in favor of using an adjacent healthy tooth as the abutment, even though the span is increased one tooth by doing so.

The most common application of the use of multiple abutments is the splinting of two premolars or a first premolar and a canine (Fig. 15.11). Mandibular premolars generally have round and tapered roots that are easily loosened by rotational as well as by tipping forces. They are the weakest of the posterior abutments. Maxillary premolars also often have tapered roots, which may make them poor risks as abutments, particularly when they will be called on to resist the leverage of a distal extension base. Such teeth are best splinted by casting or soldering two crowns together. When a first premolar to be used as an abutment has poor root form or support, it is best that it be splinted to the stronger canine.

Anterior teeth on which lingual rests are to be placed often must be splinted together to avoid orthodontic movement of individual teeth. Mandibular anterior teeth are seldom used for support, but if they are, splinting of the teeth involved is advisable. When splinting is impossible, individual lingual rests on cast restorations may be slightly inclined apically to avoid possible tooth displacement, or lingual rests may be used in conjunction with incisal rests, slightly engaging the labial surface of the teeth.

Lingual rests should always be placed as low on the cingulum as possible, and single anterior teeth, other than canines, should not be used for occlusal support. Where lingual rests are used on central and lateral incisors, as many teeth as possible should

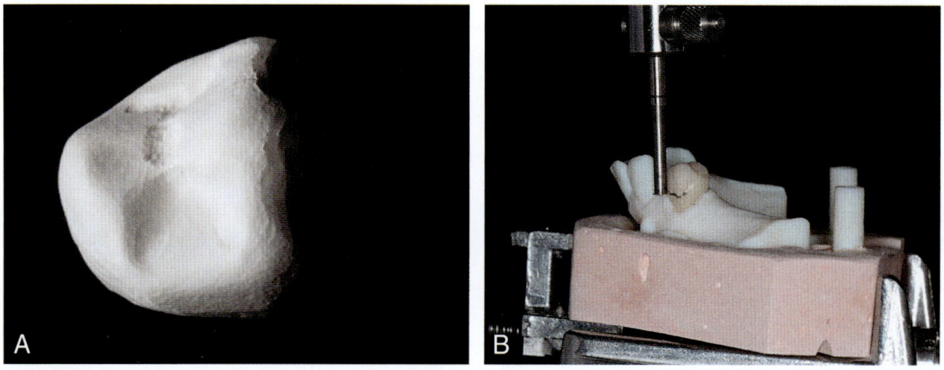

Fig. 15.10 **A,** An unsintered crown clearly shows the rest seat. **B,** After sintering the crown should be seated on the printed cast and mounted onto a surveyor to inspect the designed undercut and guide plane. Any adjustment should be completed before the patient appointment. (Courtesy of Ahmed Mahrous Copyright © 2024. All rights reserved.)

be included to distribute the load, thereby minimizing the force on any one tooth. Even so, some movement of individual teeth is likely to occur, particularly when they are subjected to the forces of indirect retention or when bone support is compromised. This is best avoided by splinting several teeth with united cast restorations. The condition of the teeth and cosmetic considerations will dictate whether complete crowns, three-quarter crowns, pin ledge inlays, resin-bonded retainers, or composite restorations will be used for this purpose.

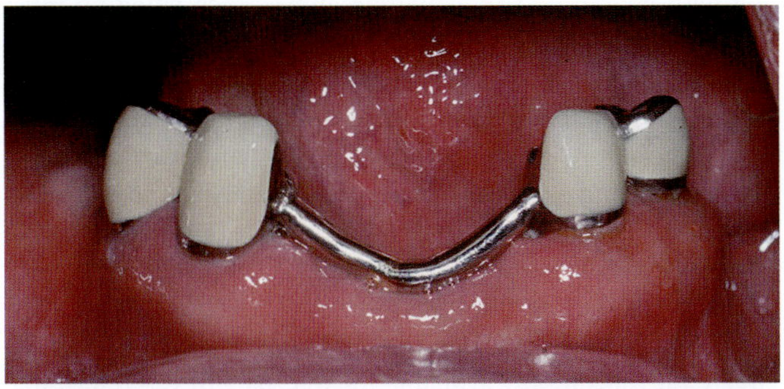

Fig. 15.11 First premolars and canines have been splinted in this Class I, modification 1, partially edentulous arch. The splint bar was added to provide cross-arch stabilization for the splinted abutments and to support and retain the anterior segment of the removable restoration. The prospective longevity of the abutments has been enhanced.

Splinting of molar teeth for multiple abutment support is less frequently used because they are generally multirooted. A two- or three-rooted tooth that is not strong enough alone is probably a poor abutment risk. However, there may be notable exceptions when a molar abutment would benefit from the effect of splinting, as in a hemisected molar root (Fig. 15.12).

USE OF ISOLATED TEETH AS ABUTMENTS

The average abutment tooth is subjected to some distal tipping, rotation, torquing, and horizontal movement, all of which must be held to a minimum by the quality of tissue support and the design of the removable partial denture. The isolated abutment tooth, however, is also subjected to mesial tipping caused by lack of proximal contact. Despite indirect retention, some lifting of the distal extension base is inevitable, causing torque to the abutment tooth.

In a tooth-supported prosthesis, an isolated tooth may be used as an abutment by including a fifth abutment for additional support. Thus rotational and horizontal forces are resisted by the additional stabilization obtained from the fifth abutment. When two such isolated abutments exist, a sixth abutment should be included for the same reason. Thus the two canines, the two isolated premolars, and two posterior teeth are used as abutments.

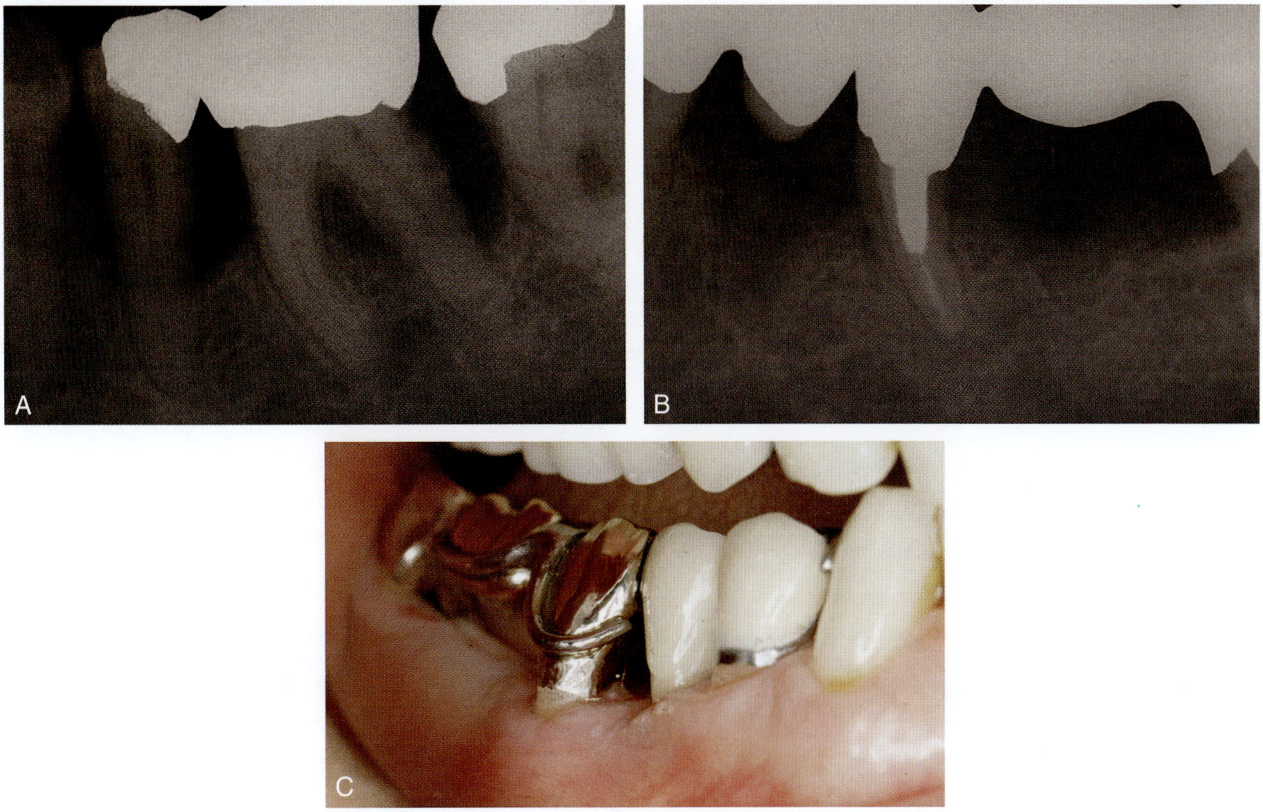

Fig. 15.12 A, Periodontal disease required removal of #30 distal and #31 mesial roots. **B,** The first premolar and hemisected roots were splinted using a five-unit fixed partial denture. **C,** Fixed prosthesis provided cross-arch support, stability, and retention to a Kennedy Class II removable partial denture.

In contrast, in most cases, an isolated anterior abutment adjacent to a distal extension base should be splinted to the nearest tooth by means of a fixed partial denture. The effect is twofold: (1) the anterior edentulous segment is eliminated, thereby creating an intact dental arch anterior to the edentulous space, and (2) the isolated tooth is splinted to the other abutment of the fixed partial denture, thereby providing multiple abutment support. Splinting should be used here only to gain multiple abutment support rather than to support an otherwise weak abutment tooth.

Although splinting is advocated for abutment teeth that are considered too weak to risk being used alone, a single abutment tooth standing alone in the dental arch anterior to a distal extension basal seat generally requires the splinting effect of a fixed partial denture (Fig. 15.13). Even though the form and length of the root and the supporting bone seem to be adequate for an ordinary abutment, the fact that the tooth lacks proximal contact endangers the tooth when it is used to support a distal extension base removable partial denture.

A second factor that may influence the decision to use an isolated tooth as an abutment is an esthetic consideration. However, neither esthetics nor economics should deter the dentist from recommending to the patient that an isolated tooth to be used as a terminal abutment should be given the advantage of splinting by means of a fixed partial denture. If compromises are necessary, the patient must assume responsibility for use of the isolated tooth as an abutment.

The economic aspect of the use of fixed restorations as part of the mouth preparations for a removable partial denture is essentially the same as that for any other splinting procedure—the best design of the fixed partial denture that will ensure the longevity of its service makes the additional procedure and expense necessary. Although it must be recognized that economic considerations, combined with a particularly favorable prognosis of an isolated tooth, may influence the decision to forego the advantages of using a fixed partial denture, the original treatment plan should include this provision, even though the alternative method may be accepted for economic reasons.

MISSING ANTERIOR TEETH

When a removable partial denture is used to replace missing posterior teeth, especially in the absence of distal abutments, any additional missing anterior teeth are best replaced by means of fixed restorations rather than included in the removable partial denture. In any distal extension situation, some anteroposterior rotational action results from the addition of an anterior segment to the denture. The ideal treatment plan, which considers the anterior edentulous space separately, may result in conflict with economic and esthetic realities. Each situation must be treated according to its own merits. Often the best esthetic result can be obtained by replacing missing anterior teeth and tissues with the removable partial denture rather than with a fixed restoration. From a biomechanical standpoint, however, it is generally advisable that a removable partial denture should replace the missing posterior teeth only after the remainder of the anterior arch has been made intact by fixed restorations.

Although the need for compromise is recognized, the decision to include an anterior segment on the denture depends largely on the support available for that part of the removable partial denture. The greater the number of natural anterior teeth remaining, the better is the available support for the edentulous segment. If definite rest seats can be prepared on multiple abutment teeth, the anterior segment may be treated as any other tooth-bounded modification space. Sound principles of rest support apply just as much as elsewhere in the arch. Inclined tooth surfaces should not be used for occlusal support, nor should rests be placed on unprepared lingual surfaces. The best possible support for an anterior segment is multiple support extending, if possible, posteriorly across prepared lingual rest seats on the canine teeth to mesio-occlusal rest seats on the first premolars. Such support would permit the missing anterior teeth to be included in the removable partial denture, often with some cosmetic advantages over fixed restorations.

In some instances, the replacement of anterior teeth by means of a removable partial denture cannot be avoided. However, without adequate tooth support, any such prosthesis

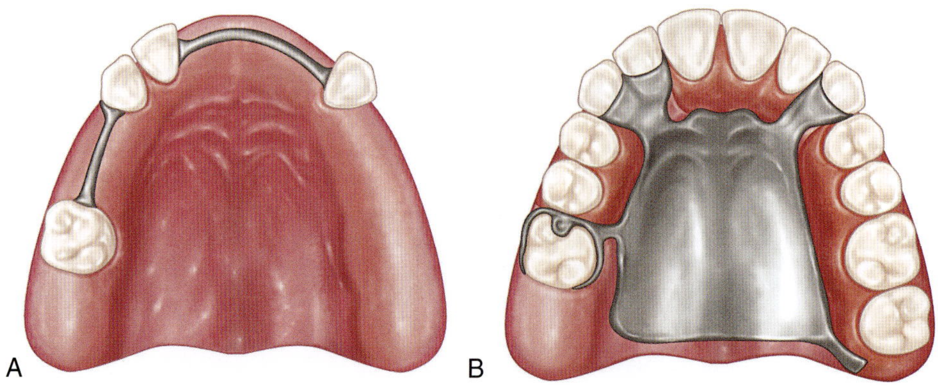

Fig. 15.13 A, Isolated abutments have been splinted using splint bars. **B,** The removable partial denture is more adequately supported by the splinting mechanism shown in **(A)** than could be realized with isolated abutments.

lacks the stability that results from replacing only the posterior teeth with the removable partial denture and the anterior teeth with fixed restorations. When anterior teeth have been lost through accident or have been missing for some time, resorption of the anterior residual ridge may have progressed to the point that neither fixed nor removable pontics may be butted to the residual ridge. In such instances, for reasons of esthetics and orofacial tissue support, the missing teeth must be replaced with a denture base supporting teeth that closely approximate original natural tooth positions that could be anterior to the residual ridge. Creating ideal contours and characterization of the denture base material can be esthetically pleasing based on artistic efforts of both the dentist and the technician. Such a removable partial denture, both from an esthetic and a biomechanical standpoint, is one of the most difficult of all prosthetic restorations. However, a splint bar, connected by abutments on both sides of the edentulous space, will provide much-needed support and retention to the anterior segment of the removable partial denture. Because the splint bar will provide vertical support, rest seats on abutments adjacent to the edentulous area need not be prepared, thus simplifying an anterior restoration to some extent.

The concept of a dual path of placement to enhance the esthetic replacement of missing anterior teeth with a removable partial denture is recognized. Sources of information on this concept are made available in the Reference section of this chapter.[6–8]

TEMPORARY CROWNS WHEN A REMOVABLE PARTIAL DENTURE IS BEING WORN

Occasionally, an existing removable partial denture must remain serviceable while the mouth is being prepared for a new prosthesis. In such situations, temporary crowns must be made that will support the old removable partial denture and will not interfere with its placement and removal. Digitally fabricated crowns are ideal in this situation as they allow the copying of the contours of the existing crown onto the new crown; however, if this is not available, acrylic-resin temporary crowns that duplicate the original form of the abutment teeth must be made.

The technique for making temporary crowns to fit direct retainers is similar to that used for other types of acrylic-resin temporary crowns. The principal difference is that an impression, made with an elastic impression material, must be made of the entire arch with the existing removable partial denture in place. It is necessary that the removable partial denture remains in the impression when it is removed from the mouth. If it remains in the mouth, it must be removed and inserted into the impression in its designated position. The impression with the removable partial denture in place is disinfected, wrapped in a wet paper towel (if irreversible hydrocolloid was used as the impression material) or placed in a plastic bag, and set aside while the tooth or teeth are being prepared for new crowns.

After the preparations are completed and the impressions and jaw relation records have been made, the prepared teeth are dried and lubricated. The original impression is trimmed to eliminate any excess, undercuts, and interproximal projections that would interfere with the replacement of the impression in the mouth.

The methyl methacrylate acrylic resins, composites, copolymers, and fiber-reinforced resins may serve as excellent materials for temporary crowns in conjunction with removable partial dentures. Making temporary crowns requires a small mixing cup or dappen dish; a cement spatula; and a small, disposable, plastic syringe. Autopolymerizing acrylic resin of the appropriate tooth color is placed in the cup or dappen dish, and monomer is added to make a slightly viscous mix. The volume should be slightly more than the amount estimated to fabricate the temporary restorations. The mix should be spatulated to a smooth consistency and the mix immediately poured into the barrel of the disposable syringe. A small amount of the mix should be injected over and around the margins of the prepared teeth. The remaining material should be injected into the impression of the prepared teeth. The impression is seated into the mouth, where the dentist holds it in place until sufficient time has elapsed for it to reach a stiff, rubbery stage, or a consistency recommended by the manufacturer. This again must be based on experience with the particular resin used. At this time, the impression is removed. The crowns may remain in the impression. If so, they are stripped out of the impression, all excess is trimmed away with scissors, and the crowns are reseated on the prepared abutments. The removable partial denture is then removed from the impression and reseated in the mouth onto the temporary crowns, which should be in a stiff-rubbery state. The patient may bring the teeth into occlusion to reestablish the former position and occlusal relationship of the existing removable partial denture.

After the resin crown or crowns have polymerized, the removable partial denture is removed, and the crowns remain on the teeth. These are then carefully removed, contoured to accommodate oral hygiene access, trimmed, polished, and temporarily cemented. The result is a temporary crown that restores the original abutment contours and allows the removable partial denture to be placed and removed without interference while temporarily providing the same support to the denture that existed before the teeth were prepared.

Cementation of Temporary Crowns

Cementation of temporary crowns may require slight relief of the internal surface of the crowns to accommodate the temporary cement and to facilitate removal. The temporary cement should be thin and applied only to the inside gingival margin of the crowns to ensure complete seating. As soon as the temporary cement has hardened, the occlusion should be checked and adjusted accordingly. Regardless of the type of temporary cement used, any excess that might irritate the gingivae should be removed.

FABRICATING RESTORATIONS TO FIT EXISTING DENTURE RETAINERS

It is often necessary that an abutment tooth be restored with a complete crown (or other restoration) that fits the inside of the clasp of an otherwise serviceable removable partial denture. This can be accomplished using the digital workflow as it allows for the duplication of the existing crown contours onto the new crown that would fit the old prosthesis perfectly. In the absence of this technology, one technique requires that an indirect-direct pattern be made and therefore justifies a fee for this complex planning above that required for the usual restoration.

The technique for making a crown to fit the inside of a clasp[1] is as follows: An irreversible hydrocolloid impression of the mouth is made with the removable partial denture in place. This impression, which is used to make the temporary crown, is wrapped in a wet paper towel or placed in a plastic bag and set aside while the tooth is being prepared. Even though several abutment teeth are to be restored, it is usually necessary that each temporary restoration be completed before the next one is begun. This is necessary so that the original support and occlusal relationship of the removable partial denture can be maintained as each new temporary crown is being made. During preparation of the abutment tooth, the removable partial denture is replaced frequently to ascertain that enough tooth structure has been removed to allow for the casting's thickness. When the preparation is completed, an individual impression of the tooth is obtained from which a stone die is made. A temporary crown is then made in the original irreversible hydrocolloid impression, as outlined in the preceding paragraphs. It is trimmed, polished, and temporarily cemented, and the removable partial denture is returned to the mouth. The patient is dismissed after the excess cement has been removed.

On the stone die made from the individual impression, a thin, autopolymerizing resin coping will be formed with a brush technique. The stone die should first be trimmed to the finishing line of the preparation, which is then delineated with a pencil, and the die painted with a tinfoil substitute. A separating material, such as a tinfoil substitute, should be used and will form a

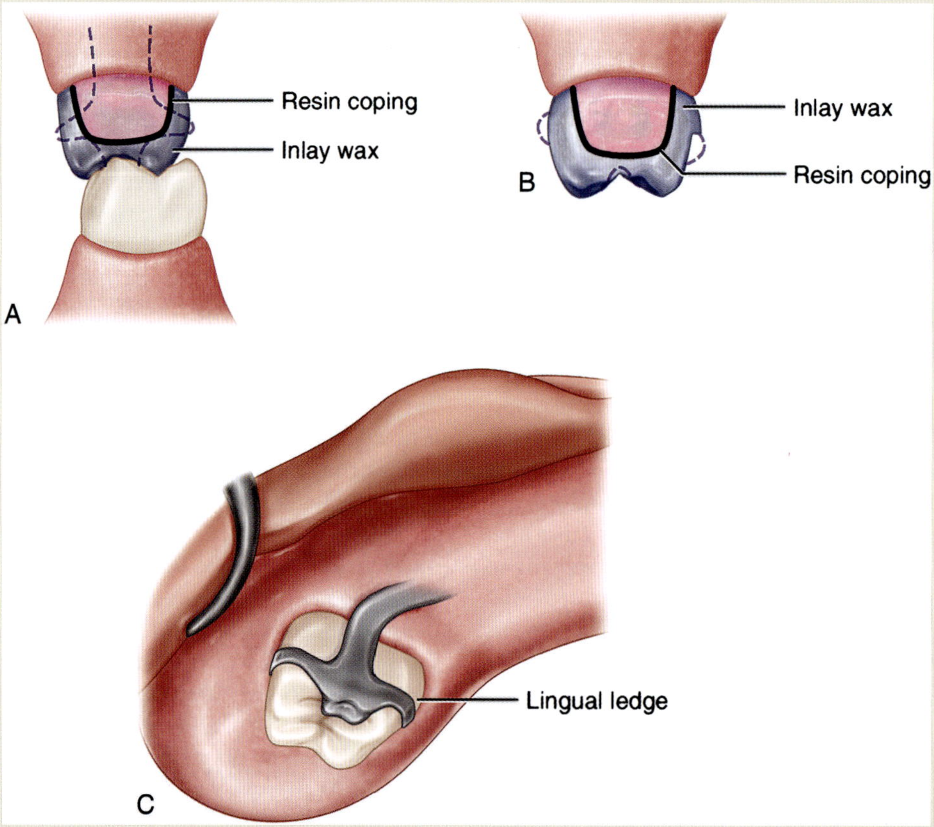

Fig. 15.14 Making of the cast crown to fit an existing removable partial denture clasp. **A,** Thin acrylic-resin coping is made first on the individual die of a prepared tooth. Inlay wax is then added and coping placed onto the prepared tooth where occlusal surfaces and contact relations are established directly in the mouth. The clasp assembly is warmed with a needlepoint flame only enough to soften the inlay wax, the removable partial denture is placed into the mouth, and it is guided gently into place by the opposing occlusion. This step must be repeated several times and excess wax removed or wax added until full supporting contact with the underside of the clasp assembly has been established, with the denture fully seated. Usually, the wax pattern withdraws with the denture and must be gently teased out of the clasp each time. **B,** The wax pattern is then placed back onto the individual die to complete the occlusal anatomy and refine the margins. Excess wax remaining below the impression of the retentive clasp arm must be removed, but the wax ledge may be left below the reciprocal clasp arm. **C,** Finished casting in the mouth. The terminus of the retentive clasp is then readapted to engage the undercut. It is frequently necessary to remove some interference from casting, as indicated by articulating paper placed between the clasp and the crown, until the clasp is fully seated.

thin film on a cold, dry surface. Not all tinfoil substitutes are suitable for this purpose. With autopolymerizing resin powder and liquid in separate dappen dishes and a fine brush, a coping of resin of uniform thickness is painted onto the die. This should extend not quite to the pencil line representing the limit of the crown preparation. After hardening, the resin coping may be removed, inspected, and trimmed if necessary. The thin film of foil substitute should be removed before the coping is reseated onto the die.

The wax pattern buildup on the resin coping is usually not begun until the patient returns. A sequence using a functional chew-in technique for occlusion would be followed, establishing proximal contact and contours appropriate for the clasp assembly as outlined in the following paragraphs.

First, the occlusal portion of the wax pattern is established by having the patient close into maximum intercuspation, followed by excursive movements (Fig. 15.14, *A*). The wax pattern is returned to the cast, and additions are made to dull areas as required. The process is repeated until a smooth occlusal registration has been obtained. Except for narrowing of the occlusal surface and carving of grooves and spillways, this will be the occlusal anatomy of the finished restoration.

The second step is the addition of sufficient wax to establish contact relations with the adjacent tooth. At this time, the occlusal relation of the marginal ridges also must be established. Next, wax is added to buccal and lingual surfaces where the clasp arms will contact the crown, and the wax pattern is again reseated in the mouth. The clasp arms, minor connectors, and occlusal rests involved in the removable partial denture are carefully warmed with a needlepoint flame, carefully avoiding any adjacent resin, and the removable partial denture is positioned in the mouth and onto the wax pattern (see Fig. 15.14, *B*). Several attempts may be necessary until the removable partial denture is fully seated and the components of the clasp are clearly recorded in the wax pattern. Each time the removable partial denture is removed, the pattern will draw with it and must be teased out of the clasp.

When contact with the clasp arms and the occlusal relation of the removable partial denture have been established satisfactorily, the temporary crown may be replaced and the patient dismissed. The crown pattern is completed on the die by narrowing the occlusal surface buccolingually, adding grooves and spillways, and refining the margins. Any wax ledge remaining below the reciprocal clasp arm may be left to provide some of the advantages of a crown ledge described earlier in this chapter. Excess wax remaining below the retentive clasp arm, however, must be removed to permit the adding of a retentive undercut later (see Fig. 15.14, *C*).

If a veneer material is to be added, the veneer space must now be carved in the wax pattern. In such situations, the contour of the veneer may be recorded by making a stone matrix of the buccal surface, which can be repositioned on the completed casting to ensure the proper contour of the composite veneer.

The wax pattern must be sprued with care so that essential areas on the pattern are not destroyed. After casting, the crown should be subjected to a minimum of polishing because the exact form of the axial and occlusal surfaces must be maintained.

Because it is impossible to withdraw a clasp arm from a retentive undercut on the wax pattern, the casting must be made without any provision for clasp retention. After the crown has been tried in the mouth with the denture in place, the location of the retentive clasp terminal is identified by scoring the crown with a sharp instrument. Then the crown may be ground and polished slightly in this area to create a retentive undercut. The clasp terminal then may be carefully adapted into this undercut, thereby creating clasp retention on the new crown.

An alternate method for making crowns to fit existing retainers uses mounted casts with the removable prosthesis adapted to the working cast to develop occlusal surfaces for the involved crowns.

Ideally, all abutment teeth would best be protected with complete crowns before the removable partial denture is fabricated. Except for the possibility of recurrent caries caused by defective crown margins or gingival recession, abutment teeth so protected may be expected to give many years of satisfactory service in support, stabilization, and retention of the removable partial denture. Economically, a policy of insisting on complete coverage for all abutment teeth may well be justified from the long-term viewpoint. It must be recognized, however, that in practice, complete coverage of all abutment teeth is not always possible at the time of treatment planning. Many factors influence the future health status of an abutment tooth, some of which cannot be foreseen. The dentist must be able to treat abutment teeth that later become defective so that their service as abutments may be restored and the serviceability of the removable partial denture maintained. Although not part of the original mouth preparations, this service accomplishes much the same objective by providing support, stability, and retention, and the dentist must be technically capable of providing this removable partial denture service when it becomes necessary.

REFERENCES

1. Diaz-Arnold AM, Langenwalter EM, Hatch LK. Cast restorations made to existing removable partial dentures. *J Prosthet Dent.* 1989;61:414–417.
2. Johnston JF, et al. Construction and assembly of porcelain veneer gold crowns and pontics. *J Prosthet Dent.* 1962;12:1125–1137.
3. Dixon DL, Breeding LC, Swift EJ. Use of a partial coverage porcelain laminate to enhance clasp retention. *J Prosthet Dent.* 1990;63:55–58.
4. Dixon DL, et al. Wear of I-bar clasps and porcelain laminate restorations. *Int J Prosthet.* 1992;5:28–33.
5. Maroso DJ, Schmidt JR, Blustein R. A preliminary study of wear of porcelain when subjected to functional movements of retentive clasp arms. *J Prosthet Dent.* 1981;45:14.
6. Byron Jr R, Frazer RQ, Herren MC. Rotational path removable partial denture: an esthetic alternative. *Gen Dent.* 2007;55:245–250.
7. Jacobson TE, Krol AJ. Rotational path removable partial denture design. *J Prosthet Dent.* 1982;48:70–376.
8. Jacobson TE. Rotational path partial denture design: a 10-year clinical follow-up. Parts I and II. *J Prosthet Dent.* 1994;71:271–282.

16

Impression Materials and Procedures for Removable Partial Dentures

Ahmed Mahrous, Berna Saglik, Wendy Clark, and Audrey Marie Selecman

CHAPTER OUTLINE

Making an impression is an essential skill that is utilized in various phases of removable partial denture (RPD) fabrication. The technique used when making an impression can be accomplished using traditional, analog methods and various impression materials or using an intraoral scanner for a digitally generated image.

Intraoral support for an RPD can be from both the abutment teeth and supporting tissues. The morphology of the residual alveolar ridge consists of intraoral mucosal tissues and the underlying osseous structures with variances from maxilla to mandible and unique from patient to patient. Changes in these tissues are time dependent, progressive, and highly variable. The support and stability of an RPD, as well as the patient's comfort and function, are closely tied to the anatomical features and quality of residual ridge soft and hard tissues.

The primary mandibular support area is the buccal shelf. The mandibular buccal shelf area is bound by the external oblique line and the crest of the alveolar ridge where the cortical bone is covered by relatively firm, dense, fibrous connective tissue. In most instances, this anatomical area exhibits a more horizontal pitch than other regions of the residual ridge, providing the best foundation to resistant occlusal forces. Unlike cortical bone, the trabeculated structure of cancellous bone often found at the crest of the ridge after tooth loss is an irritant to overlying, poorly keratinized soft tissues which under persistent occlusal load can result in chronic inflammation. The inflammatory condition accelerates ridge resorption as well as contributes to patient discomfort. Therefore designing a mandibular RPD should incorporate the anatomy of the buccal shelf to support a mandibular distal extension prosthesis.

The crest of the maxillary residual ridge often consists of cancellous bone. Unlike in the mandible, the overlying oral mucosa of the maxillary residual alveolar is firm and dense in nature, similar to the mucosa of the hard palate. Much like the buccal shelf, the hard palate consists of cortical bone covered by firm, dense, fibrous connective tissue, lending itself to an excellent supporting structure. Unfortunately, the hard palate is only utilized for support if the major connector of the partial denture makes contact in this area. Consequently, the crestal area of the residual ridge on which the prosthetic teeth are positioned to achieve function and esthetics often bears the impact of occlusal forces. Some resistance to occlusal forces generated may be obtained by the buccal and palatal slopes of the residual ridge. The glandular palatal tissues between the medial palatal raphe and the lingual slope of the posterior edentulous ridge are readily displaceable and cannot be considered as stress-bearing sites.

Impression materials are classified as rigid, thermoplastic, or elastomeric in physical properties. Rigid impression materials are those set to a rigid consistency. Thermoplastic impression materials are those that become plastic at higher temperatures and resume their original form when cooled. Elastomeric impression materials are those that remain in an elastic or flexible state after setting and retain flexibility after removal from the mouth.

Although rigid impression materials may be capable of recording tooth and tissue details accurately, they cannot be removed from the mouth without fracture and reassembly. Thermoplastic materials cannot record minute details accurately because they undergo permanent distortion during withdrawal from tooth and tissue undercuts. Elastomeric materials are the only ones that can be withdrawn without permanent deformation and therefore are used generally for making impressions for RPDs, immediate dentures, crowns, and fixed partial dentures when tooth and tissue undercuts and surface detail must be recorded with accuracy. Intraoral scanners can be used to make impressions when fabricating an RPD as well as for diagnostic purposes. Challenges can occur in certain circumstances since intraoral scanners may not capture movable soft tissue nor the extent to which soft tissues can be manipulated manually.

ELASTOMERIC IMPRESSION MATERIALS*

Reversible Hydrocolloids

Reversible (agar-agar) hydrocolloids, which are fluid at higher temperatures and gel on reduction in temperature, are used primarily as impression materials for fixed restorations. They demonstrate acceptable accuracy when properly used; however, the reversible hydrocolloid impression materials offer few advantages over the irreversible (alginate) hydrocolloids when used as an RPD impression material. Present-day irreversible hydrocolloids are sufficiently accurate for making master casts for RPDs. However, control of the border width and length of impressions made with these materials is difficult. The use of reversible hydrocolloid clinically has decreased in recent years due to concerns over disinfection.

Irreversible Hydrocolloids

Irreversible hydrocolloids are used for making diagnostic casts, orthodontic treatment casts, and master casts for RPD procedures. Because they are made of colloid materials, neither reversible nor irreversible hydrocolloid impressions can be stored for any length of time, but must be poured immediately.

These materials have low tear strength, provide less surface detail than other materials (e.g., mercaptan rubber base), and are not as dimensionally stable as other materials. They can, however, be used in the presence of moisture (saliva); are hydrophilic; pour well with stone; have a pleasant taste and odor; and are nontoxic, nonstaining, and inexpensive. The combination reversible-irreversible hydrocolloids have demonstrated a tendency to separate and should be used with that understanding. The hydrocolloids can be acceptably disinfected with a spray solution of 2% acid glutaraldehyde, stored in 100% humidity, and poured within 1 hour.

Polysulfide Impression Materials

Polysulfide impression material, often referred to as "rubber base," can also be used for RPD impressions and especially for altered or corrected cast impressions. To be accurate, the impression must have a uniform thickness that does not exceed 3 mm (⅛ inch). This necessitates the use of a carefully made individual impression tray of acrylic resin or some other material possessing adequate rigidity and stability. Those materials that are highly cross-linked (medium and heavy body) do not recover well from deformation and should not be used when large or multiple undercuts are present. The long-term dimensional stability of these materials is poor due to loss of water after setting. The material must be held still during the impression-making procedure because it does not have a snap set; it should be allowed to rebound for 7 to 15 minutes after it is removed from the mouth and should then be poured immediately. Many of these materials have an unpleasant odor and can stain clothes. These materials are moderately inexpensive; have high tear strength, long working and setting times (8–10 minutes); and can be disinfected in liquid, cold-sterilizing solutions. The accuracy of mercaptan rubber base is acceptable for making impressions for RPDs; however, as with hydrocolloid impression materials, certain precautions must be taken to avoid distortion of the impression. The polysulfide impression materials do have an advantage over hydrocolloid materials in that the surface of an artificial stone poured against them is of a smoother texture and therefore appears to be smoother and harder than one poured against a hydrocolloid material. This is probably so because the rubber base material does not have the ability to retard or etch the surface of the setting stone. Despite their accuracy, this has always been a disadvantage of all hydrocolloid impression materials. Rubber-based impression materials possess a longer setting time than the irreversible hydrocolloid materials and lend themselves to border molding with a tray design for material support, that is, a custom tray.

Polyether Impression Materials

Polyether impression material is an elastic-type material. These materials have demonstrated good accuracy in clinical evaluations and are thixotropic, which provides good surface detail and makes them useful as a border molding material. It should be noted, however, that these materials are not compatible with the addition-reaction silicone impression materials and should not be used to border mold custom trays when the silicone impression materials are to be used as the final impression material. The polyethers are also hydrophilic, which provides good wettability for easy cast forming.

Polyether impression materials have low-to-moderate tear strength, shorter working and setting times, which can limit the usefulness of the material, and an unpleasant taste. The flow characteristics and flexibility of the polyether materials are the lowest of any of the elastic materials. These characteristics can limit the use of polyethers in RPD impression procedures. The

*Some of the historical parts of this discussion have been quoted or paraphrased from McCracken WL. Impression materials in prosthetic dentistry. *Dent Clin North Am.* 1958;2:671–684.

stiffness of the material can result in cast breakage when removal of the cast from a custom tray is attempted. These materials have a higher permanent deformation than the addition-reaction silicones and cannot be immersed in disinfecting solutions or stored in high humidity for any extended period of time since the material will absorb moisture. Polyether impression material should be poured within 2 hours; however, manufacturers claim that if the impression is kept dry, clinically acceptable casts can be poured for up to 7 days.

Silicone Impression Materials

The silicone impression materials are more accurate and easier to use as compared to elastomeric impression materials. The condensation silicones have a moderate working time (5–7 minutes) that can be altered by adjusting the amount of the accelerator. They have a pleasant odor, moderately high tear strength, and excellent recovery from deformation. These materials can be used with a compatible putty material to form a custom tray. Silicone impression materials are hydrophobic, which can make cast formation a problem. These materials can be disinfected in any of the disinfecting solutions with no alteration in accuracy. Ideally, these materials should be poured within 1 hour.

The addition-reaction silicones are the most accurate of the elastic impression materials. They have less polymerization shrinkage, low distortion, fast recovery from deformation, and moderately high tear strength. These materials have a working time of 3 to 5 minutes, which can be easily modified with the use of retardants and temperature controls. They are available in both hydrophilic and hydrophobic forms, have no smell or taste, and come in a putty form to assist in form fitting the impression tray at the chairside. Most of the addition-reaction silicones are available in automixing devices, can be poured up to 1 week after impression making with acceptable clinical results, and are stable in most sterilizing solutions. Sulfur in latex gloves and in ferric and aluminum sulfate retraction solutions may inhibit polymerization. Many of the hydrophobic types are difficult to pour with stone, and adhesion to acrylic-resin trays is not good. The putties for these materials have a relatively short shelf life, and they are more expensive than the other elastic impression materials.

RIGID MATERIALS[1]

Plaster of Paris

Historically, plaster of Paris impression material was the only material available for RPD impressions, but with the advent of elastomeric impression materials, impression plasters are no longer used in this phase of prosthetic dentistry. Due to its rigidity, plaster can be used for making accurate transfers of abutment castings or copings in the fabrication of fixed restorations and internal attachment dentures or used when making rigid indexes and matrices for various purposes in prosthetic dentistry. Modified impression plasters may be used to record maxillomandibular relationships.

Metallic Oxide Paste

Metallic oxide paste is a rigid impression material and consists of zinc oxide and eugenol (ZOE). Due to its rigidity, ZOE impression material is not indicated for use as a primary impression material in a patient with remaining natural teeth and not for use in stock impression trays.

Metallic oxide pastes are usually dispensed from two tubes and mixed on a mixing pad. Border molding with metallic oxide impression pastes is not recommended due to the presence of "wrinkles" that occur when movement occurs as the material sets.

As with all impression techniques, the accuracy of the primary impression and of the impression tray has a great influence on the final impression. In general, metallic oxide pastes and plaster of Paris impression materials should not be disturbed during setting.

Metallic oxide paste can be used when making an altered or corrected cast impression for a distal extension base of an RPD with a carefully designed custom impression tray segment attached to the RPD framework to avoid having the material flow into hard and soft tissue undercuts (see Chapter 17).

THERMOPLASTIC MATERIALS*

Modeling Plastic Compound

Modeling plastic compound is among the oldest impression materials used in prosthetic dentistry. This material is most often used for border correction, often referred to as border molding of custom impression trays for Kennedy Class I and Class II RPD bases. The material is available in several colors; the variation in colors indicates the thermodynamic behavior of the compound and its workability as an indication of the fusing temperature range. A common error while using modeling plastic is that it is often subjected to higher temperatures than intended by the manufacturer. It then becomes too soft and loses some of its favorable working characteristics. If a temperature-controlled water bath is not used, a thermometer should be used to maintain the water temperature associated with the color of the material. If modeling plastic is softened at a temperature above that recommended by the manufacturer, the material becomes brittle and unpredictable. Also, there is the ever-present danger of burning the patient when the temperature used in softening the modeling plastic is too high.

The most commonly used modeling plastic for corrected impressions of extension base areas is the red (red-brown) material, in cake form, that softens at about 132°F. It should never be softened at temperatures much above this. Neither it nor any other modeling plastic should be immersed in the water bath for an indefinite period. It should be dipped and kneaded until soft and subjected to no more heat than necessary before the tray is loaded and placed in the mouth. Then it may be flamed with an alcohol torch for the purpose of border molding, but it should always be tempered by placing it into the water bath to avoid burning the patient before returning the material intraorally. After using border molding techniques, sometimes referred to as muscle trimming, the tray with modeling plastic should be chilled using a water spray before removal from the

* Some of the historical parts of this discussion have been quoted or paraphrased from McCracken WL. Impression materials in prosthetic dentistry. *Dent Clin North Am.* 1958;2:671–684.

mouth, although this is not necessary if care is used in removing the impression. During sectional flaming and border molding, the modeling plastic should be chilled in ice water after each removal from the mouth; then it may be trimmed with a sharp knife without danger of fracture or distortion.

Red, gray, and green modeling plastics are obtainable in stick form for use in border molding an impression or an impression tray. The green material is the lowest-fusing modeling plastic, while the red and gray sticks have a higher and broader temperature working range than do the cakes of the same color. Unlike the cake form, the stick form may be flamed without harming the material.

Impression Waxes and Natural Resins

A second group of thermoplastic impression materials consists of impression waxes and resins commonly spoken of as mouth-temperature waxes. The most familiar of these have been the Iowa wax (Kerr Co., Romulus, MI) and the Korecta waxes (D-R Miner Dental, Concord, CA), all of which were developed for specific techniques.

Knowledge of the characteristics of mouth-temperature waxes is important if they are to be used correctly.

The Iowa wax was developed for use in recording the functional or supporting form of an edentulous ridge. It may be used as an altered/corrected cast impression material or as an impression material for relining the finished RPD to obtain support from the underlying tissues. The mouth-temperature waxes lend themselves for use in all relining techniques because of the flow of material intraorally which avoids tissue displacement. As with any relining technique, it is necessary that sufficient relief and venting be provided to give the material the opportunity to flow.

The difference between impression wax and modeling plastic is that impression waxes have the ability to flow as long as they are in the mouth and thereby permit equalization of pressure and prevent displacement. The use of modeling plastics with heating using the flame and tempering is possible outside of the mouth but material flow does not continue when the modeling plastic reaches mouth temperature. The principal advantage of mouth-temperature waxes is that, given sufficient time, they permit a rebound of those tissues that may have been forcibly displaced.

Impression waxes also may be used to correct the borders of impressions made of more rigid materials, thereby establishing optimum contact at the border of the denture. All mouth-temperature wax impressions have the ability to record border detail accurately and include the correct width of the denture border. They also have the advantage of being correctable.

Mouth-temperature waxes vary in their working characteristics. They are designed primarily for impression techniques that attempt to record the tissues under an occlusal load. In such techniques, the occlusion rim or the arrangement of the artificial teeth is completed first. Mouth-temperature wax is then applied to the tissue side of the denture base, and the final impression is made under functional loading by using various movements to simulate functional activity. These mouth-temperature materials also may be used successfully in open-mouth impression techniques. Iowa wax will not distort after removal from the mouth at normal room temperatures, but the more resinous waxes must be stored at much lower temperatures to avoid flow when they are out of the mouth.

INTRAORAL SCANNERS

Intraoral scanning has become a popular method for impressioning in recent years. The reason for its popularity can be attributed to it providing a more comfortable alternative to using impression materials especially with patients with a heightened gag reflex. Another advantage is the convenience of sending and saving models with relative ease and finally the increased accuracy over stone models due to bypassing any possible deformation caused by the impression material, impression technique, or stone. Because of all those reasons, intraoral scanning has become the dominant technique of choice when it comes to fixed restorations. Adoption of intraoral scanners for RPD and complete denture cases remains less pronounced. The reason for this can be attributed mainly to the capacity of a scanner to record movement that occurs with soft tissues of the vestibule and other border tissues, a critical limitation for a successful removable partial or complete denture impression. Because scanners work by capturing multiple still images and then triangulating them to create a three-dimensional model, scanners work best when all the images captured are static. Any movement of the tissues will result in stitching errors and tearing in the generated model. Despite the listed limitations, digital impressions present significant advantages for RPD cases. The first advantage is the ability to capture jaw relation records

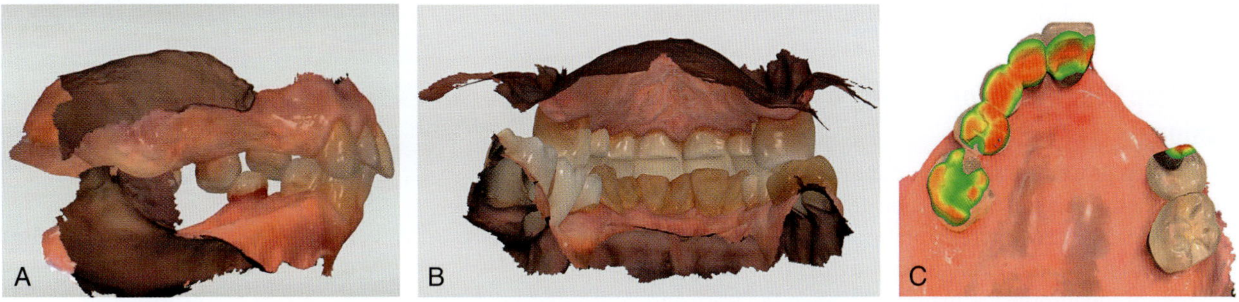

Fig. 16.1 **A,** Intraoral scanning allows for the recording of a patient's jaw relation record in the absence of all but one occlusal stop. **B,** Another benefit is the ability to inspect adequate rest seat clearance during the patient's clinical appointment. **C,** This can also be done by generating an occlusal contact map to evaluate the relationship of the occlusal contact with the rest seats.

without the use of record bases in situations where the patient has a limited number of occlusal stops (Fig. 16.1, *A*).

The second advantage is that it provides a means of inspecting and verifying that sufficient clearance exists between the prepared rest seats and the opposing arch especially on the anterior rest seat preparations in cases where the incisal overlap is excessive (see Fig. 16.1, *B* and *C*).

Intraoral scanning can be predictable with tooth-bounded extension bases, like Kennedy Class III cases. However, distal extension cases can be challenging, especially if the patient presents with the following conditions:

1. Compressible, movable, loose, or flabby residual alveolar ridges: any soft tissue movement of the ridges will cause a stitching error in the impression making. Such tissues also need to be recorded in the compressive state, and intraoral scanners are incapable of such techniques.
2. Increased salivation: moisture contamination of the soft tissue interferes with the accuracy of the scan as it induces reflections and refractions that ultimately distort the images captured by the scanner.
3. Poor neuromuscular control: during intraoral scanning, patients are frequently asked to open, maintain, or move their jaw or tongue into certain positions to allow for access to hard-to-reach areas like the lingual vestibule and hamular notch. If the patient cannot follow such instructions, this will cause additional challenges and frustration to the dentist and the patient and might also ultimately affect the impression's quality.

IMPRESSIONS OF THE PARTIALLY EDENTULOUS ARCH

Impression making for RPDs can be classified into two broad categories: (1) preliminary or diagnostic impressions and (2) final impressions.

Preliminary or diagnostic impressions

Preliminary impressions are made as part of the patient's diagnostic records. Diagnostic records need to accurately record the teeth and tissue to provide sufficient information to aid in the proper diagnosis and treatment planning of the patient. Irreversible hydrocolloid in stock trays is commonly used for this purpose. Alternatively, intraoral scanning can be done, which allows for digital surveying and design or printing of the diagnostic model and the subsequent physical surveying and design.

Step-by-Step Procedure for Making a Hydrocolloid Impression

The step-by-step procedure and important points to observe in the making of a hydrocolloid impression are as follows:

1. Select a suitable, sterilized, perforated, or rim-lock impression tray that is large enough to provide a 4- to 5-mm thickness of the impression material between the teeth and tissues and the tray.
2. Build up the palatal portion of the maxillary impression tray with wax or modeling plastic to ensure even distribution of the impression material and to prevent the material from slumping away from the palatal surface (Fig. 16.2, *A*). At this time, it is also helpful to pack the palate with gauze that has been sprayed with a topical anesthetic. This serves to anesthetize the minor salivary glands and mucous glands of the palate and thus prevent secretions as a response to smell or taste or to the physical presence of the impression material. If gelation occurs next to the tissues while the deeper portion is still fluid, a distorted impression of the palate may result, which cannot be detected in the finished impression. This may result in the major connector of the finished casting not being in contact with the underlying tissues. The maxillary tray frequently has to be extended posteriorly to include the tuberosities and the vibrating line region of the palate. Such an extension also aids in correctly orienting the tray in the patient's mouth when the impression is made.
3. The lingual flange of the mandibular tray may need to be lengthened with wax in the retromylohyoid area or to be extended posteriorly, but it rarely ever needs to be lengthened elsewhere. The wax may need to be added inside the distolingual flange to prevent the tissues of the floor of the mouth from rising inside the tray (see Fig. 16.2, *B*).
4. Place the patient in an upright position, with the arch to be impressed nearly parallel to the floor.
5. When irreversible hydrocolloid is used, place the measured amount of water (at 70°F) into a clean, dry, rubber mixing bowl (600-mL capacity). Add the correct amount of powder, then spatulate rapidly against the side of the bowl using a short, stiff spatula. This should be accomplished in less than 1 minute. The patient should rinse his or her mouth with cool water to eliminate excess saliva, while the impression material is being mixed and the tray is being loaded.
6. In placing the material in the tray, avoid entrapping air. Have the first layer of the material lock through the perforations of the tray or rim-lock to prevent any dislodgment after gelation.

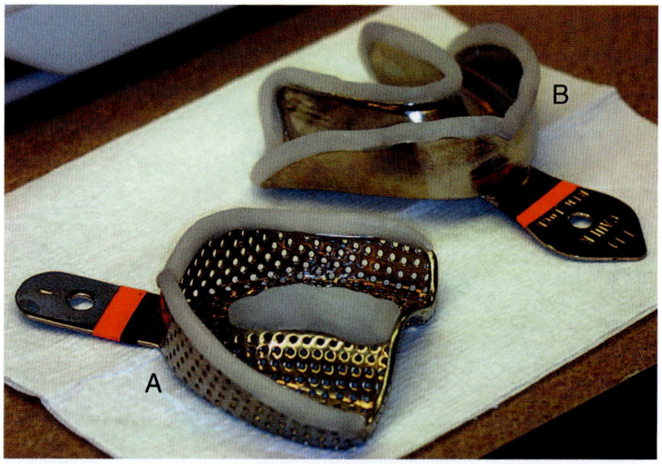

Fig. 16.2 A, Maxillary impression tray with a palatal portion built up with baseplate wax to prevent the impression material from sagging away from the palatal surface. **B,** Mandibular impression tray with periphery wax added to lingual flanges to prevent tissues of the floor of the mouth from rising inside the tray. The posterior end of the tray is extended with the periphery wax to cover the retromolar pad regions.

7. After loading the tray, remove the gauze with the topical anesthetic and quickly place (rub) some of the impression material on any critical areas using your finger (areas such as rest preparations and abutment teeth). If a maxillary impression is being made, place the material in the highest aspect of the palate and over the rugae.
8. Use a mouth mirror or index finger to retract the cheek on the side away from you as the tray is rotated into the mouth from the near side.
9. Seat the tray first on the side away from you, next on the anterior area, while reflecting the lip, and then on the near side using the mouth mirror or finger for cheek retraction. Finally, make sure that the lip is draping naturally over the tray.
10. Be careful not to seat the tray too deeply, leaving room for an adequate thickness of material over the occlusal and incisal surfaces.
11. Hold the tray immobile for 3 minutes with light finger pressure over the left and right premolar areas. To avoid internal stresses in the finished impression, do not allow the tray to move during gelation. Any movement of the tray during gelation will produce an inaccurate impression. If, for example, you allow the patient or the assistant to hold the tray in position at any time during the impression procedure, some movement of the tray will be inevitable during the transfer, and the impression will probably be inaccurate. Do not remove the impression from the mouth until the impression material has completely set.
12. After releasing the surface tension, remove the impression quickly in line with the long axis of the teeth to avoid tearing or other distortion.
13. Rinse the impression free of saliva with slurry water, or dust it with plaster, and rinse gently; then examine it critically. Spray the impression thoroughly with a suitable disinfectant and cover it immediately with a damp paper towel.

A cast should be poured immediately into a disinfected hydrocolloid impression to avoid dimensional changes and syneresis. Circumstances often necessitate some delay, but this time, lapse should be kept to a minimum. A delay of 15 minutes will satisfy the disinfection requirements and should not be deleterious if the impression is kept in a humid atmosphere.

Step-by-Step Procedure for Making a Stone Cast from a Hydrocolloid Impression

The step-by-step procedure for making a stone cast from the impression is as follows:

1. A more abrasion-resistant Type IV stone should be used to form RPD casts. Have the measured dental stone at hand, along with the designated amount of room temperature water, as recommended by the manufacturer. A clean 600-mL rubber mixing bowl, a stiff spatula, and a vibrator complete the preparations. A No. 7 spatula also should be within reach.
2. First, pour the measured water into the mixing bowl, and then add the measured stone. Spatulate thoroughly for 1 minute, remembering that a weak and porous stone cast may result from insufficient spatulation. Mechanical spatulation under vacuum is preferred. After any spatulation other than in a vacuum, place the mixing bowl on the vibrator and knead the material to allow any trapped air to escape.
3. After removing the impression from the damp towel, gently shake off excess moisture and hold the impression over the

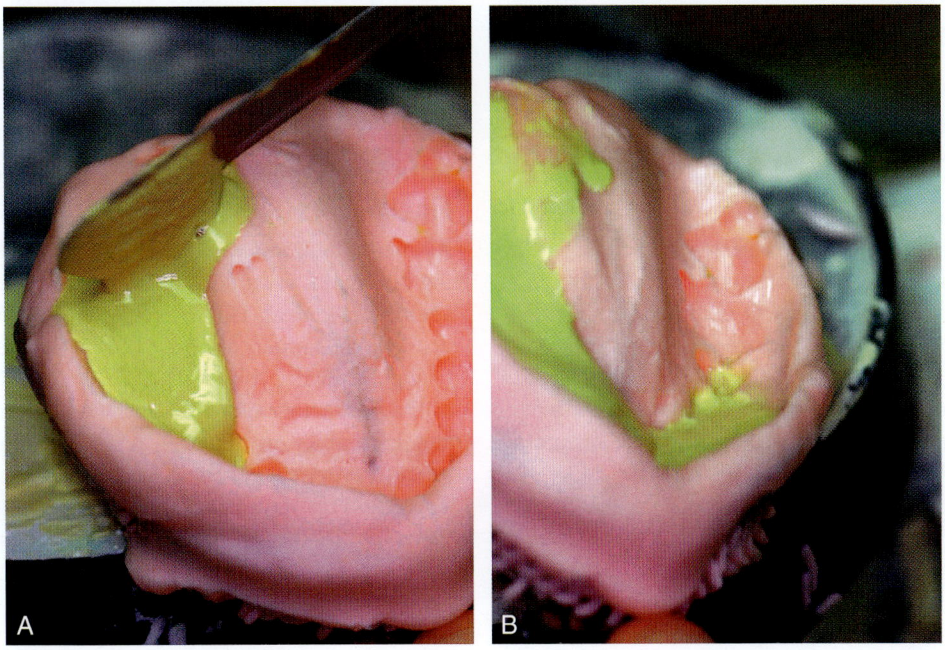

Fig. 16.3 A, Stone is introduced at one posterior region of the impression, with care taken to trace the stone moving into each tooth as it rounds the arch. **B,** Additional stone is not needed until the stone has reached the most posterior tooth on the opposite side.

vibrator, impression side up, with only the handle of the tray contacting the vibrator. The impression material must not be placed in contact with the vibrator because of possible distortion of the impression.

4. With a small spatula, add the first cast material to the distal area away from you. Vibrate this initial material around the arch from tooth to tooth toward the anterior part of the impression (Fig. 16.3). Continue to add small increments of the material to the same distal area, with each portion of added stone pushing the material ahead of it. This avoids entrapment of air. The weight of the material causes any excess water to be pushed around the arch and ultimately to be expelled at the opposite end of the impression. Discard this fluid material. When the impressions of all teeth have been filled, continue to add the artificial stone in larger portions until the impression is filled completely.
5. The filled impression should be placed so that its weight does not distort the hydrocolloid impression material. The base of the cast can be completed with the same mix of stone. The base should be 16 to 18 mm (⅔ to ¾ inch) at its thinnest portion and should be extended beyond the borders of the impression so that buccal, labial, and lingual borders will be recorded correctly in the finished cast. A distorted cast may result from an inverted impression.
6. As soon as the cast material has developed sufficient body, trim the excess from the sides of the cast. Wrap the impression and cast in a wet paper towel or place it in a humidor until the initial set of the stone has taken place. This prevents the impression from losing water by evaporation, which might deprive the cast material of sufficient water for crystallization. Chalky cast surfaces around the teeth are often the result of the hydrocolloid acting as a sponge, absorbing the water needed for proper crystallization of the cast material.
7. After the cast and impression have been in the humid atmosphere for 30 minutes, separate the impression from the cast. Thirty minutes is sufficient for initial setting. Any stone that interferes with separation from the tray must be trimmed away with a knife.
8. Clean the impression tray immediately while the used impression material is still elastic.
9. Trimming of the cast should be deferred until final setting has occurred. The sides of the cast may then be trimmed to be parallel, and any blebs or defects resulting from air bubbles in the impression may be removed. If this is a cast for a permanent record, it may be trimmed to orthodontic specifications to present a neat appearance for demonstration purposes. Master casts and other working casts are ordinarily trimmed only to remove excess stone.

Possible Causes of an Inaccurate and/or a Weak Cast of a Dental Arch

The possible causes of an inaccurate cast are as follows:

1. Distortion of the hydrocolloid impression (a) by use of an impression tray that is not rigid; (b) by partial dislodgment from the tray; (c) by shrinkage caused by dehydration; (d) by expansion caused by imbibition (this will be toward the teeth and will result in an undersized rather than oversized cast); and (e) by attempting to pour the cast with stone that has already begun to set.
2. The ratio of water to powder is too high. Although this may not cause volumetric changes in the size of the cast, it will result in a weak cast.
3. Improper mixing. This also results in a weak cast or one with a chalky surface.
4. Trapping of air, either in the mix or in pouring, because of insufficient vibration.
5. Soft or chalky cast surface that results from the retarding action of the hydrocolloid or the absorption of necessary water for crystallization by the dehydrating hydrocolloid.
6. Premature separation of the cast from the impression.
7. Failure to separate the cast from the impression for an extended period.

FINAL IMPRESSIONS

The purpose of the final impression is to capture the state of the teeth and jaw to fabricate the framework as well as the final RPD. The final impressions are made after all mouth preparations and fixed restorations have been completed according to a well-constructed plan. Intraoral scans, irreversible hydrocolloid, and elastomeric impression materials can all be used for making the final impression. Final impressions usually require the fabrication of a custom/individualized tray. The choice of technique and material will vary depending on the Kennedy classification and the compressibility and the displaceability of the supporting tissues.

Final impressions for Kennedy Class III arches and short-span Kennedy Class IV arches can be completed using an intraoral scan or by using any impression material listed above and seldom require border molding of the movable tissue. Extension base partial dentures, however, usually require border molding in the extension base area. Thus the use of a custom/individualized tray is advisable. Intraoral scanning can still be achieved if the patient exhibits firm tissue, low or normal salivary flow, and good neuromuscular control.

Intraoral Scanning Technique for Preliminary or Final Impressions

As mentioned, intraoral scanning has the benefit of minimizing distortion, potentially caused by impression material warpage or stone wear. However, digital scans are not immune to distortion. Scanners are designed to acquire digital images and triangulate their position in space to create a 3D model. Because of this, any movement of the structures during scanning creates inaccuracy in the final model. Throughout the scanning process, every effort should be made to keep hard and soft tissue structures stationary. This might be impossible to do with patients with flabby or compressible tissues. Extension base cases are more challenging to scan but not impossible if the practitioner takes meticulous care when scanning soft tissue areas. It is sometimes helpful to use a retraction device to assist in maintaining constant tissue retraction (Fig. 16.4). It is important to attempt to scan beyond the depth of the vestibule as this ensures the capture of the depth of the vestibule during digital model creation (Fig. 16.5).

Step-by-Step Procedure for Making an Intraoral Scan of a Bounded Case, Maxillary Case

1. Before starting the scan, it is advisable to place a cheek and lip retractor in the patient's mouth to maintain the border tissues and prevent their movement.

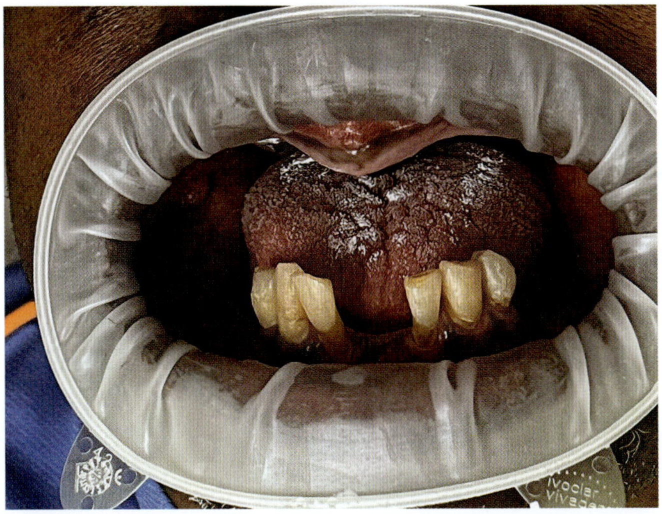

Fig. 16.4 A retractor in place assists in scanning by maintaining constant and even tension on the buccal and labial tissues. (Courtesy of Ahmed Mahrous Copyright © 2024. All rights reserved.)

2. The scan is best started on an occlusal surface of a tooth. Continue the scan of all occlusal surfaces of all teeth. It might be necessary to scan some occlusal portions of the ridge if there are missing teeth. When doing so, make sure not to move the soft tissues. When scanning the anterior teeth, the scanner should be angled slightly to the lingual aspect (Fig. 16.6, *A–C*).
3. The scanner is then moved to the facial surface, and scanning is completed across the arch at a 45-degree angle to the facial surface (see Fig. 16.6, *D–F*).
4. The scanner is then directed to the facial surface and moved across the arch; while moving the scanner across the arch, it is important to move the scanner wand in an occluso-gingival direction to capture as much soft tissue and vestibular data as possible. It is also important not to disturb the tension on the soft tissue so as not to change the shape of the soft tissue while scanning (see Fig. 16.6, *G–I*).
5. The wand is then directed to the lingual aspect of the teeth, and the arch scan is completed.
6. It is important to make sure that the scan is intact and that there are no artifacts or stitching errors (see Fig. 16.6, *J–L*).

Step-by-Step Procedure for Making an Intraoral Scan of an Extension Base, Mandibular Case

1. It is particularly helpful to place a cheek and lip retractor when scanning extension base cases.

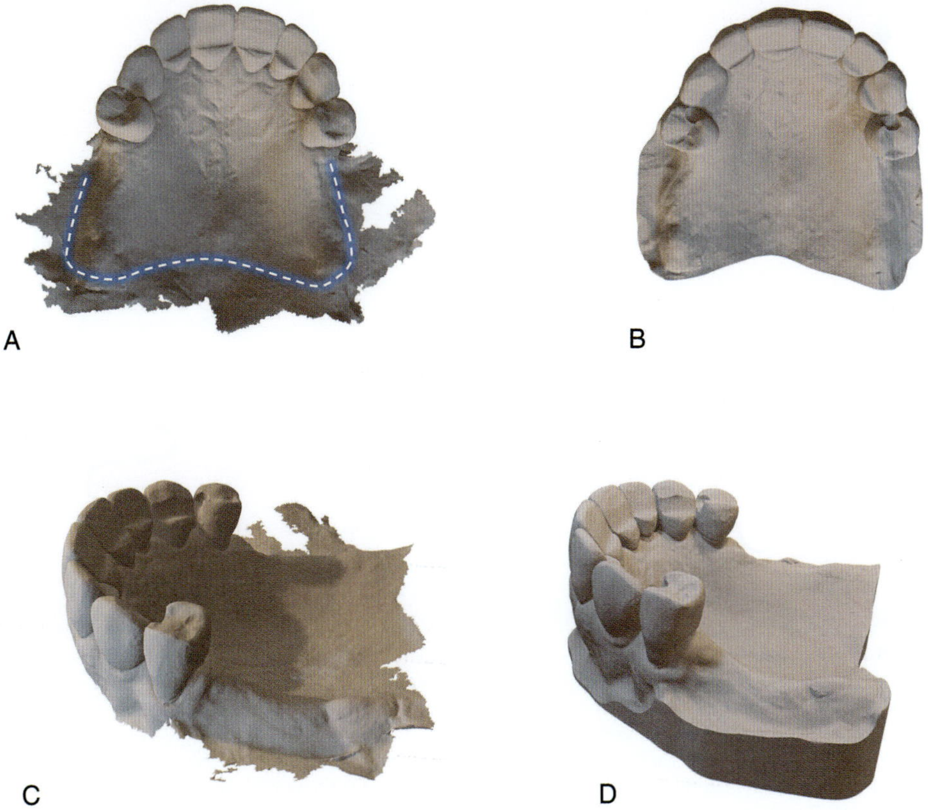

Fig. 16.5 A and **C,** When scanning, it is advisable to *overextend* the area of scanning. **B** and **D,** During cast preparation, any uneven surface will be preferably removed in order to maintain a smooth and sealed edge for the final model. (Courtesy of Ahmed Mahrous Copyright © 2024. All rights reserved.)

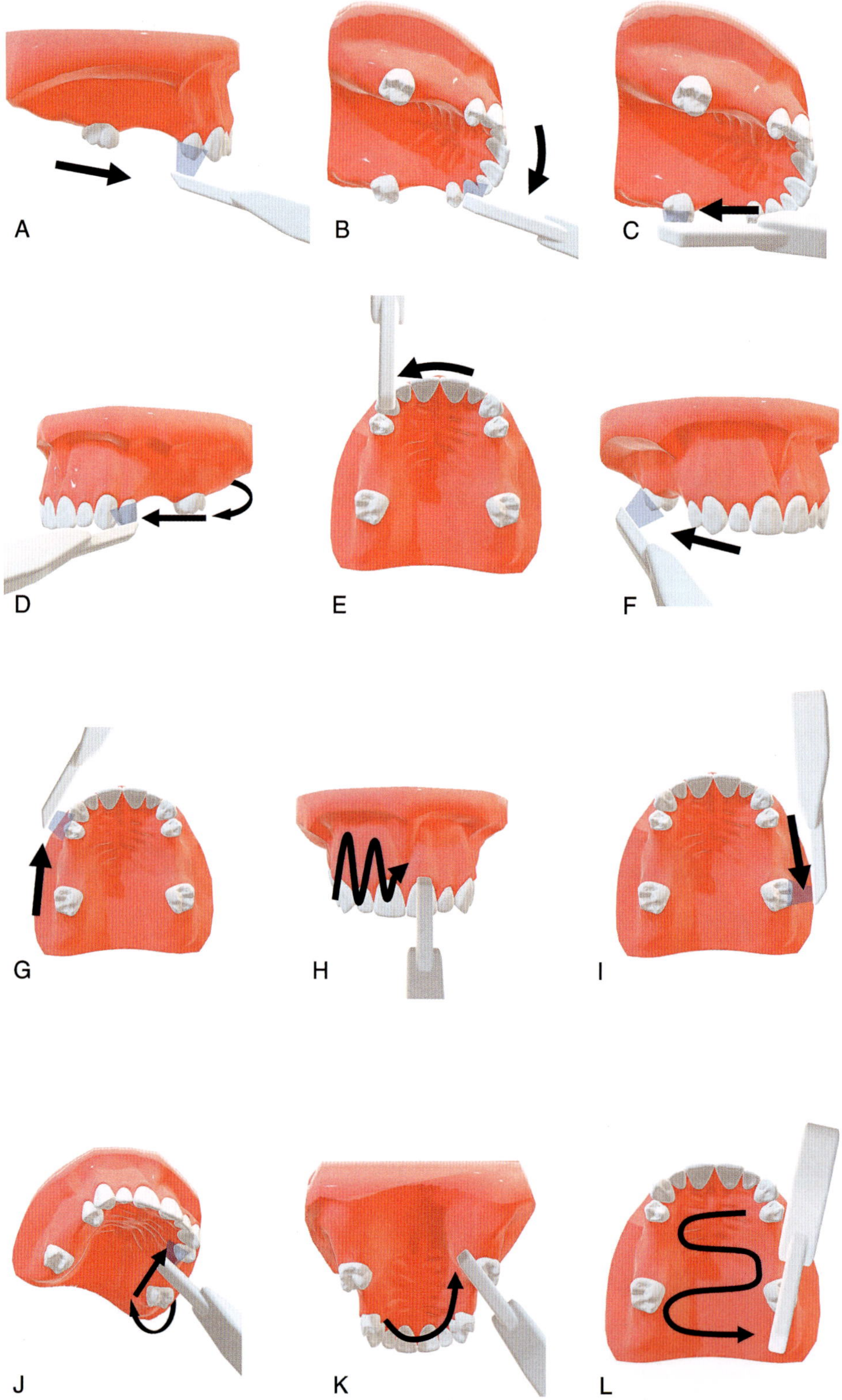

Fig. 16.6 **A,** The scan is best started on an occlusal surface of the tooth. **B** and **C,** Continue the scan of all occlusal surfaces of all teeth. **D–F,** The scanner is then moved to the facial surface and scanning is completed across the arch at a 45-degree angle to the facial surface. **G–I,** The scanner is directed to the facial surface and moved across the arch. **H,** It is important to move the scanner wand in an occluso-gingival direction to capture as much soft tissue and vestibular data as possible. **J,** The wand is then directed to the lingual aspect of the teeth and the arch scan is completed. **K,** The lingual aspect of the teeth is scanned. **L,** The palate is scanned by going in an S pattern joining the previously scanned portions of the arch. (Courtesy of Ahmed Mahrous Copyright © 2024. All rights reserved.)

2. Scanning should start as it was described in the previous step-by-step scanning for bounded saddles with occlusal scanning followed by a 45-degree scan of the remaining teeth.
3. The next step involves scanning the distal extension portion of the arch. Maintain constant and even tension on the tongue with the mouth mirror and the cheek and lip retractor to avoid any possible movement of the scanned soft tissue. It is also important that the user scan the distal extension area in one continuous motion. After scanning the teeth, the scanner should be positioned distal to the most posterior abutment, to begin scanning the ridge and the facial side of the residual ridge, continuing to the retromolar pad (Fig. 16.7, *A*). Without pausing the scan, the scanner is moved over the retromolar pad and to the lingual side of the residual ridge (see Fig. 16.7, *B*). The scanner is then moved deeper into the retromolar space and pulled anteriorly back to the abutment teeth (see Fig. 16.7, *C*).
4. The lingual side of the anterior teeth can be scanned with constant retraction being applied to the tongue (see Fig. 16.7, *D*).
5. The steps outlined in Step 3 can be repeated on the contralateral side if another distal extension exists (see Fig. 16.7, *E*). It may be necessary to have a dental assistant retract the tongue in order to maintain the scanner in the user's dominant hand.
6. Finally, the vestibule associated with any dentate areas can be scanned by moving the scanner in an occluso-gingival direction as it is moved anteriorly (see Fig. 16.7, *F*). It may be helpful to ask the patient to slightly close their mouth to decrease the tension of the lower lip and facilitate access to the facial vestibule.

It is often impossible to capture the full extent of the extension base in a scan. In such situations, it is recommended to use a final impression using the impression material; however, it is possible to carry out a "corrected cast procedure" during the framework try-in stage on a printed model (Fig. 16.8; see Chapter 17).

After all scans are complete, most scanner systems will ask for a maxillo-mandibular record to be made. This may be possible in situations where the patients still retain at least one occlusal stop. If no occlusal stops exist, then occlusion rims will need to be fabricated on printed models and used to relate the two models. Virtual mounting is beneficial as it allows for the inspection of clearance for rest seat preparations, especially for cases with a deep overbite (see Fig. 16.1).

FINAL IMPRESSION USING IMPRESSION MATERIAL

The most used elastomeric impression material for RPD final impression making is additional silicone. A stock tray must be sufficiently rigid to avoid distortion during the impression and

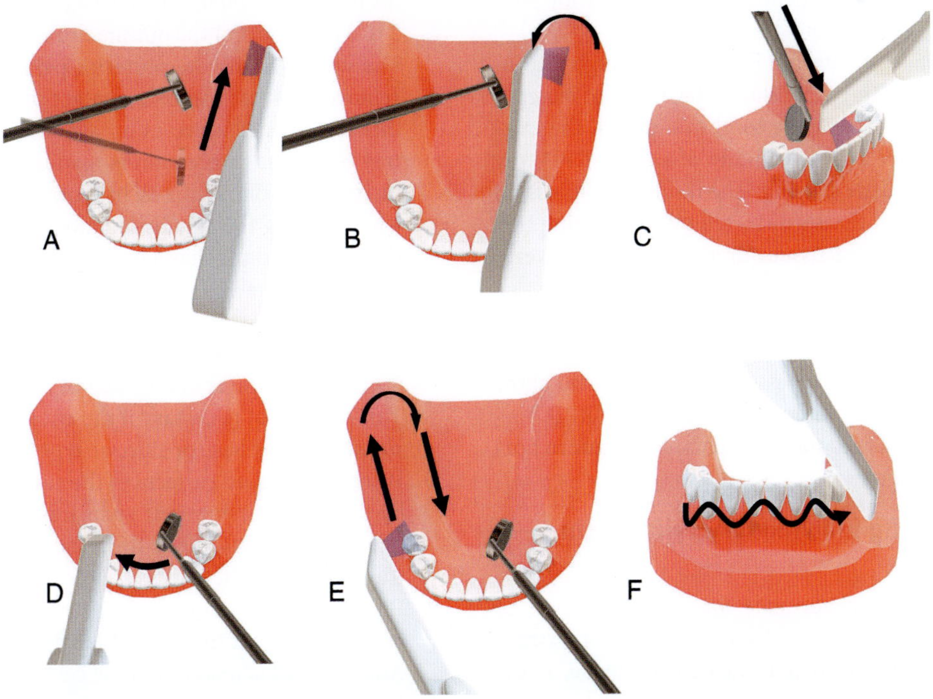

Fig. 16.7 Scanning should start as it was described in the previous step-by-step scanning for bounded extensions with occlusal scanning followed by a 45-degree scan of the remaining teeth (see Fig. 16.6). **A,** The next step involves scanning the distal extension portion of the arch. **B,** Without pausing the scan, the scanner is moved over the retromolar pad and to the lingual side of the residual ridge. **C,** The scanner is then moved deeper into the retromolar space and pulled anteriorly back to the abutment teeth. **D,** The lingual side of the anterior teeth can be scanned with constant retraction being applied to the tongue. **E,** Contralateral side is completed. **F,** Finally, the vestibule associated with any dentate areas can be scanned by moving the scanner in an occluso-gingival direction as it is moved anteriorly. (Courtesy of Ahmed Mahrous Copyright © 2024.)

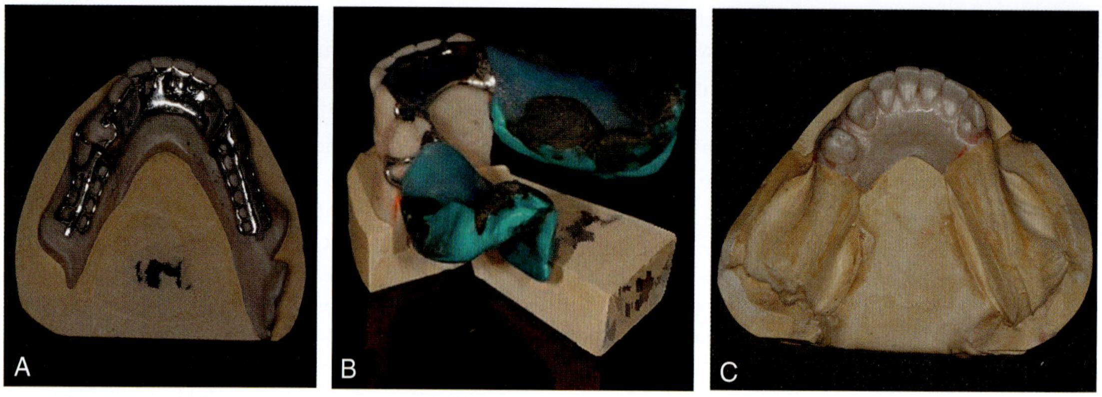

Fig. 16.8 **A,** Underextended model resulting from an intraoral scan of this Kennedy Class I partial denture. **B,** A corrected cast impression was made, and the cast was trimmed in the distal extension area. **C,** The poured and completed cast showing seamless borders and correct extension to the border tissues. (Courtesy of Ahmed Mahrous Copyright © 2024. All rights reserved.)

cast forming procedures and should fit the mouth with about 4 to 5 mm clearance for the impression material without interfering with the teeth or bordering tissues; otherwise, an individual, custom tray made of acrylic resin or a light-cured urethane dimethacrylate resin tray material should be used for the final anatomical impression.

Most stock or disposable RPD trays are of the rim-lock or perforated varieties. Both are made in a limited selection of sizes and shapes. Wide selections of trays are available that can be used for partially edentulous patients, including trays for both bilateral and unilateral edentulous areas.

All of these trays have reinforced borders. Although a complete denture impression tray is, or should be, made of material that permits trimming and shaping to fit the mouth, the existence of a beaded border and the rigidity of a stock RPD tray allow no trimming and little shaping. The resulting impression is often a record of border tissues distorted by an ill-fitting tray rather than an impression of tissues draping naturally over a slightly underextended impression tray.

An individual acrylic-resin tray, on the other hand, can be made with sufficient clearance for the impression material and can be trimmed just short of the vestibular reflections to allow the tissues to drape naturally without distortion. The RPD borders may then be made as accurately as complete denture borders with equal advantages.

Technique for Making Individual Acrylic-Resin Impression Trays

The diagnostic cast is often adequate for the preparation of the individual tray. However, if extensive surgery or extractions were performed after the diagnostic cast was made, a new impression in a rigid stock tray and a new cast must be made.

A duplicate of the diagnostic cast, on which the individual tray can be fabricated, should be made because the cast on which an individual tray is made is often damaged or must be mutilated to separate the tray from the cast.

Several techniques may be used to make individual impression trays; traditionally they have been made manually with either autopolymerizing acrylic resin or visible light-cured (VLC) material; however, it is becoming popular for practitioners to virtually design and print the individualized trays.

The technique for making an individual maxillary tray with light-polymerized resin is as follows (Fig. 16.9).

1. Outline the extent of the tray on the cast with a pencil. The tray must include all the teeth and tissues that will be involved in the RPD.
2. Adapt one layer of the baseplate wax over the tissue surfaces and two layers over the teeth of the cast to serve as a spacer for impression material. The wax spacer should be trimmed 2 to 3 mm short of the outline drawn on the diagnostic cast. The wax covering the posterior palatal seal area should be removed so that intimate contact of the tray and tissue in this region may serve as an aid in correctly orienting the tray when the impression is made. Expose portions of the incisal edges of the central incisors to serve as anterior stops when placing the tray in the mouth. Bevel the wax so that the completed tray has a guiding incline that helps position the tray on the anterior stop. Other cast undercuts should be blocked out with wax or modeling compound. Note: Adapt an additional layer of baseplate wax over the teeth if the impression is to be made in irreversible hydrocolloid. This step is not necessary if the choice of impression material is a rubber base or silicone type of material.
3. Paint the exposed surfaces of the cast that may be contacted by the light-polymerized resin tray material with a model release agent to facilitate the separation of the polymerized tray from the cast.
4. Remove the VLC tray material from the light-proof pouch and carefully cut the desired length with a knife or scalpel. Adapt the VLC material to the cast and trim it with a knife. Be sure not to thin the material over the teeth or the posterior border area.
5. Attach a handle by molding excess VLC material into the desired shape and blend it into the tray material in the cast. With some materials, a paper clip or similar wire may be shaped and used to reinforce the handle. Alternatively, some manufacturers make prefabricated metal custom tray handles that may be easily adapted.

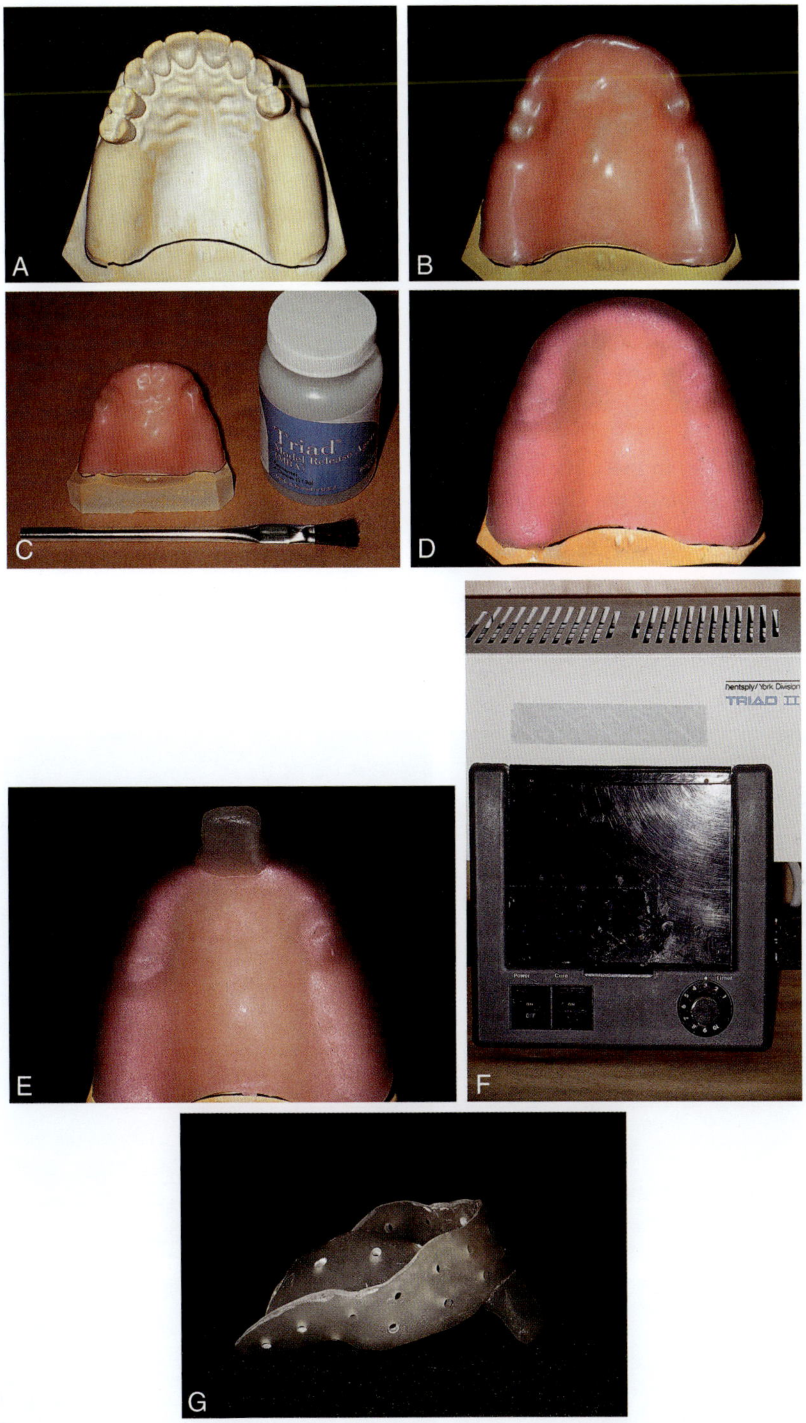

Fig. 16.9 **A,** The desired outline of the tray is drawn on the diagnostic cast. The tray must include all teeth and tissues that will be involved in the removable partial denture. **B,** One thickness of baseplate wax is adapted to the cast and is trimmed to the penciled outline, which is 2 to 3 mm short of the desired border. The posterior palatal seal region is not covered by wax but will be included in the finished tray. Two thicknesses of baseplate wax cover the teeth. A window is created in the wax spacer over the incisal edges. **C,** A model release agent is painted on the stone surfaces of the cast that will be contacted by the resin. **D,** The visible light-cured resin tray material is removed from the light-proof wrap and shaped into the desired outline in a uniform manner. **E,** A handle is added to provide a means to place and remove the tray, as well as to pass the tray from assistant to dentist. Its form should consider the lip length and need to manipulate the perioral region. **F,** Before the tray is placed in the curing oven, an air barrier coating is painted on the surface. The tray is then polymerized as per manufacturer's recommendations. **G,** As soon as the tray material has hardened, the tray is removed from the cast, and the wax spacer is removed from the rough tray. An acrylic-resin trimmer in the lathe is used to rough finish the tray. Holes are drilled through the tray, spaced approximately 4.5 mm apart. These holes serve to lock the impression material in the tray. In addition, excess impression material is forced out of the holes when the impression is made, thereby minimizing displacement of soft oral tissues. These two features assist in correctly orienting the individualized impression tray in the mouth.

6. Place the cast with the adapted tray in the light-polymerizing unit and process according to the manufacturer's directions—usually a maximum of 1 minute.
7. Remove the cast from the unit and gently remove the tray from the cast. Peel the softened wax out of the tray while the wax is still warm.
8. Paint the entire impression tray with the manufacturer's air barrier coating material and return the tray to the unit's turnstile for additional polymerizing, with the tissue side up.
9. When the polymerizing cycle is completed, remove the tray from the unit and clean it with a brush and water.
10. Perfect the borders of the tray with rotary instruments (vulcanite burs, acrylic-resin trimmers, etc.), and slightly polish the external surface of the tray.
11. Place perforations (No. 8 bur size) in the VLC resin tray at 5-mm intervals, with the exception of the alveolar groove areas, if an irreversible hydrocolloid impression material is to be used (see Fig. 16.9).
12. The finished tray must be sanitized and tried in the mouth so that any necessary corrections to the tray can be accomplished before the impression is made.

The following details the step-by-step process of making individualized custom trays using digital methods. Only general guidelines will be given as many software systems may be used with comparable results (Figs. 16.10 and 16.11).

1. The model is imported into the software, and the model is trimmed (see Fig. 16.10, *A*).
2. The custom tray is designed by extruding the shape of the model and creating the appropriate occlusal stops and clearance (see Fig. 16.10, *B*).
3. The handle is added as a separate mesh and customized (see Fig. 16.10, *C*).
4. The tray is finalized, and any rough or sharp areas are modified (see Fig. 16.10, *D*).
5. The .stl is exported into a 3D-printer nesting software (see Fig. 16.11, *A*).
6. The tray is printed (see Fig. 16.11, *B*).
7. The tray is cleaned and cured (see Fig. 16.11, *C*), and the supports are subsequently removed and smoothed.

In cases where an extension base partial denture is to be made on a mandibular case, the buccal shelf regions are not covered by the wax spacer because these areas provide the primary

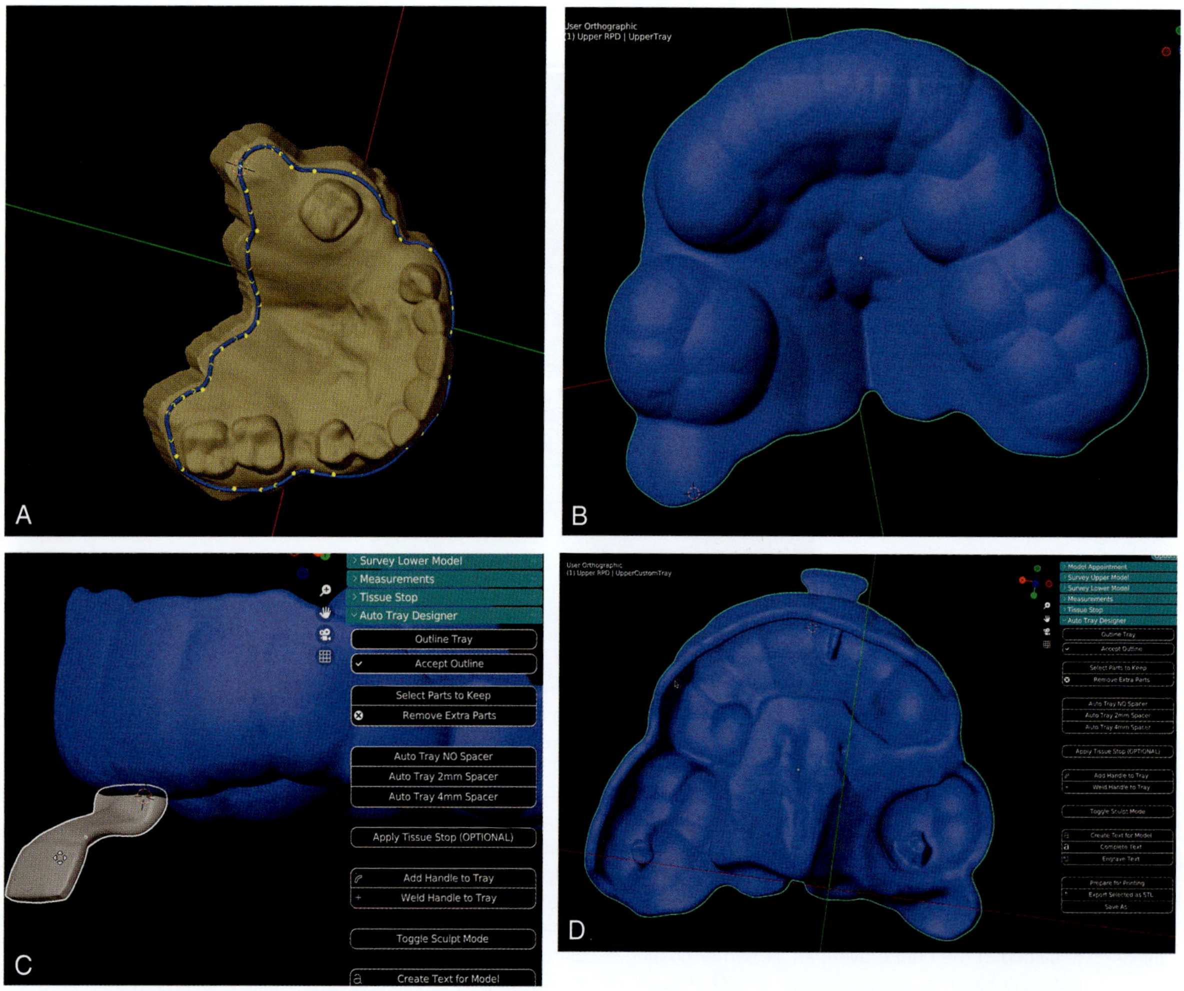

Fig. 16.10 A, The model is imported into the software, and the model is trimmed. **B,** The custom tray is designed by extruding the shape of the model and creating the appropriate occlusal stops and clearance. **C,** The handle is added as a separate mesh and customized. **D,** The tray is finalized, and any rough or sharp areas are modified.

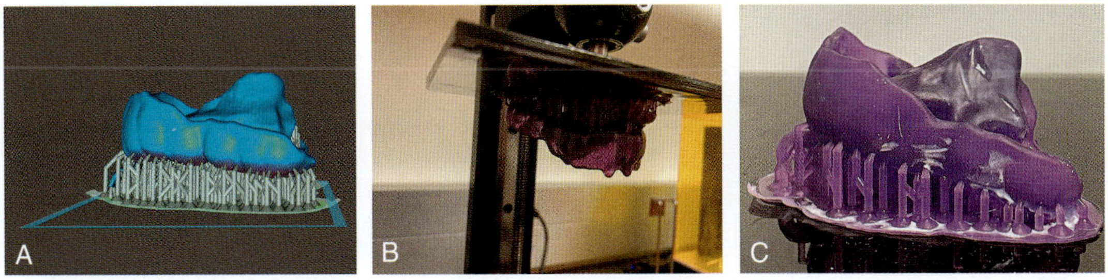

Fig. 16.11 A, The .stl is exported into a 3D-printer nesting software. **B,** The tray is printed. **C,** The tray is cleaned and cured, and the supports are subsequently removed and smoothed.

support for the mandibular RPD and serve as posterior stops in orienting the tray in the patient's mouth. During impression making, these areas permit selective placement of tissues in the mandibular stress-bearing areas.

A series of perforations are necessary in the median palatal raphe and incisive papilla areas of the maxillary tray so that excess impression material will escape through them, thus providing relief of the tissues in this area. For the same reasons, perforations are placed in the alveolar groove of the mandibular tray. With the use of adhesives, the impression material is not easily removed from the tray should a faulty impression have to be remade, but this is an inconvenience common to all newer elastic materials and does not prevent reuse of the impression tray.

Master casts made from impressions in individual acrylic-resin trays are generally more accurate than those made in rigid stock trays. The use of individual trays should be considered a necessary step in making the majority of RPDs, when an altered or corrected cast impression technique is not to be used.

FINAL IMPRESSION TECHNIQUE

Various techniques exist for making a final impression for RPDs. The morphology of the supporting oral mucosa is not static. Free of external forces, the contours of the soft tissue are in anatomic form. Perhaps, the only technique capable of capturing the oral mucosa in the undisturbed, anatomic form is by intraoral scanning. Depending on the contour and quality of these soft tissues, the anatomic form may or may not be the desired profile to achieve maximum support of the distal extension base. Because external forces such as the masticatory load on a distal extension base can displace the oral mucosa, capturing the functional form of the supporting tissue may be necessary to obtain broad stress distribution through abutment teeth and soft tissue.

The impression method and materials selected are greatly influenced by the determination of the support potential of the residual ridge mucosa. Mucosa that is firm and minimally displaceable provides a different support potential than mucosa that is more easily displaced. The *selective pressure impression technique* indicates designing custom trays that selectively compress areas of the residual ridge that can withstand additional stress and at the same time relieve the tissues of the residual ridge that cannot withstand functional loading. Choosing the appropriate viscosity of the impression material can further facilitate the desired pressure within the tray.

Advocates of the *McLean physiologic impression technique* recognized the need to record tissues that support a distal extension RPD base in their functional form. This method utilizes a custom tray formed on the distal extension tissues of the diagnostic cast. The tray is border molded and washed in an elastomeric impression material. During the set of the impression material, finger pressure is exerted on the distal extension to mimic a functional load. A subsequent "overimpression" made in alginate captures the remaining hard and soft tissues.

The technique described here uses additional silicone and modeling compound to be used with extension base cases. The technique is as follows:

1. Check the tray extension intraorally by instructing the patient to relax their muscles, pulling the patient's cheek downwards and outwards, and inspecting the space between the tray and the patient's vestibule. The space should be 2 to 3 mm short of the depth of the vestibule. If the partial denture extends onto the labial frenum, the lips are extended in a similar manner. The only exception is the buccal shelf area, where the practitioner should extend the area as far as possible to maximize support for the partial denture. This is done by palpating the outside of the patient's face to make sure that the tray does not create an outwards protrusion over the extension of the buccal shelf area.
2. It is advisable to start border bolding on the buccal shelf of a mandibular extension base partial denture as those provide the tray with additional support.
3. The modeling compound is heated until plastic; it is then tempered and applied to the tray as an approximately 2 mm even layer. The layer can be molded slightly by hand if it does not conform to the intended shape.
4. The tray is carefully inserted in the patient's mouth while it is still plastic, the mandibular buccal vestibule requires only that the practitioner make sure the soft tissue is not caught under the tray, and the cheek is moved inwards and upwards as the buccinator muscles attach horizontally onto the external oblique ridge. The maxillary buccal border molding is to be done, and the buccal tissue is moved in a downwards, inwards, and outwards direction. If the mandibular lip is to be border molded, then the lip tissue is moved in an outwards, upwards, and inwards direction.
5. A small, heated portion of the modeling compound is softened and placed on the distal portion, and the retromolar area is border molded. The patient is instructed to

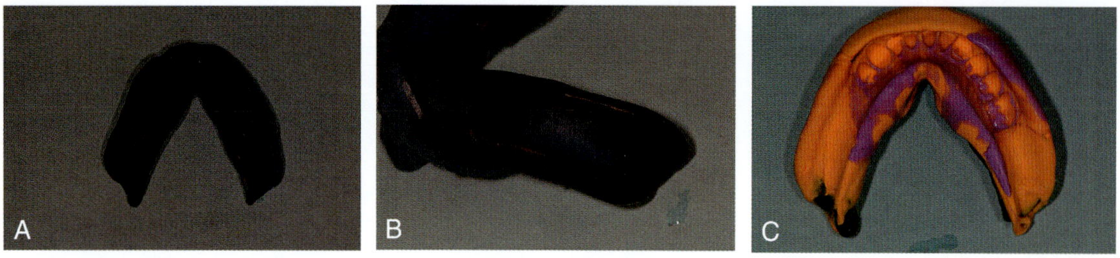

Fig. 16.12 A, The completed border molding on a Kennedy Class II partial denture. **B,** The modeling compound is trimmed using a #25 blade so that it is flush with the tray. **C,** The completed impression. (Courtesy of Ahmed Mahrous Copyright © 2024. All rights reserved.)

open wide that causes the pterygomandibular raphe to be brought forward into the modeling compound, and the patient is instructed to thrust the tongue forward and then close the mouth. Closing the mouth activates the masseter muscle that marks the masseteric groove.

6. The lingual flange is border molded by adding a softened portion of modeling compound on the lingual flange portion of the tray. Care must be taken when inserting the tray into the patient's mouth to avoid colliding the modeling compound with the abutment teeth, which can cause folding of the modeling compound before being fully seated. Once fully seated, the patient is instructed to protrude the tongue, which activates the genioglossus and raises the sublingual fold. The tongue is then pushed against the front part of the palate, which activates the mylohyoid and the superior constrictor. The inferior edge of both posterior lingual flanges is border molded by pushing the tongue into the opposite cheek, which activates the palatoglossus.
7. For maxillary cases, care must be taken when border molding the distobuccal region, and the patient should be instructed to move the mandible sideways as this causes the coronoid process of the mandible to mold the distobuccal border of the modeling compound.
8. The border molding may be tested for proper extension by asking the patient to move the tongue and cheeks with the tray in position. Minimal movement should be experienced during such movements. A properly border-molded modeling compound should demonstrate a matte finish look with no shiny areas (Fig. 16.12, *A*).
9. After border molding is complete, a #25 blade is used to trim the inside of the modeling compound to be flushed with the tray (see Fig. 16.12, *B*). This allows easier removal of the solidified cast.
10. The tray and modeling compound are lined with tray adhesive and allowed to dry.
11. Prior to making the impression, it might be recommended to inspect the patient for any wide interdental spaces or pontics that might prevent removal of the impression. If those areas are identified, soft wax may be used to occlude those areas if they are not to be directly contacted by areas of the metal framework.
12. A medium viscosity impression material is loaded onto the tray, and a light viscosity material is injected into all areas of the mouth where metal framework contact is expected, the tray is seated, and border molding movements are done and repeated until the impression material sets.
13. The impression is removed and inspected for any bubbles, distortions, or tears (see Fig. 16.12, *C*).

In some situations, an additional altered or corrected cast impression may be needed after the framework is made; such techniques will be described in detail in Chapter 17.

REFERENCE

1. McCracken WL. Impression materials in prosthetic dentistry. *Dent Clin North Am*. 1958;2:671–684.

17

Framework Try In

Audrey Marie Selecman and Ahmed Mahrous

CHAPTER OUTLINE

FRAMEWORK FITTING

The finished cast metal framework is the culmination of an appropriate design, adequately prepared abutment teeth, and meticulous laboratory techniques that yield a substructure of the removable partial denture (RPD) that can withstand functional loads without detriment to the supporting tissues. Despite the quality and fit of the framework, poor design or inadequate abutment tooth preparations will result in damage to the oral structures and/or prosthesis. Conversely, ideal design, preparations, and laboratory techniques prove successful only when the framework components are adjusted to achieve the appropriate fit to the abutment teeth and oral mucosa. Studies indicate that nearly all frameworks returned from the dental laboratory require adjustment to achieve complete seating, passivity, and physiologic relief. Fitting the framework involves the following steps:

1. Identifying and removing interferences obstructing the complete seating of the RPD framework.
2. Evaluating and eliminating inappropriate contact(s) of the framework components in the designated terminal position.
3. Evaluating opposing occlusal contacts and adjusting to achieve occlusal harmony.

The framework must be evaluated to ensure complete seating and full contact with the remaining dentition for stabilization, support, and retention as planned, as illustrated in Fig. 17.1. Several types of disclosing media may be used depending on the intraoral location of the assessment. Framework-to-tooth contact (e.g., components of the clasp assembly) can be evaluated with disclosing wax or aerosolized articulating spray (Fig. 17.2). The three-dimensional nature of disclosing wax has the added advantage of revealing areas of excessive framework contact and areas of framework deficiency. Pressure-indicating paste can be used to evaluate framework-to-tissue contacts. After applying a disclosing media, the framework is inserted with mild pressure onto dry abutment teeth. Incomplete seating is seen when any portion of the framework binds to the abutment teeth. It is imperative that the framework is not forcefully placed at this initial seating, as this could result in tooth or restoration damage, inability to readily retrieve the framework, or distortion of the disclosing media.

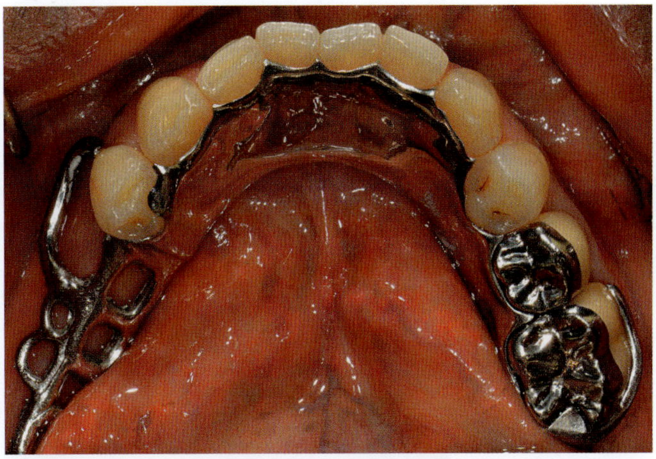

Fig. 17.1 Properly fitting framework seated during the framework try-in appointment. All components of the framework should show close adaptation to their intended position, rests should be adapted to their respective rest seats, and no gaps should exist between the lingual plate and the teeth. The retentive clasp should be inspected and checked for proper positioning. (Courtesy of Ahmed Mahrous Copyright © 2024. All rights reserved.)

Intraoral visual verification of metal interference or residual disclosing media on the hard and soft tissues will facilitate the adjustment procedure. Excessive show through of the metal through the disclosing media indicates binding and may require relief by adjusting the metal interference. Common areas of interference include the apical third of the proximal plates, interproximal extension of the lingual plate, clasp shoulders (junction of the clasp assembly with the proximal plate or major connector), or other sites adjacent to areas of the

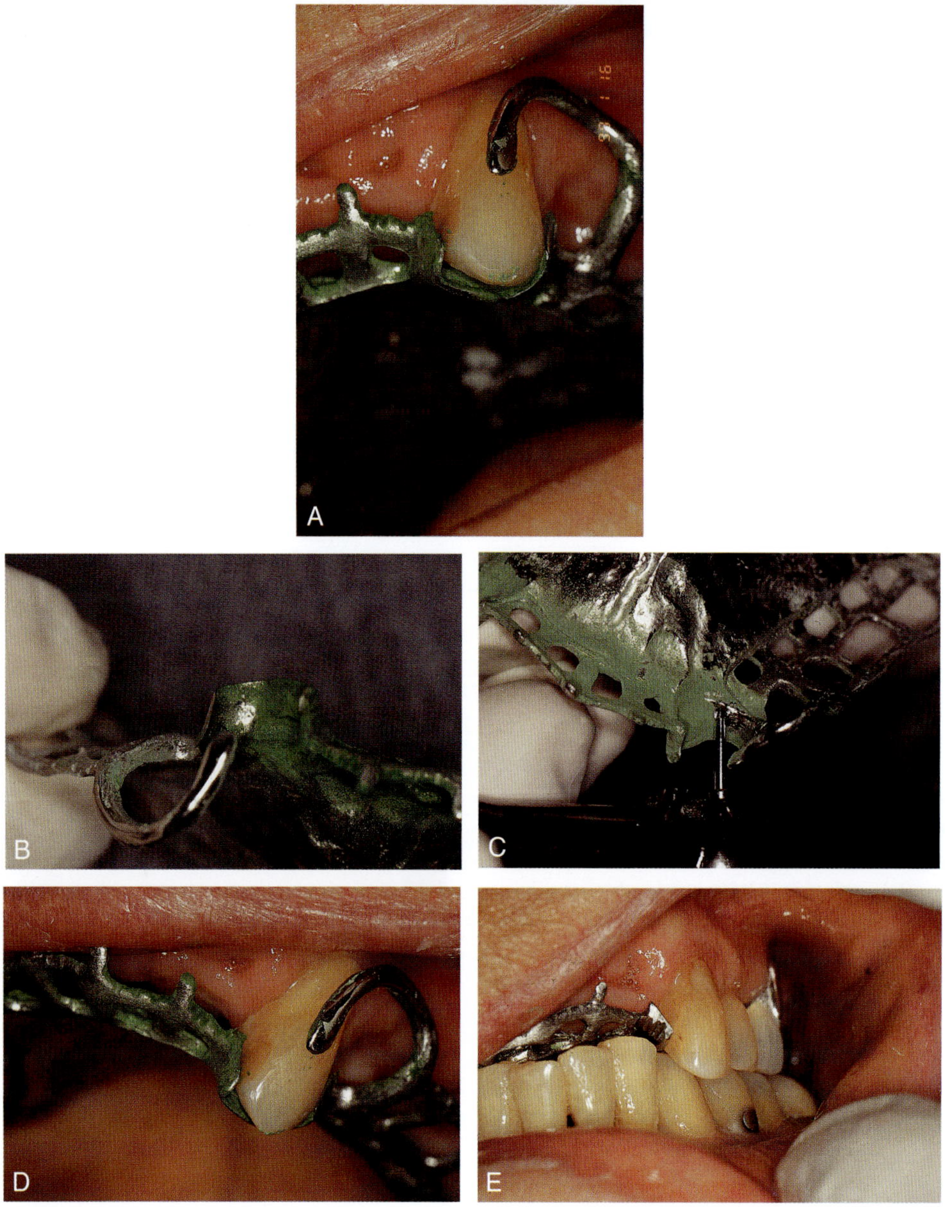

Fig. 17.2 The framework must be evaluated to assure complete seating and full contact with the remaining dentition for stabilization, support, and retention as planned and to allow full natural tooth contact. Several types of disclosing media may be used, such as stencil correction fluid, and disclosing fluids, pastes, and waxes. **A,** Spray-disclosing medium has been applied, and the framework is placed with mild pressure. Incomplete seating is seen when the framework binds. It is imperative that the framework is not forcefully placed at this initial seating. **B,** A portion of the proximal plate is preventing complete seating. **C,** The framework is carefully adjusted as overadjustment can result in a poorly adapted framework. **D,** The framework seats completely after adequate adjustment. This may require repeated disclosing and careful adjustment; however, if improvement is not seen with each framework modification, there should be concern regarding framework accuracy. **E,** Following complete seating and verification of appropriate tooth contacts by component parts (i.e., rests, proximal plates, and stabilizing components), the occlusion must be checked and the framework must be adjusted until natural tooth contacts that exist without the framework seated are achieved with the framework in place. All adjusted regions can be carefully polished with rotary rubber points.

master cast subject to deformation or abrasion during laboratory procedures.

The framework is carefully adjusted using either a carbide or finishing bur with either a slow-speed handpiece or high-speed handpiece. Polishing stones in a slow-speed handpiece can be used in sequential order to return the metal to a high shine. Careful identification of interferences caused by the framework is important and limited to areas of interference; avoid adjusting areas intended to have tooth contact such as the components of the direct retainer or major connectors. Adjustments of the components of the direct and indirect retainers require careful inspection and minimal adjustment to prevent accidental removal of the metal surfaces intended to intimately contact the abutment teeth, as overadjustment can result in a poorly adapted framework. If improvement is not seen with each modification, there should be concern regarding master cast and/or framework accuracy that may require an additional impression for the fabrication of a new framework. The clasps or retentive arms should always be adjusted last. Tight or binding clasps may allow full seating of the framework under pressure, but the framework will rebound when the pressure is released. Cast clasp interferences are evaluated and adjusted like any other portion of the framework, by meticulous evaluation with a disclosing media and minimal removal of the interfering metal with a carbide or finishing bur. Bending a cast clasp is not recommended, as it work-hardens the metal and may result in further distortion of the clasp. If the cast clasp does not adequately contact the tooth, a remake of the framework is indicated. Wrought wire clasps may be modified by slight adjustments with a 2- or 3-prong plier, although this is best accomplished after processing in the event clasp distortion is worsened by additional laboratory procedures. Grasping the midsection of the clasp arm, the 2-prong plier should be used to make bodily movements. Adjustments to the terminus are best accomplished with the 3-prong plier.

Following complete seating of the framework intraorally and verification of the appropriate tooth and tissue contact of all components (i.e., rests, proximal plates, and stabilizing components), the framework must be adjusted to achieve harmonious occlusion with the opposing dentition, whether the patient is in maximum intercuspal position (MIP) or the treatment plan includes restoration to achieve contact at centric relation position. If the patient is to remain in MIP, the framework must not interfere with established occlusal contacts. To verify MIP, the most anterior tooth contact is identified with articulating paper. Shimstock is placed in this location and the patient is instructed to close the mouth. If the shimstock is securely held at this position of closure, the contact should be reevaluated with the framework in the mouth. Occlusal interference will allow shimstock to slip through the identified contact. Interference can be evaluated with articulating paper or by spraying aerosolized articulating spray on the components of concern. While rests are often the offending component, clasps and major connector finish lines may also contribute to occlusal interferences. Opposing contacts on the framework that do not create an occlusal interference or obstruct occlusion do not require adjustment. If RPDs are planned for both the maxilla and mandible, each framework should be fitted individually, beginning with the framework that opposes the most teeth; repeat fitting procedures for the opposing framework individually. After all occlusal interferences are eliminated, both frameworks should be evaluated simultaneously to identify framework-to-framework interferences that prevent natural tooth intercuspation where possible.

SPECIAL CONSIDERATION OF THE DISTAL EXTENSION FRAMEWORK

In a tooth-supported RPD, direct transfer of occlusal forces to the abutment teeth occurs through the occlusal rests. Although the denture base of the modification space(s) in a Kennedy Class III RPD must intimately contact the underlying residual ridge for hygiene and esthetics, forces are transferred to the supporting metal substructure (e.g., structs, mesh, and base) of the rigid metal framework and dispersed to the abutment teeth through the rests. However, the framework must be rigid and designed to broadly distribute the occlusal load through occlusal rests that are properly formed, positioned, and seated into healthy abutment teeth along the span of the framework.

Support for a distal extension RPD emanates from both the abutment teeth and soft tissues covered by the denture base distal to the most posterior abutment(s). Failure to provide adequate tissue support would allow rotational movement of the RPD around the posterior-most rests, resulting in both potential tooth and soft tissue damage. Therefore the support of the distal extension RPD relies not only on the aforementioned considerations of the framework and abutment teeth but also on the intimate contact and maximum vestibular extension of the denture base(s) located on the posterior edentulous residual ridges. Hence additional factors contribute to the support of the distal extension including contour and quality of the residual ridge (see Chapter 16), prosthesis design, and fit of the distal extension base(s).

PROSTHESIS DESIGN

Rotational movement of a distal extension base around the fulcrum line is inevitable under functional loading with the presence of soft tissue that is compressible under occlusal function. Therefore the design of the distal extension framework must include stress-breaking direct retainers, indirect retainers, and a denture base that can adequately resist tissue-ward movement.

It is important to note that the extent to which abutments are subjected to rotational and torquing forces that result from masticatory function is directly related (but not limited) to the position and resistance of the food bolus. The greatest movement takes place at the most posterior extent of the denture base. The retromolar pad region of the mandibular residual ridge and the maxillary tuberosity region of the maxillary residual ridge, therefore, are subjected to the greatest movement of the denture base. Therefore the design of the denture base must provide broad coverage within the physiologic limits of the border structures to disperse occlusal loads (Fig. 17.3), especially to primary stress-bearing tissues as captured by the appropriate impression material and technique as discussed further in Chapter 16.

FIT OF THE DENTURE BASE

The extent of support generated by the distal extension base is dependent on the accuracy of its fit to the underlying tissues. The desired form of the soft tissue is achieved by using the appropriate impression material and technique. The impression or scan must then be poured or printed, respectively, to yield an accurate final analog model to which the base will be processed. Evaluation of the supporting soft tissues in conjunction with the framework of a distal extension RPD is imperative to providing

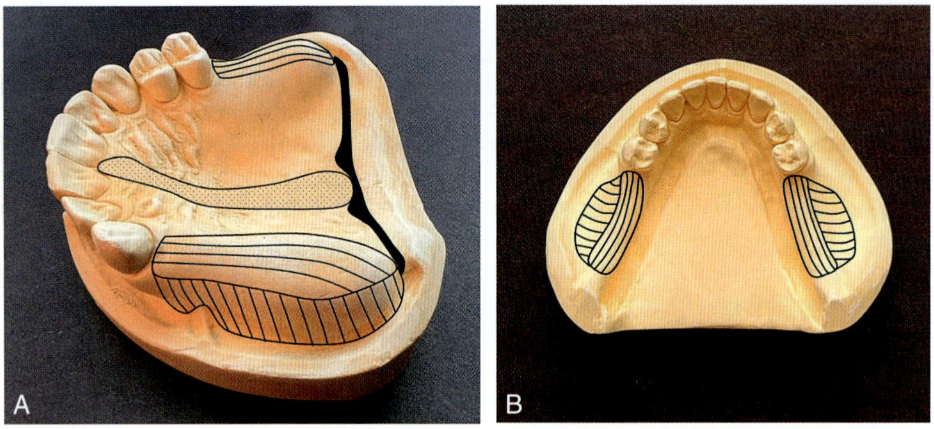

Fig. 17.3 A, The crest of the maxillary residual ridge (anteroposterior lines) is the primary supporting region for the maxillary distal extension denture base. Buccal and lingual slopes (vertical lines) may furnish limited vertical support to the denture base. It seems logical that their primary role is to counteract the horizontal rotational tendencies of the denture base. The dotted portion outlines the incisive papilla and the median palatal raphe. Relief must be provided for these regions, especially if tissues covering the palatal raphe are less displaceable than those covering the crest of the residual ridge. **B,** In the mandible, the buccal shelf (mediolateral lines) provides primary support for the distal extension base while the crest of the ridge (anteroposterior lines) offers secondary support.

optimal support of the final prosthesis. If the contours of the soft tissue or extension of the vestibular borders in the master cast are not conducive to broad coverage to maximize support (see Fig. 17.3), a special impression procedure to register the tissues in the functional form must be utilized to modify the master cast before processing the acrylic base. This is called the altered cast or corrected cast impression.

The altered cast impression technique is a well-accepted procedure to capture tissue in the functional form for the mandibular distal extension partially edentulous arch after framework construction (Kennedy Class I and Class II arch forms). A common clinical finding in these situations is greater variation in tissue mobility and tissue distortion or displaceability, which requires some selective tissue placement to obtain the desired support from these tissues. This variability in tissue mobility is related to the pattern of mandibular residual ridge resorption. Altered cast impression methods are seldom used in the maxillary arch because of the nature of the masticatory mucosa and the amount of firm palatal tissue present to provide soft tissue support. If excessive tissue mobility is present, removing this tissue by surgical resection to improve the support of the final prosthesis is recommended.

ASSESSMENT OF THE DISTAL EXTENSION SUPPORT TISSUES

While an ideal ridge form of firm, keratinized tissue over a broad base of cortical bone lends to negligible tissue-ward movement under normal functional loads, most ridges are not ideal. Hypermobile or redundant soft tissue covering resorbed ridges may have discernable displacement under the same load. Therefore the propensity for change in the supporting soft tissues under a functional load must be considered for the fabrication of the final contours of the acrylic resin base.

There are many accepted impression techniques and materials, including intraoral scanning, to capture the supporting soft tissues of the distal extension base. While efforts can be made to selectively compress or relieve soft tissue through impression tray construction and material selection, the soft tissue ridge form in the resultant cast is unpredictable and can only be evaluated for support when a record or final acrylic resin base is added to the framework and assessed intraorally.

It is important to understand that all Kennedy Class I and II and some long-span Kennedy Class IV frameworks are susceptible to displacement in a tissue-ward direction when force is applied to the distal extension retention lattice which is constructed with intaglio surface relief to accommodate the final acrylic resin contours of the RPD base. The only component of the metal framework to contact the supporting tissue is the "cast stop," which is an approximately 2 mm in diameter vertical stop added to the struts or mesh to prevent framework movement during acrylic resin processing by compression molding (Fig. 17.4). The crestal location and small size of the cast stop cannot prevent intraoral framework movement and should not be used to assess support. Rather a simple technique utilizing a record base applied to the retention lattice of the extension base will provide a suitable clinical assessment.

To evaluate the ridge contours of the master cast, the framework must first be fully adjusted to seat intraorally in its terminal position. Next the undercuts of the extension base must be minimally blocked out with wax on the master cast. A thin coat of model-releasing agent is then applied to all areas of the cast that will contact the visible light-cured (VLC) record base material. On the master cast a sheet of VLC material is placed over the distal extension retention lattice and lightly compressed until contact is made with the cast. The VLC base must extend to cover the full extent of the edentulous ridge. The border of the record base should be trimmed with a blade approximately 2 mm (about 0.08 in.) shy of the myostatic outline. Once the material

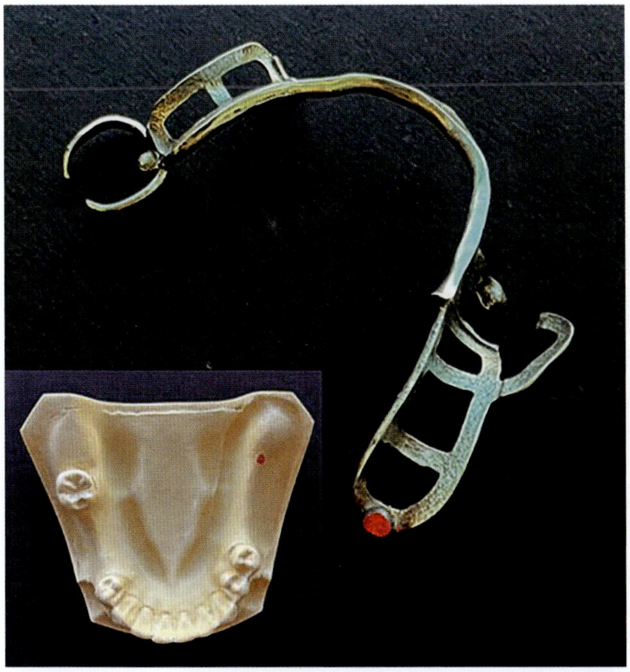

Fig. 17.4 The cast stop (red mark) represents the only portion of the metal framework that contacts the tissue on Kennedy Class I and II removable partial dentures.

is cured and the borders are finished with an acrylic bur, the framework is returned to the patient's mouth. Finger pressure is then applied to the distal extension base. If the framework rotates toward the tissue, as evidenced by the unseating of the most anterior rests, the cast contours of the soft tissue require modification by the altered cast method. This assessment technique can also be used to evaluate the acrylic resin base of a completed RPD where rotational movement would indicate the need for a reline of the distal extension base (see Chapter 23).

If the master cast soft tissue contours prove to provide adequate support, compulsory modification of the cast by the altered cast method is not necessary. Rather, wax rims may be added to the record base to register the interocclusal record as discussed in Chapter 18.

ALTERED CAST TECHNIQUE

A custom tray is fabricated on the distal extension portion of the framework to facilitate the altered cast impression (Fig. 17.5). The record base used to assess the distal extension can also be used as the custom tray for the impression technique for the altered cast method. The following is a step-by-step technique of performing the altered cast technique

1. Fully seat the framework into its terminal position in the mouth and evaluate the border extension of the affixed trays to ensure adequate space is available for border molding material.
2. Compound or vinyl polysiloxane (VPS) can then be applied to the borders of the tray and trimmed to register the vestibular tissues at maximum extension (Fig. 17.6).
3. Using a medium-body elastomeric impression material, fill the tray and cover the border molding material.
4. Reinsert the framework, ensuring all rests are fully seated, and maintain this position with finger pressure in an open mouth position. During the working phase, the impression material should also be muscle trimmed to form a thin wash over the border molding material to prevent overextension and improve cast surface accuracy (see Fig. 17.6).
5. When the impression material has set, remove the framework and trim away all excess impression material that has flowed onto the clasp assembly components or major connector. The impressed trays should look and function exactly like the intended contours of the distal extension base, so much so that when reevaluated in the mouth, the impressed distal extension tray provides adequate support against rotational movement of the framework and the patient should express satisfaction with the fit.
6. The reevaluation process is critical to confirm the support and stability of the proposed acrylic base design, as processing laboratory procedures will yield a base that fits like the impression.

If rotational movement was not eliminated, the impression or contours of the tray should be assessed and remade to achieve appropriate support. Highly redundant tissue may require modification on the master cast to achieve a sufficient impression tray design. In addition, heavy body impression materials can be used to selectively increase pressure. If excessive show through of the impression material is evident or the framework unseats when finger pressure is discontinued, a light-body elastomeric or zinc-oxide paste may be the impression material of choice in combination with tray relief when repeating the impression.

In the laboratory the master cast is now altered to represent the new altered cast impression made on the framework. The following is a step-by-step procedure of preparing and pouring the altered cast (Fig. 17.7).

1. The edentulous ridge distal to the most posterior abutment tooth must be removed sufficiently enough to seat the framework without the impressed base contacting the master cast. This can be accomplished with a die saw, acrylic bur, or large disc on a lathe using extreme caution.
2. Vertical grooves should be added to the prepared surfaces to improve retention.
3. Using sticky wax or hot glue, the position of the metal components of the framework must be secured to the trimmed master cast.
4. The impression borders are beaded to create a vestibular roll in the altered cast.
5. The base is formed by boxing wax secured at the appropriate height to the periphery of the beading wax.
6. Wetting the cast strictly on the prepared surfaces will improve the retention of the stone. Excessive wetting, such as soaking the cast, may separate the sticky wax or hot glue from the metal components, thereby potentially dislodging the framework from its correct position. Preserving the position of the framework on the master cast is critical through the pouring procedure.

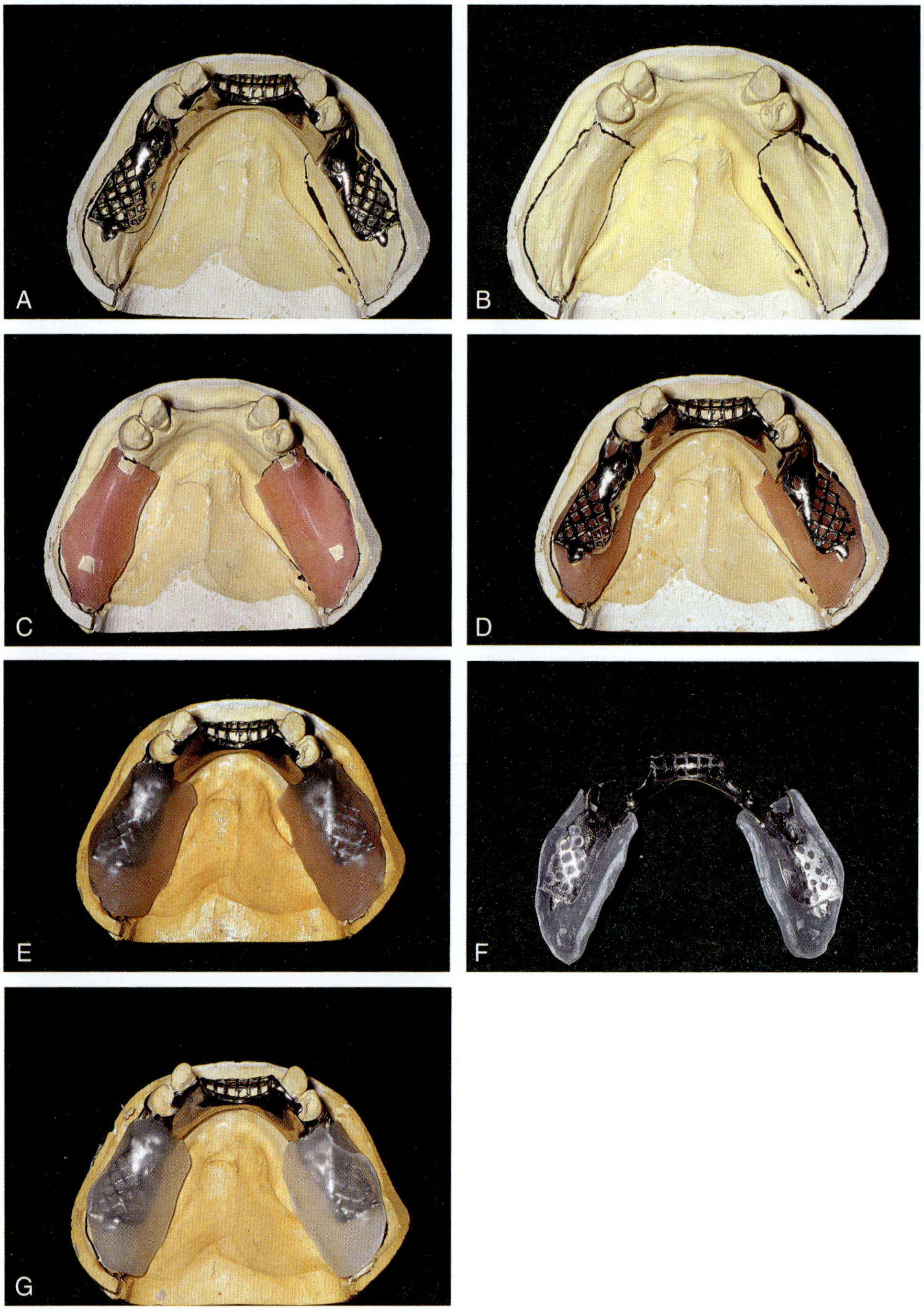

Fig. 17.5 **A,** If a secondary impression, an altered cast impression, is needed to correct the cast inaccuracies of the distal extension portion(s) of the master cast, the fitted framework is reseated back on the master cast and the outline for the tray borders is drawn on the cast. **B,** The outline of the impression tray borders after removal of the removable partial denture (RPD) framework. The outline of acrylic-resin trays is marked with a pencil on the cast. **C,** A secondary impression for the distal extension mandibular RPD is made in individual trays attached to the removable partial denture framework. One thickness of baseplate wax is adapted to outlines to act as spacers so that room for the impression material exists in the finished trays. Windows are cut in the wax spacers corresponding to regions on the cast contacted by minor connectors (tissue stops) for denture bases. **D,** The framework is warmed and pressed to position on the relieved master cast. All regions of the cast that will be contacted by autopolymerizing acrylic resin or visible light-cured resin are painted with tinfoil substitute (e.g., Alcote) or model release agent. **E,** Acrylic-resin material is adapted to the cast and over the framework with a finger. Excess material over the borders of the cast is removed with a sharp knife while the material is still soft. **F,** Polymerized acrylic-resin trays and framework are removed from the cast, and trays are trimmed to outline the wax spacer. **G,** Borders of the trays will be adjusted to extend 2 mm short of the tissue reflections. Holes will be placed in the trays corresponding to the crest of the residual ridge and retromolar pads to allow escape of excess impression material when an impression is made.

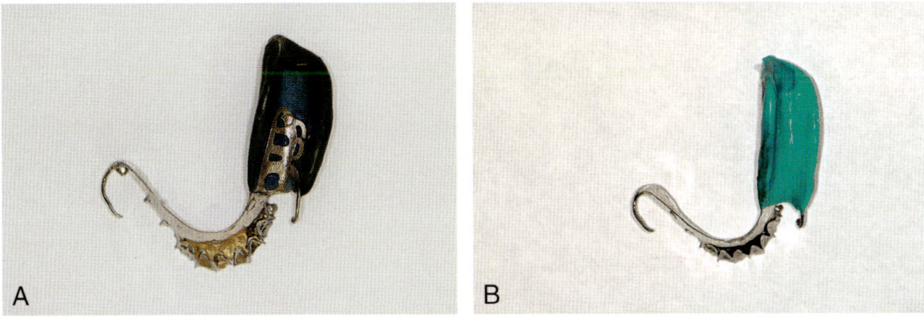

Fig. 17.6 **A,** The trays are border molded in the mouth with compound. **B,** The impression is made. (Courtesy of Ahmed Mahrous Copyright © 2024. All rights reserved.)

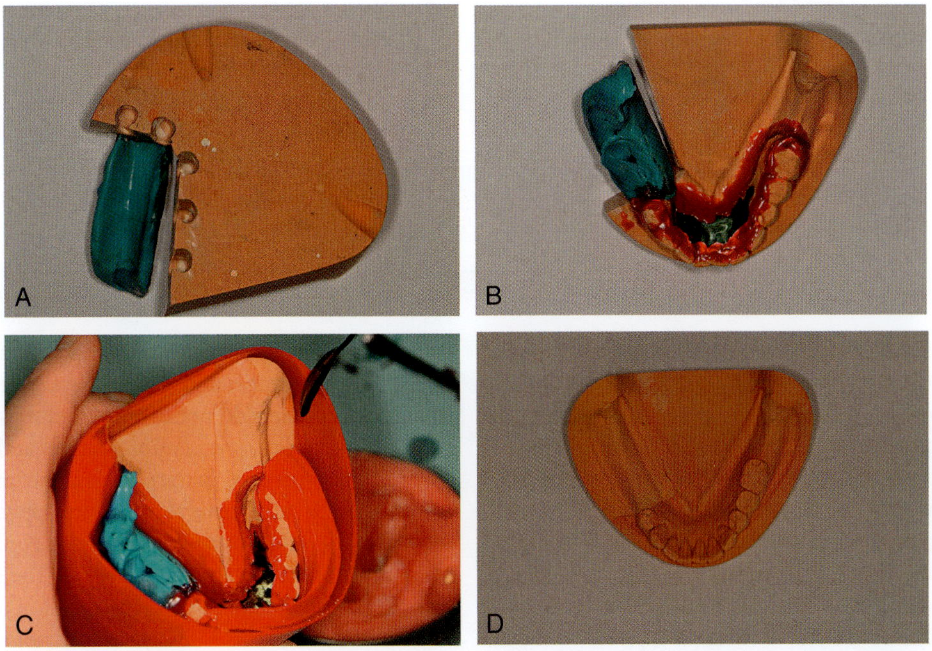

Fig. 17.7 **A,** The edentulous ridge distal to the most posterior abutment tooth has been reduced to allow proper seating of the framework, with the impression base positioned on the master cast. **B,** The metal components of the framework are secured to the trimmed master cast using sticky wax, ensuring proper alignment for the altered cast process. **C,** The impression borders are beaded with wax, and the base is formed using boxing wax at the appropriate height, ready for pouring the altered cast. **D,** The completed altered cast, trimmed to match the master cast's height, with a preserved vestibular roll and proper land area width. (Courtesy of Ahmed Mahrous Copyright © 2024. All rights reserved.)

7. The impression should be poured in vacuum-mixed, type III stone, brushing the surface of the impression with the stone and slowly filling the base to avoid entrapping air bubbles. Vibrating the stone should be avoided as it might unseat the framework from the master cast.
8. After the stone is set, the beading and boxing wax and the framework are removed from the master cast and altered cast base. The altered cast base is trimmed to attain the same height as the master cast, to preserve 2 mm of vertical vestibular roll, and to create 3–4 mm in width in the land area.
9. The impressed trays are then removed from the framework, and the framework is reseated on the altered master cast. If the cast stop is no longer in contact with the functional form of the distal extension, a new cast stop fabricated with autopolymerizing acrylic resin should be added to the retention lattice.

18

Occlusal Relationships for Removable Partial Dentures

Lisa A. Lang, Lily T. García, and Ahmed Mahrous

CHAPTER OUTLINE

Occlusal harmony between a removable partial denture and the opposing dentition (remaining natural teeth or a removable prosthesis) is a major factor in the preservation of the health of their surrounding structures. In the treatment of patients with complete dentures, the inclination of the condyle path is the only factor not within the control of the dentist. All other factors may be altered to obtain occlusal balance and harmony in eccentric positions to conform to a particular concept or philosophy of occlusion.

Balanced occlusion is desirable with complete dentures because unbalanced occlusal stresses may cause instability of the dentures and trauma to the supporting structures. These stresses can reach a point that causes movement of the denture bases. In removable partial dentures, however, because of the attachment of the removable partial denture to the abutment teeth, occlusal stresses can be transmitted directly to the abutment teeth and other supporting structures, resulting in sustained stresses that may be more damaging than those transient stresses found in complete dentures. Failure to provide and maintain adequate occlusion on the removable partial denture is primarily a result of (1) lack of support for the denture base, (2) the fallacy of establishing occlusion to a single static jaw relation record, and (3) an unacceptable occlusal plane.

In establishing occlusion on a removable partial denture, the influence of the remaining natural teeth is usually such that the occlusal forms of the teeth on the removable partial denture must be made to conform to an already established occlusal pattern. Occlusal adjustment or restoration may have altered this pattern. However, the pattern present at the time the removable partial denture is made will dictate the occlusion on the removable partial denture. The only exceptions are those in which an opposing complete denture can be made to function harmoniously with the removable partial denture or in which only anterior teeth remain in both arches and the incisal relationship can be made so that tooth contacts do not disturb denture stability or retention. In these situations, jaw relation records and the arrangement of the teeth may proceed in the same manner as with complete dentures, and the same general principles apply.

With all other types of removable partial dentures, the remaining teeth dictate the occlusion. The dentist should strive for planned contacts in centric occlusion and no interferences in lateral excursions. Although a functional relationship of the removable partial denture to the natural dentition sometimes may be adjusted satisfactorily in the mouth, extraoral adjustment is often easier for both dentist and patient, is more accurate, and can be accomplished in a more comprehensive manner.

Establishment of a satisfactory occlusion for the removable partial denture patient should include the following: (1) analysis of the existing occlusion, (2) correction of existing occlusal disharmony, (3) recording of centric relation or an adjusted centric occlusion, (4) harmonizing of eccentric jaw movements for a functional eccentric occlusion, and (5) correction of occlusal discrepancies created by the fit of the framework and during processing of the removable partial denture.

DESIRABLE OCCLUSAL CONTACT RELATIONSHIPS FOR REMOVABLE PARTIAL DENTURES

The following occlusal arrangements are recommended to develop a harmonious occlusal relationship among removable partial dentures and to enhance the stability of the removable partial dentures:

1. Simultaneous bilateral contacts of opposing posterior teeth must occur in centric occlusion.
2. Occlusion for tooth-supported removable partial dentures may be arranged similarly to the occlusion seen in a harmonious natural dentition because the stability of such removable partial dentures results from the effects of direct retainers at both ends of the denture base.
3. Bilateral balanced occlusion in eccentric positions should be formulated when a maxillary complete denture (Fig. 18.1) opposes the removable partial denture. This is accomplished primarily to promote the stability of the complete denture. However, simultaneous contacts in a protrusive relationship do not receive priority over appearance, phonetics, and/or a favorable occlusal plane.
4. Working side contacts should be obtained for the mandibular distal extension denture (Fig. 18.2). These contacts should occur simultaneously with working side contacts of the natural teeth to distribute the stress over the greatest possible area. The masticatory function of the denture is improved by such an arrangement.
5. Simultaneous working and balancing contacts should be formulated for the maxillary bilateral distal extension removable partial denture whenever possible (Fig. 18.3). Such an arrangement will compensate in part for the unfavorable position that the maxillary artificial teeth must occupy in relation to the residual ridge, which is usually lateral to the crest of the ridge. However, this desirable relationship often must be compromised when the patient's anterior teeth have an excessively steep vertical overlap with little or no horizontal overlap. Even in this situation, working side contacts can be obtained without resorting to excessively steep cuspal inclinations.
6. Only working contacts need to be formulated for the maxillary or mandibular unilateral distal extension removable partial denture (Fig. 18.4). Balancing side contacts would not enhance the stability of the denture because it is entirely tooth supported by the framework on the balancing side.
7. In the Kennedy Class IV removable partial denture configuration, contact of opposing anterior teeth in the planned intercuspal position is desired to prevent continuous eruption of the opposing natural incisors, unless they are otherwise prevented from extrusion by means of a lingual plate or auxiliary bar or by splinting. Contact of the opposing anterior teeth in eccentric positions can be developed to enhance incisive function but should be arranged to permit balanced occlusion without excursive interferences.
8. Artificial posterior teeth should not be arranged farther distally than the beginning of a sharp upward incline of the mandibular residual ridge or over the retromolar pad

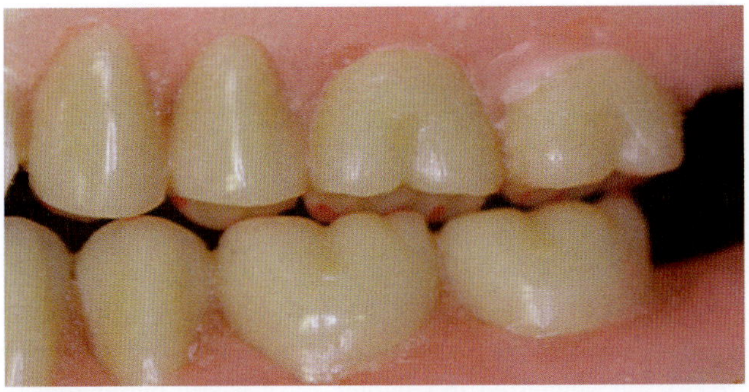

Fig. 18.1 Posterior occlusion of a maxillary complete denture opposing a Kennedy Class I mandibular removable partial denture. The stability of the maxillary complete denture can be promoted by developing a balanced occlusion as shown.

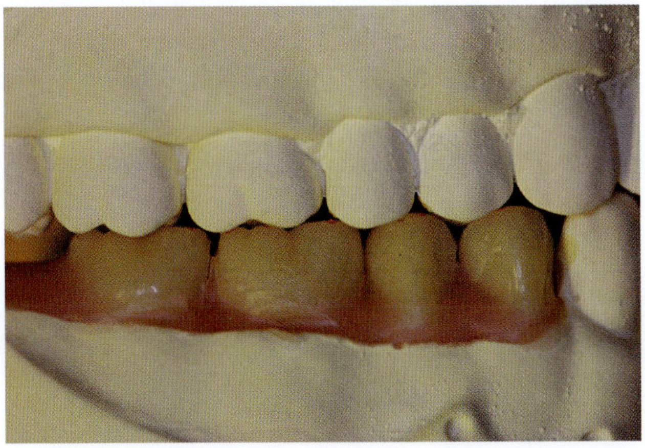

Fig. 18.2 Bilateral distal extension mandibular removable partial denture opposed by natural dentition in the maxillary arch. Working contacts are achieved, balancing contacts are purposefully avoided because they would not enhance the stability of the restoration, and protrusive balance is avoided in favor of an acceptable appearance and a favorable occlusal plane.

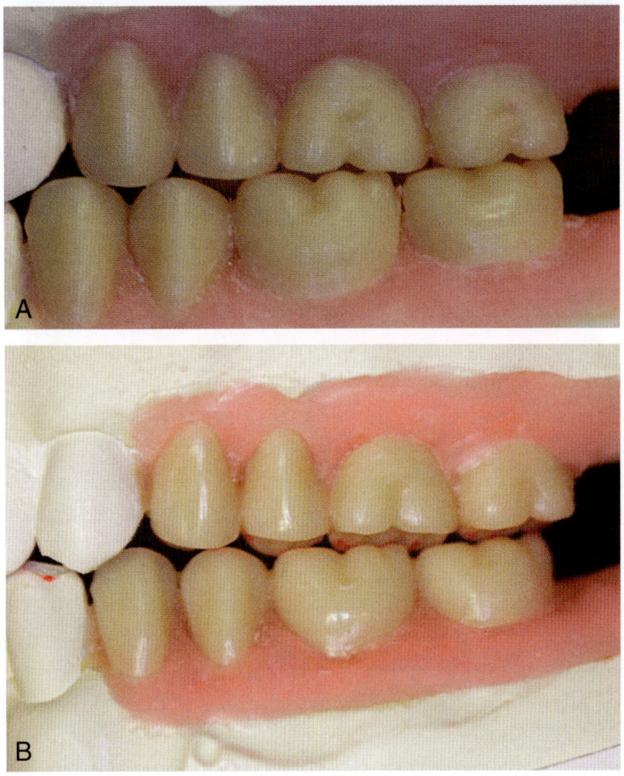

Fig. 18.3 Opposing Kennedy Class I partially edentulous arches arranged to allow working side contacts of opposing posterior teeth **(A)** with balancing contact **(B)** arranged to minimize tipping of the maxillary removable partial denture and to broadly distribute forces accruing to its supporting structures (abutments and residual ridges).

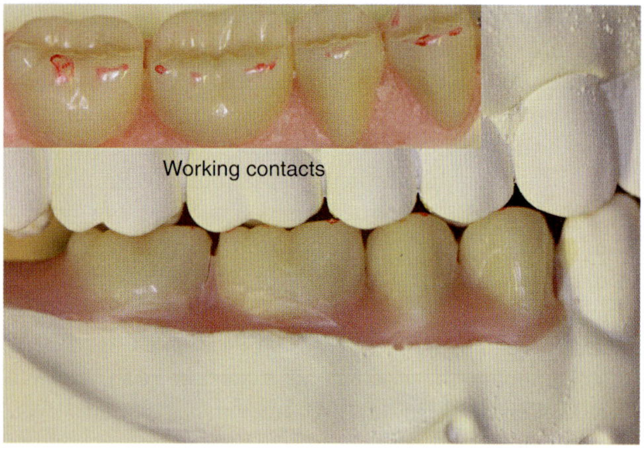

Fig. 18.4 When occlusion is developed for a Kennedy Class II removable partial denture (maxillary or mandibular), only working side contacts are necessary because the cross-arch framework stability gained from tooth engagement provides resistance to movement. Balancing side contacts does not enhance stability beyond that provided by the contralateral teeth.

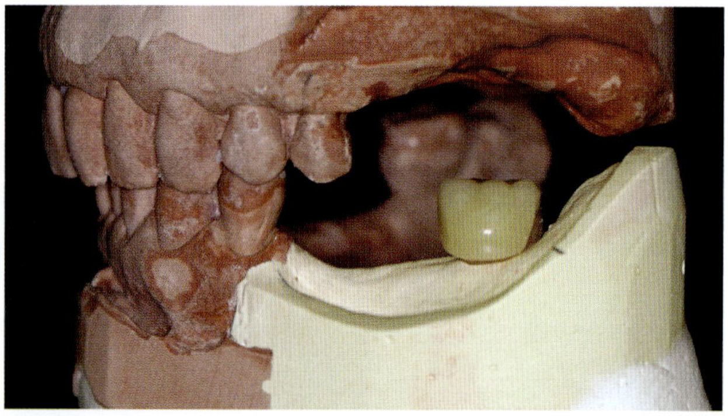

Fig. 18.5 Mandibular posterior teeth should not be arranged distal to the ascending ramus (upward incline) (ascending ramus) of the residual ridge. The molar tooth has been placed just anterior to a mark on the cast land area designating the beginning incline.

(Fig. 18.5). To do so would have the effect of shunting the denture anteriorly.

A harmonious relationship of opposing occlusal and incisal surfaces alone is not adequate to ensure the stability of distal extension removable partial dentures. In addition, the relationship of the teeth to the residual ridges must be considered. Bilateral eccentric contact of the mandibular distal extension removable partial denture need not be formulated to stabilize the denture. The buccal cusps, however, must be favorably placed to direct stress toward the buccal shelf, which is the primary support area in the mandibular arch. In such positions, the removable partial denture is not subjected to excessive tilting forces (Fig. 18.6). On the other hand, the artificial teeth of the bilateral, distal extension, maxillary removable partial denture often must be placed lateral to the crest of the residual ridge (Fig. 18.7). Such an unfavorable position can cause tipping of the removable partial denture, which is restrained only by direct retainer action on the balancing side. To enhance the stability of the removable partial denture, it seems logical to provide simultaneous working and balancing contacts in these situations if possible.

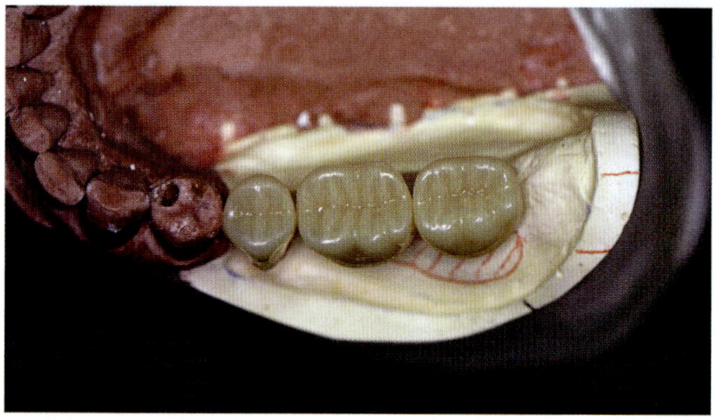

Fig. 18.6 The posterior teeth with a narrower buccal-lingual width than the original teeth have been selected in this distal extension, and they are placed relative to the primary support (buccal shelf) to distribute the functional load to the most anatomically favorable location in a manner that reduces leverage effects.

METHODS FOR ESTABLISHING OCCLUSAL RELATIONSHIPS

Five methods of establishing interocclusal relations for removable partial dentures will be briefly described. Before any of these are described, it is necessary that the use of a facebow mounting of the maxillary cast and pertinent factors in removable partial denture occlusion be considered. The technique for applying the facebow has been described briefly in Chapter 13.

Although a hinge axis mounting may be desirable for complete oral rehabilitation procedures, any of the common types of facebow will facilitate mounting of the maxillary cast in relation to the condylar axis in the articulating instrument with reasonable accuracy and are acceptable for a removable partial denture. As was suggested in Chapter 13, it is still better that the plane of occlusion be related to the axis-orbital plane. Because the dominant factor in removable partial denture occlusion is the remaining natural teeth and their proprioceptive influence on occlusion, a comparable radius at the oriented plane of occlusion in an acceptable instrument will allow reasonably valid mandibular movements to be reproduced.

Semiadjustable articulators can simulate but not duplicate jaw movement. Realization of the limitations of a specific instrument and knowledge of the procedures that can overcome these limitations are necessary if an adequate occlusion is to be created.

The recording of occlusal relationships for the partially edentulous arch may vary from the simple apposition of opposing casts (by occluding sufficient remaining natural teeth) to the recording of jaw relations in the same manner as for a completely edentulous patient. If some natural teeth remain in contact, the cuspal influence that those teeth will have on functional jaw movements dictates the placement of the artificial teeth and the occlusal scheme.

The horizontal jaw relation (planned intercuspal position or centric relation) in which the restoration is to be fabricated should have been determined during diagnosis and treatment planning. Mouth preparations also should have been

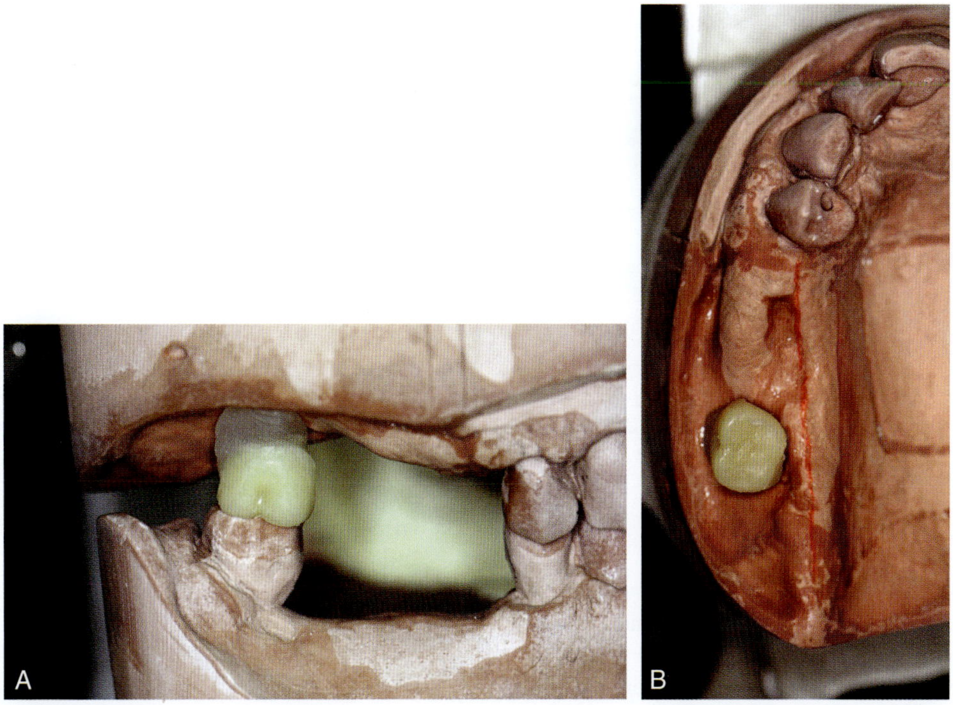

Fig. 18.7 A, Maxillary molar occluded in a normal horizontal relationship to the opposing molar. **B,** The resultant position is lateral to the supporting crest of the residual ridge. This position is functionally unfavorable because of the potentially unstable leverage effects; however, stability can be improved by arranging simultaneous working and balancing contacts in the occlusal scheme.

accomplished in keeping with this determination, including occlusal adjustment of the natural dentition, if such was indicated. Therefore one of the following conditions should exist: (1) centric relation and planned intercuspal position coincide with no evidence of occlusal pathologic conditions; therefore the decision should be to fabricate the restoration in centric relation; (2) centric relation and the planned intercuspal position do not coincide, but the planned intercuspal position is clearly defined and the decision has been made to fabricate the restoration in the planned intercuspal position; (3) centric relation and the planned intercuspal position do not coincide and the intercuspal position is not clearly defined; therefore the decision should be made to fabricate the restoration in centric relation; and (4) posterior teeth are not present in one or both arches, and the denture will be fabricated in centric relation.

Occlusal relationships may be established by using the most appropriate of the following methods to fit a particular partially edentulous situation.

Direct Apposition of Casts

The first method is used when sufficient opposing teeth remain in contact to make the existing jaw relationship obvious, or when only a few teeth are to be replaced on short denture bases and no evidence of occlusal abnormalities is found. With this method, opposing casts may be occluded by hand. The occluded casts should be held in apposition with rigid supports attached with sticky wax to the bases of the casts until they are securely mounted in the articulator.

At best, this method can only perpetuate the existing occlusal vertical dimension and any existing occlusal disharmony present between the natural dentition. Occlusal analysis and the correction of any existing occlusal disharmony should precede the acceptance of such a jaw relation record. The limitations of such a method should be obvious. Yet, such a jaw relation record is better than an inaccurate interocclusal record between the remaining natural teeth. Unless a record is made that does not influence the closing path of the mandible because of its bulk and/or the consistency of the recording medium, direct apposition of opposing casts at least eliminates the possibility that the patient may have a faulty jaw relationship.

Interocclusal Records With Posterior Teeth Remaining

A second method, which is a modification of the first, is used when sufficient natural teeth remain to support the removable partial denture (Kennedy Class III or IV) but the relation of opposing natural teeth does not permit the occluding of casts by hand. In such situations, jaw relations must be established as for fixed restorations with some type of interocclusal record.

The least accurate of these methods is the interocclusal wax record. The bulk, consistency, and accuracy of the wax will influence the successful recording of centric relation with an interocclusal wax record after chilling. Excess wax that contacts the mucosal surfaces may distort soft tissue, thereby preventing accurate seating of the wax record onto the stone casts. Distortion of wax during or after removal from the mouth may also interfere with accurate seating. Therefore a definite procedure for making interocclusal wax records is given as follows:

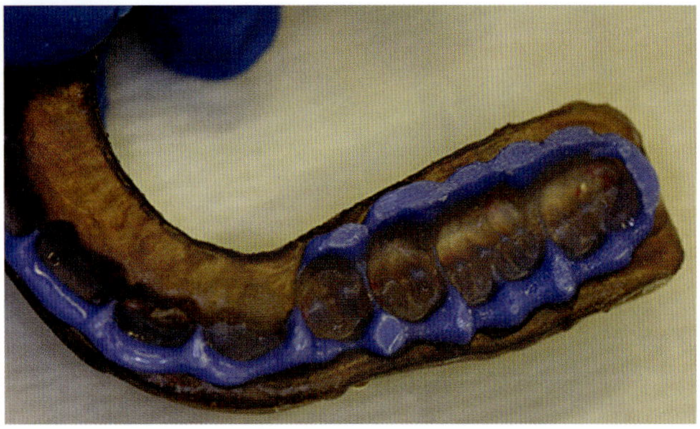

Fig. 18.8 A wax wafer softened in a water bath is used to register an interocclusal position. Once removed and cooled, it is corrected with a more rigid and accurate registration material. Before it is used for mounting, the registration is trimmed to allow complete seating of the cast without distortion of the material.

- A uniformly softened, metal-reinforced wafer of the baseplate or setup wax is placed between the teeth, and the patient is guided to close in centric relation (Fig. 18.8). Correct closure should have been rehearsed before placement of the wax so that the patient will not hesitate or deviate in closing. The wax is then removed and immediately chilled thoroughly in room-temperature water. It should be replaced a second time to correct the distortion that results from chilling and then chilled again after removal.
- All excess wax should now be removed with a sharp knife. It is most important at this time that all wax that contacts mucosal surfaces be trimmed free of contact. The chilled wax record should be replaced again to make sure that no contact with soft tissue occurs.

A wax record can be further corrected with a freely flowing occlusal registration material, such as a metallic oxide paste, which is used as the final recording medium. In making such a corrected wax record, the opposing teeth, the patient's lips, and the dentist's gloves should first be lightly coated with petroleum jelly or a silicone preparation. The occlusal registration material is then mixed and applied to both sides of the metal-reinforced wax record. It is quickly placed, and the patient is assisted with closing in the rehearsed path, which will be guided by the previous wax record. After the occlusal registration material has set, the corrected wax record is removed and inspected for accuracy. Any excess projecting beyond the wax matrix should be removed with a sharp knife until only the registration of the cusp tips remains. Such a record should seat on accurate casts without discrepancy or interference and will provide an accurate interocclusal record. When an intact opposing arch is present, the use of an opposing cast may not be necessary. Instead, a hard stone may be poured directly into the occlusal registration material record to serve as an opposing cast. However, although this may be an acceptable procedure in the fabrication of a unilateral fixed partial denture, the advantages of having casts properly oriented in a suitable articulator contraindicate the practice. The only exception to this occurs if the maxillary cast on which the removable partial denture is to be fabricated has been mounted previously with the aid of a facebow. In such an instance, an intact mandibular arch may be reproduced in stone by pouring a cast directly into the interocclusal record.

Some of the advantages of using a metallic oxide paste over wax as a recording medium for occlusal records include (1) uniformity of consistency, (2) ease of displacement on closure, (3) accuracy of occlusal surface reproduction, (4) dimensional stability, (5) the possibility of some modification in an occlusal relationship after closure if it is made before the material sets, and (6) reduced likelihood of distortion during mounting procedures.

Three important details to be observed when one uses such a material are as follows:

- Make sure that the occlusion is satisfactory before making the interocclusal record.
- Be sure that the casts are accurate reproductions of the teeth being recorded.
- Trim the record with a sharp knife wherever it engages undercuts, soft tissue, or deep grooves.

Occlusal Relations Using Occlusion Rims on Record Bases

A third method is used when one or more distal extension areas are present, when a tooth-supported edentulous space is large, or when opposing teeth do not meet. In these instances, occlusion rims on accurate jaw relation record bases must be used. Simple wax records of edentulous areas are never acceptable. Any wax, however soft, will displace soft tissue. It is impossible to accurately seat such a wax record on a stone cast of the arch.

With this method, the recording proceeds much the same as with the second method, except that occlusion rims are substituted for missing teeth (Fig. 18.9). It is essential that accurate bases be used to help support the occlusal relationship. Visible light-cured (VLC) bases may be adapted to the casts through the technique described in Chapter 16 for making impression trays. Utilizing the master cast, block out undesirable undercuts. However, do not add any wax for spacing. Paint a thin layer of the model release agent on the cast and the relief wax to aid in the removal of the base from the cast after the designated time of polymerization recommended by the manufacturer. Carefully, adapt the VLC base material to the cast. Do not thin the material, and do not adapt the VLC base material over the remaining teeth. Process the base in the polymerization to set the material, and then separate the record base from the cast and remove any remaining blockout wax. Clean the base, apply the air barrier coating over the entire record base, and process (tissue side up) as directed.

Record bases may also be made entirely of autopolymerizing acrylic resin. Those materials used in dough form lack sufficient accuracy for this purpose unless they are corrected by relining. An acrylic-resin base may be formed by sprinkling monomer and polymer into a shallow matrix of wax or clay after any undercuts are blocked out. If the matrix and blockout have been formed with care, interference with removal will not occur, and little trimming will be necessary. When the sprinkling method is used and sufficient time is allowed for progressive polymerization to occur, such bases are stable and accurate. Other record

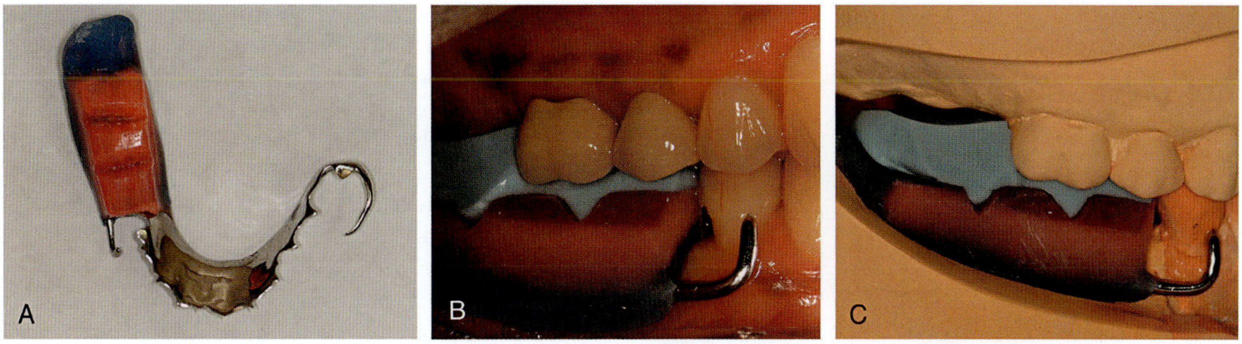

Fig. 18.9 Relationship and distribution of remaining teeth for this patient require that record bases and occlusion rims be used for accurate mounting of casts. **A,** Acrylic-resin record bases and hard baseplate wax occlusion rims adapted to the final metal framework for a Kennedy Class II mandibular arch. **B,** The patient has remaining occlusal contacts; thus a space is maintained between the rims, and V indices are shaped onto the wax rims. Polyvinyl siloxane *(PVS)* bite registration material is used to record the jaw relation record. **C,** The wax rim PVS records are used to relate the casts. (Courtesy of Ahmed Mahrous Copyright © 2024. All rights reserved.)

bases include the use of cast metal and compression molded or processed acrylic-resin bases for jaw relation records.

Relative to the third method, some mention must be made of the ridge on which the record bases are formed. If the prosthesis is to be tooth supported or if a distal extension base is to be made on the anatomic ridge form, the bases will be made to fit that form of the residual ridge. But if a distal extension base is to be supported by the functional form of the residual ridge, it is necessary that the recording of jaw relations be deferred until the master cast has been corrected to that functional form.

Record bases must be as nearly identical as possible to the bases of the finished prosthesis. Jaw relation record bases are useless unless they are made on the same cast or a duplicate cast on which the removable partial denture will be processed or are themselves the final denture bases on metal frameworks.

Jaw relation records made by this method accomplish the same purpose as the two previous methods. The fact that record bases are used to support edentulous areas does not alter the effect. In any method, the skill and care used by the dentist in making occlusal adjustments on the finished prosthesis will govern the accuracy of the resulting occlusion.

Digital Interocclusal Records

When patients have remaining occlusal surfaces in contact, an intraoral scan can capture the relationship of the ridges accurately without the need for record bases. Care must be taken to make sure the patient does not deviate from their planned maximum intercuspation during the recording (Fig. 18.10).

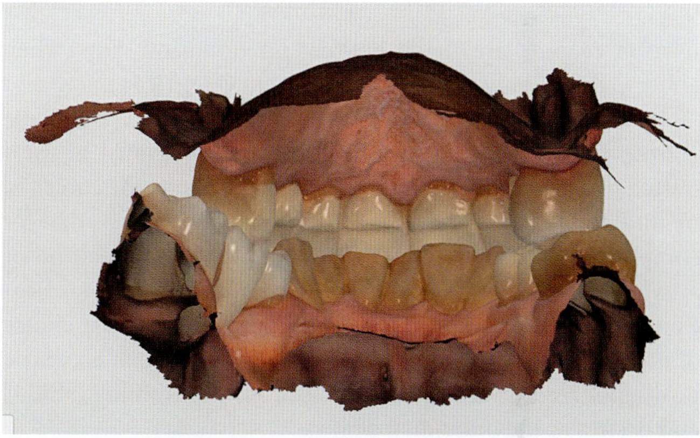

Fig. 18.10 A digital jaw relation made for this Kennedy Class 1 maxillary partial denture allows for the accurate positioning of the scanned models despite the patient having only two occlusal contacts, which would otherwise possibly need a record base to ensure proper stability of the occluded casts. (Courtesy of Ahmed Mahrous Copyright © 2024. All rights reserved.)

Methods for Recording Centric Relation on Record Bases

Centric relation may be recorded in many ways when record bases are used. The least accurate is the use of softened wax occlusion rims. Modeling plastic occlusion rims, on the other hand, may be uniformly softened by flaming and tempering, resulting in a generally acceptable occlusal record. This method is time proven, and when competently done, it is equal in accuracy to any other method.

When wax occlusion rims are used, they should be reduced in height until just out of occlusal contact at the desired vertical dimension of occlusion. A single stop is then added to maintain their terminal position as a jaw relation record is made in some uniformly soft material, which sets to a hard state. Quick-setting impression plaster, bite registration paste, or autopolymerizing resin may be used. With any of these materials, opposing teeth must be lubricated to facilitate easy separation. Whatever the recording medium, it must permit normal closure into centric relation without resistance and must be transferable with accuracy to the casts for mounting purposes.

Jaw Relation Records Made Entirely on Occlusion Rims

The fourth method is used when no occlusal contact occurs between the remaining natural teeth, such as when an opposing maxillary complete denture is to be made concurrently with a mandibular removable partial denture. It may also be used in those rare situations in which the few remaining teeth do not occlude and will not influence eccentric jaw movements. Jaw

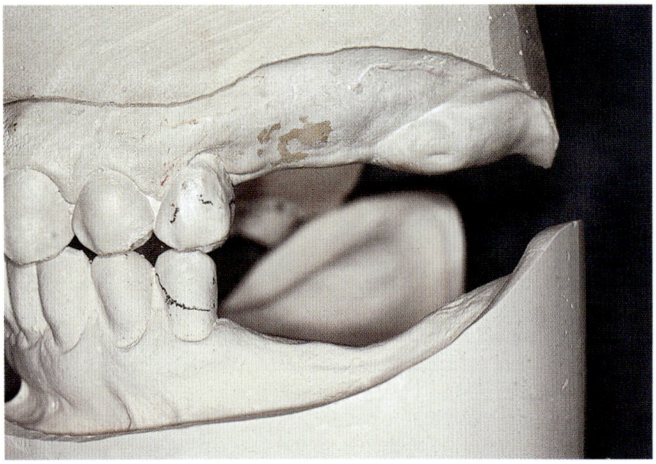

Fig. 18.11 Opposing Kennedy Class I dental arches with remaining anterior teeth only. Recording of maxillomandibular relations was accomplished by using stable record bases and occlusion rims.

relation records are made entirely on occlusion rims when either arch has only anterior teeth present (Fig. 18.11).

In any of these situations, jaw relation records are made entirely on occlusion rims. The occlusion rims must be supported by accurate jaw relation record bases. Here, the choice of method for recording jaw relations is much the same as that for complete dentures. Either some direct interocclusal method or a stylus tracing may be used. As with complete denture fabrication, the use of a facebow, the choice of articulator, the choice of method for recording jaw relations, and the use of eccentric positional records are optional, based on the training, ability, and desires of the individual dentist.

Establishing Occlusion by the Recording of Occlusal Pathways

The fifth method of establishing occlusion on the removable partial denture is the registration of occlusal pathways and the use of an occluding template rather than a cast of the opposing arch. When a static jaw relation record is used, with or without eccentric articulatory movements, the prosthetically supplied teeth are arranged to occlude according to a specific concept of occlusion. On the other hand, when a functional occlusal record is used, the teeth are modified to accept every recorded eccentric jaw movement.

These movements are made more complicated by the influence of the remaining natural teeth. Occlusal harmony on complete dentures and in complete mouth rehabilitation may be obtained by using several different instruments and techniques. Schuyler has emphasized the importance of establishing first the anterior tooth relation and incisal guidance before proceeding with any complete oral rehabilitation. Others have shown the advantages of establishing canine guidance as a key to functional occlusion before proceeding with any functional registration against an opposing prosthetically restored arch. This is done on the theory that the canine teeth serve to guide the mandible during eccentric movements when the opposing teeth come into functional contact. It also has been pointed out that canine teeth transmit periodontal proprioceptor impulses to the muscles of mastication and thus influence mandibular movement even without actual contact guidance. However, if the occlusal surfaces of unrestored natural teeth remain in contact, as in many a partially dentulous mouth, these teeth will always provide the primary influence on mandibular movement. The degree of occlusal harmony obtained on a fixed or removable restoration depends on the occlusal harmony between these teeth.

Regarding occlusion, Thompson has written, "Observing the occlusion with the teeth in static relations and then moving the mandible into various eccentric positions is not sufficient. A dynamic concept is necessary to produce an occlusion that is in functional harmony with the facial skeleton, the musculature, and the temporomandibular joints."[1] By adding "and with the remaining natural teeth," the requirements for removable partial denture occlusion are more completely defined.

Some of the methods described previously may be applied to the fabrication of removable partial dentures in both arches simultaneously, whereas the registration of occlusal pathways necessitates that an opposing arch be intact or restored to the extent of planned treatment. A diagnostic wax-up of both maxillary and mandibular arches will facilitate visualization of the proposed mouth preparation and restorative procedures required to accommodate the planned occlusal scheme, correct orientation of the occlusal plane, correct arch form, and complete tooth modifications to accommodate the removable partial denture design—all at the desired vertical dimension of occlusion. If removable partial dentures are planned for both arches, a decision is necessary as to which denture is to be made first and which is to bear a functional occlusal relation to the opposing arch. Generally, the mandibular arch is restored first, and the maxillary removable partial denture is occluded to that restored arch. If the maxillary arch is to be restored with a complete denture or a fixed partial denture or crowns, a full diagnostic wax-up must be done before occlusion is established on the opposing removable partial denture. If opposing fixed partial dentures or opposing occluding crowns are to be fabricated, it may be advantageous to develop the occlusion and fabricate them simultaneously to ensure optimal positioning, cuspal relationship, and functional integrity.

Registering Occlusal Pathways for RPDs

Restoring a patient's occlusion using a functionally generated path technique is primarily used by specialists and more experienced clinicians so it is included here only for completeness. When registering a functional pathway, after the framework has been adjusted to fit the mouth, the occlusal pathways are registered using a stable record base that has the same degree of accuracy and stability as the finished denture base. The occlusal pathways are captured in a registration medium as the patient manipulates their jaw through all extremes of jaw movement. The occlusal paths, thus recorded, will represent each tooth in its three-dimensional aspect. Recording occlusal paths in this way eliminates the need to reproduce mandibular movement on an articulating instrument.

Occlusion thus established on the removable partial denture will have more complete harmony with the opposing natural or artificial teeth than can be obtained by adjustments in the mouth alone because occlusal adjustment to accommodate voluntary movement does not necessarily prevent occlusal disharmony in all postural positions or during periods of stress. Furthermore, occlusal adjustment in the mouth without occlusal analysis is limited by the dentist's ability to correctly interpret occlusal markings made intraorally, whether by articulating ribbon or by other means.

Regardless of the method used for recording jaw relations, when one arch is completely restored first, that arch is treated as an intact arch even though it is wholly or partially restored by prosthetic means. The dentist must consider at the time of treatment planning the possible advantages of establishing the final occlusion to an intact arch.

MATERIALS FOR ARTIFICIAL POSTERIOR TEETH

Double cross-linked resin teeth have high wear resistance and compressive strength compared to traditional poly(methyl methacrylate) (PMMA) teeth that result in a longer service life. They are generally preferred to porcelain teeth because they are more readily modified and are thought to resemble enamel more nearly in their abrasion potential against opposing teeth (Fig. 18.12). Resin teeth with gold occlusal surfaces are preferably used in opposition to natural teeth restored with gold occlusal surfaces, whereas porcelain teeth are generally used in opposition to other porcelain teeth.

Acrylic resin tooth surfaces, however, may in time become impregnated with abrasive particles, thereby becoming an abrasive substance themselves. This may explain why acrylic-resin teeth are sometimes capable of wearing opposing gold surfaces. An evaluation of occlusal contact or lack of contact, however, should be meticulously accomplished at each 6-month recall appointment, regardless of the choice of material for posterior tooth forms.

Although some controversy may continue regarding the use of porcelain or acrylic-resin artificial teeth, there is broad agreement that narrow (reduced buccolingual) occlusal surfaces are desirable. Posterior teeth that will satisfy this requirement should be selected, and the use of tooth forms that have excessive buccolingual dimensions should be avoided.

Acrylic-resin teeth are easily modified and readily lend themselves to the construction of cast gold surfaces on their occlusal portions. A simple procedure for fabricating gold occlusal surfaces and attaching them to acrylic-resin teeth is described in Chapter 19 under posterior tooth forms.

Arranging Teeth to an Occluding Template

The occlusal surface of the artificial teeth (porcelain or resin) must be modified to occlude with the template. With this method, there are a few materials from which an occlusal surface is developed that are in harmony with an existing occlusal pattern. Therefore the teeth must be occluded too high and then modified to fit the template at the established vertical dimension of occlusion.

Teeth arranged to an occluding template ordinarily should be placed in the center of the functional range. Whenever possible,

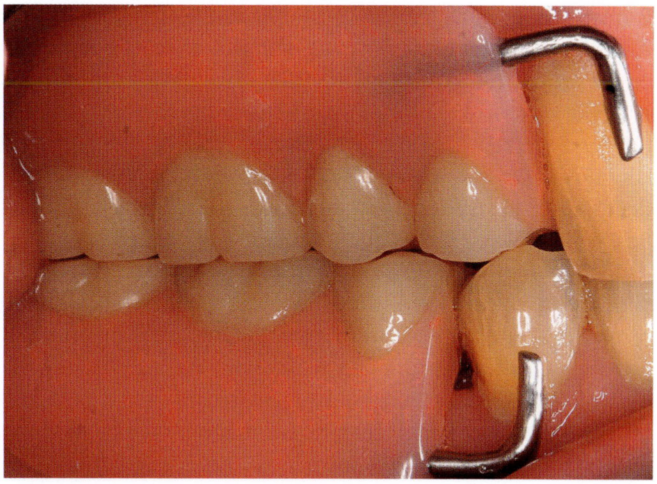

Fig. 18.12 Opposing Kennedy Class I dental arches with remaining anterior teeth only. Double cross-linked resin teeth used in this case will closely match the wear characteristics of natural teeth. (Courtesy of Ahmed Mahrous Copyright © 2024. All rights reserved.)

the teeth should be arranged buccolingually in the center of the template. If some artificial occlusion in the opposing arch has been recorded, such as that of an opposing denture, the teeth should be arranged in a favorable relation to their foundation, even if this means arranging them slightly buccally or lingually from the center of the template.

The teeth are usually arranged for intercuspation with the opposing teeth in a normal cuspal relationship. Whenever possible, the mesiobuccal cusp of the maxillary first molar should be located in relation to the buccal groove of the mandibular first molar and all other teeth arranged accordingly. The opposing teeth in a dental arch that is not contiguous may not be in normal alignment, and intercuspation may be difficult to accomplish. The occlusal surfaces will need to be modified so that they will function favorably regardless of their anteroposterior position. Because cusps modified to fit an occlusal template will be in harmony with the opposing dentition, it is not necessary that the teeth themselves be arranged to conform to the usual concept of what constitutes a normal anteroposterior relationship.

ESTABLISHING JAW RELATIONS FOR A MANDIBULAR REMOVABLE PARTIAL DENTURE OPPOSING A MAXILLARY COMPLETE DENTURE

It is common for a mandibular removable partial denture to be made to occlude with an opposing maxillary complete denture. The maxillary denture may already be present, or it may be made concurrently with the opposing removable partial denture. In any event, the establishment of jaw relations in this situation may be accomplished by one of several previously outlined methods.

If an existing maxillary complete denture is satisfactory and the occlusal plane is oriented to an acceptable anatomic, functional, and esthetic position (which rarely occurs), then the complete denture need not be replaced, and the opposing arch is treated as an intact arch as though natural teeth were present. A facebow transfer is made of that arch, and the cast is mounted on the articulator. To accomplish this, a facebow record is made with the complete denture in place. After the facebow apparatus has been removed from the patient, the complete denture is removed, and an irreversible hydrocolloid impression of the denture is made. When the impression material has set, the denture is removed, cleaned, and returned to the patient. A cast is formed in the impression and then mounted on the articulator with the facebow record. Maxillomandibular relations may be recorded on accurate record bases attached to the mandibular removable partial denture framework with the use of a suitable recording medium. Centric relation is recorded and is transferred to the articulator. Eccentric records can then be made to program the articulator.

In rare instances, when the mandibular removable partial denture replaces all posterior teeth and the anterior teeth are noninterfering, a central bearing point tracer may be mounted in the palate of the maxillary denture, and centric relation recorded by means of an intraoral stylus tracing against a stable mandibular base. If a stylus jaw relation recording method is used, the stylus must be carefully removed from the denture and attached to the same palatal location of the stone cast that was transferred to the articulator via the facebow. The mandibular cast can then be oriented by way of the horizontal jaw relation record and attached to the articulator.

When an existing complete denture is opposing the arch on which a removable partial denture is fabricated, a cast of the complete denture may be used during the fabrication procedures. However, when the occlusion is corrected after processing and the removable partial denture is finalized during initial placement, the complete denture should be retrieved and mounted on the articulator with a centric relation record at the desired vertical dimension of occlusion. This will ensure a more accurate cuspal relationship and will prevent abrasion of the cusp contacts that would occur if a stone cast of the denture is used. This procedure is completed when the patient is in the office so as not to deprive the patient of the use of the existing complete denture.

More often than not, the existing maxillary complete denture will not be acceptable to use because of poor tooth position. The denture will have been made to occlude with malpositioned mandibular teeth, which have since been lost, or the teeth will have been arranged without consideration for the future occlusal relation with a mandibular removable partial denture. Too often, one sees a maxillary complete denture with posterior teeth arranged close to the residual ridge without regard for the interarch relationship and with an occlusal plane that is too low. Usually, however, a new maxillary complete denture must be made concurrently with the mandibular removable partial denture, and jaw relations may be established in one of two ways.

If the mandibular removable partial denture is tooth supported (a Kennedy Class III arch accommodating a bilateral removable prosthesis), the mandibular arch is restored first. The same applies to a mandibular arch that is restored with fixed partial dentures. In either situation, the mandibular arch is completely restored first, and jaw relations are established, as they would be to a full complement of opposing teeth. Thus the maxillary complete denture is made to occlude with an intact arch.

On the other hand, as is more often the situation, the mandibular removable partial denture may have one or more distal extension bases. The situation then necessitates that the occlusion be established on both dentures simultaneously.

All mouth preparations and restorative procedures required to correctly orient the occlusal plane, correct the arch form, accommodate the desired occlusal scheme, and accommodate the removable partial denture design must be accomplished on the remaining natural teeth. In addition, all supporting *tissue* must be in an acceptable state of health before the final impression is made. After final impressions, which include the altered cast impression or the corrected cast impression, are made, the maxillary occlusion rim is contoured, occlusal vertical relation with the remaining lower teeth is established, and a facebow transfer of the maxillary arch is made. The maxillomandibular relations may be recorded by any of the several methods previously outlined and the articulator mounting completed. Occlusion for complete dentures may be established with care for a favorable tooth-to-ridge relationship in both arches, an optimum occlusal plane, and cuspal harmony between all occluding teeth.

After try-in, several methods may be used to complete the restorations. Both dentures may be processed concurrently and remounted for occlusal correction, or the removable partial denture may be processed first. After the dentures are completed and remounted, the teeth—still in wax on the complete denture—are adjusted to any discrepancies that are occurring.

Occlusal discrepancies created during processing must be corrected before the patient is permitted to use the denture(s). Methods by which these discrepancies may be corrected are discussed in Chapter 19.

REFERENCE

1. Thompson JR. Temporomandibular disorders: diagnosis and dental treatment in the temporomandibular joint. In: Sarnat B, ed. *The Temporomandibular Joint*. 2nd ed. Bernard G. Sarnat and Charles C. Thomas; 1964:146–184.

19

Work Authorizations for Removable Partial Dentures

Ahmed Mahrous, David L. Botsko, and Berna Saglik

CHAPTER OUTLINE

WORK AUTHORIZATION

A work authorization contains the written directions for laboratory procedures to be performed for fabrication of dental restorations. The responsibility of a dentist to the public and to the dental profession to safeguard the quality of prosthodontic services is controlled in part through meaningful work authorizations. If work authorizations are properly completed, they provide a means for increased professional quality assurance and satisfaction in a removable partial denture service.

A work authorization completed by a dentist is similar to granting power of attorney. It grants authority for others to act on the dentist's behalf and specifically prescribes what is authorized.

When properly executed, work authorizations are effective channels of communication. They enhance the quality of the completed restorations by providing instructions for individually and scientifically considered prostheses.

Content

Information contained in a work authorization should include the following: (1) the name and address of the dental laboratory, (2) the name and address of the dentist who initiates the work authorization, (3) the identification of the patient, (4) the date of work authorization, (5) the desired completion date of the request, (6) specific instructions, (7) the signature of the dentist, and (8) the registered license number of the dentist. Work authorizations have traditionally been written on paper (Fig. 19.1). However, in recent years, they have increasingly shifted toward a digital format. Physical lab authorization is usually accompanied by casts, impressions, or a prosthesis. Digital lab prescriptions are usually accompanied by a standard triangle (tessellation) language (.stl) scan, pictures, or diagrams.

Function

The following four essential functions are performed by a work authorization:

- It furnishes definite instructions for laboratory procedures to be accomplished and implies an expectation of a level of acceptable quality for the services rendered.
- It provides a means of protecting the public from the illegal practice of dentistry.
- It is a protective legal document for both the dentist and the dental laboratory technician.
- It completely delineates the responsibilities of the dentist and the dental laboratory technician.

Characteristics

A work authorization must be legible, clear, concise, and readily understood. It is unreasonable to assume that laboratory technicians are decoding experts. Sufficient information must be included in a work authorization to enable the technician to understand and execute the request. Many dentists are overly presumptive in assuming that a request can be acceptably fulfilled without proper directions.

It is sound practice to provide the dental laboratory technician with adequate written instructions for each laboratory service required in the fabrication of a restoration. Therefore a new work authorization should accompany the material returned to the laboratory for continuing progress to complete the restoration.

No single work authorization form is adequate to furnish detailed instructions for accomplishing the laboratory phases in the fabrication of removable partial dentures, crowns, and fixed partial dentures or complete dentures or for accomplishing orthodontic laboratory procedures. Inherent differences in the many types of restorations themselves and differences in

Removable Partial Prosthodontics

Patient name:____________________ Patient number:________

Student name:____________________ Student number:________

☐ Treatment plan ☐ Laboratory instructions

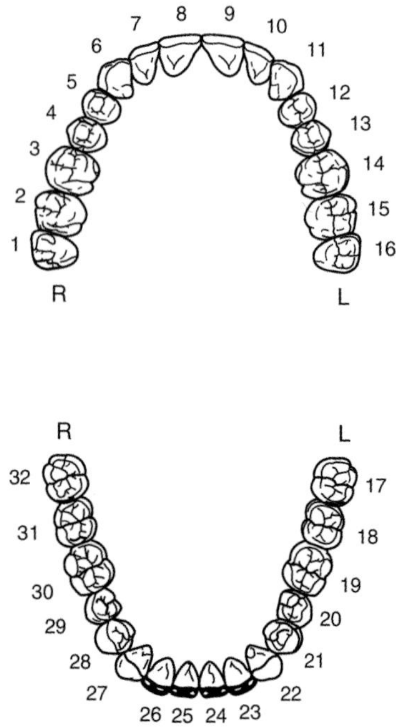

Design specifications:

1. Rests
2. Retention
3. Reciprocation
4. Major connector
5. Indirect retention
6. Guide planes
7. Base retention
8. Areas to be modified or contoured

Color code:

Blue: Cast metal
Red: Resin base and wrought wire
Green: Areas to be contoured

Instructor:________________

Approval to send to laboratory:________________________ Date:__________

Fig. 19.1 Work authorization form, designed specifically for removable partial dentures, to furnish detailed information to the laboratory technician. Form used to specifically plan framework design and to designate mouth alterations and preparations.

the laboratory phases necessary for their fabrication establish a requirement for individual work authorization forms.

DEFINITIVE INSTRUCTIONS BY WORK AUTHORIZATIONS

Work authorization forms may be designed so that only a minimum of input is necessary to provide thorough instructions (Fig. 19.2). The form can contain listings of materials and specifications that require either a check mark or a fill-in for authorization of their use.

A reminder space is included to designate the choice of material for the framework. The type of denture base material may also be indicated by a check mark.

Space is reserved on the work authorization form to furnish the technician with information on the dentist's selection of teeth. The responsibility for tooth selection must remain with the dentist. The success of the removable partial denture depends in part on the consideration given to the size, number,

Removable Partial Prosthodontics

Patient name: *John Doe* Patient number: *158390*

Student name: *Joe Smith* Student number: *1234*

☐ Treatment plan ☐ Laboratory instructions

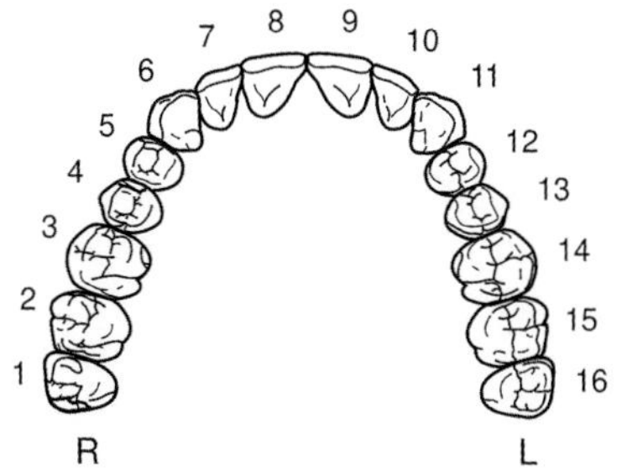

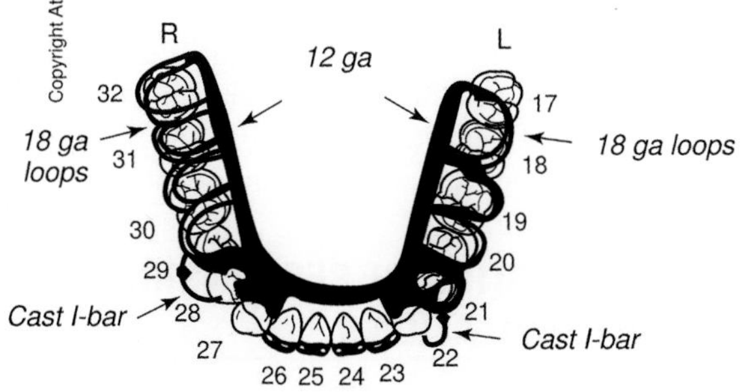

Design specifications:

1. Rests
   Cingulum rests #22, #27
   MO occlusal rest #20
   MO occlusal rest #28
2. Retention
   I-bar clasp #28
   I-bar clasp #22
3. Reciprocation
   Lingual plate #22, #27, #28
4. Major connector
   Lingual bar
5. Indirect retention
   Cingulum rest #22, #27
6. Guide planes
   Distal #20, #22, #27
   Mesial #20
7. Base retention
   18 ga. loops, 12 ga. inferior border
8. Areas to be modified or contoured
   Metal tooth to replace #21

Color code:

Blue: Cast metal
Red: Resin base and wrought wire
Green: Areas to be contoured

Instructor:__________

Approval to send to laboratory:__________ Date: *2/15/09*

Fig. 19.2 This work authorization accompanies a master cast on which the dentist has designed and drawn an outline for a removable partial denture framework. It is simple and is not time consuming to execute, yet it furnishes detailed information so the request can be properly fulfilled.

and placement of the artificial teeth and to the material from which they are made.

'A display of courtesy and a demonstration of respect for the laboratory technician are indicated. The general request is prefaced by "please," and the specific instructions end with "thank you."

A quality work authorization form not only ensures clarity but also simplifies correct execution. Figures can be provided on which diagrams may be drawn to enhance written descriptions when necessary and drawings on physical (duplicate or diagnostic) casts may be submitted as well to give instruction on the exact intended dimensions and extensions of the metal framework and other components (Fig. 19.3).

A color-code index can be used to explain the markings on the master cast when it is submitted to the laboratory for the fabrication of a framework. For example, a green pencil can be used to outline the framework, red to designate the desired location of finishing lines on the framework, and black to denote the height of contour on teeth and soft tissue created during the survey of the cast. The color code

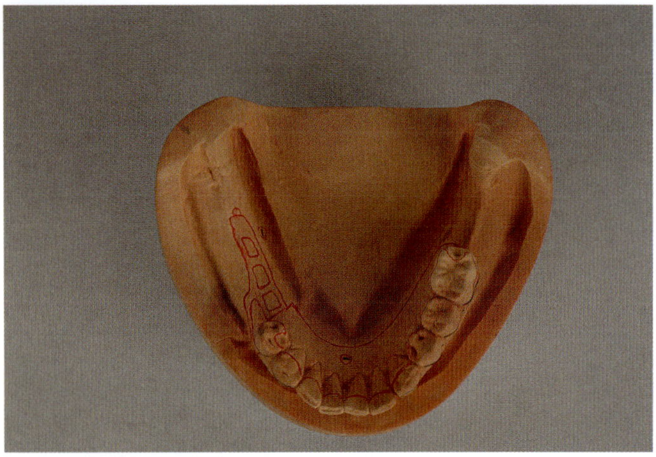

Fig. 19.3 The completed design on a master cast. (Courtesy of Ahmed Mahrous Copyright © 2024. All rights reserved.)

eliminates confusion in interpreting the markings on the master cast.

DIGITAL WORK AUTHORIZATIONS

Digital work authorizations offer advantages such as bypassing physical pickup or delivery to the laboratory, reducing risk of breakage of casts and damage to impressions during transit, and increasing overall efficiency. All the requirements of a good work authorization must exist in the digital work authorization as well; however, special consideration needs to be given to how sufficient instruction can be sent to the laboratory through a digital portal. Many modern laboratories will have their own digital portal for filling out digital lab authorizations, and there are more universal digital laboratory portals that specialize in sending to a variety of laboratories (Fig. 19.4). It is important that the laboratory system is cybersecured related to patient health information and meets the necessary regulatory controls and guidelines for transfer of patient information. All systems usually operate in a similar manner; they allow the input of patient information, followed by a specific work request, a space for specific written instructions, and a method to upload relevant files. The layout of most digital work authorizations will provide different drop-down menus depending on the type of work authorization ordered, for example, allowing a space to input the shade and type of prosthetic tooth to be used if processing of a final removable partial denture is selected as the work request. One of the most critical components of digital work authorization is the process of uploading relevant information to the work authorization. An ideal digital work authorization would be accompanied by the following items (Fig. 19.5):

- The digital scan, usually in an .stl format (see Fig. 19.5, *A*).
- A depiction of the design of the framework. This can be a scan of a hand-drawn design or a digitally made design (see Fig. 19.5, *B*).
- A design cast, which could be an image of a physical drawing, but ideally would be a colored digital model (see Fig. 19.5, *C*).

LEGAL ASPECTS OF WORK AUTHORIZATIONS

Although the National Association of Dental Laboratories (NADL) provides guidelines for statutory regulation, it is the inherent right of each state to implement its own regulation. Fortunately, all states exercise this control. Interpretations of acts that constitute the practice of dentistry are moderately uniform. However, statutory restrictions on dental laboratory operations vary from state to state. Properly executed work authorizations serve to document communication and protect the professional relationship between the dentist and the dental laboratory.

Many states require that work authorizations be made in duplicate and that both the dentist and the dental laboratory technician retain a copy for a specified period from the date of work authorization. Thus documents are available to substantiate or refute claims and counterclaims that concern the illegal practice of dentistry or to aid in the settlement of misunderstandings between a dentist and a dental laboratory technician.

DELINEATION OF RESPONSIBILITIES BY WORK AUTHORIZATIONS

The dentist is responsible for all phases of a removable partial denture service in the strict sense of the word, although the dental laboratory technician may be requested to perform certain technical phases of the service. However, the laboratory technician is responsible only to the dentist and never to the patient. A dentist who relegates the design of a removable partial denture to a less qualified individual accepts the possibility of and responsibility for an inferior removable partial denture service.

A dentist may delegate much of the laboratory phase of a removable partial denture service. Work authorizations help fulfill the moral obligation to supervise and direct those technical phases that can be accomplished by dental laboratory technicians. Substantial indications suggest that many members of the dental profession either are not cognizant of the rewards of writing good work authorizations or are not proficient in their execution. It is not a secret that some dentists do not submit instructions when availing themselves of commercial dental laboratory services.

If the practice of prosthodontics is to remain in the control of dentists, each member of the dental profession must avoid delegating responsibility to those who are less qualified to accept the responsibility.

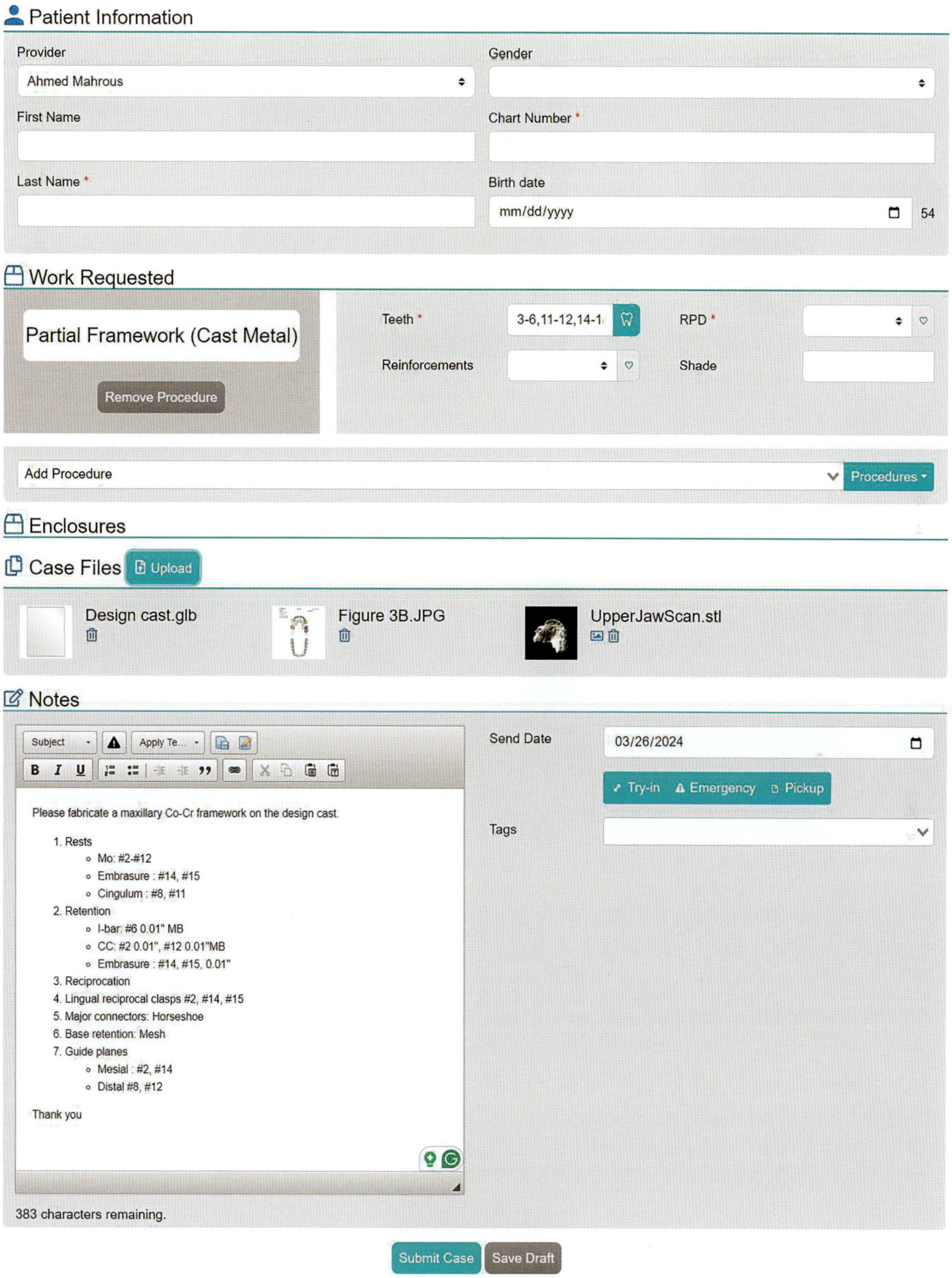

Patient Information

Provider: Ahmed Mahrous

Gender:

First Name:

Chart Number *

Last Name *

Birth date: mm/dd/yyyy 54

Work Requested

Partial Framework (Cast Metal)

Remove Procedure

Teeth *: 3-6,11-12,14-1

RPD *

Reinforcements

Shade

Add Procedure | Procedures

Enclosures

Case Files | Upload

Design cast.glb

Figure 3B.JPG

UpperJawScan.stl

Notes

Subject | Apply Te...

Please fabricate a maxillary Co-Cr framework on the design cast.

1. Rests
   - Mo: #2-#12
   - Embrasure : #14, #15
   - Cingulum : #8, #11
2. Retention
   - I-bar: #6 0.01" MB
   - CC: #2 0.01", #12 0.01"MB
   - Embrasure : #14, #15, 0.01"
3. Reciprocation
4. Lingual reciprocal clasps #2, #14, #15
5. Major connectors: Horseshoe
6. Base retention: Mesh
7. Guide planes
   - Mesial : #2, #14
   - Distal #8, #12

Thank you

383 characters remaining.

Send Date: 03/26/2024

Try-in | Emergency | Pickup

Tags

Submit Case | Save Draft

Fig. 19.4 A digital lab authorization completed for the fabrication of a removable partial denture framework attached to the lab authorization is the .stl of the preparation arch, the design created using an automatic designer, and a design cast with a virtual drawing. (Courtesy of Ahmed Mahrous)

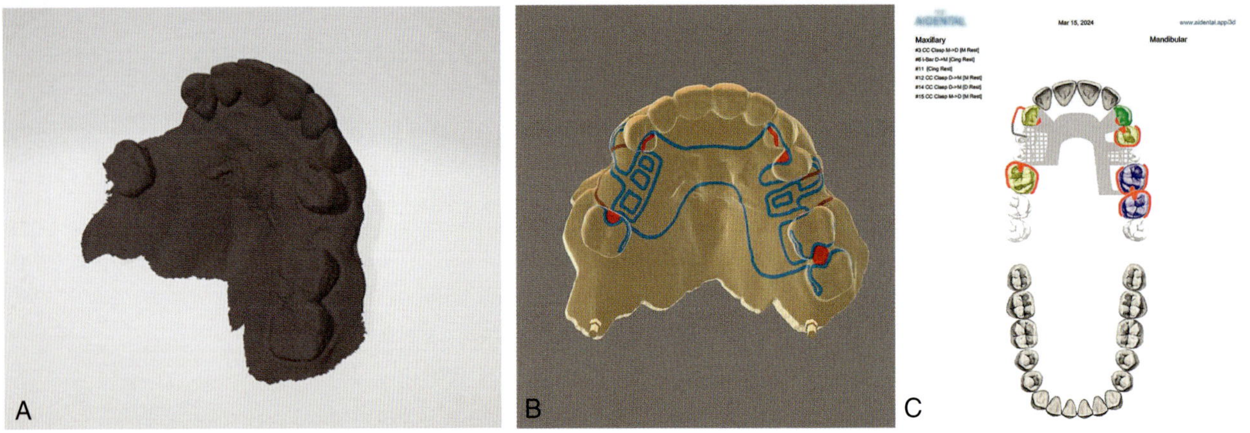

Fig. 19.5 The attachments used as part of a digital lab authorization include **(A)** the .stl of the final scan, **(B)** the design cast with a drawn design, and **(C)** the design diagram PDF designed through an automated design software. (Courtesy of Ahmed Mahrous Copyright © 2024. All rights reserved.)

20

Laboratory Procedures

Ahmed Mahrous, Heba Elkassaby, Craig Joseph Holland, Matt Tait, and Leila Jahangiri

CHAPTER OUTLINE

Dental laboratory procedures utilized in the fabrication of a removable partial denture (RPD) prosthesis are presented. Detailed information regarding laboratory procedures relative to making fixed restorations and removable complete dentures is available through multiple references. Knowledge of the principles and techniques for mounting casts, articulating teeth, waxing, processing, and polishing complete dentures is a necessary background for the laboratory phases of RPD fabrication. Digital technology has revolutionized the manufacture of dental prostheses, so different digital techniques that have been developed to design and fabricate RPDs are described as well.

ANALOG LABORATORY PROCEDURES

Blocking out the Master Cast

After the path of insertion and the location of undercut areas have been established on the master cast, any undercut areas that will be crossed by rigid components of the RPD (which includes every part of the framework but the retentive clasp terminals) must be eliminated by blockout.

In the broader sense of the term, *blockout* includes areas crossed by the RPD framework during seating and removal. *Blockout* also includes areas on the cast not involved in the denture design that are blocked out for convenience, ledges on which prefabricated clasp patterns are to be placed, relief beneath connectors to avoid soft tissue impingement, and relief to allow for attachment of the denture base to the framework.

Ledges or shelves (shaped blockout) for locating clasp patterns may or may not be used (Fig. 20.1). However, this should not be confused with the actual blocking out of undercut areas that would interfere with placement of the RPD framework. Only the latter is made on a surveyor, with the surveyor blade or diagnostic stylus used as a paralleling device.

Hard inlay wax may be used satisfactorily as a blockout material. It is easily applied and is easily trimmed with the

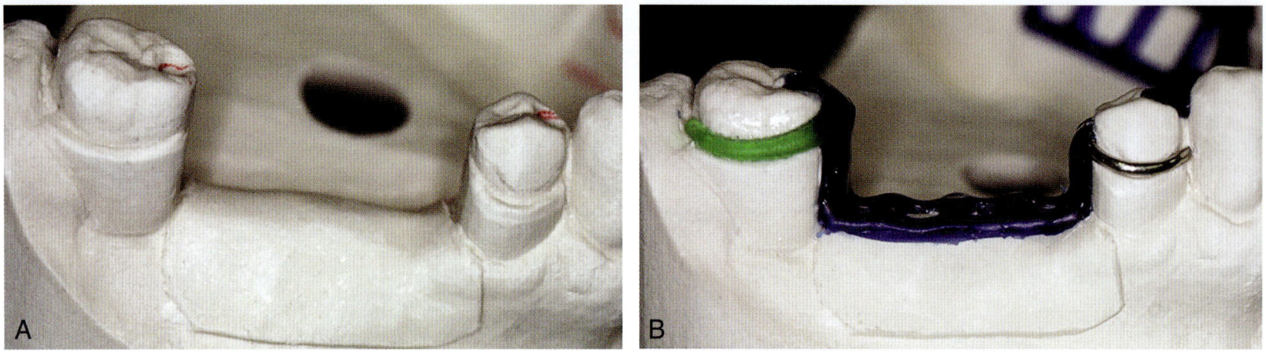

Fig. 20.1 TA, The wax ledge on the buccal surface of the molar abutment will be duplicated in a refractory cast **A** for for exact placement of the clasp pattern **B**. Note that the ledge has been carved slightly below the penciled outline of the clasp arm. This allows the gingival edge of the clasp arm to be polished and still remain in its planned relationship to the tooth when the denture is seated. It should also be noted that the wax ledge definitively establishes planned placement of the direct retainer tip into the measured undercut.

surveyor blade. Trimming is facilitated by a slight warming of the surveyor blade with an alcohol torch. Whereas it is true that any wax will melt more readily than a wax-clay mixture if the temperature of the duplicating material is too high, it should be presumed that the duplicating material will not be used at such an elevated temperature. If the temperature of the duplicating material is high enough to damage a wax blockout, other distortions resulting in an inaccurate duplication will likely occur.

Paralleled blockout is necessary for areas that are cervical to guide plane surfaces and over all undercut areas that will be crossed by major or minor connectors. Other areas that are to be blocked out for convenience and for the avoidance of difficulties in duplication should be blocked out with hard baseplate wax or oil-base modeling clay (artist's modeling clay). Such areas include the labial surfaces and labial undercuts not involved in the denture design and the sublingual and distolingual areas beyond the limits of the denture design. These are blocked out arbitrarily with hard baseplate wax or clay, but because they have no relation to the path of insertion, they do not require the use of the surveyor. Modeling clay that is water soluble should not be used when duplication procedures are involved.

Areas to be crossed by rigid connectors should be trimmed with the surveyor blade or some other surveyor tool parallel to the path of insertion (Fig. 20.2). This imposes a considerable responsibility on the technician. If the blockout is not sufficiently trimmed to expose guide plane surfaces, the effects of these guide planes, which were carefully established by the dentist, will be nullified. At times, paralleling the blockout can abrade the stone cast by heavy contact with the surveyor blade. Although the resulting cast framework would seat onto the master cast without interference, an interference along the guide plane to placement in the mouth would result. If this results, it would necessitate relieving the framework casting chairside, which is a time-consuming operation and one that may have the additional effect of obliterating guide plane surfaces.

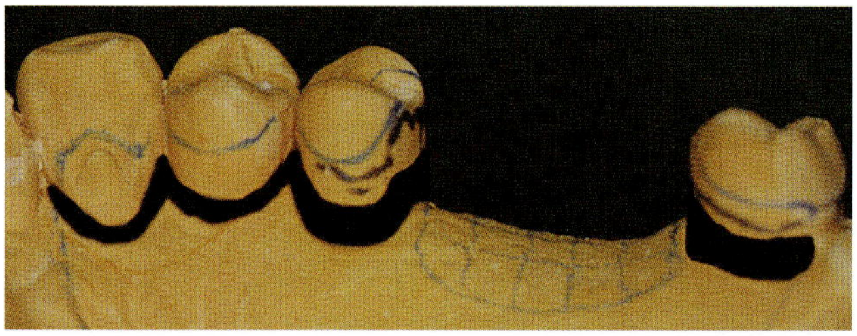

Fig. 20.2 All guide plane areas must be parallel to the path of placement, and all other areas that will be contacted by rigid parts of the denture framework must be made free of the undercut by parallel blockout. Relief must also be provided for the gingival crevice and gingival margin. *Black regions* designate parallel blockout at proximal guide plane surfaces and relief along the palatal marginal gingiva.

Relieving the Master Cast

Tissue undercuts that must be blocked out are paralleled in much the same manner as tooth undercuts. The difference between blockout and relief must be clearly understood (Figs. 20.3 and 20.4). For example, tissue undercuts that would offer interference to the seating of a lingual bar connector are blocked out with blockout wax and trimmed parallel to the path of insertion. This does not in itself necessarily afford relief to avoid tissue impingement. In addition to such blockout, a relief of varying thickness must sometimes be used, depending on the location of the connector, the relative slope of the alveolar ridge, and the predictable effect of denture rotation. It must be assumed that indirect retainers, as such, or indirect retention is provided in the design of the denture to prevent rotation of the lingual bar inferiorly. A vertical downward rotation of the denture bases around posterior abutments places the bar increasingly farther from the lingual aspect of the alveolar ridge when this surface slopes inferiorly and posteriorly (Fig. 20.5). Adequate relief of soft tissues adjacent to the lingual bar is obtained by the initial finishing and polishing of the framework in these instances. However, excessive upward vertical rotation of a lingual bar will impinge on lingual tissues if the alveolar ridge is nearly vertical or undercut to the path of insertion (Fig. 20.6). The region of the cast involving the proposed placement of the lingual bar should, in this situation, be relieved first by parallel blockout and then by a 32-gauge wax strip. Low-fusing casting wax (such as green casting wax) should not be used for this purpose; it is too easily thinned during adapting and may be affected by the temperature of the duplicating material. A pressure-sensitive, adhesive-coated casting wax is preferred because it adapts readily and adheres to the cast surface. Any wax, even the adhesive type, should be sealed all around its borders with

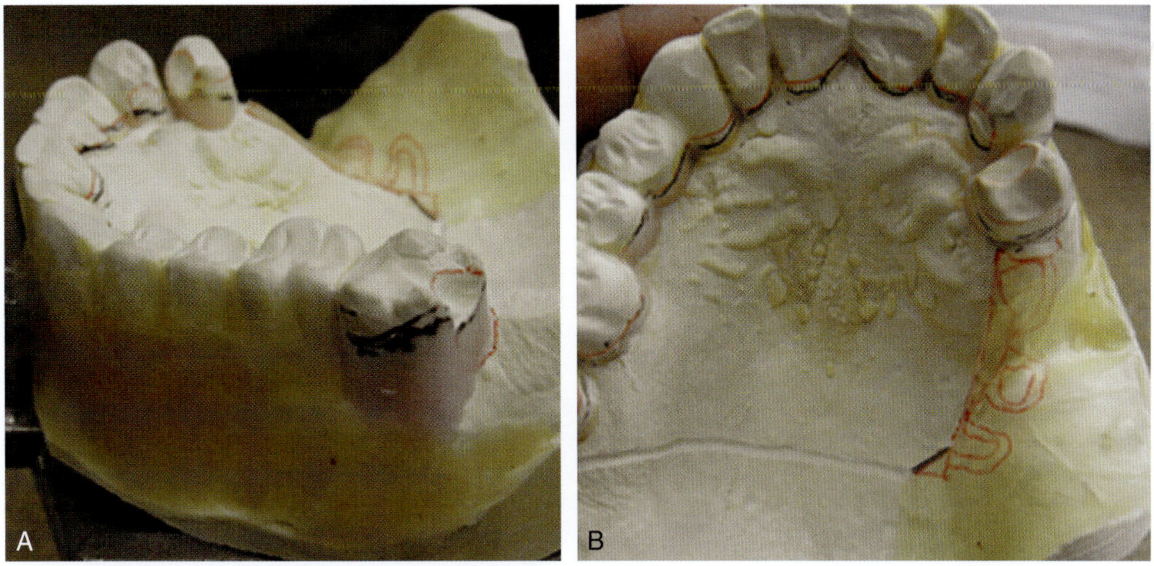

Fig. 20.3 Parallel blockout. **A,** Labial surfaces of all teeth and gingivae to the retentive clasp on tooth #2. **B,** Relief at marginal gingivae of palatal surfaces of teeth and at distal minor connector in preparation for framework casting. These spaces allow planned seating of the framework without tissue trauma while accommodating the addition of acrylic resin beneath the distal extension minor connector for base support without metal contact.

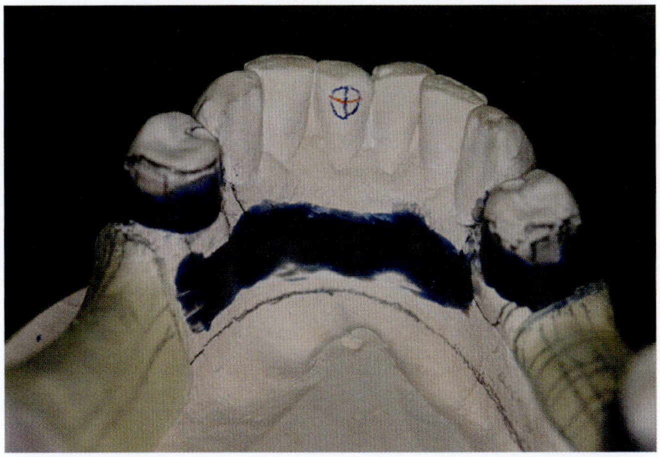

Fig. 20.4 Relief and blockout of the master cast before duplication. All undercuts involved in the denture design have been blocked out with blue wax parallel to the path of placement, except the retentive tips of the retainer clasps. Residual ridges have been provided 20-gauge relief for denture base material.

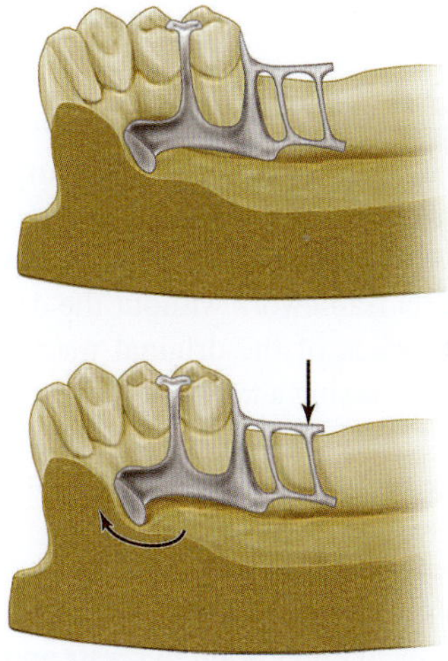

Fig. 20.5 Sagittal section of the cast and denture framework. The lingual alveolar ridge slopes inferiorly and posteriorly *(upper figure)*. When the force is directed to displace the denture base downward, the lingual bar rotates forward and upward but does not impinge on the soft tissue of the alveolar ridge *(lower figure)*. Therefore in such instances, adequate relief to avoid impingement is gained when the tissue side of the lingual bar is highly polished during the finishing process.

a hot spatula to prevent its lifting when the cast is moistened before or during duplication.

The tendency of a mandibular distal extension RPD for horizontal rotation may account for tissue irritation seen adjacent to a lingual mandibular major connector. These soft tissue irritations can usually be avoided by blocking out all undercuts adjacent to the bar parallel to the path of insertion and then including adequate stabilizing components in the design of the framework to resist horizontal rotation. Judicious relief of the tissue side of the lingual bar with rubber wheels at the site of irritation most often corrects the discrepancy. Under no circumstances should the rigidity of the major connector be jeopardized by grinding any portion of it.

Still, other areas requiring relief are the areas where component parts cross the gingiva and gingival crevices. All gingival areas bridged by the denture framework should be protected from impingement resulting from the rotation of the denture framework. Hard inlay wax may be used to block out gingival crevices.

Paralleled Blockout, Shaped Blockout, Arbitrary Blockout, and Relief

Table 20.1 differentiates between paralleled blockout, shaped blockout, arbitrary blockout, and relief. The same factors apply to both maxillary and mandibular arches, except that relief is ordinarily not used beneath palatal major connectors, as it is with mandibular lingual bar connectors, except when maxillary tori cannot be circumvented or when resistive median palatal raphes are encountered.

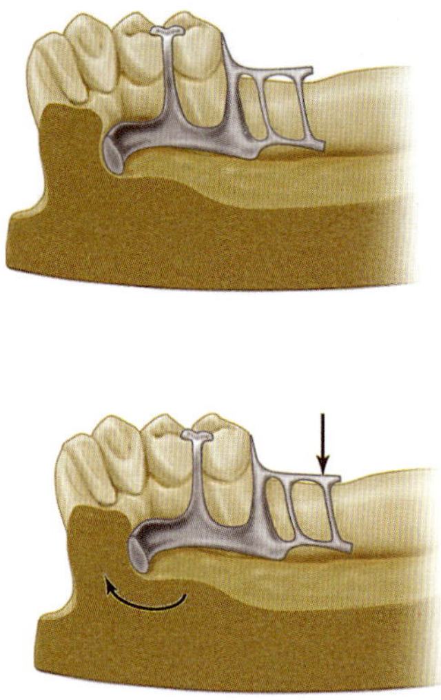

Fig. 20.6 An undercut alveolar ridge was blocked out parallel to the path of placement in fabricating the lingual bar *(upper figure)*. Application of vertical force to cause rotation of the lingual bar upward can cause impingement of lingual tissue on the alveolar ridge *(lower figure)*. To avoid impingement in these instances, not only should the master cast be blocked out parallel to the path of placement, but an additional relief of 32-gauge sheet wax should be used to block out the cast in such undercut areas.

DUPLICATING A STONE CAST

A stone cast can be duplicated for several purposes. One purpose is the duplication in stone of the original or corrected master cast to preserve the original. A second purpose of such a cast is for fitting an RPD framework without the danger of fracture or abrading the surface of the original master cast. Another use might be for processing a temporary prosthesis, where wax relief and blockout on the original cast allow the production of a duplicate, which, following processing, will make insertion of the prosthesis easier.

Another purpose of duplicating a cast is to create an investment cast used in framework fabrication. Careful preparation of the master cast prior to duplication to create an investment cast involves consideration of the defined path of insertion, heights of contour, and retentive and stabilization areas designed into the mouth preparations. The framework produced should be carefully evaluated on the cast for fit (Fig. 20.7).

Blockout should be accomplished on the master cast before an investment cast is made. On this investment cast, the wax or plastic pattern is formed. The use of preformed plastic patterns eliminates some of the danger of damaging the surface of the investment cast in the process of forming the pattern. With freehand waxing, considerable care must be taken not to score or abrade the investment cast. The metal framework is ultimately cast against its surface, and the finished casting and the original cast are then returned to the dentist after all fitting has been completed on the duplicate cast.

Duplicating Materials and Flasks

Duplicating materials include both colloidal and silicone materials. Colloidal materials are made fluid by heating and return to a gel while cooling. The cast to be duplicated must

TABLE 20.1 Differentiation Between Parallel Blockout, Shaped Blockout, Arbitrary Blockout, and Relief

Site	Material	Thickness
Parallel Blockout		
Proximal tooth surfaces to be used as guiding planes	Hard baseplate wax or blockout material	Only undercut remaining below contact of the surveyor blade with tooth surface
Beneath all minor connectors	Hard baseplate wax or blockout material	Only undercut remaining below contact of the surveyor blade with tooth surface
Tissue undercuts to be crossed by rigid connectors	Hard baseplate wax or blockout material	Only undercut remaining below contact of the surveyor blade with surface of the cast
Tissue undercuts to be crossed by the origin of bar clasps	Hard baseplate wax or blockout material	Only undercut remaining below contact of the surveyor blade with surface of the cast
Deep interproximal spaces to be covered by minor connectors or lingual plates	Hard baseplate wax or blockout material	Only undercut remaining below contact of the surveyor blade with surface of the cast
Beneath bar clasp arms to gingival crevice	Hard baseplate wax or blockout material	Only undercut area involved in attachment of the clasp arm to the minor connector
Shaped Blockout		
On buccal and lingual surfaces to locate plastic or wax patterns for clasp arms	Hard baseplate wax	Ledges for location of reciprocal clasp arms to follow height or convexity so that they may be placed as cervical as possible without becoming retentive
		Ledges for location of retentive clasp arms to be placed as cervical as tooth contour permits; point of origin of clasp to be occlusal or incisal to height of the convexity, crossing the survey line at fourth terminal, and to include undercut area previously selected in keeping with flexibility of the clasp type being used
Arbitrary Blockout		
All gingival crevices	Hard baseplate wax	Enough to just eliminate gingival crevice
Gross tissue undercuts situated below areas involved in the design of denture framework	Hard baseplate wax or oil-based clay	Leveled arbitrarily with a wax spatula

TABLE 20.1 Differentiation Between Parallel Blockout, Shaped Blockout, Arbitrary Blockout, and Relief—cont'd

Site	Material	Thickness
Tissue undercuts distal to the cast framework	Hard baseplate wax or oil-based clay	Smoothed arbitrarily with a wax spatula
Labial and buccal tooth and tissue undercuts not involved in denture design	Hard baseplate wax or oil-based clay	Filled and tapered with spatula to within the coronal third of the crown
Relief		
Beneath lingual bar connectors or the bar portion of the lingual plates when indicated (see text)	Adhesive wax sealed to the cast; should be wider than the major connector to be placed on it	32-gauge wax if the slope of the lingual alveolar ridge is parallel to the path of insertion; 32-gauge wax after parallel blockout of undercuts if the slope of the lingual alveolar ridge is undercut to the path of insertion
Areas in which major connectors will contact thin tissue, such as hard areas so frequently found on lingual of mandibular ridges and elevated palatal raphes	Hard baseplate wax	Thin layer flowed on with hot wax spatula; however, if the maxillary torus must be covered, the thickness of the relief must represent the difference in the degree of displacement of the tissues covering the torus and the tissues covering the residual ridges
Beneath framework extensions onto ridge areas for attachment of resin bases	Adhesive wax, well adapted to and sealed to the cast beyond the involved area	20-gauge wax

be placed in the bottom of a suitable flask, called a *duplicating flask*. A duplicating flask should contain the fluid material to facilitate its cooling, to support the mold while it is being filled with the cast material, and to facilitate the removal of the cast from the mold without permanent deformation or damage to the mold. Numerous duplicating flasks are available on the market.

The technique for duplicating is the same for any cast, whether or not blockout is present. However, if wax or clay blockout is present, the temperature of the duplicating material must not be any higher than that recommended by the manufacturer, to prevent melting and distortion of the blockout material.

Ordinary baseplate wax can be used for paralleled blockout and ledges, but care must be taken to avoid overheating the duplicating material to avoid melting the wax. The use of the prepared blockout material, such as Ney blockout wax, is preferred.

Duplicating Procedure

The equipment needed and the steps required for duplication using a silicone material are described in Figs. 20.8 through 20.12.

WAXING THE REMOVABLE PARTIAL DENTURE FRAMEWORK

When preformed plastic patterns are used (Fig. 20.13), parts of the denture framework must be waxed freehand to prevent excessive bulk and to create the desired contours for a satisfactory custom-made RPD framework (Fig. 20.14).

Although most dentists do not fabricate their own RPD castings, it is essential that they understand the dental laboratory procedures involved. This enables them to design the RPD framework, complete a laboratory work authorization that communicates the desired design and authorizes its fabrication, and evaluate the quality of the framework (Fig. 20.15). Understanding and evaluation of the key features required in a completed RPD framework ensures the patient of a chance to function comfortably with the finished product (Fig. 20.16). The contrary is also true.

Forming the Wax Pattern for a Mandibular Class II Removable Partial Denture Framework

Examples that illustrate many of the essentials of waxing an RPD framework are presented in Figs. 20.17 through 20.26. This exercise includes the waxing of three types of direct retainers (circumferential, combination, and bar type), a mandibular lingual bar major connector, a maxillary anterior-posterior palatal strap major connector, both distal extension and tooth-bound modification spaces, and adaptation of round, 18-gauge, wrought-wire retentive arms for combination-type direct retainers.

Attaching Wrought-Wire Retainer Arms by Soldering

Wrought-wire retainers may be attached to an RPD framework after it has been cast and finished (Figs. 20.27 and 20.28). The soldering procedure may be accomplished by electric soldering or by a direct-heat method with an oxygen-gas flame. With either method, care must be taken to use compatible alloys, appropriate solders, and flux in conjunction with the careful application of controlled heat.

Readers are encouraged to review the Chapter 12 discussion of the selection of metal alloys to enhance their understanding of the properties of solder, flux, the effects of heat on metal alloys, and the necessity for quality control in soldering procedures.

Waxing Metal Bases

A technique for forming the retentive framework for the attachment of acrylic resin bases has been given. Two basic types of metal bases may be used instead of the resin base. The

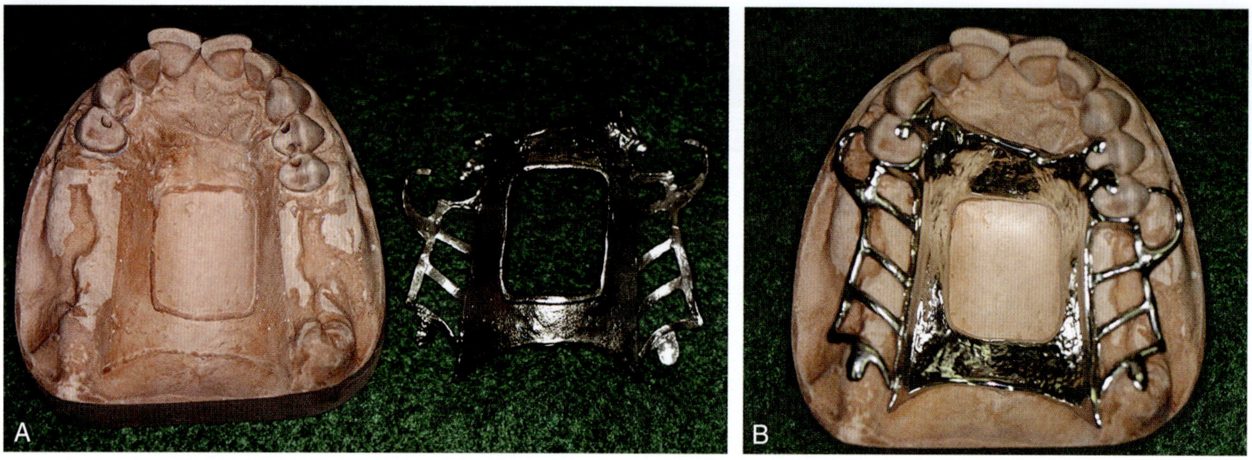

Fig. 20.7 **A,** Framework returned from the laboratory with the master cast. **B,** Replacement on the cast reveals areas of contact that can erode the cast surface. Careful fitting to the cast allows determination of potential framework adjustment regions before fitting in the mouth. If the framework is indiscriminately finished in the laboratory or before intraoral placement, critical tooth contact regions may be lost, resulting in a poorly retained and stabilized prosthesis. Most often, such an overly adjusted framework is poorly stabilized, not poorly retained.

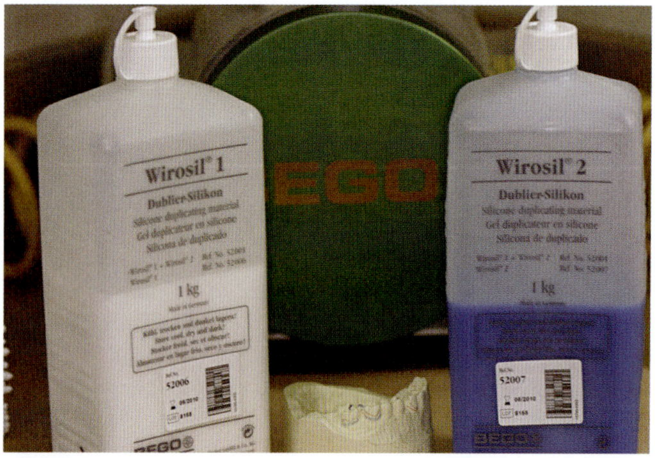

Fig. 20.8 Duplicating material with a vacuum curing unit in the background, which is used to ensure a dense mold.

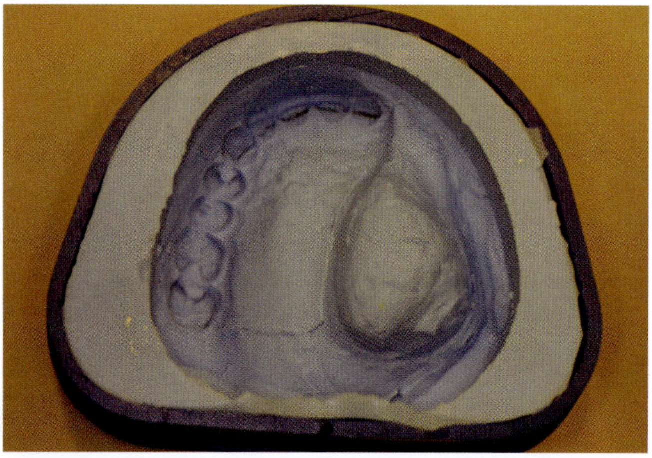

Fig. 20.9 Duplicating mold following removal of the relieved and blockout cast.

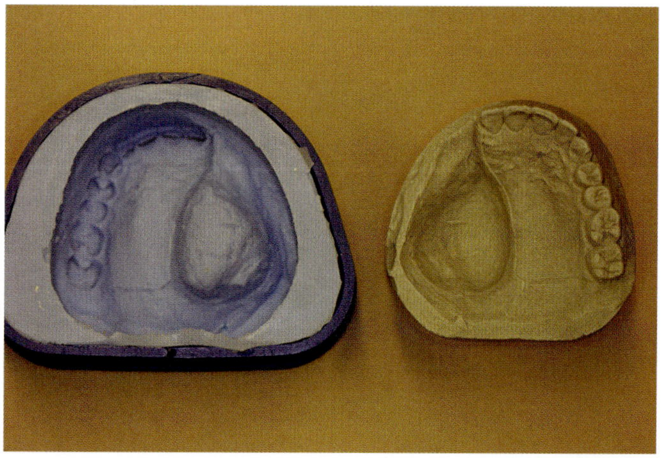

Fig. 20.10 Refractory cast *(right)* following removal from the duplication mold *(left)*. This cast incorporates all the features of the relieved and blockout master cast generated from the clinical framework impression.

advantages of cast metal bases in preference to acrylic resin bases have been discussed in Chapter 9. The type of base to be used must be determined before blockout and duplication so that the relief over each edentulous ridge may be provided or eliminated as required.

For an acrylic resin base, relief for the retentive framework must be provided. No relief over the residual ridge is used for a complete metal base. For a partial metal base, the junction between metal and acrylic resin must be clearly defined by trimming the relief along a definite, previously determined line.

One type of metal base is the complete base with a metal border to which tube teeth, cast copings, or an acrylic resin superstructure may be attached. Whether porcelain or acrylic tube teeth or grooved teeth are used, the prosthetic teeth must be positioned first, then the pattern is waxed around the teeth to form a coping. The teeth are then attached to the metal base by cementation or, with the use of resin teeth, are attached with additional acrylic resin under pressure, a so-called pressed-on method of attaching acrylic resin teeth to a metal base. Another method of attaching teeth is to wax the base to form a coping for each tooth, either by carving recesses in the wax or by waxing around artificial teeth. Rather than attaching a stock tooth,

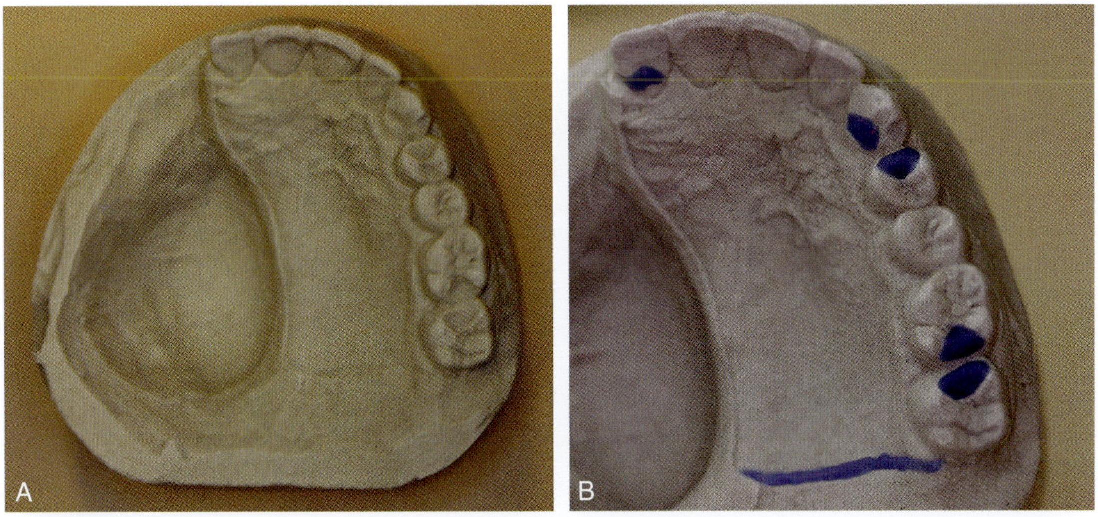

Fig. 20.11 **A,** Close-up of the refractory cast. **B,** Initial wax added to rests and the posterior bead line of the refractory cast.

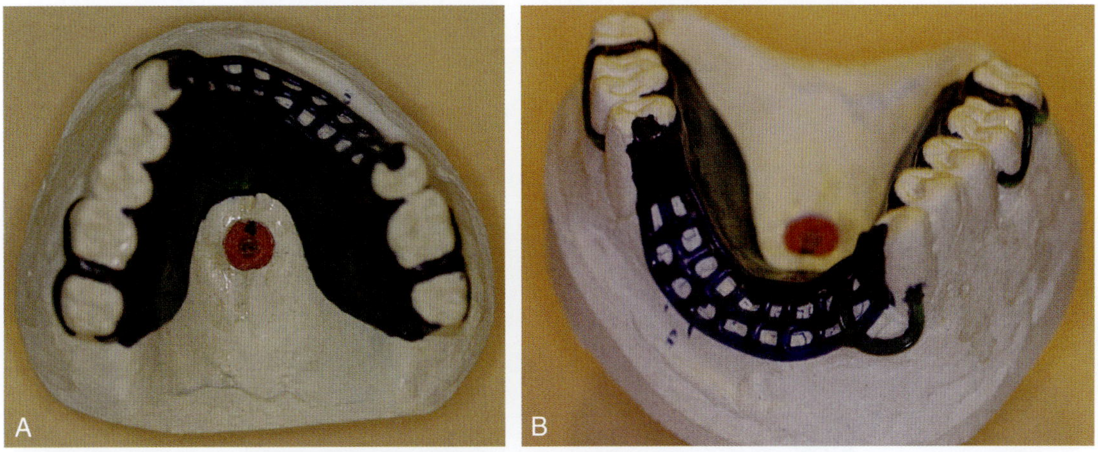

Fig. 20.12 Example of a completed maxillary waxed framework on a refractory cast with the sprue access positioned. **A,** From occlusal. **B,** From anterior.

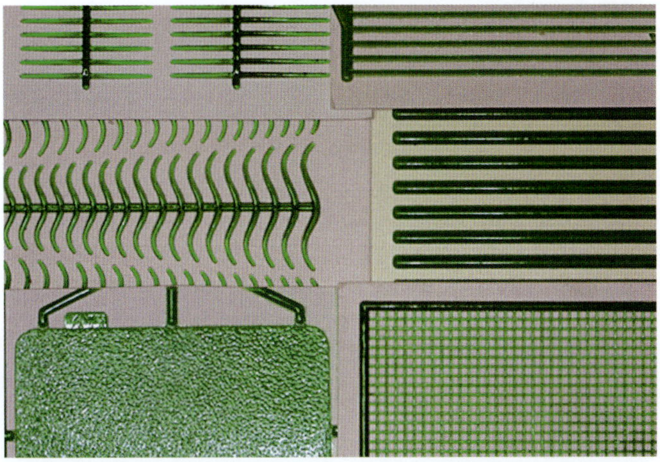

Fig. 20.13 Preformed plastic patterns are available in many shapes and sizes for clasps, for minor connectors connecting to teeth, or for distal extension bases, bars, mesh, and palatal coverage. Because they are made of soft plastic material, they tend to stretch on removal from their backing. Therefore care must be exercised when removing patterns. Their use generally requires that tacky liquid be applied first to the investment cast at their area of placement.

the full tooth may be waxed into occlusion, the base invested, and the wax patterns replaced with heat-polymerized acrylic resin. This method permits some variation in the dimension and form of the supplied teeth that is not possible with stock teeth. It is particularly applicable to abnormally long or short spaces or when a stock tooth of desired width is not available. With modern cross-linked acrylic resins, such processed teeth are durable; however, adding gold occlusal surfaces is an option.

When artificial teeth are to be arranged to occlude with an opposing cast or an opposing template, the metal base must be formed for attachment of the tissue-colored denture resin supporting the teeth. This is the most common method of attaching teeth to a metal base. The wax pattern for the base is formed from one thickness of 24-gauge casting wax, which is then reinforced at the border and forms the retention of the acrylic resin superstructure. Because metal borders are more difficult to adjust than acrylic resin, they are usually made somewhat short of the area normally covered with an acrylic resin base. Also, because border thickness adds objectionable weight to the denture, it is made with only a slight border roll. This is one

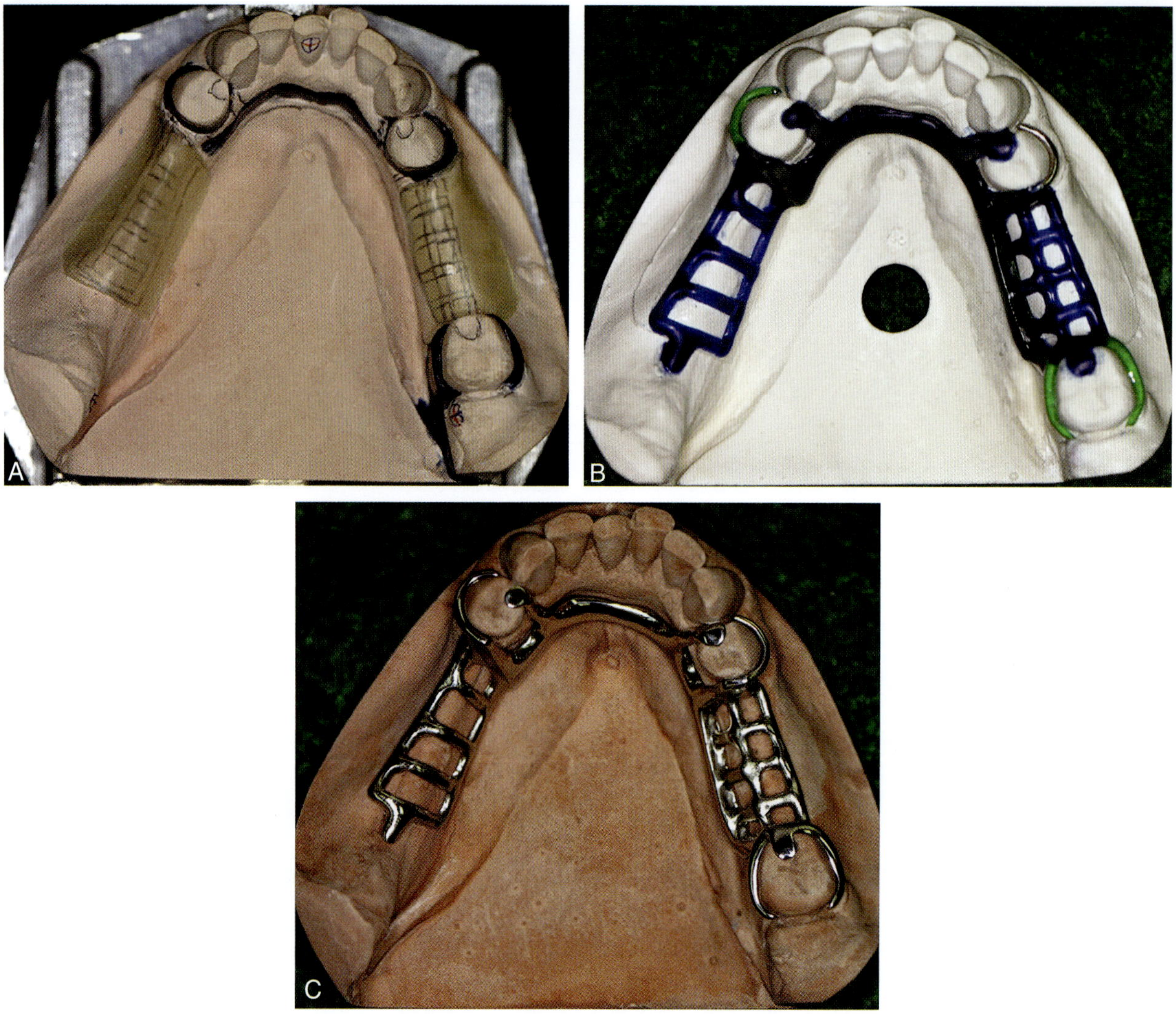

Fig. 20.14 Three steps are involved in making a denture framework by using relief, blockout ledges, and ready-made pattern forms. **A,** Master cast with relief, blockout of undercuts at posterior right and anterior lingual regions, and shaped blockout ledges for location of retentive and nonretentive clasp arms. **B,** Completed pattern using lingual bar major connector pattern, plastic clasp forms resting on investment ledges, wrought wire, and open retention mesh. **C,** Finished casting returned to master cast.

disadvantage of the complete metal base, because the border accuracy of the impression registration cannot be used to its fullest advantage and contouring of facial and lingual surfaces cannot be as effective as with an acrylic resin base, in which added bulk can sometimes be used to advantage.

The border is first penciled lightly on the investment cast, and then the 24-gauge sheet casting wax is smoothly adapted. Considerable care must be taken not to stretch and thin the sheet wax in adapting it to the cast. To prevent wrinkling, the wax should be adapted in at least two longitudinal pieces and joined and sealed together at the ridge crest. The wax is then trimmed along the penciled outline with a warm, dull instrument to prevent the scoring of the investment cast.

A single piece of 14-gauge round wax is adapted around the border over the sheet wax. With a hot spatula, the round wax must be sealed to the cast along its outer border. Sufficient wax is flowed onto the round wax to blend it smoothly into the sheet wax, thus completing a border roll. The inner half of the round wax form remains untouched. Wax is added when needed to facilitate carving without trimming the original 24-gauge thickness. The result should be a rounded border that blends smoothly into the sheet wax.

The boxing for the resin, which will in turn support the artificial teeth, is now added, again with 14-gauge round wax. The proposed outline for the boxing is identified by lightly scoring the sheet wax. On this scored line, the 14-gauge round wax is adapted, thus forming the outline of the boxing.

With additional wax, the ditch between the sheet wax and the outer border of the round wax is filled in and blended smoothly onto the sheet wax. This is done in the same manner as the border, with sufficient wax added to allow for smoothing and carving. As was mentioned previously, the pattern should not be flamed or polished with a cloth. Instead, the pattern must be smoothed by carving.

The result thus far should be a pattern reinforced at the border and at the boxing and slightly concave in between, with

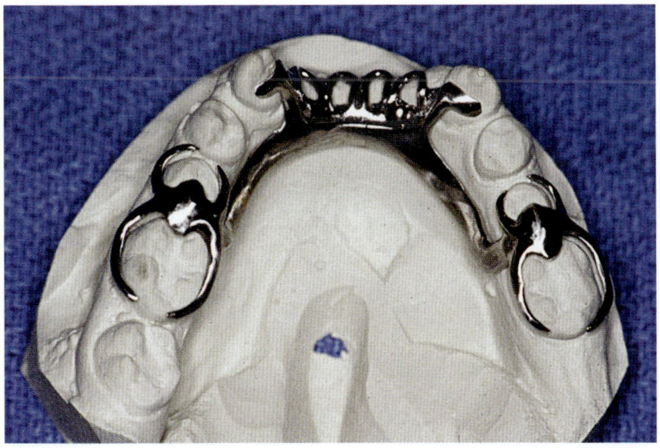

Fig. 20.15 Evaluation of the framework by the clinician is as important for removable partial denture frameworks as it is for implant and/or fixed partial denture castings. Careful scrutiny and attention to detail in following the design specifications are necessary, as is evaluation of the fit of the framework to the cast. On this cast, initial seating of the framework reveals interference with complete seating bilaterally from the embrasure clasps. Only minor adjustment should be required to completely seat the framework. If major adjustment is needed, or if after complete seating of the framework the clasp assemblies do not contact the teeth as prescribed, the framework should be remade.

some of the original sheet wax exposed. The inside of the boxing is not sealed to the sheet wax, thus leaving a slight undercut for the attachment of the acrylic resin. With a sharp blade, the margins of the boxing are then carved to a knife-edge finishing line. With the backside of the large end of the No. 7 wax spatula, this margin may be lifted slightly, further deepening the undercut beneath the finishing line.

In addition to the undercut finishing line, retention spurs, loops, or nail heads are added for retention of the acrylic resin to be added later. Spurs are usually made of 18-gauge or smaller round wax attached at one end only at random acute angles to the sheet wax. Loops are small-gauge round (wax, resin, or metal) circles attached vertically or horizontally with space beneath for the acrylic resin attachment. Nail heads are made of short pieces of 18-gauge round wax attached vertically to the sheet wax, with the head flattened by a slightly warmed spatula. Any method of providing retention is acceptable if it permits positive attachment of the acrylic resin and will not interfere with the placement of artificial teeth.

A metal base waxed as described provides optimum contours with a minimum of bulk and weight and with adequate provision for the attachment of artificial teeth to the metal base. If properly designed, the more visible portions of the metal base will be covered with the acrylic resin supporting the supplied teeth.

SPRUING, INVESTING, BURNOUT, CASTING, AND FINISHING OF THE REMOVABLE PARTIAL DENTURE FRAMEWORK

Factors that influence the quality of a dental casting are listed in Box 20.1.

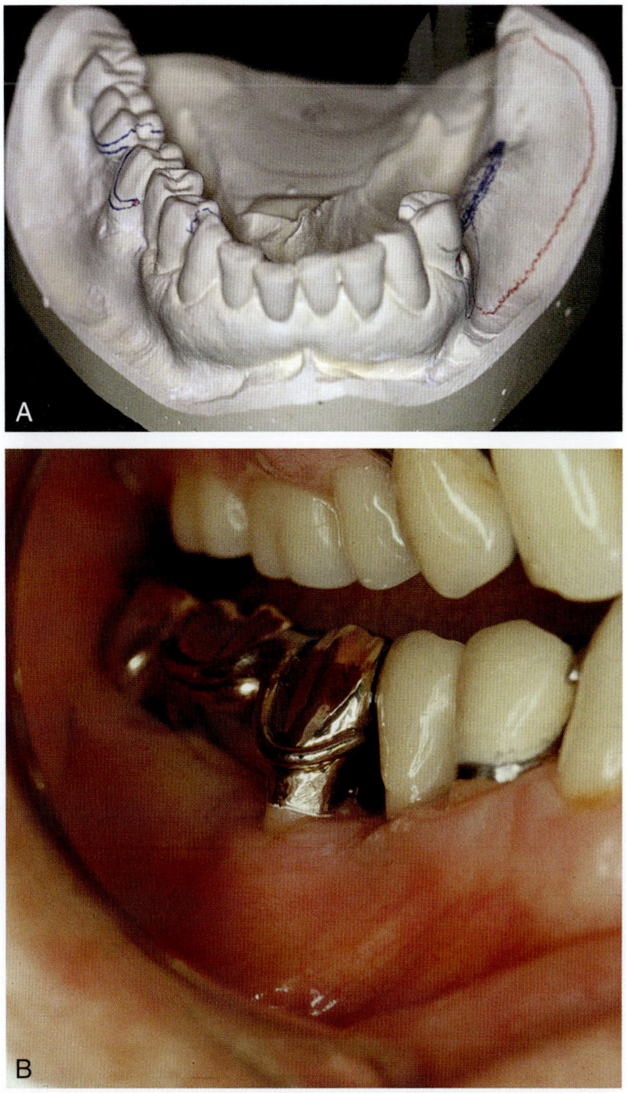

Fig. 20.16 **A,** Design of a mandibular removable partial denture framework is outlined on the master cast for the technician to follow in waxing and casting the framework. **B,** Cast framework as returned from the laboratory is evaluated intraorally, revealing sufficiently accurate adaptation and design identical to the embrasure clasp and mesio-occlusal rest #28, as shown on the design cast in **(A)**.

Spruing

As mentioned previously, familiarity with dental laboratory procedures used in fabricating fixed prostheses was presumed. This helps in understanding the use of a sprue and creating a sprue channel for traditional lab fabrication of an RPD cast framework. As a reminder, use of a sprue creates a channel into the cavity in which the framework is cast. The sprue channel allows molten metal to flow from the crucible into the mold cavity similar to a fixed casting using the lost-wax technique. In casting an RPD framework, the sprue should be large enough and shaped to allow molten alloy with the least amount of turbulence. A sprue allows for a reservoir of molten metal, from which the casting may draw during solidification, thus preventing porosity caused by shrinkage.

Spruing the wax pattern on a cast can be summarized with the following general principles:

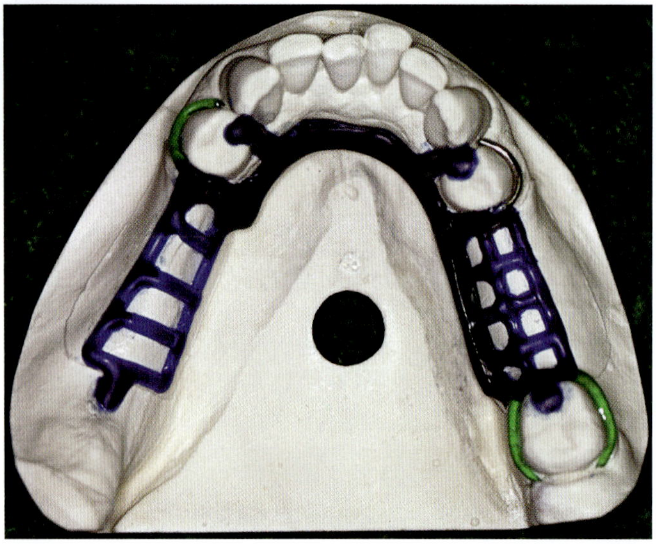

Fig. 20.17 Occlusal view of mandibular Kennedy Class I, modification 1 wax pattern on a refractory cast. The lingual bar major connector joins three clasp assemblies (rest, proximal plate, and Akers clasp, wrought wire, and cast circumferential).

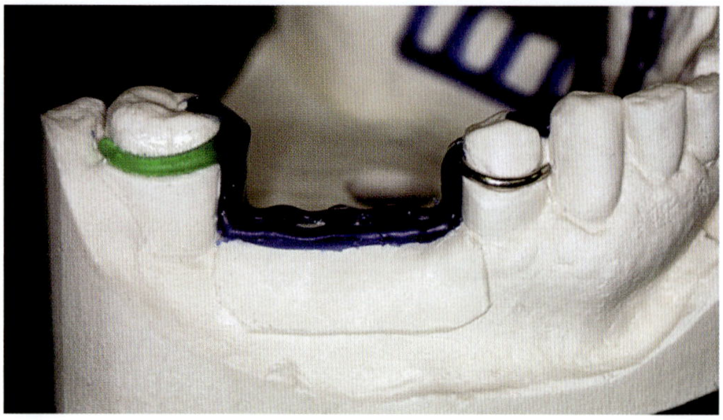

Fig. 20.19 Buccal view of modification space of the pattern shown in Fig. 20.17. A wrought-wire clasp is contoured at the anterior extent of the modification space. Such a retainer will not overly stress the tooth if opposite denture base movement causes rotation across the fulcrum (see Fig. 20.17, occlusal rests at #21 and #31). A tapered cast circumferential clasp follows the shaped ledge to a distal buccal 0.01-inch undercut. Both proximal plates have been waxed with sufficient bulk to provide a complete casting. If thickness presents a problem with tooth placement, some finishing can be done at a later time.

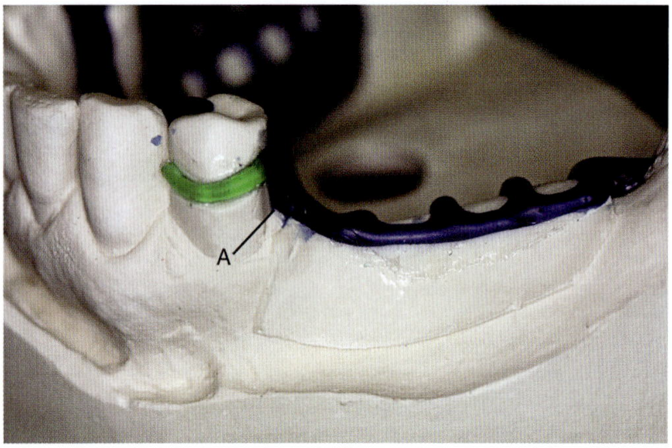

Fig. 20.18 Buccal view of the left side of the pattern shown in Fig. 20.17. A tapered retainer clasp pattern is placed on the refractory cast ledge produced by duplication of shaped blockout ledges. The cast illustrates relief provided beneath the minor connector, which retains the denture base resin. The tissue index at the gingival region of the proximal plate (*A*) will provide an easily identifiable finish line for resin finishing and future trimming of altered cast impression.

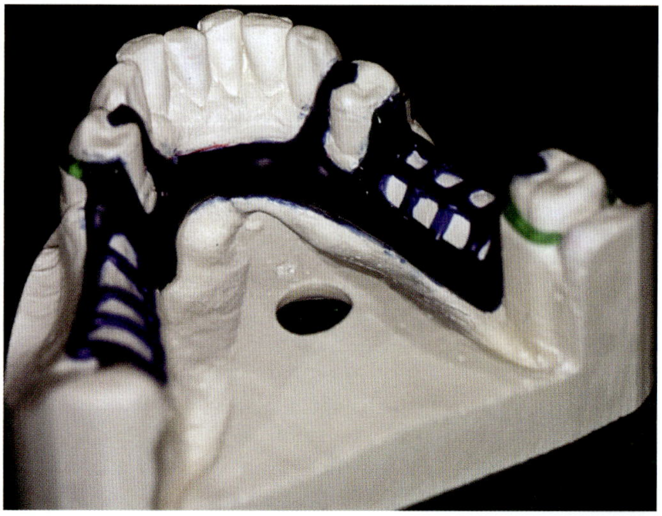

Fig. 20.20 Lingual view of the pattern shown in Fig. 20.17. The lingual bar major connector rigidly connects components cross-arch. The minor connector for resin retention on the left has buccal and lingual struts to allow unimpeded tooth placement. The tapered proximal plate on the right (tooth #28) is thicker on the lingual and thinner on the buccal, to allow close placement of the buccal surface of the denture tooth to #28. The finish line of the modification space is positioned below adjacent tooth-gingival margins to allow normal lingual contouring of the resin matrix.

1. Sprues should be large enough such that the molten metal reservoir does not solidify initially but rather until after the molten alloy in the casting proper has set (8- to 12-gauge round wax is usually used for multiple sprues in RPD framework castings).
2. Sprue design should be made as a smooth channel configuration to minimize turbulence in the stream of molten alloy.
3. Sprues are designed to exit from a common point and attached to the bulkier sections of the wax pattern; it is important to avoid attaching sprues, leaving thin sections of casting between two bulky, unsprued portions.

The configuration of the sprues, from their point of attachment at the crucible until they reach the mold cavity, may be influential in reducing turbulence. One possible complication in casting is the entrapment of gases in the mold cavity without allowing gases to escape. If the sprue channels contain sharp right-angle turns, turbulence during flow of molten alloy is induced, which can entrap such gases and result in faulty castings. Sprue channels should be designed with smooth, long curves from a direction designed to prevent turbulence or "splashing" at this point.

As was previously stated, the sprues should be attached to the bulky points of the mold pattern. If two bulky points exist with a thin section between them, each of the bulky spots should be

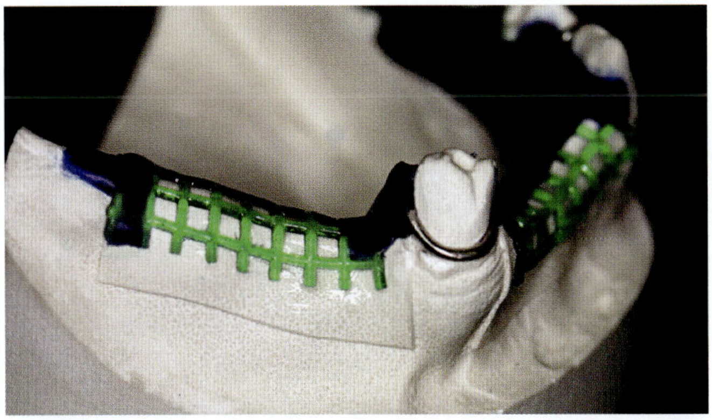

Fig. 20.21 Another example of a wax pattern for a mandibular framework. A wrought wire has been adapted to tooth #27. The clasp demonstrates an appropriate circlet shape, allowing maximum length. The circlet shape also allows the undercut to be approached from below; this improves retention—push retention is more efficient than pull retention. Ridge relief is evident beneath the resin minor connector, and the proximal plate housing the wire has been waxed with bulk to facilitate casting. The plate may require adjustment at a later time.

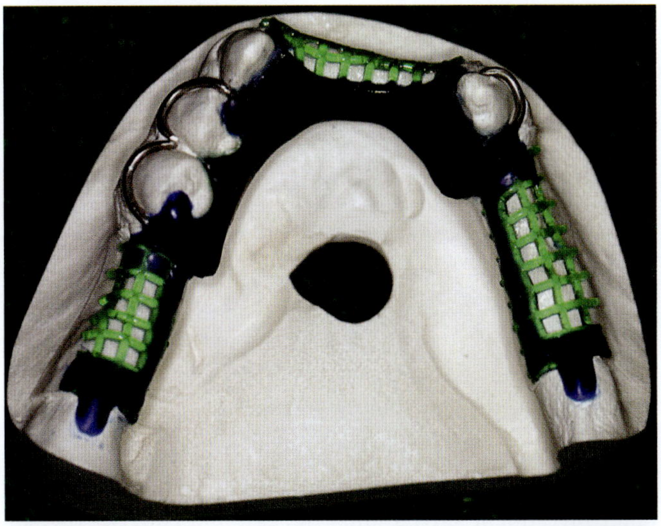

Fig. 20.22 Same pattern as shown in Fig. 20.21. Includes a lingual plate major connector design. The external finishing line at the anterior modification space is lingual to the anticipated tooth and resin position, allowing a natural contour to be developed in the completed prosthesis. The posterior denture base minor connector patterns have been reinforced with additional wax to add stiffness at the junction with the proximal plate and major connector. Because of the potential for repeated flexure in this region under function, such reinforcement is critical to long-term success with patterns such as this. Because the wrought-wire retainers are not cast, it is important that they be contoured to contact the teeth as accurately as possible, as shown.

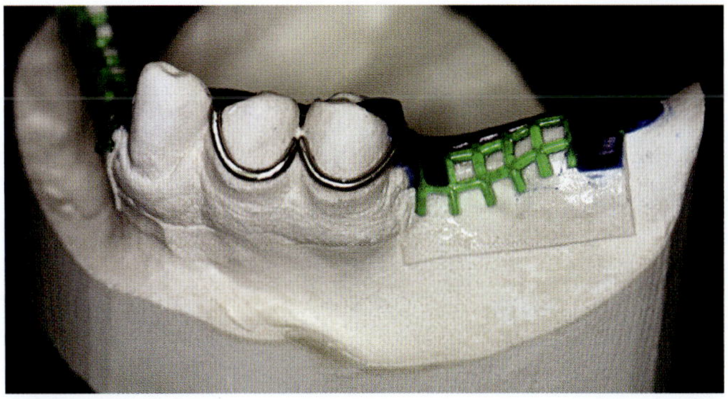

Fig. 20.23 Buccal view of the pattern shown in Fig. 20.22. Double wrought wires are contoured to follow the ledges, the tissue stop at the posterior of the ridge relief is shown, and an occlusal rest distal of #20 will require finishing following completion of casting.

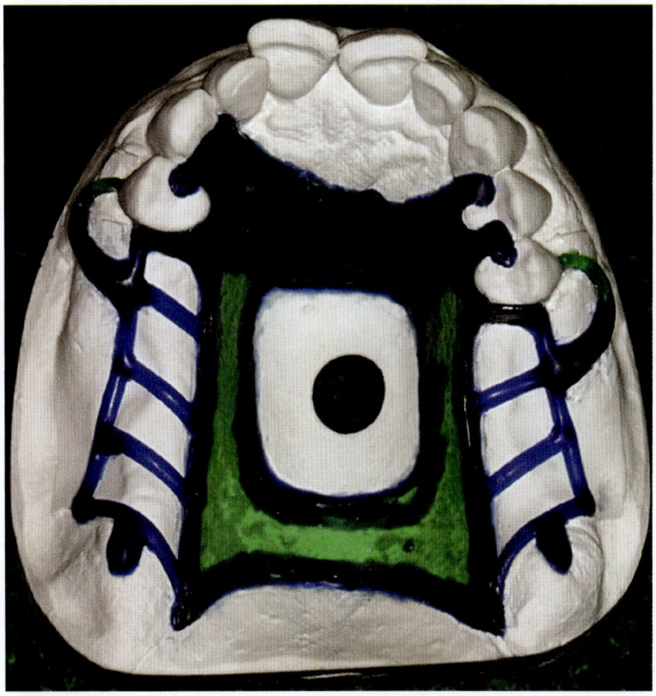

Fig. 20.24 Occlusal view of the maxillary refractory cast with a wax pattern. An anatomic replica has been used to develop an anterior-posterior palatal strap major connector with beading evident at the anterior, posterior, and internal edges. Bilateral, tapered I-bar retainers have been waxed as extensions of the resin-retaining minor connectors, and double rests were incorporated into the design on each side.

sprued. The points of attachment should be flared out and local constrictions avoided. If this protocol is followed, the sprue, which is bulky enough to freeze after the case framework has frozen, will continue to feed molten metal to the framework until it has entirely solidified. The intent is to provide sound metal in the casting proper with all shrinkage porosity forced into the sprue rod, which is later discarded.

The laboratory procedure for multiple spruing is essentially the same for all mandibular and maxillary castings, except those with a palatal plate. Typical examples are illustrated in Figs. 20.29 and 20.30.

Two basic types of sprues are used: multiple and single. Most RPD castings require multiple sprues, with the use of 8- to 12-gauge round wax shapes for main sprues and 12- to 18-gauge round wax shapes for auxiliary sprues. Occasionally, however, a single sprue is preferred for cast palates and cast metal bases for the mandibular arch when these are used as complete denture bases. With RPDs, the use of a single sprue is limited to those maxillary frameworks in which—because of the presence of a palatal plate—it is impossible to locate multiple sprues centrally. In such situations, the single sprue may

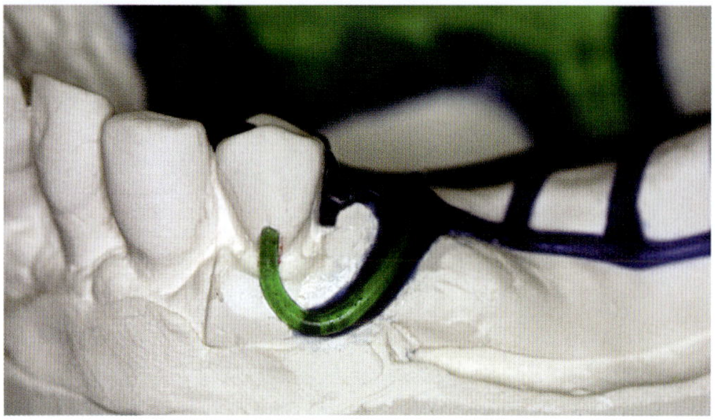

Fig. 20.25 Buccal view of right I-bar shown in Fig. 20.24. The tissue index is demonstrated gingival to the proximal plate, tissue relief is provided beneath the denture base minor connector, and the I-bar shows a taper as it approaches the mid-buccal 0.01-inch undercut.

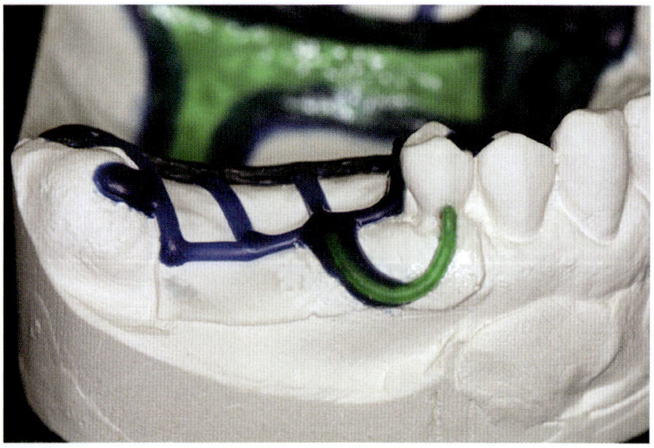

Fig. 20.26 Buccal view of I-bar opposite to that shown in Fig. 20.25. Many of the same features seen in Fig. 20.25 are evident in this example. The tissue stop distal to the ridge relief is shown, and the palatal external finishing line continues distal to the junction of the hard and soft palate (which is the terminus of the posterior palatal strap).

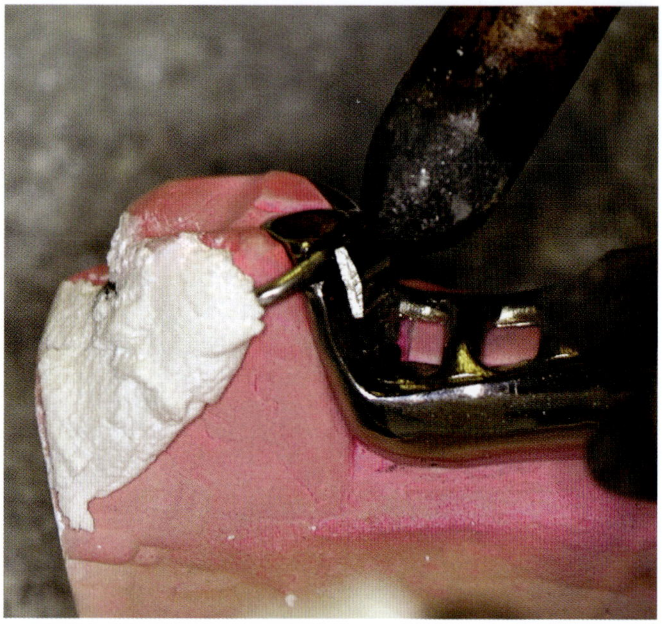

Fig. 20.27 Wrought wire can be soldered to cast frameworks as an alternative method to incorporating in the wax pattern and casting procedure. Electric soldering is a common method for soldering and does not require heating of the entire framework. Following preparation of the minor connector where the wire will be soldered, an 18-gauge, round, wrought-wire clasp is carefully adapted and then secured to the framework and the duplicate stone cast with the use of refractory investment. In this situation, a distolingual molar undercut will be used bilaterally for retention. The flux is placed at the proximal plate, followed by placement of sufficient solder, and the electric heat element tip is placed into contact with the solder while the framework is grounded at another location.

be used advantageously. A single sprue must be attached to the wax pattern so that the direction of flow of the molten metal will be parallel to the long axis of the single sprue. In some instances, the investment cast may have to be cut away anteriorly to make room for the attachment of the sprue; in others, the sprue may be attached posteriorly. One disadvantage of using a single sprue for large castings is that an extra-long investment ring must be used.

Some important points to remember using multiple sprued are as follows:

1. Use a few sprues of large diameter rather than several smaller sprues.
2. Keep all sprues as short and direct as possible.
3. Avoid abrupt changes in direction; avoid T-shaped junctions as much as possible.
4. Reinforce all junctions with additional wax to prevent constrictions in the sprue channel and to prevent V-shaped sections of investment that might break away and be carried into the casting.

Investing the Sprued Wax Pattern

The investment for an RPD casting consists of two parts: the investment cast on which the pattern is formed, and the outer investment surrounding the cast and pattern. The latter is confined within a metal ring, which may or may not be removed after the outer investment has been set. If the metal ring is not to be removed, it must be lined with a layer of cellulose, asbestos substitute, or ceramic fiber paper to allow for both setting and thermal expansion of the mold in all directions.

The investment must conform accurately to the shape of the pattern and must preserve the configuration of the pattern as a cavity after the pattern itself has been eliminated through vaporization and oxidation. The casting investment:

- Provides the strength necessary to hold the forces exerted by the entering stream of molten metal until this metal has solidified into the form of the pattern.
- Provides a smooth surface for the mold cavity so that the final casting will require as little finishing as possible; in some situations, a deoxidizing agent is used to keep surfaces bright.
- Provides an avenue of escape for most of the gases entrapped in the mold cavity by the entering stream of molten alloy.

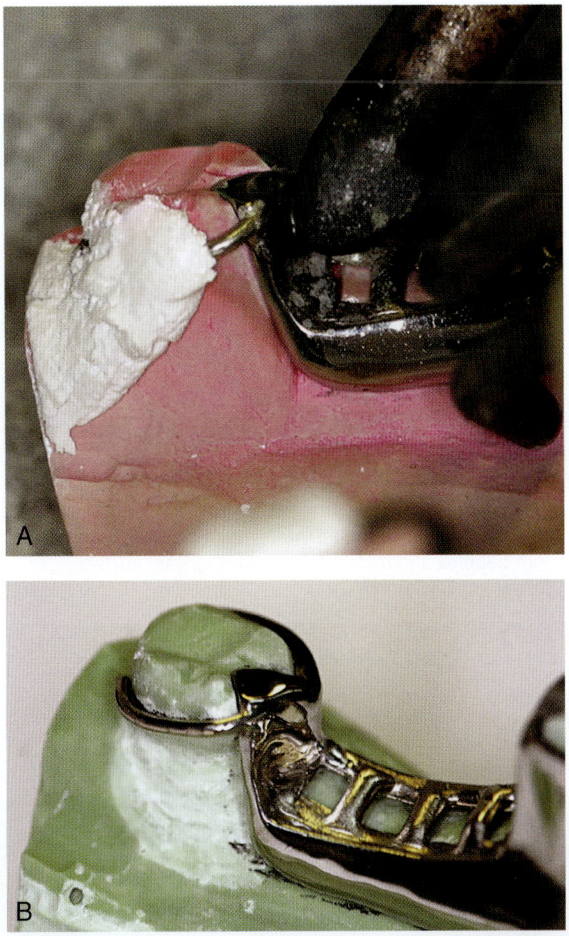

Fig. 20.28 A, An electric soldering technique has been used to solder the wrought wire. The solder has flowed into the space between the framework and the wire, and around the wire itself to ensure its secure attachment to the framework. **B,** Finished and polished wrought-wire retainer.

- Together with other factors, provides necessary compensation for the dimensional changes of the alloy[1] from the molten to the solid, set state.

The investment for casting gold alloys is a plaster-bound silica material, compounded in such a way that the total mold expansion will offset the casting shrinkage of the alloy, which varies from 1% to 1.74% (the highest figure being the shrinkage of pure gold). Generally, the higher the percentage of gold in the alloy, the greater the contraction of the casting on solidifying.

Only one cobalt-chromium alloy has a sufficiently low melting temperature to be cast into a plaster-silica investment mold. According to Peyton,[1] for the other alloys that have a higher melting temperature, an investment that contains quartz powder held together by an ethyl silicate or sodium silicate binder is generally used. Expansion to offset casting shrinkage for cobalt-chromium alloys is accomplished primarily through thermal expansion of the mold and must be sufficient to offset their greater casting shrinkage, which is on the order of 2.3%. For this reason, the casting ring is usually removed after the mold has hardened to allow for the greater mold expansion necessary with these alloys. Because the investments for cobalt-chromium alloys are generally less porous, there is a greater danger that gases will be entrapped in the mold cavity by the molten metal. Spruing must be done with greater care, and in some instances, provision for venting the mold is necessary to prevent defective castings.

BOX 20.1 Factors That Influence the Excellence of a Dental Casting

1. Care and accuracy with which the cast is reproduced
2. Intelligence with which the framework is designed and proportioned
3. Care and cleanliness in waxing up the cast
4. Consideration of the expansion of the wax caused by temperature
5. Size, length, configuration, points of attachment, and manner of attachment of the sprues
6. Choice of investment
7. Location of the pattern in the mold
8. Mixing water: amount, temperature, and impurities
9. Spatulation of the investment during mixing
10. Restraint offered to expansion of the investment caused by the investment ring
11. Setting time
12. Burnout temperature and time
13. Method of casting
14. Gases: adhered, entrapped, and absorbed
15. Force used in throwing the metal into the mold
16. Shrinkage on cooling
17. Removal from the investment after casting
18. Scrubbing, pickling, and so on
19. Polishing and finishing
20. Heat handling

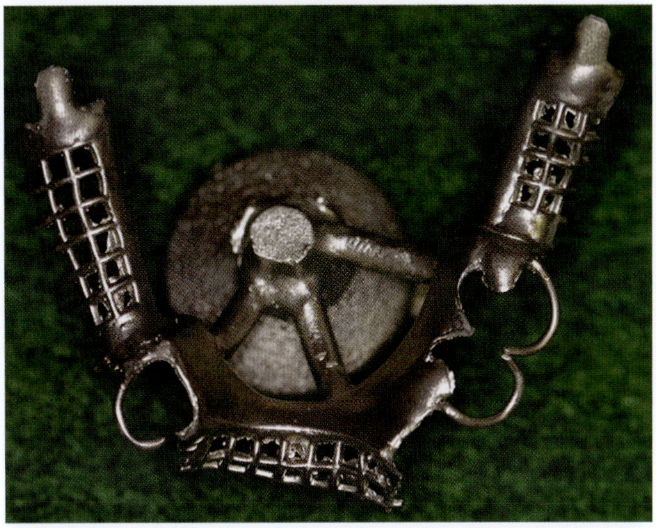

Fig. 20.29 Mandibular cast framework with sprue intact, showing three 8-gauge sprues attached to the lingual bar. If one is concerned about completely filling distal extension base minor connectors, 12-gauge sprues can be attached to the minor connector.

[1]Note the substitution of the word alloy, as the same principles apply whether the metal is a precious metal alloy or a cobalt-chromium alloy. In some of the latter alloys, the cobalt is partially replaced by nickel; such alloys are sometimes described as Stellite alloys.

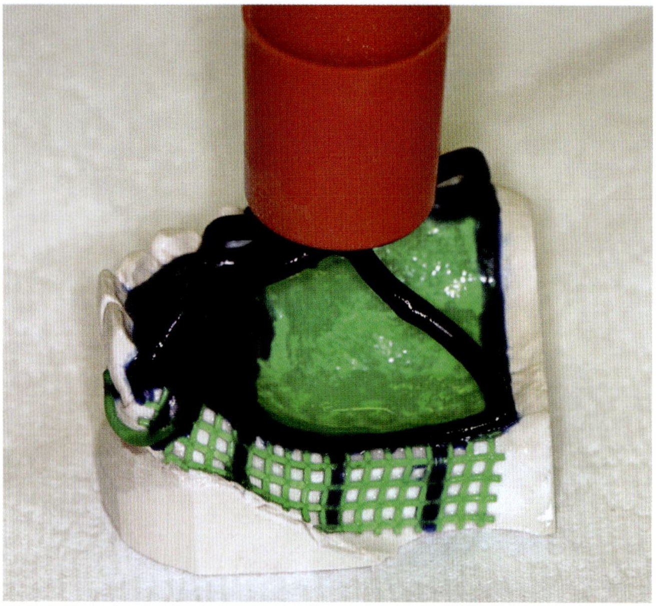

Fig. 20.30 For a maxillary framework, multiple 8-gauge sprues or a single main sprue located posteriorly can be used. When a single main sprue is used, additional sprues can feed critical regions for casting completeness.

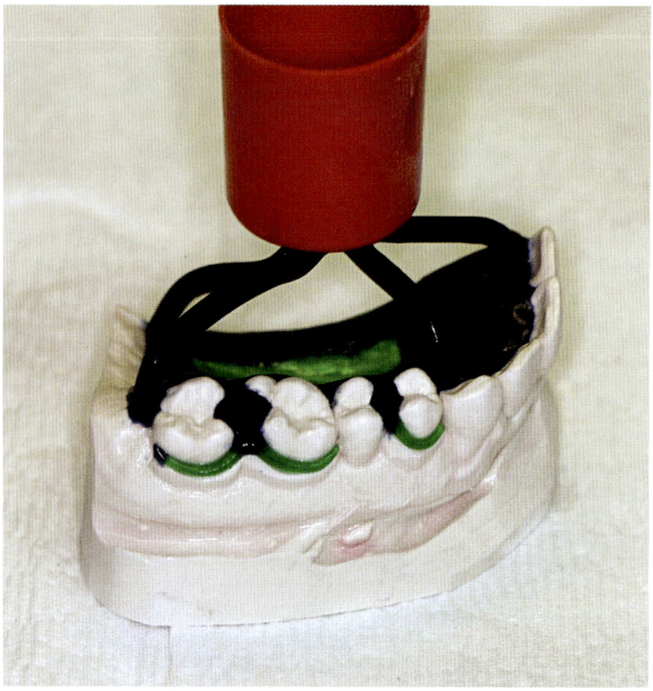

Fig. 20.31 Wax pattern sprued and ready to invest.

Step-by-Step Procedure

The technique for applying the outer investment is usually referred to as *investing the pattern*. However, the cast on which the pattern is formed is part of the investment also. This investment technique is presented in Figs. 20.31 through 20.33.

Burnout

The burnout operation serves three purposes: it drives off moisture in the mold; it vaporizes and thus eliminates the pattern,

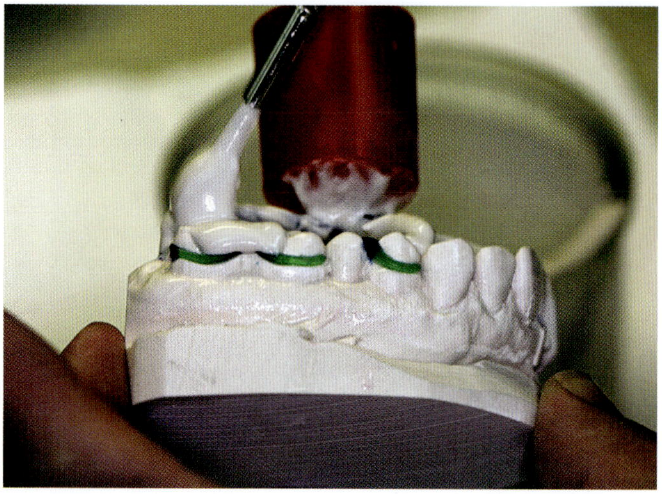

Fig. 20.32 Applying the investment with a soft moistened brush to ensure complete adaptation of the investment. This helps reduce the number of bubbles and makes for a smoother cast surface.

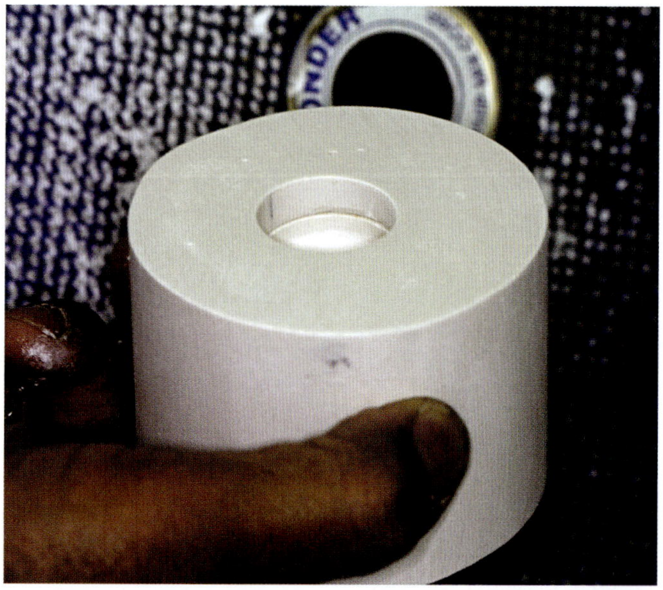

Fig. 20.33 Investment mold has been trimmed to prepare the sprue end for burnout and subsequent complete adaptation to the casting machine.

leaving a cavity in the mold; and it expands the mold to compensate for the contraction of the metal on cooling.

For the investment to heat uniformly, it should be moist at the start of the burnout cycle. Steam will then carry the heat into the investment during the early stages of burnout. Therefore if the investment is not burned out on the same day that it is poured, it should be soaked in water for a few minutes before it is placed in the burnout furnace.

Just before it is placed in the furnace, the mold should be placed in the casting machine to balance the weight against the weight of the mold. At this time, the mold should be properly oriented to the machine and its crucible, and a scratch line should be made at the top for later repositioning of the hot mold.

The mold should be placed in the oven with the sprue hole down and the orientation mark forward. Burnout should be started with a cold oven, or nearly so. Then the temperature of the oven should be increased slowly to a temperature recommended by the manufacturer. This temperature should be maintained for the period recommended by the manufacturer to ensure uniform heat penetration. More time must be allowed for plastic patterns, particularly palatal anatomic replica patterns. It is important that the peak temperature recommended by the manufacturer is not exceeded during the burnout period. (When a high-heat investment is used, follow the manufacturer's instructions as to burnout temperature.)

Casting

The method of casting varies widely with the alloy and equipment used. All methods use force to quickly inject the molten metal into the mold cavity. This force may be centrifugal or air pressure; the former is more commonly used. In any case, too much or too little force is undesirable. If too little force is used, the mold is not fully filled before the metal begins to freeze. If too much force is used, excessive turbulence may result in the entrapment of gases in the casting. With centrifugal casting machines, this is regulated by the number of turns put on the actuating spring.

The metal may be melted with a gas-oxygen blowtorch or by an electric muffle surrounding the metal. In some commercial casting procedures and in some dental laboratories, the induction method may be used (Fig. 20.34); this provides a rapid and accurate method of melting the metal. Currently, available casting machines include those that are electrically controlled to heat alloys to a specified temperature and to release the molten metal at precisely the correct casting temperature. These machines are costly and primarily located in commercial laboratories or institutions where casting volume is high.

Removing the Casting from the Investment

Cobalt-chromium alloys are allowed to cool in the mold, divested (Fig. 20.35), and should not be cleaned by pickling. Finishing (Fig. 20.36) and polishing (Fig. 20.37), which are done with special high-speed equipment, such as a high-speed lathe, require technical skill in the use of bench lathes. Just before they are polished (high-shine), cobalt-chromium castings are electropolished; this is a controlled deplating process (Fig. 20.38).

Finishing and Polishing

The sprues should not be removed from the casting until polishing is near completion, suggesting that leaving the sprue may prevent distortion; this is difficult to accomplish and may not be practical. Instead, reasonable care should be exercised to prevent distortion resulting from careless handling. A specific precaution is to prevent bending a cast clasp arm. It is more predictable to wax the clasp to minimize the need for finishing to maintain the clasp fit to the abutment (Fig. 20.39).

Actual polishing procedures vary widely according to personal preference for certain abrasive shapes and sizes. However, the following several rules for finishing the casting are important:

1. *High speeds are preferable to low speeds.* Not only are they effective, but in experienced hands, there is less danger of the casting being caught and thrown out of the hands by the rotating instrument.
2. *The wheels or points and the speed of their rotation create the finish.* Excessive pressure generates heat, crushes the abrasive

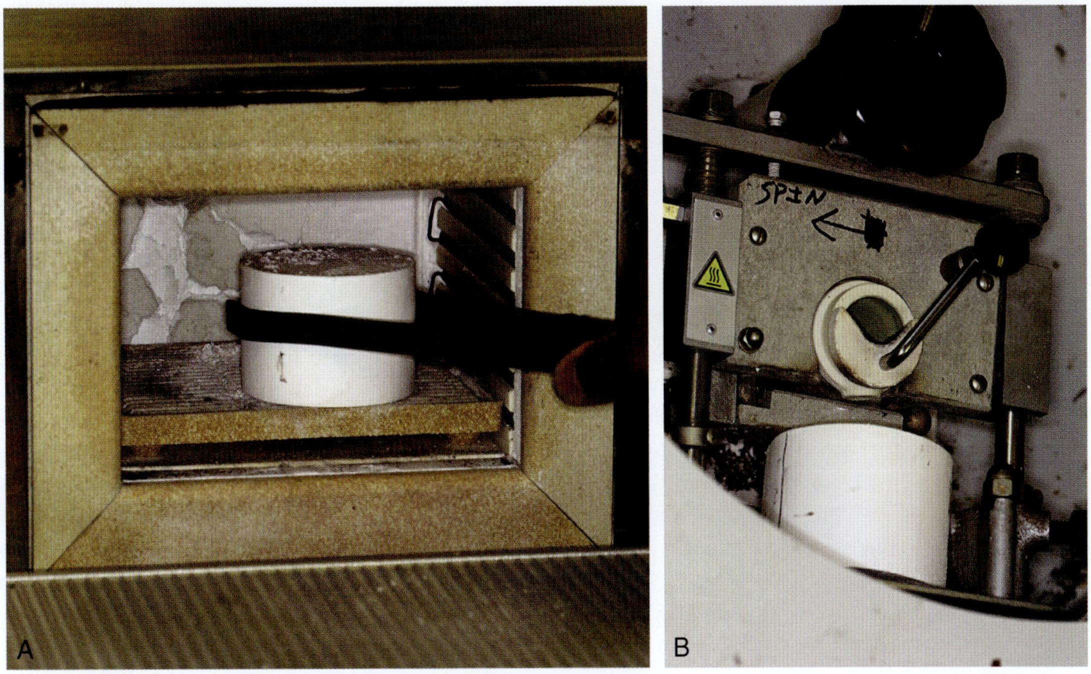

Fig. 20.34 A, An invested pattern is removed from the burnout oven following complete elimination of the wax pattern. **B,** An investment mold is placed into the casting machine. The induction casting process provides consistency to the casting procedure.

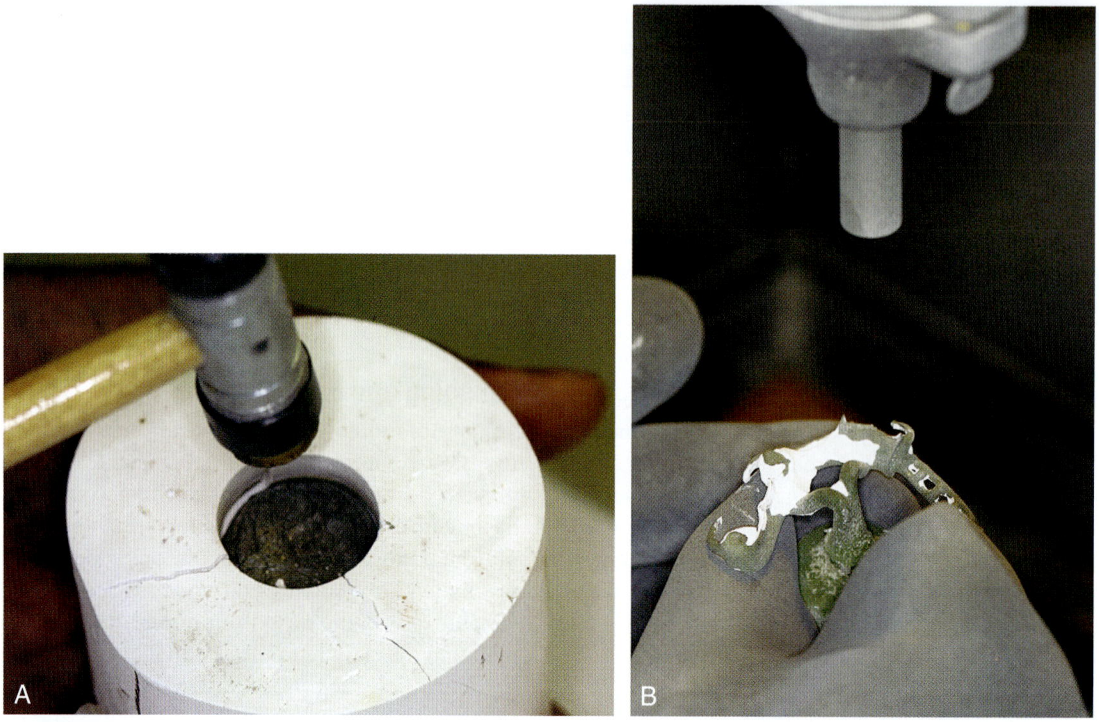

Fig. 20.35 A, Divesting of the framework involves bulk removal of the investment. **B,** The framework is divested with aluminum oxide.

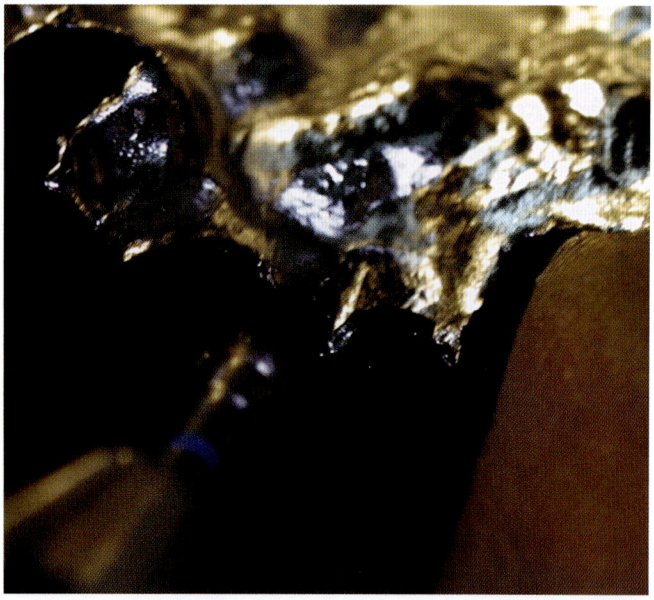

Fig. 20.36 Gross finishing is accomplished with metal finishing burs, abrasive stones, or sintered diamonds (except at contact areas).

particles, causes the wheels to clog and glaze, and slows the cutting.

3. *A definite sequence for finishing should be adopted and followed for every framework.*
4. *Clean polishing wheels should be used.* If contaminated wheels are used, foreign particles may become embedded in the surface, which will lead to later discoloration.
5. *Be sure that each finishing operation completely removes all "scratches" caused by the preceding abrasive material.* Each successive finishing step uses a finer abrasive and therefore cuts more slowly and requires more time to accomplish.

MAKING RECORD BASES

Use materials that provide accurately fitting bases for jaw relation records or a material that can be relined to provide accuracy. Relining may be accomplished in a laboratory setting by placing the previously adapted base onto the cast; be certain to adapt tinfoil or lubricate the cast prior to adding a mix of zinc oxide–eugenol paste or autopolymerizing acrylic resin. An elastomeric impression material can be used but the use of lining jaw relation record bases is questionable. If rigid liner materials are used for this purpose, any undercuts on the cast must be blocked out with wax or clay to facilitate their removal without damage to the cast.

The ideal jaw relation record base is well adapted to fit the master cast, either processed or cast, and is incorporated into the permanent base of the completed prosthesis. Cast metal bases for complete dentures or RPDs offer this advantage, as do acrylic resin bases that are processed directly to the master cast, thus becoming the permanent denture base. When undercuts are present, the master cast will be destroyed during removal of the base. In this situation, existing undercuts must be blocked out on the intaglio surface of the denture base before dental stone is poured into it to make a cast for articulator mounting, a remount cast. A second cast, which includes the undercuts, must be poured against the entire base to support it when the overlying acrylic resin is processed. With both the processed base and the overlying acrylic resin, some care must be taken to prevent visible junction lines between the original acrylic resin

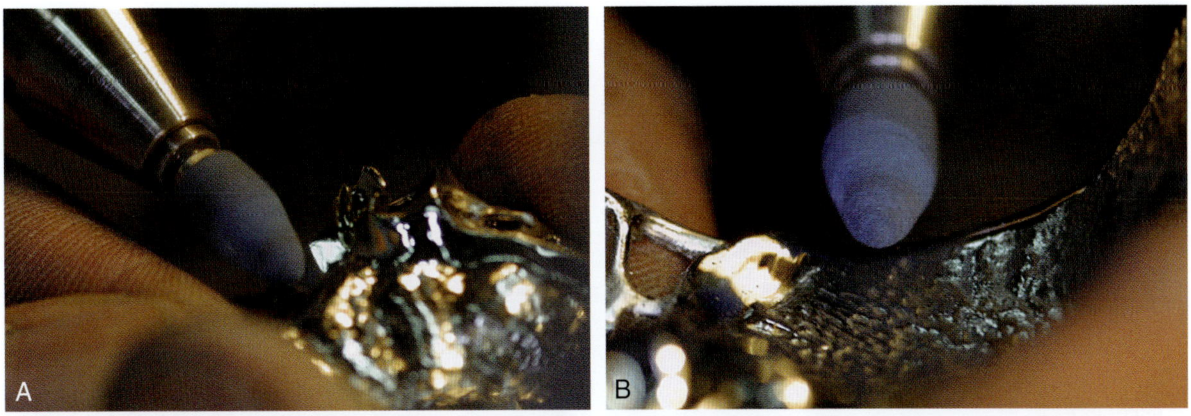

Fig. 20.37 **A,** The framework is finished with a rubber polishing point before final "high-shine" polish in a region adjacent to the teeth and **(B)** at the periphery of a major connector.

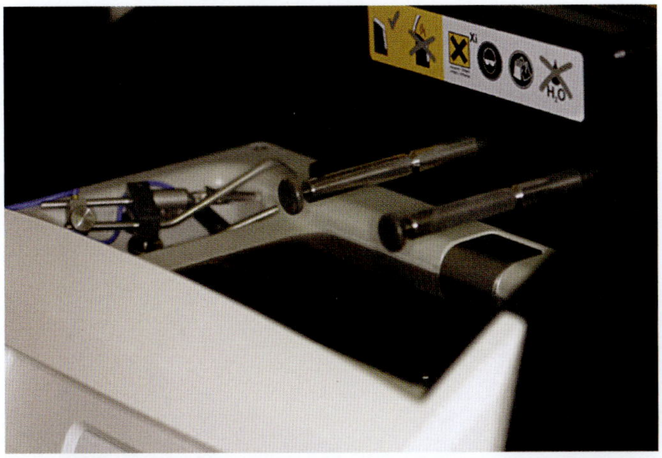

Fig. 20.38 Electropolishing unit used for the final surface polish of frameworks in a heated polishing liquid.

base and the acrylic resin that supports the teeth and establishes facial contours.

Autopolymerizing acrylic resin materials can be used as a jaw relation base. These are used with a sprinkling technique, which, when properly done, permits the formation of a base that compares favorably with a processed base or a visible light polymerized base. A material must be selected that will polymerize in a reasonable time (usually a 12-minute monomer) and will retain its form during the sprinkling process. Because polymerization with typical shrinkage toward the cast begins immediately, alternate addition of monomer and polymer in small increments results in reduced overall shrinkage and greater accuracy. Another option is to use visible light-cured (VLC) denture base materials, which employ a technique for making custom impression trays similar to that described in Chapter 16.

Technique for Making a Sprinkled Acrylic Resin Record Base

The technique for sprinkling a record base is described here because the techniques used for the VLC impression tray and record bases were presented in Chapter 16 and elsewhere in this chapter. Some blockout and lubrication of the cast are necessary (Fig. 20.40). Relief of undercut areas on the cast is best accomplished with a water-soluble modeling clay or baseplate wax. Modeling clay is easily formed and shaped on the cast and is easily removed from the cast or the base with a natural bristle toothbrush under warm running water. Wax must be flushed off the cast with hot water and removed from the inside of the base before use.

Bases for jaw relation records must have maximum contact with the supporting tissue. The accuracy of the base will be proportionate to the contact provided to the total area of intimate tissue. Those areas are most often undercut and require blockout of the distolingual and retromylohyoid areas of the mandibular cast, the distobuccal and labial aspects of the maxillary cast, and, frequently, small multiple undercuts in the palatal rugae. These areas and any other undercuts are blocked out with a minimum of clay or wax to obliterate as little of the surface of the cast as possible. A close-fitting base may then be made that will have the necessary accuracy and stability and yet may be lifted from and returned to the master cast without abrading it.

The cast and the blockout or relief are coated with a separating medium. Following this, the cast is wet with the monomer from a dropper bottle. After the surface has been wetted with the monomer, the polymer is sprinkled or dusted onto the wet surface until all the monomer has been absorbed. Sprinkling is best accomplished with a large-mouthed bottle with a single hole in the lid near the rim. This facilitates the placement of the polymer without excess in any one area. A flexible bottle with a suitable applicator tip also may be used. The objective should be to apply polymer uniformly over the entire ridge rather than allowing excess to accumulate at the border to be trimmed later. An autopolymerizing acrylic resin material must be used that will retain its form during the sprinkling procedure without objectionable flow into low areas (Figs. 20.41–20.43).

Once the polymer has been sprinkled in slight excess, the monomer is again added. Flooding must be prevented; therefore the monomer must be directed over the entire surface gradually until the polymer has just absorbed the monomer. A few seconds delay before the addition of excess monomer allows the mass to reach a tacky consistency and prevents it from flowing

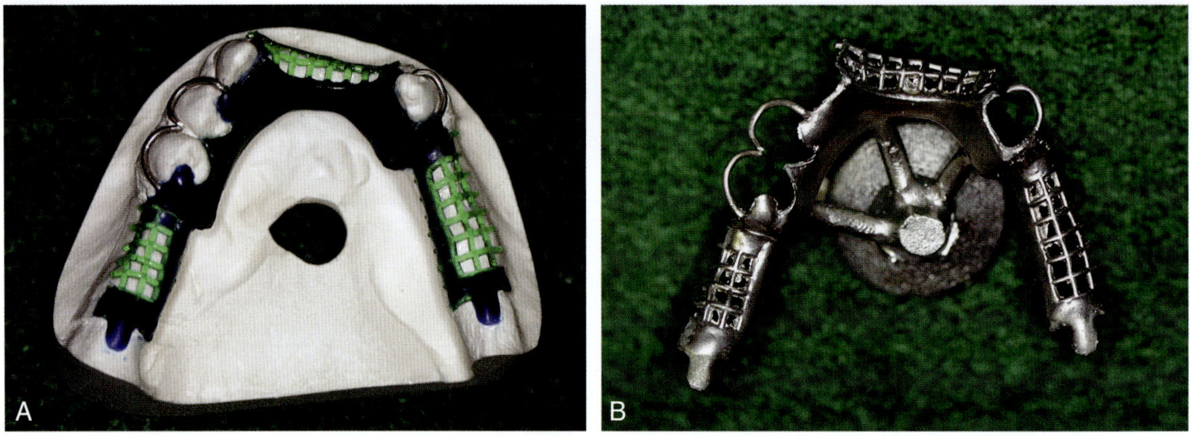

Fig. 20.39 Attention to detail in forming the wax pattern not only ensures the quality of the framework, but it also saves time in finishing and polishing the resultant casting. **A,** Wax pattern of the mandibular framework, which incorporates three wrought-wire retainers. **B,** The same framework following casting shows a smooth casting surface and attention to detail regarding casting completeness and clasp form.

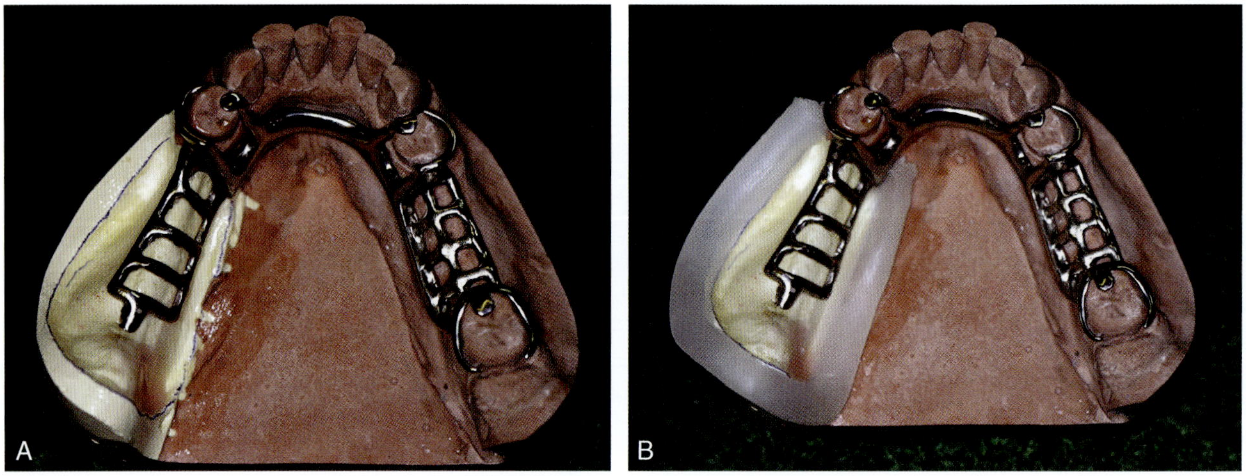

Fig. 20.40 A, Preparation of Kennedy Class I, modification 1 distal extension for sprinkle-on record base technique. Cast undercuts are blocked out with wax, and the cast is coated with separator. **B,** Peripheral extent of the base (the same as the peripheral extent of the prosthesis captured during border molding and an impression-making procedure for this altered cast) is outlined with rope wax to contain resin.

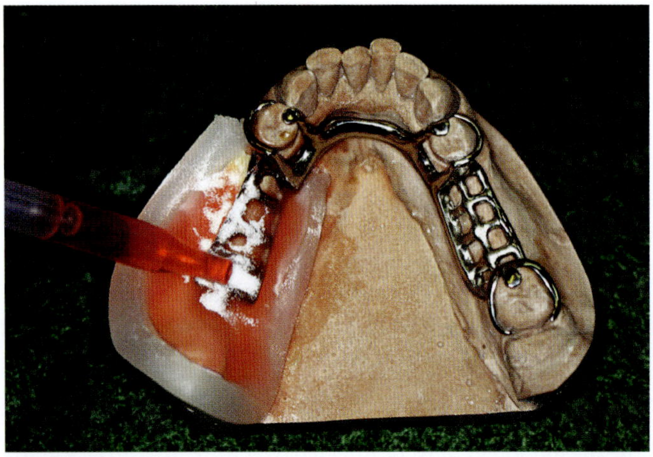

Fig. 20.41 The cast is wetted with monomer, and polymer resin is added in increments to uniformly control thickness. Use of a typical eyedropper may be difficult if the monomer addition cannot be controlled. Use of peripheral rope wax helps in this regard.

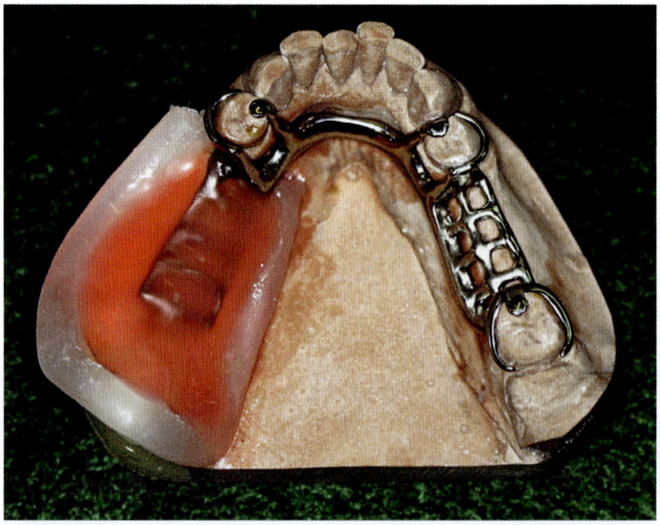

Fig. 20.42 The record base is complete when a uniform thickness is created that provides strength and accuracy. The completed unpolymerized resin is covered to ensure polymerization without loss of surface monomer.

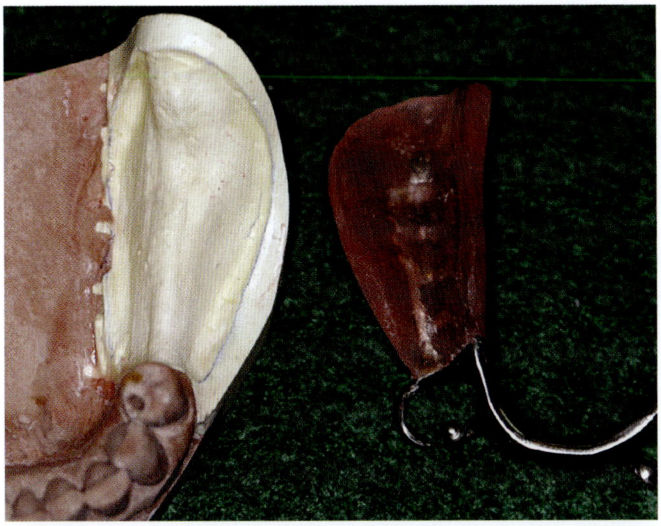

Fig. 20.43 Once completely polymerized, the record base and the framework can be removed from the cast, finished, and prepared for addition of the record base. The tissue side of the record base (intaglio) should possess similar accuracy and stability as are seen with the completed prosthesis. Such a record base provides a significant advantage for jaw relation records when minimal teeth remain and ridge configurations along with extensive base areas place a premium on base accuracy and stability.

when more monomer is added. Then the monomer may be added in excess and is immediately absorbed by the application of more polymer, as before. This process is repeated selectively until a uniform layer has been built up that is just thick enough so that none of the underlying cast or relief may be seen.

The final step in sprinkling is the addition of a monomer sufficient to leave a wet surface. Immediately, the cast should be placed in a covered glass dish or covered with an inverted bowl. This permits final polymerization in a saturated atmosphere of monomer and prevents evaporation of surface monomer. The cast should not be placed in water, nor any attempt be made to accelerate polymerization. Slow polymerization is necessary so that shrinkage toward the cast will occur. Only then will overall shrinkage be negligible and accuracy of fit ensured. This is of little consequence in making an impression tray, but it is essential in making a sprinkled acrylic resin base.

Although polymerization will be about 90% complete within an hour and an impression tray may even be lifted within a half-hour, it is critical that a sprinkled denture base should be left overnight before it is separated from the cast. It should be lifted dry or under lukewarm tap water. It should not be immersed in hot water because some warping may occur.

A sprinkled acrylic resin base made with the precautions outlined previously will retain its accuracy for days, or even for an indefinite period, similar to a heat-polymerized resin base (see Fig. 20.43) or a VLC base.

OCCLUSION RIMS

The jaw relation records for RPDs always should be made on accurate bases that may be part of the denture casting or may be attached to it in exactly the same relation as the final denture base will be. Although the use of the final denture base is best for jaw relation records, a sprinkled or corrected acrylic resin base may be used satisfactorily. In any case, the accuracy of the base supporting a maxillomandibular record must be ensured before the function of occlusion rims is considered.

Occlusion rims may be made of several materials. The material that is most commonly used to establish static occlusal relationships is the hard baseplate wax rim. However, the use of a wax occlusion rim can be inaccurate when the occlusal portion of the rim is mishandled. When some soft material that sets to a rigid state, such as impression plaster or bite registration paste, is used in conjunction with wax rims to record static occlusal relations, many of the errors common to wax rims are eliminated—provided some space for the material exists between the occlusion rims, the opposing teeth, or both, at the desired vertical dimension to be recorded. Jaw registrations made on wax occlusion rims with the use of a wax registration material must be handled carefully and mounted immediately.

Occlusion rims for static jaw relation records should be so shaped that they represent the lost teeth and their supporting structures (Fig. 20.44). An occlusion rim that is too broad and is extended beyond where prosthetic teeth will be located is unnecessary. Such rims will substantially alter the shape of the palatal vault and the arch form of the mandibular arch, will crowd the patient's tongue, will have an unwelcome effect on the patient, and will offer more resistance to jaw relation recording media than will a correctly shaped occlusion rim.

Modeling plastic (compound) has several advantages and may be used rather than wax for occlusion rims. It may be softened uniformly by flaming, yet when chilled it becomes rigid and sufficiently accurate. It may be trimmed with a sharp knife to expose the tips of the opposing cusps to recheck or position an opposing cast into the record rim. Opposing occlusion rims of modeling plastic may be keyed with greater accuracy than opposing wax rims. Even those should be trimmed short of contact at the vertical dimension of occlusion, and bite registration paste should be interposed for the final record. As with wax rims, an adjustable frame may be used to support the final record.

Occlusion rims made of extra hard baseplate wax or modeling plastic may be used to support intraoral central bearing devices, intraoral tracing devices, or both. Because of its greater stability, modeling plastic is preferable for this purpose when the edentulous situation permits the use of flat plane tracings. An example of such a situation occurs when an opposing complete denture is made concurrently with the RPD. In such a situation, modeling plastic occlusion rims provides greater stability than wax rims, with a corresponding improvement in the predictable accuracy of such a jaw relation record. Although sealing opposing occlusion rims or using clips for complete denture jaw relation records may be acceptable, particularly for an initial articulator mounting, the existence of an RPD framework makes this practice hazardous. The framework with attached base should be seated accurately on its cast before the opposing cast is repositioned in occlusion to it, because it is necessary for the dentist to be able to see the RPD framework is in its designed terminal relation to the supporting teeth before articulating the casts.

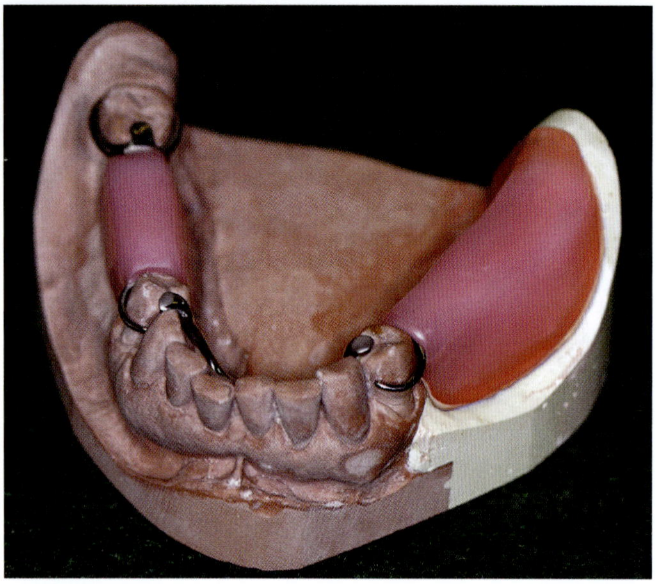

Fig. 20.44 Occlusion rims are added to allow recording of jaw relation records. Placement of the wax record is dictated by the opposing tooth position and the supporting ridge characteristics. When possible, the occlusion rim should allow recording of the jaw position within the primary bearing area of the ridge.

ARRANGING POSTERIOR TEETH TO AN OPPOSING CAST OR TEMPLATE

Whether posterior teeth are to be arranged to occlude with an opposing cast or with an occlusal template, the denture base on which the jaw relation record has been made must not be entirely supported by the tissue. Because record bases that are entirely tissue supported have no place in recording occlusal relations for RPDs, the bases must be attached to the denture framework. Auto- or heat-polymerized acrylic resin bases attached to the framework may be used to make the record. Metal bases that are part of the prosthesis present no problem. If entirely tissue-supported record bases were used in making the occlusal registration, and an adjustable articulator has been used to develop the occlusion, then the trial dentures must have been evaluated, the articulator mounting has been approved, and the articulator has been programmed for eccentric positions. If this is the case, the acrylic record base should be discarded prior to setting the posterior teeth. Unless occlusal relations are recorded on final acrylic resin bases, autopolymerizing acrylic resin bases attained by the sprinkling method or VLC bases are the most accurate and stable of bases that may be used for this purpose. In either situation, the denture cannot be completed on these bases; neither can the bases be removed conveniently from the retentive framework during the boil out after flasking. Therefore the metal framework must be lifted from the cast, and the original record base removed by flaming its underside. Care must be taken not to allow the acrylic resin to burn, or the cast framework will become discolored with carbon. The framework is repolished and is then returned to its original position on the master cast and secured there with sticky wax before the artificial teeth are arranged. The teeth may be arranged in wax or placed directly on the metal base, depending on the type of posterior tooth used, and these must be occluded directly to the opposing cast or template.

Posterior Tooth Forms

Posterior tooth forms for RPDs should not be selected arbitrarily. One should remember that the objective of RPD occlusion is harmony between natural and artificial dentition. Whether the teeth are arranged to occlude with an opposing cast or to an occlusal template, they should be modified to harmonize with the existing dentition. In this respect, RPD occlusion may differ from complete denture occlusion. In the latter case, posterior teeth may be selected and articulated according to the dentist's concept of what constitutes the most favorable complete denture occlusion, whereas RPD occlusion must be made to harmonize with an existing occlusal pattern. Thus the occlusal surfaces on the finished RPD may bear little resemblance to the original occlusal surfaces of the teeth as manufactured.

Artificial tooth forms should be selected to restore the space and fulfill the esthetic demands of the missing dentition. Manufactured tooth forms usually require modification to satisfactorily articulate with an opposing dentition. The original occlusal form, therefore, is of little importance in forming the posterior occlusion for the RPD.

The posterior teeth are most often made of resin (including all resin forms—composite, interpolymer network, cross-link, double cross-link, and so on). An advantage of resin teeth is that they are more easily modified and subsequently reshaped for masticating efficiency by the addition of grooves and spillways. Resin teeth are also more easily narrowed buccolingually to reduce the size of the occlusal table without sacrificing strength or esthetics. They may be more easily ground to fit minor connectors and irregular spaces and to avoid retentive elements of the RPD framework. However, when resin teeth are used, the occlusion must be evaluated periodically to make sure that the occlusal surfaces have not worn out of contact.

Arranging Teeth to an Occluding Surface

The procedure for arranging teeth to a static relationship with an opposing cast is essentially the same as for arranging teeth to an occluding template. On the other hand, articulation of artificial teeth on an adjustable instrument, which reproduces to some extent mandibular movement, will follow more closely the customary pattern for complete denture occlusion. The procedure for arranging posterior teeth to an occluding template was presented in Chapter 18.

TYPES OF ANTERIOR TEETH

Anterior teeth on RPDs are concerned primarily with esthetics and the function of incising. These are best arranged when the patient is present because an added appointment for try-in would be necessary anyway. They may be arranged arbitrarily on the cast and then tried in, but a stone index of their labial surfaces should be made on the master cast after the final arrangement has been established to preserve the arrangement that the patient saw and approved.

From a purely mechanical standpoint, all missing anterior teeth are best replaced with fixed restorations rather than with the RPD. However, for cosmetic or economic reasons, or in situations in which several missing anterior teeth are involved—such as in a Class IV partially edentulous arch—their replacement with the RPD may be unavoidable.

Some types of anterior teeth used in RPDs are as follows:

1. *Porcelain or resin teeth, attached to the framework with acrylic resin.*
2. *Ready-made resin teeth processed directly to retentive elements on the metal framework with a matching resin.* This is called a *pressed-on method* and has the advantage of permitting previous selection and evaluation of the anterior teeth, plus the advantage of the use of ready-made resin teeth for labial surfaces. These are then hollowed out on the lingual surface to facilitate their permanent attachment to the denture framework with the resin of the same shade.
3. *Resin teeth processed to a metal framework in the laboratory.* Tooth forms of wax may be carved on the RPD framework and tried in the mouth, adjusted for esthetics and occlusion, and then processed in an acrylic resin of a suitable shade. There is some question as to whether the shade and durability of such teeth are comparable with those of manufactured resin teeth, but improvements in materials have led to improved quality and appearance of laboratory-made teeth. Moreover, such teeth may often be shaped and characterized to better blend with adjacent natural teeth.
4. *Porcelain or acrylic resin facings cemented to the denture framework.* These may be tried in the mouth on a baseplate wax base and adjusted for esthetics. Ready-made plastic backings may be used, which become part of the pattern for the RPD framework. The teeth are then ultimately cemented to the framework. Esthetically, these are less satisfactory than other types of anterior teeth, but because the plastic backing is cast as part of the RPD framework, they have the advantage of greater strength and are replaced easily. A record of the mold and shade of each tooth should be kept, and only the ridge lap of the replacement teeth needs to be ground to fit. When replaceability is the main reason for its use, the stock facing should not be beveled, or difficulty will be encountered in replacing it. Replacement also may be accomplished by waxing and processing a resin tooth that directly faces the metal backing. Stock tube or side-groove teeth are not ordinarily used for anterior teeth on RPDs because of the horizontal forces that tend to dislodge them.
5. *Anterior resin denture teeth can be modified to be used as resin veneers, the same as for veneer crowns and veneer pontics on fixed partial dentures(FPD).* This is most applicable when the RPD framework is to be cast in an alloy. Then labial surfaces may be waxed and the final carving for esthetics done in the mouth. A modification of this method is the waxing of the veneer coping on a previously cast metal base. These then are cast separately and are attached to the framework by soldering. Esthetically, the result is comparable with that obtained with resin veneer crowns. This method is particularly applicable when there is a desire to make the replaced teeth match adjacent veneered abutment crowns.

WAXING AND INVESTING THE REMOVABLE PARTIAL DENTURE BEFORE PROCESSING ACRYLIC RESIN BASES

Waxing the Removable Partial Denture Base

Waxing the RPD base before investing differs little from waxing a complete denture. The only difference is the waxing of and around exposed parts of the metal framework. At the framework-denture base junction, undercut finishing lines should be provided whenever possible. Then the waxing is merely butted to the finishing line with a little excess to allow for finishing. Otherwise, small voids in the wax may become filled with investing plaster, or fine edges of the investment may break off during boil out and packing. In either situation, small pieces of investment may become embedded in the acrylic resin at the finishing lines. This is prevented by slightly overwaxing and then finishing the acrylic resin back to the metal finishing line with finishing burs. Abrasive wheels and disks should not be used for this purpose, because they will cut into the metal and may burn the acrylic resin. Pumice and a rag wheel should be used sparingly for polishing because they will abrade the acrylic resin more rapidly than the metal and will leave the finishing line elevated above the adjacent acrylic resin.

When waxing polished metal parts that do not possess a finishing line is done, it must be remembered that no attachment will exist and that over time, some seepage, separation, and discoloration of the acrylic resin in this area are inevitable. This may be prevented to some extent by roughening the metal whenever possible to affect some mechanical attachment by silicoating the attachment or by using one of the resin adhesives. The wax should be left 1.5 to 2.0 mm thick so that the acrylic resin will have some bulk at its junction with the polished metal. Thin films of acrylic resin over metal should be avoided. In finishing, these should be cut back to an area of bulk with finishing burs. Otherwise, any thin acrylic resin film will separate eventually and become discolored and unclean due to marginal seepage. Gingival forms should be waxed in accordance with modern concepts of esthetics and should be made to prevent the entrapment of food particles.

Artificial teeth should be uncovered fully to expose the entire anatomic crown and beyond when gingival recession is simulated. Adjacent or contralateral tooth-gingival relationships should be used as a guide to facilitate the harmonious esthetic presentation of the gingival contours. Relatively few prosthodontic patients are in an age bracket in which some gingival recession and exposed cementum would not normally be present; this should be simulated on prosthodontic restorations in proportion to the patient's age. With RPDs, gingival contours around the remaining natural teeth should be used as a guide to the gingival contours to be reproduced on the prosthesis. However, interproximal spaces are almost always filled, particularly between posterior artificial teeth.

Frush[2] has listed the following rules for varying the height of the gingival tissue at the cervical portion of the teeth:

1. Slightly below the high lip line at the central incisors.
2. Lower than the central incisor gingival margin at the lateral incisors.

3. Higher than the central or lateral incisor gingival margin at the canine.
4. Slightly lower than the canine at the premolar and variable for both premolars and molars.

The correctly formed papilla should be shaped so that it will be self-cleansing. It should be carved so that it is in harmony with the interpretation of age and will be the deciding factor in the visible outline form of the tooth. As Frush has pointed out, even a drop of wax properly placed can change the appearance of a square tooth to a tapering or ovoid appearance. A properly formed papilla further enhances the natural appearance by increasing the color in this area.

The rules for forming the papilla were given by Frush as follows:

1. The papilla must extend to the point of tooth contact for cleanliness.
2. The papillae must be of various lengths.
3. The papilla must be convex in all directions.
4. The papilla must be shaped according to the age of the patient.
5. The papilla must end near the labial face of the tooth and must never slope inward to terminate toward the lingual portion of the interproximal surface.

The denture base should be waxed and carved to create the desired form regardless of the material or the method of processing used. The fact that a split-mold technique is used for processing does not alter the fact that the form of the denture base is to be reproduced by a casting procedure. Therefore the denture pattern should be waxed with care in the same form as that desired for the finished restoration, rather than attempting to shape facial contours on the prosthesis during the polishing phase (Fig. 20.45). Polishing should consist primarily of trimming away the flash, stippling polished surfaces when desired, and polishing lightly with brush wheels and pumice, followed by final polishing with a soft brush wheel and a nonabrasive shining agent, such as whiting. Gross trimming and polishing with pumice should not be necessary if the denture has been properly waxed before investing.

Because the polished surfaces of any denture play an important part in both retention and control of the food bolus, buccal and lingual contours generally should be made concave. In most situations, the border thickness of the denture should be left as recorded in the impression. The only exceptions are the distolingual aspect of the mandibular denture base, to prevent interference with the tongue, and the distobuccal aspect of the maxillary denture base, to prevent interference with the coronoid process of the mandible. These are the only areas that cannot ordinarily be waxed to final contour before investing and may need to be thinned by the dentist at the time of final polishing.

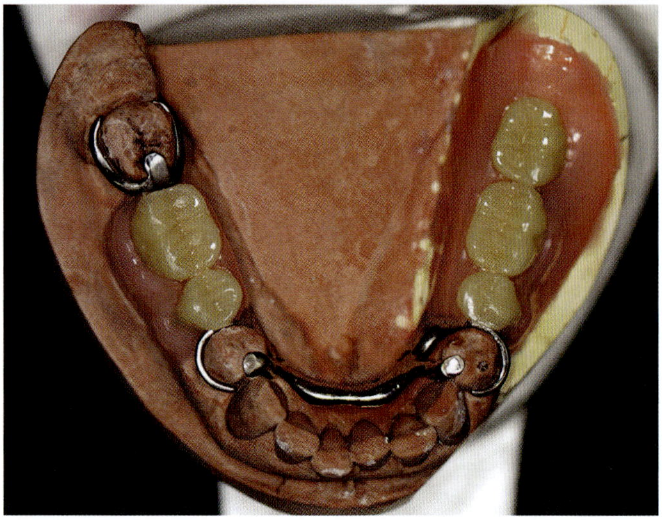

Fig. 20.45 Waxing of the removable partial denture base should reproduce anatomic contours normal for the specific patient's characteristics. This is especially important for regions where the junction of denture tooth and resin will be visible. Healthy interdental papillae are convex and extend to contact points of the teeth. Root prominence can be carved into wax to create a natural appearance. Stippling is typically accomplished after processing done with the use of an eccentric round bur. All of these features should be considered against the specific oral environment in which the prosthesis will be placed. A finished and polished prosthesis that demonstrates esthetic features not found in the patient's mouth may be considered objectionable.

Investing the Removable Partial Denture

In investing an RPD for processing an acrylic resin base, it must be remembered that the denture cast must be recovered from the flask intact for remounting. The practice of cutting the teeth off the cast to expose the connectors and retainers, which are then embedded in the upper half of the flask, is permissible only when an existing denture base is being relined and no provision has been made for remounting. (In such a situation, it seems that this practice offers no advantage over investing the denture that is being so relined upside down in the lower half of the flask.) Because in the past some increase in occlusal vertical dimension has been inevitable in any split-mold processing technique, this method results in raising the RPD framework from the supporting teeth by the amount of increase. Occlusal adjustment in the mouth may temporarily reestablish a harmonious occlusal relation with the opposing teeth, whereas the RPD framework will then settle into supporting contact with the abutment teeth at the expense of the underlying ridge.

Changes in occlusal vertical dimension may be held to a minimum by the use of acrylic denture resins, which can be placed in the mold in a fluid rather than in a doughy state or those that may be injected in a fluid state into a closed mold. Dimensional changes that occur during relining may also be held to a minimum by the use of autopolymerizing acrylic resins for this purpose, thus preventing thermal expansion of a mold subjected to elevated temperatures.

When two opposing RPDs are being made concurrently, one is sometimes processed and placed first, and then the final occlusion is established on the second denture to a fully restored arch. In such a situation, when no natural teeth are in opposition, it is not necessary for the first denture to be remounted after processing. In all other situations, remounting to correct for errors in occlusion is absolutely necessary. Flasking must be accomplished so that the cast can be recovered from the flask undamaged.

Minute voids in the base of the cast will have been reproduced in the stone mounting, and although the obvious larger blebs may be trimmed away, smaller blebs will remain. If the voids in the cast become filled with investing material, the effect is that two particles are trying to occupy the same space. Covering the base with tinfoil substitute before investing can prevent this. Coating the base and sides of the cast with petroleum jelly not only keeps the base of the cast isolated from investing material but also may allow the cast to be more easily recovered from the surrounding investment.

The entire cast, except for the wax and teeth, may then be invested in the lower half of the flask (Fig. 20.46). As with a complete denture, only the supplied teeth and wax are left exposed to be invested in the upper half. Also, as with a complete denture, the investment in the lower half must be smooth and free of undercuts and must be coated with a separator to facilitate the separation of the two halves of the flask.

An alternate and preferred procedure is to invest the cast only to the top of the tinfoil on the base, smoothing the investment and applying a reliable separator. Then a second layer of investment placed around the anatomic portion of the cast covers the natural teeth and the exposed parts of the denture framework. This is likewise smoothed and made free of undercuts and coated with a separator before the top half of the flask is poured. Recovery of the cast is thus made easier by having a shell of investment over the anatomic portion of the cast, which may be removed separately.

When the denture base is to be characterized by applying tinted acrylic resins to the mold, care should be taken not to embed the wax border in the lower half of the flask. The entire surface that is to be tinted should be reproduced in the upper half of the flask. With this precaution, tinting may be carried all the way to the border, and later removal of the flask will not mar the tinted surface. If tinting is not to be done or is to be done only at the cervical margins of the teeth and the papillae, the wax border should be embedded in the lower half, where it may be faithfully reproduced and preserved during polishing.

The use of acrylic resin materials that require trial packing is complicated by the presence of the retentive framework of the RPD. With their use, trial packing must be done with two sheets of cellophane between two layers of the resin dough; otherwise, the flask could not be opened without pulling the resin away from the teeth in one half of the flask or the metal framework in the other. Acrylic resin dough is placed in each half of the flask, the sheets of cellophane are placed between them, and the flask is closed for trial packing. The flask is then opened, the cellophane is removed, and the excess flash is trimmed away. Trial packing should be repeated until no excess is visible. Final closure is accomplished without the intervening sheets of cellophane.

Acrylic resin materials have been developed that require no trial packing. These are mixed as usual but may be poured into the mold or placed into the mold in a soft state. They offer little or no resistance to the closure of the flask, yet the finished

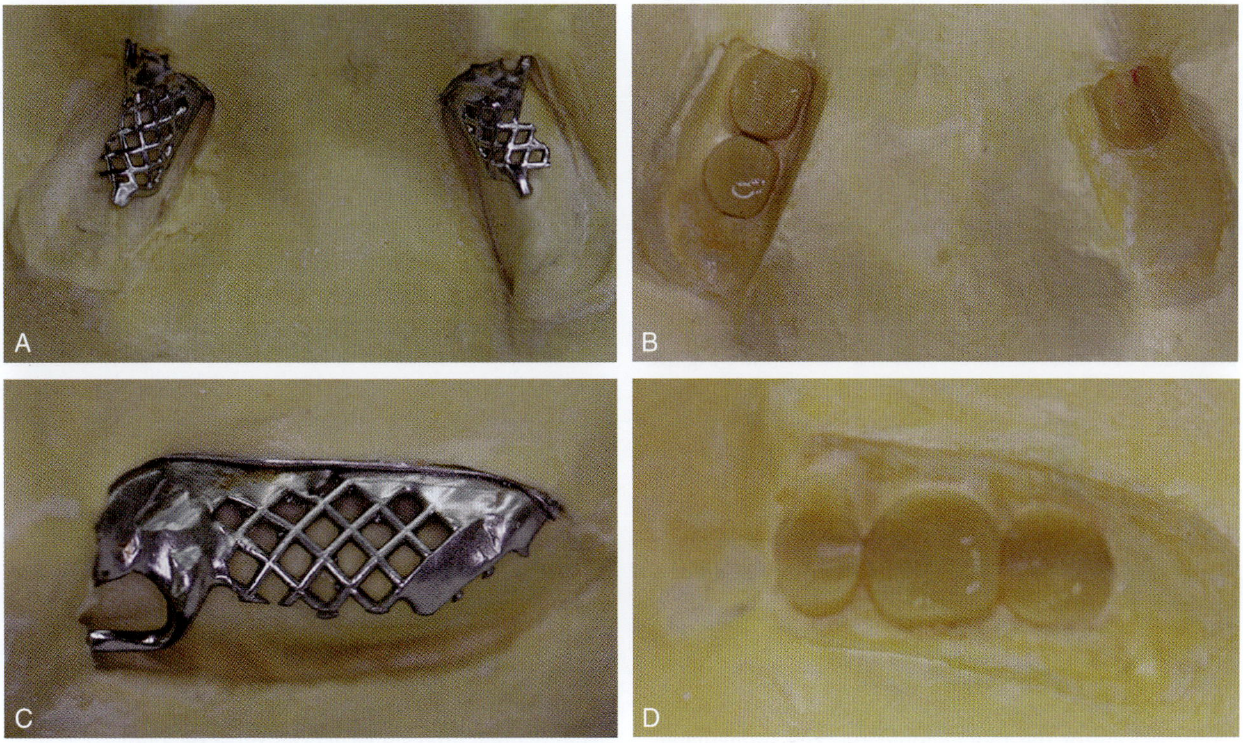

Fig. 20.46 Prostheses invested in processing flasks. **A,** Mandibular Kennedy Class I master cast with exposed minor connectors of the distal extension bases. **B,** Denture teeth for framework shown in **(A)**. **C,** Maxillary distal extension minor connector embedded in investing stone. **D,** Opposing flask unit with denture teeth for distal extension shown in **(C)**.

product is comparable with acrylic resin materials packed in a doughy state. They must be used in some excess, with the excess escaping between the halves of the flask. Although they are soft enough to allow the escape of gross excess, the use of a land space is advisable to prevent a thin film from forming on the land area. Any film that exists on the land area after deflasking may be interpreted as an opening of the flask by that amount, hence the need for some provision for an intervening space to accommodate the excess and to facilitate flow of excess material as the flask is closed.

To provide such a land space, the land area on the lower half of the flask may be painted with melted baseplate wax before the top half is poured. After wax elimination, a space then remains to accommodate any excess acrylic resin remaining after the flask has been completely closed. No plaster or wax should remain on the rim of the flask, and the flask components must make a metal-to-metal contact before the second half is poured. Only in this way is it possible to see that the flask is completely closed before it is placed in the curing unit.

Pouring of the top half of the flask follows the same procedure as that used with a complete denture. Although it is not absolutely necessary for the entire top half of the flask to be filled with stone, it is necessary for a stone cap of some type to be used to prevent tooth movement in an occlusal direction. This is so because of the inability of plaster to withstand closing pressures. All plaster remaining on the occlusal surfaces of the teeth should be removed and a separator added before the stone cap is poured to facilitate its removal during deflasking. If the use of stone investment is preferred, a shell of improved stone or die stone may be painted or applied with the fingers onto the wax and teeth and allowed to harden before the remainder of the flask is filled with plaster. If a full stone investment is preferred, some provision should be made for easy separation during deflasking. Not only should a separator stone cap be used, but metal separators or knife cuts radiating out to the walls of the flask should be placed on the partially set stone. Deflasking is then easily accomplished by removing the stone cap and inserting a knife blade between the sections of stone.

Boil out should be deferred until the investing material has set for several hours or preferably overnight. Boil out must effectively eliminate all waxy residue; an adequate source of clean hot water must be available. Immersion of a flask containing the invested denture in boiling water for 5 minutes will adequately soften the wax supporting the artificial teeth so that flask halves may be separated and the remaining wax flushed out. After wax elimination with boiling water, the invested denture should be flushed with a solution of grease-dissolving detergent and again with clean boiling water.

Immediately after boiling out, the warm mold should be painted with a thin film of tinfoil substitute, with care taken to not allow it to collect around the cervical portions of the teeth. No tinfoil substitute should be used on any part of the denture teeth. A second coat should be applied after the first coat has dried, and packing of the mold should proceed immediately after this film has dried to the touch.

When the master cast for a distal extension RPD has been repoured from a secondary impression, the supporting "foot" on the denture base retention framework may not be in contact with the cast. Closing pressure within the flask may distort the unsupported extension of the metal framework, with the subsequent rebound on deflasking. The finished denture base will then lack contact with the supporting tissue, resulting in denture rotation about the fulcrum line, similar to that which occurs after tissue resorption. To provide support for the distal extension of the metal framework during flask closure, autopolymerizing acrylic resin should be sprinkled or painted around the tissue stop at the distal end of the framework and allowed to harden before the denture resin continues to be packed.

PROCESSING THE DENTURE

Processing follows the same procedure as that used for a complete denture. Denture base characterization tinting may be added just before packing. This is most desirable if denture base material will be visible when in the mouth. Posterior acrylic resin bases alone ordinarily do not require characterization, but the dentist should select a denture base material that closely resembles the color of the surrounding tissue. The ideal acrylic resin base material for RPDs therefore is one that (1) may be used without trial packing, (2) possesses a shade that is compatible with the surrounding tissue, (3) is dimensionally stable and accurate, (4) is dense and lends itself to polishing, and (5) polymerizes completely.

There has never been any question concerning the merits of placing tinfoil over the denture before investing; this results in a tinfoil-lined matrix and eliminates the need for a separating film. The fact remains, however, that the use of a tinfoil substitute has become universal.

At best, any tinfoil substitute creates an undesirable film at the gingival margins of the teeth, resulting in microscopic separation between the teeth and the surrounding acrylic resin. This may be shown by sectioning a finished denture and by observing the marginal discoloration around the cervical portions of the teeth after several months in the mouth. To some extent, injection molding obviates this objection to the use of a tinfoil substitute; this is one of the principal advantages of injection molding over compression molding.

Because the use of compression molding is widespread and is likely to continue, methods are needed to eliminate the use of a tinfoil substitute. The layered silicone rubber method results in more complete adaptation of the acrylic resin around the cervical portions of porcelain teeth and more complete bonding to acrylic resin teeth. In addition, denture base tints may be applied directly to the mold without first applying a separating film.

A room-temperature polymerizing silicone rubber that has sufficient body and toughness for the purpose is applied to the wax surface of the denture and over the teeth. To prevent movement of the teeth during processing, the occlusal surfaces should be exposed before the upper half of the flask is poured. The manufacturer's instructions must be followed as to mixing and time elapsed before the outer stone investment is added, to ensure polymerization and bonding to the overlying investment. Boil out then is completed in the usual way.

A further advantage of the layered silicone rubber method is the ease of accomplishing deflasking. If the wax carving of the denture has been completed with care before flasking, denture tints remain unaltered by unnecessary trimming and polishing of the processed denture.

All resin base materials available up to the present time exhibit some dimensional change, both during processing and in the mouth. The fit of the denture is therefore dependent on the accuracy of the denture base material because impression and cast materials in use today are themselves accurate. To minimize dimensional changes in the denture base, materials and techniques are being improved constantly.

Denture base materials that may be poured into the mold or placed into the mold in a soft state are also popular. This technique eliminates trial packing and excessive pressures, which lead to open flasks and altered occlusal vertical dimension as is sometimes experienced with compression molding of acrylic resin base materials. Activated or autopolymerizing acrylic resins are commonly used to prevent mold expansion at higher temperatures. Materials other than acrylic resins are used with various techniques, some of which include styrene, vinyl, and experimentally epoxy resins. The main objective behind the development of newer techniques and materials is greater dimensional accuracy and stability, combined with improved strength and better appearance.

The use of injection molding or poured materials to process RPD base materials combines accuracy and efficiency to help create a well-fitting denture base. The Success Injection System (Dentsply Trubyte, York, PA) combines the accuracy of injection molding with Lucitone 199 (Dentsply Trubyte). The hardware consists of the injection unit, aluminum alloy flasks, and associated system flask components. The flasks are numbered; specifically, they are mated halves that need to be matched for more accurate results. The investment and processing techniques are as follows:

1. *The cast with the completed wax-up is embedded in the designated side "1" of the flask in the usual manner, placing the cast as close as possible to the back of the flask.* After any undercuts on the cast are eliminated, flattened wax sticks (approximately 7 mm in diameter) are used to build the injection sprues. For maxillary RPDs, attach the sprue to the posterior border, ensuring that the sprue is sufficiently wide. For mandibular RPDs, position one sprue for each base extension. Apply a separator to the investment and place the top half of the flask on the bottom half, ensuring complete intimate metal contact and closure of the halves. Secure the flask brackets to the flask and tighten. Place the flask on the leveler with side "2" up and complete the investing procedure in the usual manner.
2. *When the investment has set, loosen the bolts and remove the metal flask brackets.* Place the flask in boiling water (8–10 minutes) and complete the boil-out procedure. Place the metal injection insert into the back of the flask and slide the plastic injection socket into the metal insert as far as possible. The plastic injection socket lip should rest flush against the trim of the metal injection insert. Close the flask, position the metal flask brackets, and tighten the bolts.
3. *Use the powder/liquid vials to measure sufficient resin for the RPD.* Note that the maximum powder and/or liquid that the injection cartridge can hold is 38 g (56 mL) powder and/or 17.5 mL liquid. Stir the powder and/or liquid for approximately 15 seconds. Do not excessively mix. Cover the mixing jar until the material reaches the "soft pack" stage (approximately 6 minutes). Do not allow the material to reach the "snap set" stage.
4. *Place the resin material into the plastic injection cartridge and insert the blue plastic cartridge plug into the large open end, ribbed side out.* Push the blue cartridge plug in as far as possible to compress the material and insert the cartridge nozzle into the plastic injection socket until it seats on the injection socket's lip. Place the metal protective sleeve over the cartridge, and place the flask in the injection unit, ensuring that the bolts and the flask brackets face the operator's right side. Position the open slots on the cartridge sleeve facing out, and then push the sleeve up toward the unit's crosshead securing the sleeve around the blue rubber O-ring. Tighten the unit's hand wheel to secure the flask.
5. *Complete the injection process, ensuring the mold is completely filled by viewing the blue cartridge plug through the sleeve slots until it stops moving.* When completed, remove the flask from the unit, remove the cartridge sleeve, and pull the plastic cartridge out of the flask with a slight twist. Keep the injection socket in place inside the metal injection insert. Fit the small, blue plastic piston cap onto the end of the pressing device piston. Place the piston of the processing device into the plastic injection socket at the back of the flask and screw the pressing device onto the metal injection insert until the etched groove is visible on the pin at the top of the pressing device.
6. *Allow the flask to sit for 30 minutes before heat polymerizing to ensure a good bond between the denture resin and the teeth.* Submerge the closed flask in water at 163 ± 2°F for hours. Follow with an additional 30-minute boil. An alternate polymerization method is 9 hours in a water bath of 163 ± 2°F without boiling. Remove the flask from the polymerization tank and allow it to cool for approximately 30 minutes. Place the flask in a lukewarm water bath to cool completely.
7. *Unscrew the pressing device and loosen the bolts on the flask.* Remove the flask brackets and separate the flask. Remove the investment and divest the RPD and cast. Cut off the injection sprue(s), and finish and polish the RPD in a conventional manner.

The use of VLC denture base materials is claimed to save considerable time in providing a processed base. Manufacturers recommend the use of a light-colored cast to enhance the polymerization of the VLC material. A stone matrix must be fabricated so that the denture teeth can be positively relocated in the same position during the polymerizing process. Once the stone matrix has been completed and verified, the wax and teeth can be removed from the framework; the teeth are cleaned and silicoated, or coated with the resin bonding agent.

The ideal thickness for the VLC material requires a 1.5-mm space between the edentulous ridge and the retentive component of the framework. The ridge lap of the denture teeth should also be 1.5 mm above the retentive component of the framework, and the tissue side finishing line of the framework should be even with or slightly higher than the palatal side finishing line. If VLC denture base material is to be used, these requirements must be considered at the diagnosis and treatment planning stages.

Without the framework in place, a thin coat of model release agent is applied to the denture base areas of the cast, and the VLC material is adapted to the edentulous denture base area and is trimmed to the general outline with a sharp blade. The framework is then seated firmly by being embedded into the uncured VLC material. Make certain that the rests, tissue stops, and other components of the RPD framework are correctly positioned in their designated terminal positions on the cast. Remove any excess material that may interfere with articulation of the casts or positioning of the teeth and check to ensure that the VLC material is adapted into the tissue side finishing line of the framework on the cast. This will necessitate returning the cast with the framework to the articulator. Once this has been verified, remove the cast from the articulator and process it in the light-polymerizing unit for 2 minutes.

The denture teeth can then be secured to the stone matrix and related to the cast with the framework and the RPD base. The denture teeth may have to be adjusted before the RPD base can be fitted. To do this, trim the ridge lap areas of the teeth enough to provide the required 1.5 mm of space between the tooth and the denture base material. Remember that thin areas should be avoided between the framework and the cast (minimum of 1.5 mm) and between the framework and the denture teeth (minimum of 1.5 mm).

The denture tooth surfaces that are to be bonded to the VLC denture base must be lightly ground and cleaned. The teeth can be positioned using modeling compound or putty held in position while the bonding agent is applied to all designated surfaces to be bonded to the VLC denture base. These coated surfaces should be allowed to sit for 2 minutes and then be processed in the light polymerization unit for 1 minute.

To secure the teeth into their designated position on the VLC denture base, apply a small piece of VLC material to each tooth with the modeling tool provided by the manufacturer. With the aid of the stone matrix and by using a high-intensity light, tack each individual tooth into position on the VLC denture base.

After tacking the teeth to the VLC denture base, paint a narrow band of bonding agent on the junction line between the teeth and the denture base material. The bonding agent acts as a sealer to prevent leakage and aids bonding of the teeth to the denture base material. Allow the bonding agent to set for 2 minutes, and then process in the light unit for 1 minute. You can now complete the buccal and lingual contouring of the denture base with additional VLC material. Paint all exposed surfaces of the VLC denture base material with the air barrier coating material and process in the light polymerization unit for 2 minutes. After processing, carefully remove the RPD from the cast. Do not attempt to pry it off. Paint the tissue surfaces of the edentulous areas with the air barrier coating material and place the prosthesis in the light polymerization unit for 6 minutes with the tissue side up. Clean the RPD with water and a brush to remove all traces of the air barrier coating. Trim and polish in a routine manner to complete the RPD.

With newer materials, the future of methyl methacrylate as a denture base material is uncertain despite its acceptance as the best material available since its introduction in 1937. Although it has made possible the simulation of natural tissue color and contours combined with ease of manipulation, the fact remains that it leaves much to be desired as far as accuracy and dimensional stability are concerned. Whether other and newer materials will eventually supplant methyl methacrylate as a denture base material remains to be seen. The fact is that the denture base of the future (1) must be capable of accurately reproducing natural tissue tones faithfully through the use of characterizing stains and customizing procedures and (2) must not require elaborate processing procedures and equipment, which would make the cost prohibitive for general use.

REMOUNTING AND OCCLUSAL CORRECTION TO AN OCCLUSAL TEMPLATE

Even with improved denture base materials and processing techniques, some movement of artificial teeth will still occur because of the dimensional instability of the wax in which the artificial teeth were arranged. Remounting the RPD may be necessary. How well the occlusion may be perfected by remounting depends on how the jaw relation record was transferred to an instrument and how closely it can reproduce functional occlusion. Even with use of articulator that is limited to reproducing a static centric relation, the occlusion with that relation should be reestablished before the denture is placed.

Even with the limitations in perfecting eccentric occlusion intraorally, some believe intraoral adjustments can be accomplished more accurately than on a static, hinge instrument that is incapable of reproducing eccentric positions. It is possible to transfer centric jaw relation to an instrument with accuracy and to maintain this relation throughout fabrication of the prosthesis. If accomplished well, then centric occlusion, coinciding with centric jaw relation, with centric occlusion of the remaining natural teeth, or with both, must have been established before initial placement of the prosthesis. This means that occlusal correction to reestablish centric relation by remounting after final processing may be needed for the success of the restoration. Remounting after processing is accomplished by returning the cast to a keyed relationship with the articulator mounting.

Precautions to Be Taken in Remounting

The following precautions should be taken to ensure the accuracy of remounting to make final occlusal adjustment before polishing and initial placement of the denture. These apply to all types of occlusal relationship records but are directed particularly at remounting an occlusal template when stone vertical stops are used:

1. Make sure that the base of the cast has been reduced to fit the flask before keying and mounting so that it will not have to be altered later.

2. Bevel the margins of the base of the cast so that it will seat in a definite boxlike manner in the articulator mounting.
3. Notch the posterior and anterior aspects of the base to ensure its return to its original position. Notches at the margins are preferable to depressions within the base because the former permit a visual check of the accuracy of the remounting.
4. Lightly lubricate the base and sides of the cast before it is mounted to facilitate its easy removal from the mounting stone.
5. Add tinfoil or lightly lubricate the base and sides of the cast before flasking it so that traces of investment will not be present to interfere with remounting.
6. When remounting the cast, secure it in the articulator with sticky wax, a hot glue gun, or modeling plastic, followed by stone over both the mounting and the sides of the cast.
7. Before adjusting the occlusion, make certain that no traces of investment remain on the vertical stops.
8. Take care to avoid abrading the opposing occlusal surfaces during occlusal adjustment. The use of marking tape or inked ribbon is preferable to articulating paper. The artificial tooth is less likely to cut through and mar the opposing surface, and ink or dye will not build up a false opposing surface, as will wax from articulating paper.
9. Occlusal readjustment to an occlusal template is complete when the stone vertical stops are again in contact. With other types of articulator mountings, readjustment is complete when the vertical pin is again in contact, and any valid horizontal excursions are free of interference.

Occlusal readjustment, as with the original articulation, is done at the expense of the original tooth anatomy. Occlusal surfaces should be reshaped by adding grooves and spillways and by reducing the area of the occlusal table, thus improving the masticating efficiency of the artificial tooth. Although this may be done immediately after occlusal readjustment and before the initial placement of the denture, it may be deferred until completion of the final adjustment. In any event, it is a necessary step in the completion of any removable prosthesis.

Porcelain teeth may be reshaped with abrasive or diamond-mounted points. Resin teeth can be reshaped using small burs to restore functional anatomy. Either type should be repolished judiciously to prevent the reduction of cuspal contacts. Although cusps may be narrowed, spillways added, and the total area of contact reduced to improve masticating efficiency, critical areas of contact, both vertical and horizontal, must always be preserved.

The term *remounting* also applies to the mounting of a completed prosthetic restoration back into an instrument by using an interocclusal records. Discrepancies in occlusion resulting from processing of tooth-supported dentures may be corrected by reattaching the indexed processing cast and denture to the same instrument on which the occlusion was formulated. However, because of some instability inherent in distal extension RPDs, such dentures should be retrieved from processing investment, finished, and polished, and prepared for the performance of occlusal corrections with the use of new intraoral records. The dentist must make a remounting cast before occlusal corrections can be accomplished. This is done simply first by placing the denture in the mouth and making an irreversible hydrocolloid (alginate) impression of the denture and the remaining teeth in the arch (Fig. 20.47). When the impression is removed, the denture usually remains in the impression or can be accurately replaced. Undercuts in the denture bases are

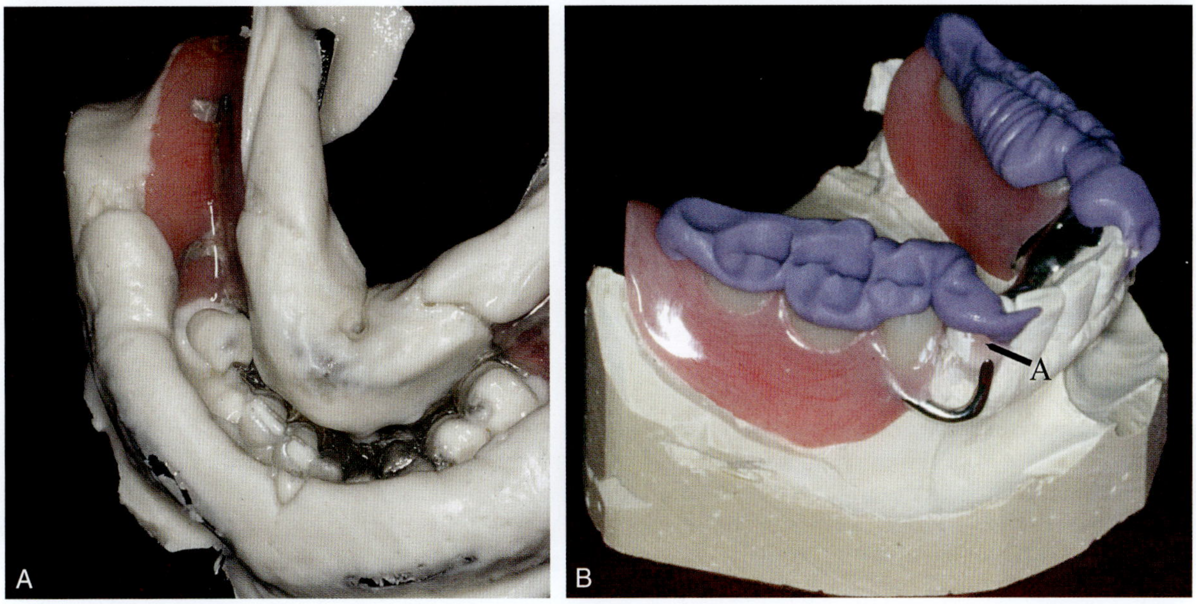

Fig. 20.47 A, A stock, perforated tray is used to make an irreversible hydrocolloid (alginate) impression of the denture and dental arch. Blockout of undercuts in the denture base and of tips of direct retainers is necessary, so the denture can be readily removed and replaced on the resultant remounting cast, as illustrated in **(B)**. **B,** Remounting cast poured in stone with the prosthesis in place and interocclusal registration for mounting against a maxillary cast. Wax placed at the retainer tip *(A)* allows the prosthesis to be readily removed and replaced on the cast for occlusal correction procedures that use an articulator.

blocked out, the retentive elements of the framework are covered with a thin layer of molten wax, and a remounting cast is poured in the impression. The remount casts are oriented in the articulator using the same type of interocclusal records that were used to orient the casts to formulate the occlusion. These procedures are covered in Chapter 21 as an integral part of the initial placement appointment.

Occlusal harmony must exist before the patient is given possession of the dentures. Delaying the correction of occlusal discrepancies until the dentures have had a chance to settle is not justifiable.

POLISHING THE DENTURE

Areas to be considered in the polishing of an RPD are (1) the borders of the denture bases, (2) the facial surfaces, and (3) the teeth and adjacent areas.

The borders on complete metal bases will have been established previously. On partial metal bases and complete acrylic resin bases, the accuracy with which the border may be finished depends on the accuracy of the impression record and how well this was preserved on the stone cast. Edentulous areas recorded from impressions in stock trays generally lack the accuracy at the borders that are found on casts made from impressions in individualized trays and by secondary impression methods. Border accuracy is determined also by whether the impression recorded a functional or a static relationship of the bordering tissue attachments.

Denture Borders

The principal objectives to be considered in making an impression of edentulous areas of a partially edentulous arch include (1) maximal support for the edentulous RPD base and (2) extension of the borders to obtain maximum coverage compatible with moving tissue. Although this second objective may be met with an adequate individualized impression tray, it is best accomplished with a secondary impression method. The extent and width of the border should be recorded accurately and preserved on the stone cast. Except for certain areas arbitrarily thinned by polishing (mentioned previously in this chapter), finishing and polishing the denture borders should consist only of removing any flash and artifact blebs. Otherwise, borders should remain as recorded in the impression.

When the impression is made in a stock tray, the tray itself will have influenced both the extent and the width of the border. Some areas will be left short of the total area available for denture support, whereas others will be extended beyond functional limits by overextension of the tray. Unfortunately, the technician may attempt to interpret the anatomy of the mouth and arbitrarily trim the denture borders. This presumes that the technician has an intimate knowledge of the anatomy of the mouth of the patient for whom the restoration is being made, which is most unlikely. The dentist must correct any overextension remaining after arbitrarily trimming the border from cast landmarks in the mouth. It is preferable for the dentist to finish the borders of dentures, having painstakingly developed them during impression procedures.

Facial Surfaces

The facial surfaces of the denture base are those polished surfaces lying between the buccal borders and the supplied teeth. Methods have been proposed for making sectional impression records of buccal contours, thereby permitting the denture base to be made to conform to the facial musculature. These have never received wide acceptance and may be considered impractical in removable partial prosthodontics.

Facial surfaces may be established in wax or may be carved into the denture base after processing. Generally, it is desirable that it be done in wax as part of the wax pattern because it is easier to do so and because contours can best be established at a time when modifications can be made if desired. Buccal surfaces should be contoured to aid in the retention of the denture by border molding, to preserve the border roll and thereby prevent food impaction, and to facilitate the return of the food bolus back onto the masticating table. Lingual surfaces should be made concave to provide tongue room and to aid in the retention of the denture. Polishing concave surfaces is always more difficult than polishing flat and convex surfaces. If such contours are established previously in wax, finishing is easily accomplished, and border and gingival areas are less likely to be altered mistakenly.

Finishing Gingival and Interproximal Areas

The contouring of gingival and interproximal areas after processing is difficult and generally unsatisfactory (Fig. 20.48). Modern cosmetic considerations demand that gingival carving be done around each tooth individually, with variations in the height of the gingival curve and in the length of the papillae. Papillae should be convex interproximally rather than concave. The gingival attachment should be free of grooves and ditches that would accumulate debris and stain and should be as free for cleansing as possible. All this precludes gross shaping and

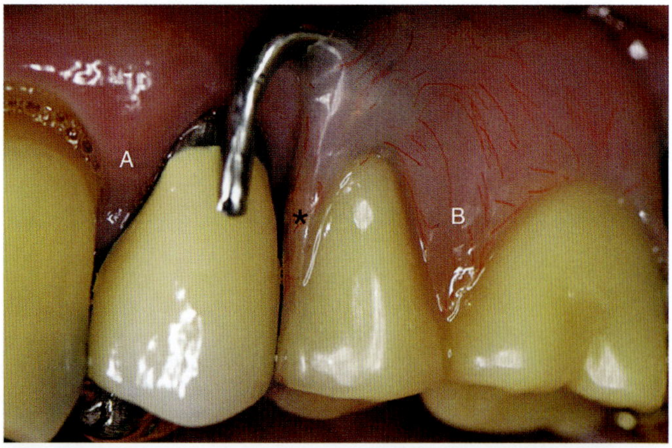

Fig. 20.48 Attention to adjacent tooth-tissue contours can facilitate the production of natural-appearing prostheses. The interproximal papilla at *(A)* demonstrates both vertical and horizontal components. In general, the horizontal component increases with age. The prosthetic interproximal papilla at *(B)* exhibits only a vertical component and appears artificial. The anterior border *(*)* contour is blunted and provides an obvious and abrupt contour change. Contouring the border to bevel into the interproximal region reduces its objectionable appearance.

trimming of gingival areas after processing. Gingival carving should be done in wax, and investing should be done with care to prevent voids, blebs, and artifacts. Finishing should consist only of trimming around the teeth and the papillae with small round burs to create a more natural simulation of living tissue, plus light stippling with an off-center round bur for the same reason. Polishing should consist only of light buffing with brush wheels and pumice, and finally with a soft brush wheel and a nonabrasive polishing agent specially made for this purpose.

Pumicing of gingival areas can only serve to polish the high spots; although it may be done lightly, its use should be limited to light buffing of areas already made as smooth as in the waxing phase. Heavy pumicing of the denture resin not only creates an unfavorable denture look but also alters the delicately carved wax surface and any plastic teeth present. If pumicing must be done, plastic teeth should be protected with adhesive masking tape during the process.

Any polishing operation on an RPD done on a lathe is made hazardous by the presence of direct retainers, which can easily become caught in the polishing wheel. Although the least damage that might occur is the distortion of a clasp arm, there is a greater possibility that the denture may be thrown forcibly into the lathe pan, with severe damage to the framework or other parts of the denture. The technician must be conscious of this possibility and must always cover any projecting clasp with the finger while it is near the polishing wheel. In addition, it is wise to keep a pumice pan well filled with wet pumice to cushion the shock should an accident occur. Any other lathe pan used in polishing should be lined with a towel or with a resilient material for the same reason. The potential hazard of retainers catching gloved fingers or hands that hold an RPD is always present. Significant injury can result, and extreme caution must be taken to prevent such an occurrence.

ADDITIONAL LABORATORY PROCEDURE USING A DENTAL SURVEYOR

Contouring Wax Patterns

If surveyed restorations are to be fabricated for the patient before RPDs, crowns must be surveyed to confirm their correctness. The surveyor blade is used as a wax carver during this phase of mouth preparation so that the proposed path of placement may be maintained throughout the preparation of cast restorations for abutment teeth (Fig. 20.49).

Guide planes on all proximal surfaces of wax patterns adjacent to edentulous areas should be made parallel to the previously determined path of placement. Similarly, all other tooth contours that will be contacted by rigid components should be made parallel. The surfaces of restorations on which reciprocal and stabilizing components will be placed should be contoured to permit their location well below occlusal surfaces and on nonretentive areas. Those surfaces of restorations that are to provide retention for clasp arms should be contoured so that retentive clasps may be placed in the cervical third of the crown and to the best esthetic advantage. Generally, a small amount of undercut from 0.01 to 0.02 inch (0.250–0.50 mm) is sufficient for retentive purposes.

Placement of Intracoronal Retainers (Internal Attachments)

In the placement of intracoronal retainers, the surveyor is used as follows:

- To select a path of placement in relation to the long axes of the abutment teeth that avoids areas of interference elsewhere in the arch.
- To cut recesses in the stone teeth on the diagnostic cast for estimating the proximity of the recess to the pulp (used in conjunction with roentgenographic information to estimate pulp size and location) and to facilitate the fabrication of metal or resin jigs to guide preparations of the recesses in the mouth.

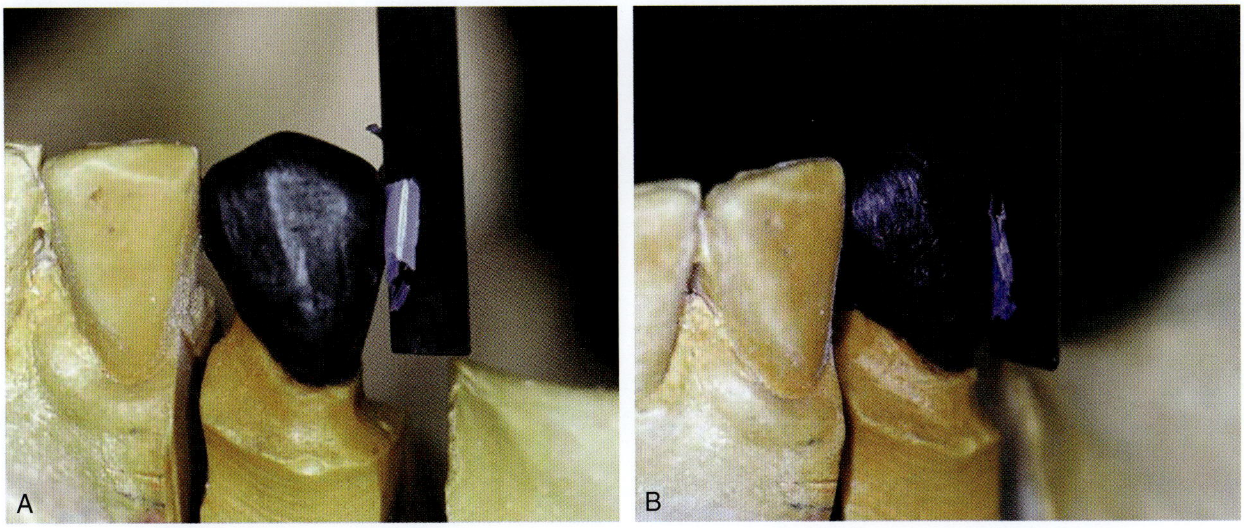

Fig. 20.49 After the cast has been oriented to the surveyor at the predetermined path of placement, designated axial surfaces of the wax pattern are altered with the surveyor blade to meet specific requirements for placement of framework components. **A,** Wax pattern is carved with the surveyor blade to produce a distal guide plane surface parallel to the selected path of insertion. **B,** The same pattern is modified from the distal guide plane along the buccal surface to align the surface with the height of contour most favorable to the direct retainer specifications.

- To carve recesses in wax patterns, to place internal attachment trays in wax patterns, or to cut recesses in castings with the handpiece holder (whichever method is preferred).
- To place the keyway portion of the attachment in the casting before investing and soldering; each keyway must be located parallel to the other keyways elsewhere in the arch.

PLACEMENT OF INTERNAL REST SEATS

The surveyor may be used as a drill press, with a dental handpiece attached to the vertical arm by a handpiece holder. Internal rest seats may be carved in the wax patterns and further refined with the handpiece after casting, or the entire rest seat may be cut in the cast restoration with the handpiece. It is best to carve the outline form of the rest seat in wax and merely refine the casting with the handpiece.

An internal rest differs from an internal attachment in that some portion of the prosthesis framework is waxed and cast to fit into the rest seat rather than a matched key and keyway attachment used. The former is usually nonretentive but provides a definite seat for an RPD or a cantilever rest for a broken-stress FPD. When they are used with FPDs, nonparallel abutment pieces may be placed separately.

The internal rest in partial denture construction provides a positive occlusal support that is more favorably located in relation to the rotational axis of the abutment tooth than the conventional spoon-shaped occlusal rest. It also provides horizontal stabilization through the parallelism of the vertical walls, thereby serving the same purpose as stabilizing and reciprocal arms placed extracoronally. More torque may be applied to the abutment tooth by an interlocking type of rest due to the distal extension base movement and be contraindicated. The ball-and-socket, spoon-shaped occlusal, or noninterlocking rest should be used in distal extension removable partial denture designs. Use of the dovetailed or interlocking internal rest should be limited to tooth-supported removable restorations, except when used with a stress breaker between the abutments and the movable base. The use of stress breakers has been discussed in Chapter 9.

Internal rest seats may be made in the form of a nonretentive box, a retentive box fashioned after the internal attachment, or a semiretentive box. In the latter, the walls are usually parallel and nonretentive, but a recess in the floor of the box prevents proximal movement of the male portion. Internal rest seats are cut with dental burs of various sizes and shapes. Tapered or cylindrical fissure burs are used to form the vertical walls, and small round burs are used to cut recesses in the floor of the rest seat.

Machining Cast Restorations

With a handpiece holder attached (Fig. 20.50), the axial surfaces of cast and ceramic restorations may be refined by machining with a suitable cylindrical carborundum point. Proximal surfaces of crowns and inlays, which will serve as guide planes, and vertical surfaces above crown ledges may be improved by machining, but only if the relationship of one crown to another is correct. Unless the seating of removable dies is accurate and they are held in place with additional stone or plaster, cast restorations should first be tried in the mouth and then transferred, by means of a plaster or acrylic resin index impression, to a reinforced stone cast for machining purposes. The new cast is then positioned on the surveyor, conforming to the path of placement of the partial denture, and vertical surfaces are machined with a true-running cylindrical carborundum point.

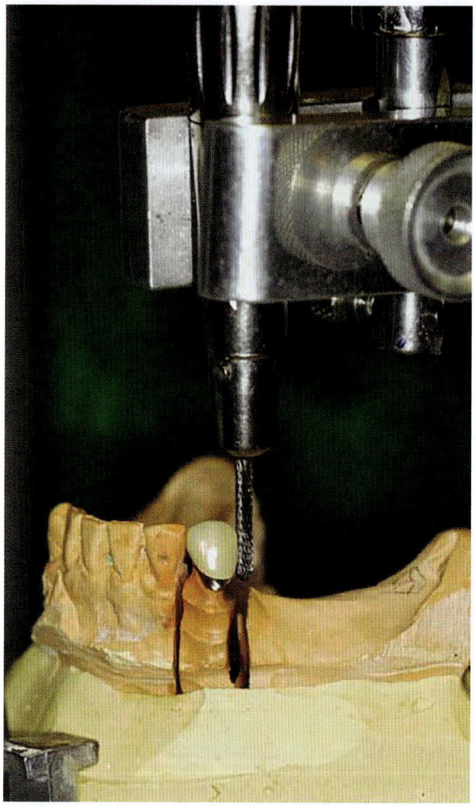

Fig. 20.50 Lab handpiece clamp. Handpiece holders attach to the vertical spindle of surveyors and may be used to create and refine any parallel surface on a surveyed crown, as a drill press to prepare internal rests and recesses in patterns and/or castings, and to establish lingual surfaces above the ledge that are parallel to the path of placement in abutment restorations.

Although machined parallelism may be considered ideal and beyond the realm of everyday application, its merits more than justify the additional steps required to accomplish it. When such parallelism is accomplished and reproduced in a master cast, it is essential that subsequent laboratory steps be directed toward the use of these parallel guide plane surfaces.

Digital Laboratory Procedures

Data acquisition via scanning, computer-aided design (CAD), and computer-aided manufacturing systems are continually improving resulting in increased accuracy and speed of manufacturing. Therefore this section is designed to explain how digital workflows work in the production of an RPD framework through to completion at the time of writing the 14th edition.

Scanning (Data Acquisition)

Scanners can be either intraoral or extraoral. Desktop scanners are extraoral scanners designed to scan casts (Fig. 20.51). Like intraoral scanners, they generate a 3D cast in a stereolithography file format known as STL. However, instead of scanning intraoral structures like intraoral scanners, desktop scanners scan a physical cast or an impression. This is done through either light projection in which the scanner projects a structured light pattern, typically consisting of stripes or grids, onto the object being scanned, or image capture in which multiple cameras placed at different angles capture images of the deformed light pattern reflected off the object's surface. Objects are placed within the scanner and secured onto a pedestal. In many cases, the desktop scanners can also scan casts in occlusion or interocclusal records.

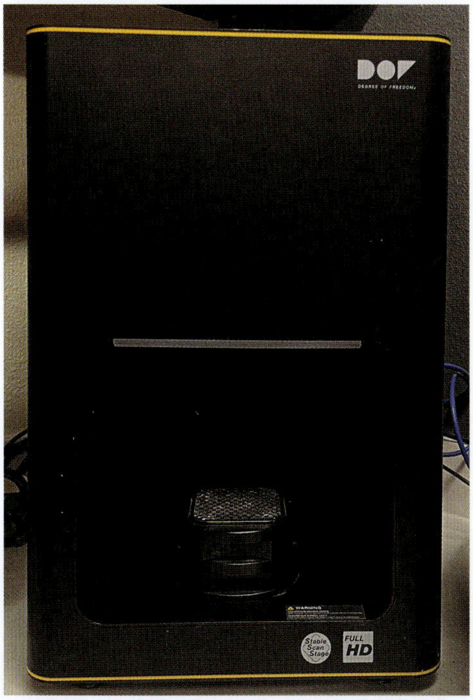

Fig. 20.51 A desktop scanner is able to scan models or impressions and transform them into an .stl file for use in design. (Courtesy of Ahmed Mahrous Copyright © 2024. All rights reserved.)

Computer-Aided Design

CAD software is an essential component of the digital design workflow. To start the design, an STL file of the intraoral structures must be imported into the software. The STL might be an intraoral scan or an extraoral desktop scan. Virtual casts might need to be trimmed or edited to the correct shape when they are initially imported into the design software system (Fig. 20.52). If a beading line is to be made, this should be added either on the physical cast or digitally after scanning. The STL file is imported into the software and set up for surveying. As was described in Chapter 11, most software systems depict the undercuts on each tooth with different colors that indicate the depth of the undercut. The path of insertion should be determined based on the angle on the provided guidelines and the tripoding provided of the diagnostic or surveyed master cast (Fig. 20.53).

The virtual blockout is done next. Most software systems have a 5° blockout angle; however, this can be set at 0° for that tooth, which prevents infrabulge clasp arms from protruding and causing discomfort for the patient (Fig. 20.54). The blockout is then trimmed to uncover the retentive undercuts to be used based on the diagnostic design. Relief is also added for any component opposing nonkeratinized or sensitive tissues such as the lingual mucosa or mid-palatine raphe.

Most software systems allow the designer to draw the outline of each component of the RPD (Fig. 20.55). The retentive latticework or mesh is usually added first followed by all other components, including the rests and the major connector. Proper component overlap must be considered for the final framework to be cohesive. The clasps, with various shapes available, are then added. Some will taper toward the tip, while others will have a uniform shape. The clasp taper and cross section can also be altered to provide adequate taper (Fig. 20.56).

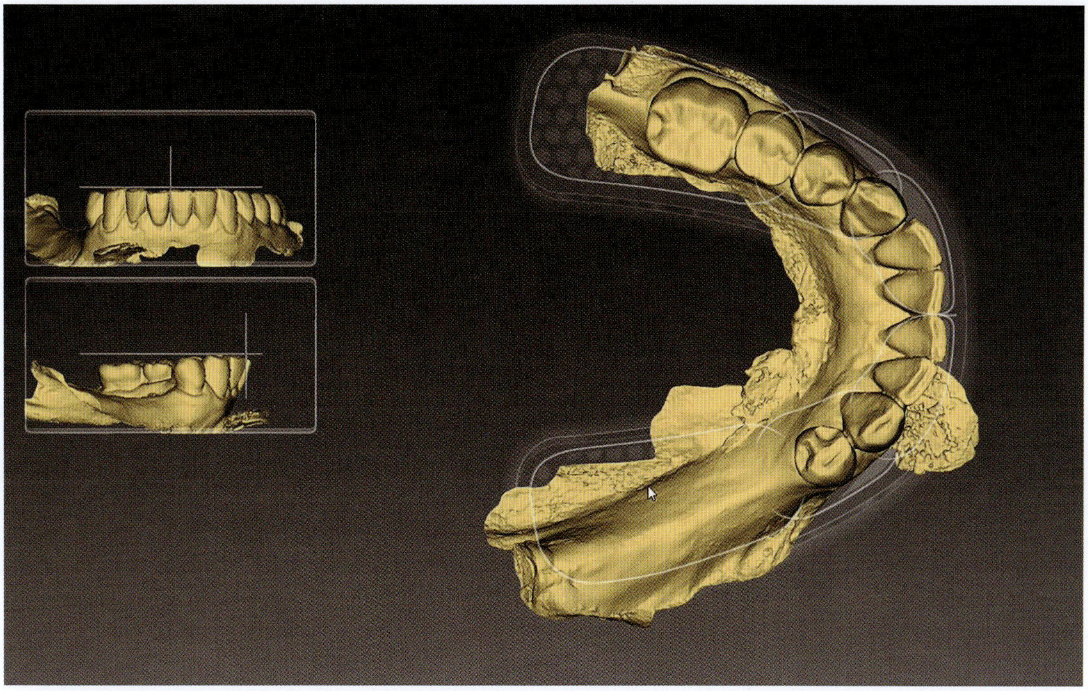

Fig. 20.52 Models are set in the proper orientation when imported into a design software, excess extension can also be trimmed off at this stage. (Courtesy of Ahmed Mahrous Copyright © 2024. All rights reserved.)

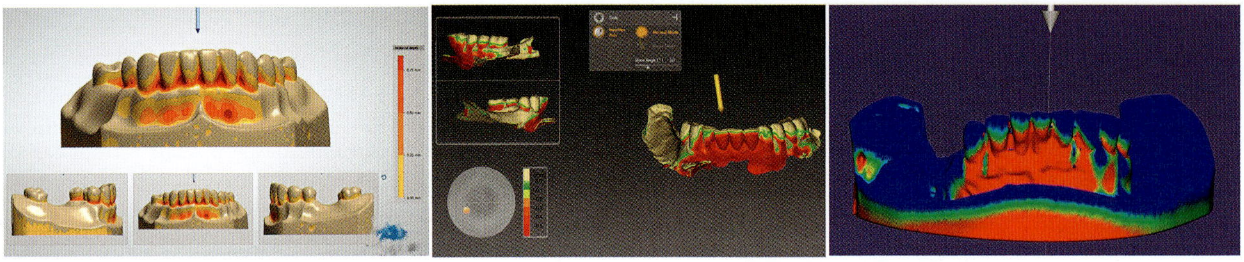

Fig. 20.53 Path of draw set on three different design software systems. Each software depicts undercuts of varying depth in different colors and shadings.

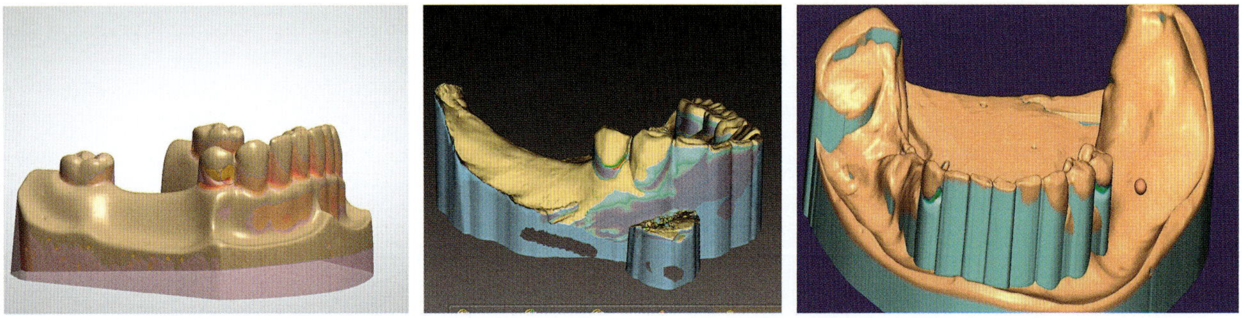

Fig. 20.54 Blockout applied on the cast after surveying in three different design software systems.

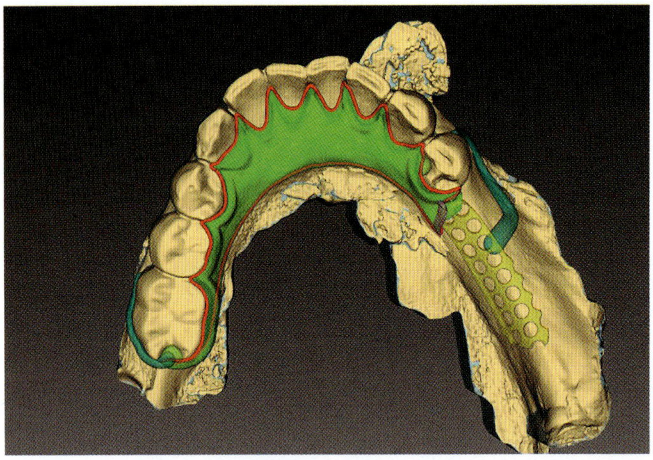

Fig. 20.55 All components are outlined and drawn separately, including rests, clasps, major connectors, minor connectors, proximal plates, and lattice. (Courtesy of Ahmed Mahrous Copyright © 2024. All rights reserved.)

After all components have been added, the different components are merged together. The framework should be evaluated for completeness and cohesion (Fig. 20.57). Any areas of discontinuity can be caused by incorrect overlap of the components from the previous steps. Thus it is recommended to return to the previous steps to ensure correct overlap. Smoothing and ensuring proper thickness and contour should be done at this step (Fig. 20.58). Posts for tube teeth can also be designed at this point. If the opposing cast was scanned, the occlusion must be checked at this stage. If the framework is going to be printed and cast, sprues are placed in the software for the casting process. After the design is complete, the framework model can be exported as an STL or saved on the local software for fabrication (Fig. 20.59).

Digital Manufacturing

Manufacturing RPDs from STL files takes place in three ways. The first method involves milling the framework from a solid block. This block can be made of resin or metal. The second method involves printing the designed model in castable resin. This castable resin is then invested and cast in a traditional lost-wax/resin technique to generate the final framework. The third method is selective laser melting (SLM) that works by fusing metallic powder particles layer by layer to produce the final framework.

Milling Frameworks

Milling utilizes a subtractive manufacturing process, where the final framework is fabricated by a computer numerical control milling machine equipped with rotating burs. The machine removes the material from a solid "*block*" or "*puck*" of metal based on the digital design, resulting in a precise and highly detailed framework (Fig. 20.60). Milling offers several advantages. It provides excellent dimensional accuracy, resulting in a well-fitting RPD framework. Milled frameworks are known for their strength and resistance to fracture.

Additionally, milling can potentially offer a faster turnaround time compared to traditional casting. However, there are also disadvantages to consider. Milling machines and materials can be more expensive compared to traditional casting techniques. While intricate designs are achievable, milling may not offer the same level of design freedom as techniques like SLM. Finally, the subtractive nature of milling generates metal scrap, contributing to considerable material waste.

Milling RPD frameworks primarily utilizes biocompatible cobalt-chromium (Co-Cr) alloys, known for their strength, durability, and biocompatibility. However, advancements have seen the introduction of titanium milling, offering a lighter weight

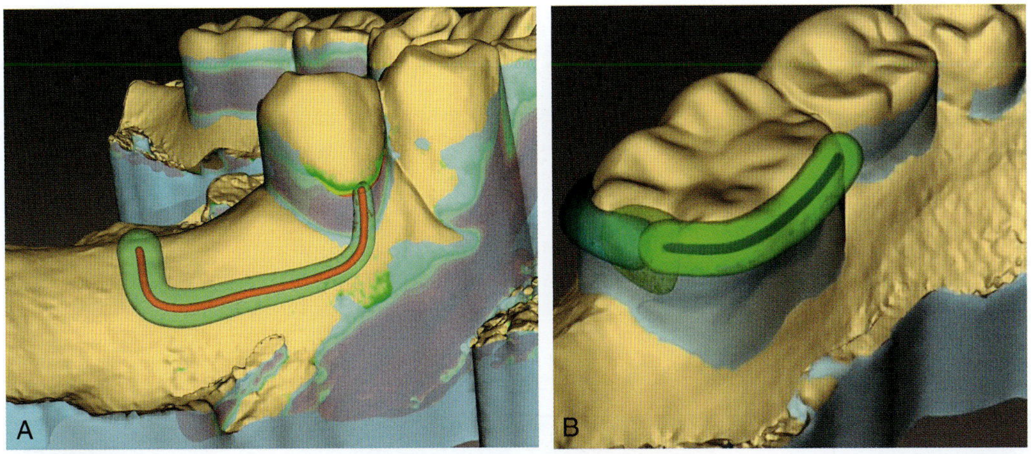

Fig. 20.56 **A,** An infrabulge clasp designed with taper toward the retentive undercut. **B,** A suprabulge clasp designed as a reciprocal clasp with minimal taper and thick diameter. (Courtesy of Ahmed Mahrous

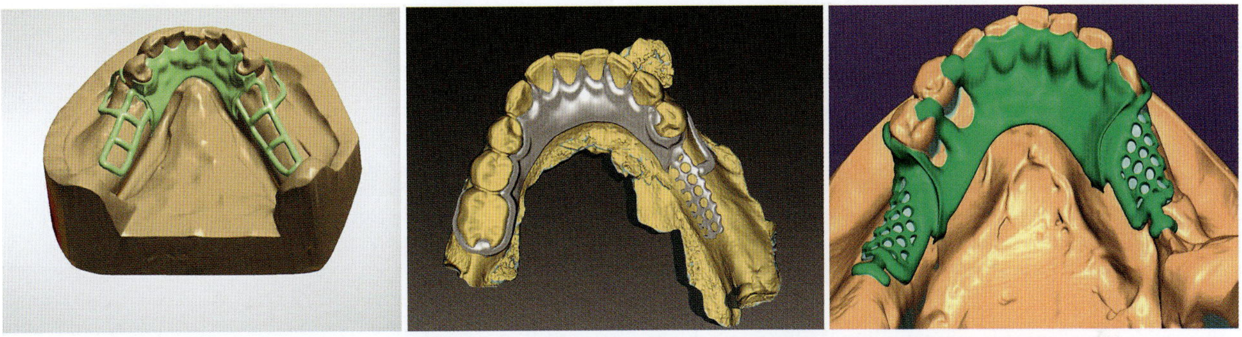

Fig. 20.57 Completed frameworks seen in three different removable partial denture design software systems, the components are cleaned up, excess is removed, and sharp edges are rounded in this stage.

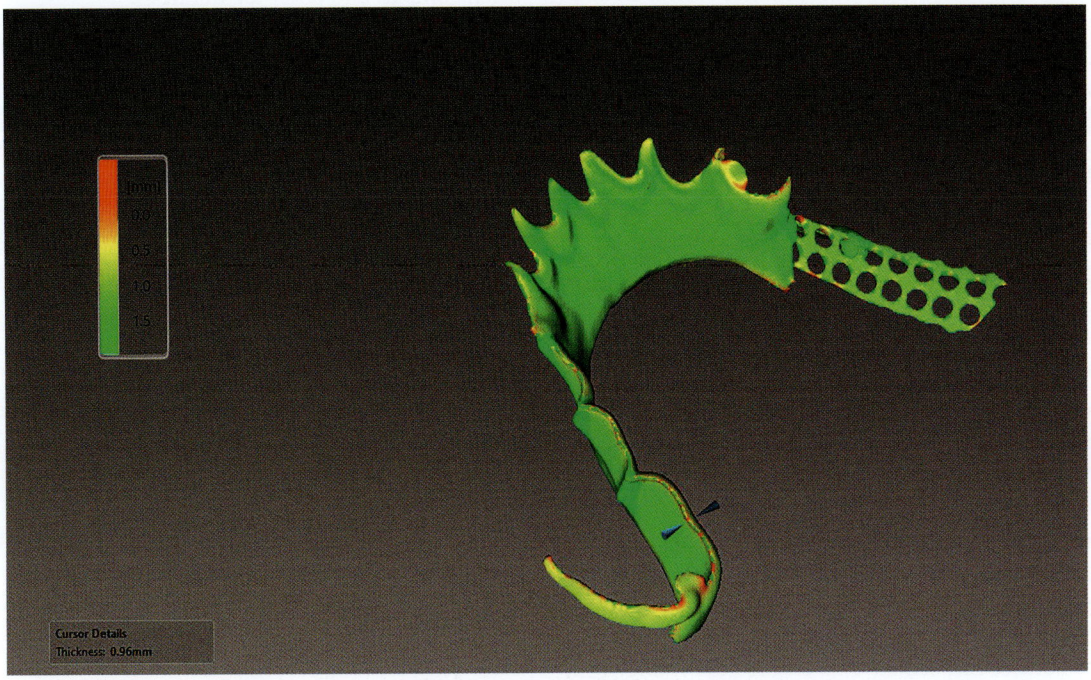

Fig. 20.58 The thickness of the removable partial denture can also be checked in this stage to confirm adequate thickness. (Courtesy of Ahmed Mahrous

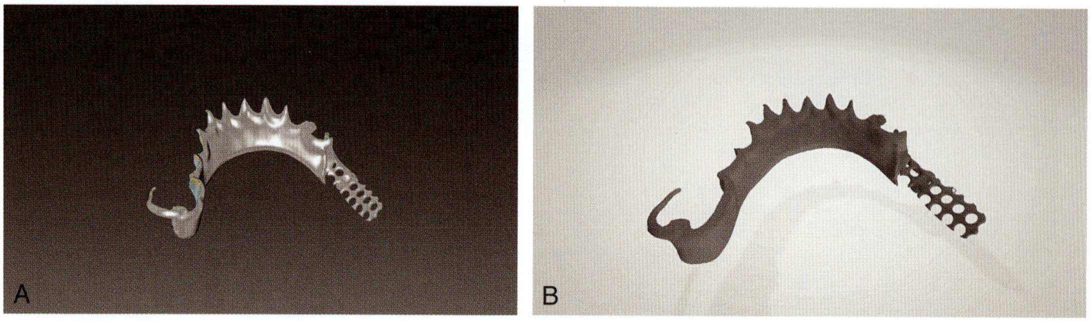

Fig. 20.59 A, The finished framework completed on the design software. **B,** The framework exported in the form of an .stl model for manufacture. (Courtesy of Ahmed Mahrous Copyright © 2024. All rights reserved.)

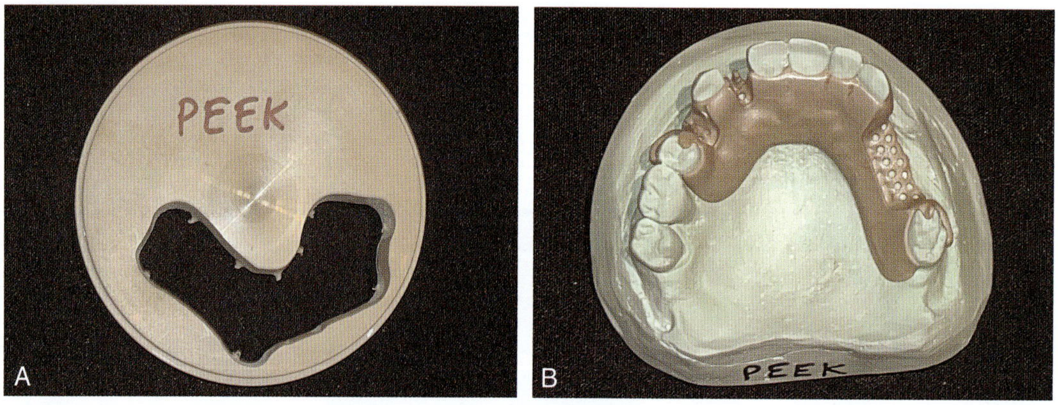

Fig. 20.60 A, The block of polyetheretherketone *(PEEK)* material after milling of a partial denture framework. **B,** The finished PEEK framework seated onto the master cast. (Courtesy of Ahmed Mahrous Copyright © 2024. All rights reserved.)

alternative with excellent biocompatibility. Milling machines specifically designed for dental applications are employed. These machines feature high-precision spindles and a variety of burs suited for various stages of the milling process. The process begins with the finalized framework design being converted into toolpaths that instruct the milling machine on the specific movements and depths of cut required to achieve the desired framework geometry.

The "*block*" or "*puck*" of a selected material is secured in the milling machine. The programmed toolpaths guide the burs to remove excess material, resulting in the creation of the RPD framework. The milled framework is then separated from the block or puck and sprues are smoothened. The surface is then meticulously inspected under magnification and any imperfections or irregularities identified during inspection may require further polishing or even remaking the framework. If the RPD design incorporates clasps or other components that require attachment, soldering with compatible metals may be performed. Depending on the chosen metal alloy, the framework may undergo heat treatment to optimize its mechanical properties. This process involves precisely controlled heating and cooling cycles that enhance strength, hardness, and resistance to fracture.

The final step involves polishing the framework to achieve a smooth, lustrous surface finish. Polishing is typically achieved using a series of progressively finer polishing wheels and pastes.

Following all postprocessing steps, the framework undergoes a final quality control inspection. This ensures the framework meets dimensional accuracy, exhibits a smooth and clean surface finish, and possesses the required strength and functionality for the intended clinical application.

Milling presents a viable alternative for fabricating RPD frameworks, offering high precision, variety of materials, and potentially faster turnaround times. However, factors like cost, design limitations, and material waste need to be considered when compared to other techniques.

Castable Resin Framework Fabrication

This method prints the final design made via the CAD software in photopolymerized castable resin to be invested and cast into the final framework. The advantage of this technique is the relatively inexpensive and fast production compared to fully analog production. However, the disadvantage is increased distortion potential of the printed framework before and during investing. This distortion potential is mainly attributed to the lack of a refractory cast as a support to the castable resin. Additionally, the resin used to create the castable patterns is photopolymerized and prone to distortion due to extraneous light sources. Nonetheless, this technique can produce accurate results if careful handling is maintained throughout the process.

Most 3D resin printers used for this purpose work by polymerizing photoactivated resin in incremental layers. Light polymerization is done using stereolithography 3D printing process, which uses UV light reflected through a mirror, or digital light processing that uses a projected light source to polymerize entire layers of the photopolymer at once. Regardless of the printer used, all 3D resin printing processes start with an STL design file that is sent to the printing software. The 3D models are "nested" in the 3D printer which is the process where the models are placed in the proper orientation and location for fabrication. Most software systems automatically generate support rods that hold the printed structure in place during the printing process. It is advisable to keep all supports on the outer surface of the printed framework to avoid possible distortion of the fitting surface (Fig. 20.61).

Depending on the technology and the material, the printed parts may require rinsing in isopropyl alcohol to remove any unpolymerized resin from their surfaces, and additional light polymerization (Fig. 20.62). Further manual work is required to remove support structures, or cleaning with compressed air, or a media blaster to remove excess powder. Before postpolymerization, the printed structure is usually relatively fragile and prone to deformation; thus care should be taken during all postprocessing steps not to distort the printed framework.

Phosphate investment is used to invest printed resin since it is strong enough to withstand the resin expansion.

Investing is done in the traditional way with measured powder and liquid. Expansion liquid is used to compensate for solidification shrinkage of the alloy per the manufacturer's instructions.

With printing and casting, it is possible to invest more than one framework in the same ring (Fig. 20.63). Once poured, the investment ring is allowed to cool, then placed in a furnace

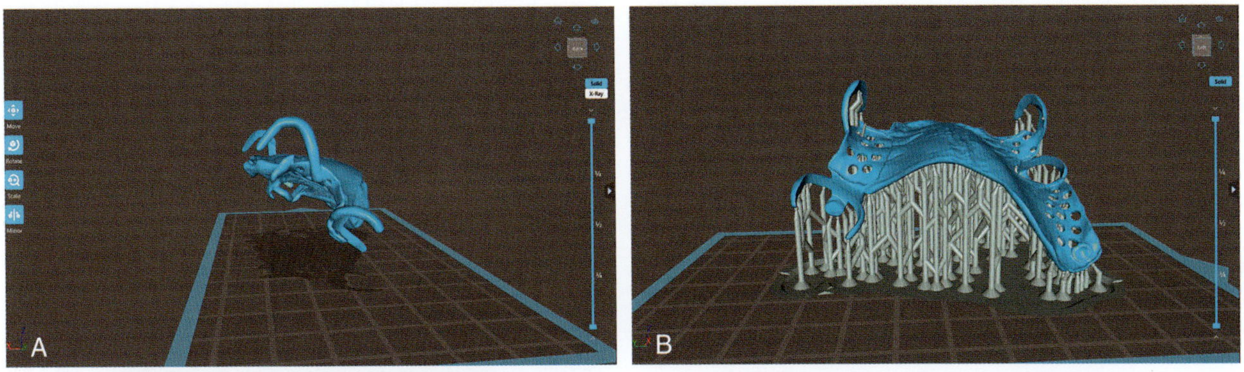

Fig. 20.61 **A,** The finished framework is nested into the printing software. **B,** The supports generated; it is important to ensure that all supports attach to the cameo surface of the framework to ensure ideal fit of the framework when completed.

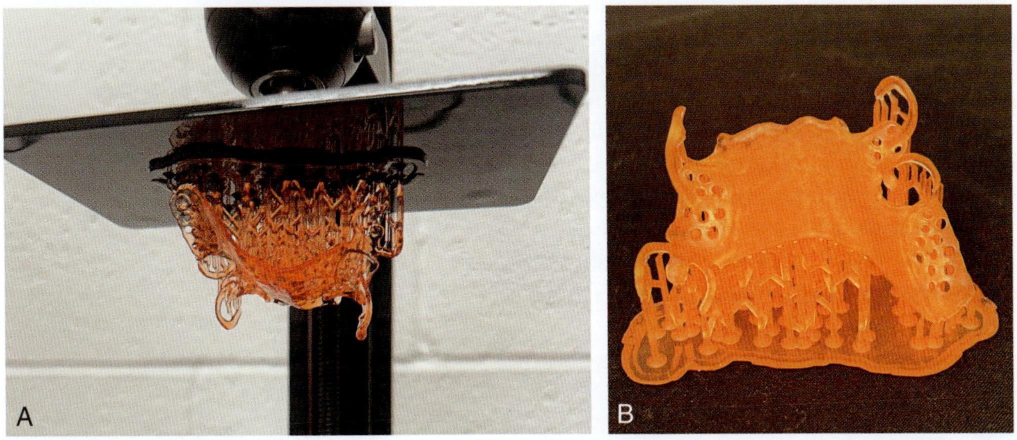

Fig. 20.62 **A,** Framework printed in castable resin. **B,** The framework is fragile during this phase and should be handled with care.

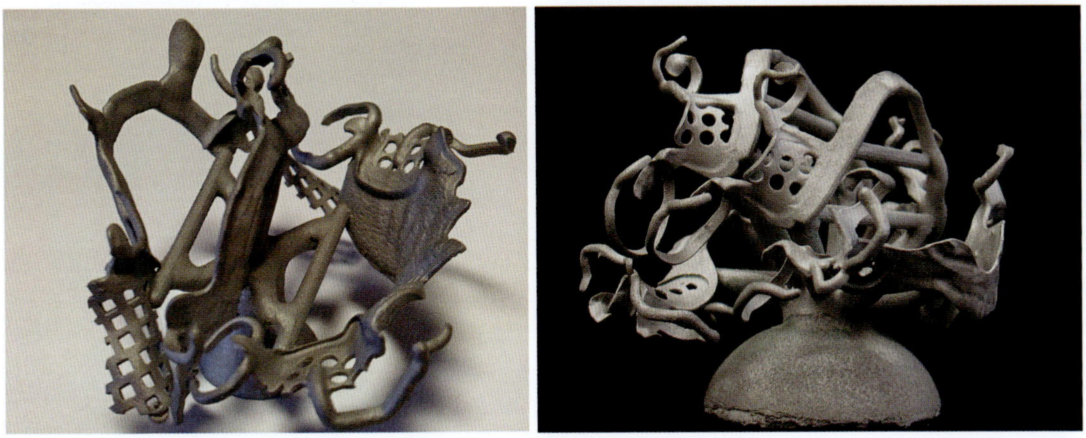

Fig. 20.63 With printing and casting, it is possible to invest more than one framework in the same ring.

and brought up to casting temperature. When the investment reaches casting temperature, additional time may be allowed to fully heat through the rings. The extra time for heating will depend on how many rings are in the oven. Rapid burnout for the castable resin is not recommended. A multistage burnout is beneficial to allow the resin to soften and melt out of the bottom of the ring before evaporation. Unlike wax, the resin is not able to evaporate completely into a gas that can escape easily through the investment. Burning out of the resin material too rapidly can cause thermal shock in the investment that may lead to cracked rings, as well as flashing and ill-fitting parts.

When at the correct temperature, the ring is taken out of the furnace and placed in the casting machine using tongs, the desired alloy is placed in the casting machine and heated to casting temperature then cast per the machine's instructions. Once the cast rings have cooled, the investment is broken away to reveal the metal frameworks. Airborne particle abrasion cleans away the investment then the framework is manually trimmed, rubber-wheeled, and polished in the usual traditional way.

Select Laser Melting

Select laser melting (SLM) is becoming the preferred method of manufacturing RPD frameworks. Cobalt-chromium dust is used in the SLM machines; the micron size is very specific and consistent. To produce the dust, cobalt-chromium is atomized in a laser chamber, and the dust is then filtered into different sizes and sold to different industries for their specific requirements.

Once the final framework design is completed and the STL file is generated, the design is imported into the SLM software for preparation. The design is then nested. A full build plate should have a combination of maxillary and mandibular frameworks to maximize space utilization. Supports are then added to the software and sent to the SLM machine for production. Care should be taken to place all supports away from the framework's intaglio surface or any delicate or critical areas such as clasps and rest seats because this might result in distortion during removal of these supports (Fig. 20.64). The frameworks should be placed at a 30-degree angle to the build plate to decrease heat generation in the metal frameworks.

To set up the machine, dust is added to the build plate, which then moves at each angle until it is leveled. There are usually three chambers that hold new dust, used dust, and the build plate; each can move upward or downward during the build process. The build plate is made of metal and its level is adjusted to hold a few microns of dust in the machine setup. Once the build starts, the dust is melted onto the metal plate starting with the supports. As the build plate moves down, the dust chamber moves upward, and the recoating arm sweeps a new dust layer over the build plate. This process is repeated until the framework has finished building, one slice at a time, while the laser melts the dust. Generally, supervision is not necessary during this process. Once the build is complete, the build plate moves upward, the dust is vacuumed off the frameworks, and the plate is removed from the build chamber and placed in a preheated furnace for annealing. SLM requires an annealing process in a furnace to enhance clasps' flexibility. Annealing, either because of cooling following casting or from using an annealing furnace, elongates the molecules in the alloy. This elongation needs to

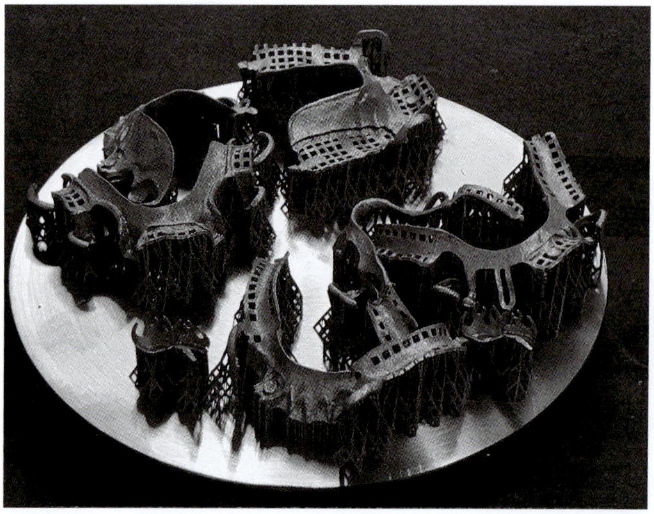

Fig. 20.64 The finished SLM-fabricated frameworks with supports still attached. It is important to keep all supports attached to the cameo surface of the frameworks to avoid interfering with the fit of the framework.

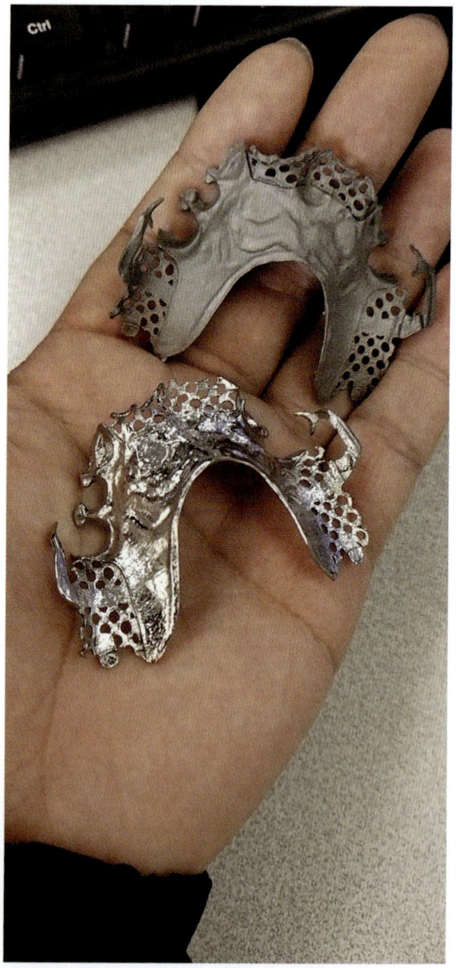

Fig. 20.65 Frameworks are manually trimmed, rubber wheeled, and polished; however, there are polishing machines that will produce a finely polished framework, reducing the technician's intervention. Comparison of a polished and unpolished framework.

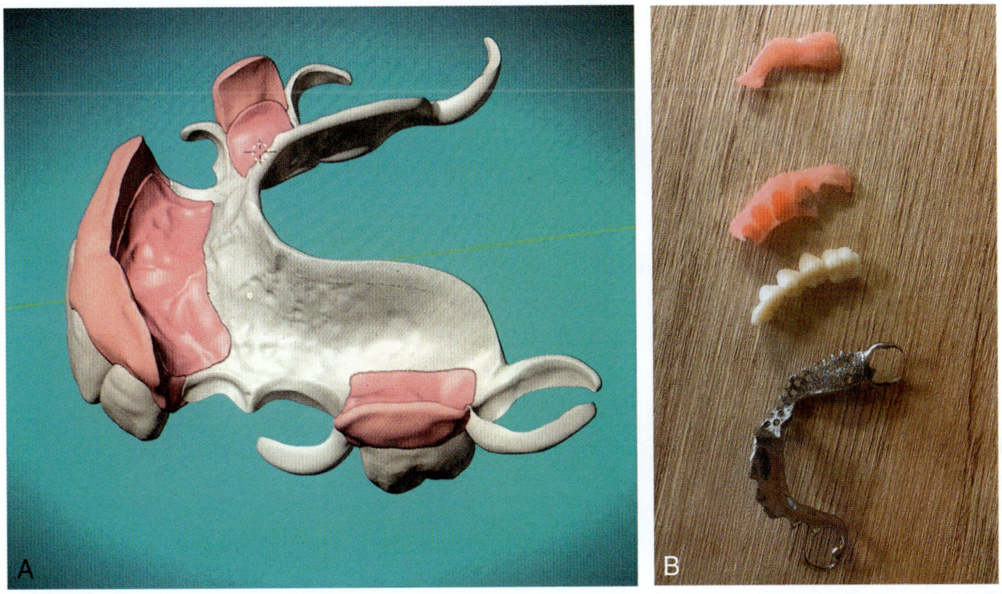

Fig. 20.66 **A,** Software used to design the teeth to be set, as well as the denture base acrylic in two halves, above and below the meshwork. **B,** The different files are printed separately and can be assembled and joined together using light polymerized resin.

be between 9% and 13%. The higher the elongation, the more flexible the clasps.

Once the build plate has cooled from the annealing furnace, the frameworks are separated from the build plate. To separate the frameworks from the build plate, the build plate is mounted on a bandsaw, and the frameworks are cut off. Once the frameworks have been separated from the build plate, all remnants of supports are removed using a hand instrument. At this point, the frameworks can be manually trimmed, rubber-wheeled, and polished; however, there are polishing machines that can produce finely polished frameworks, reducing the technician's intervention (Fig. 20.65).

Digital Acrylic Resin Printing and Incorporation Into Frameworks

With the ability to use the SLM process to fabricate frameworks, there is software that can help with the design of the RPD framework and the tooth arrangement. The software produces STL files which capture the tissue acrylic, the acrylic above the meshwork, as well as the teeth. These STL files can be used simultaneously to manufacture different components, which can then be assembled using light-polymerized acrylic resin, thereby minimizing the technician's direct workload (Fig. 20.66).

REFERENCES

1. Dootz ER, Craig RG, Peyton FA. Influence of investments and duplicating procedures on the accuracy of partial denture castings. *J Prosthet Dent*. 1965;15:679–690.
2. Frush JP. *Dentogenic Restorations and Dynesthetics*. Swissdent Foundation; 1957.

21

Initial Placement, Adjustment, and Servicing of the Removable Partial Denture

Lisa A. Lang, Lily T. García, and Ahmed Mahrous

CHAPTER OUTLINE

Initial placement of the completed removable partial denture should be a routinely scheduled appointment. All too often, the prosthesis is quickly placed and the patient dismissed with instructions to return when soreness or discomfort develops. Patients should not be given possession of removable prostheses until denture bases have been initially adjusted as required, occlusal discrepancies have been eliminated, and patient education procedures have been continued.

Many factors are part of adjusting to a removable prosthesis beyond the ability to accommodate. Other factors include how well the patient has been informed of the mechanical and biological problems involved in the fabrication and wearing of a removable prosthetic restoration and how much confidence the patient has acquired in the quality of the finished prosthesis. Knowing in advance that every step has been carefully planned and executed with skill and having acquired confidence in both the dentist and the quality of the prosthesis, the patient is better able to accept the adjustment period as a necessary but transient step in learning to wear the prosthesis. This confidence could be lost if the dentist does not approach the insertion and postinsertion phases as equally important for the success of the treatment.

The term *adjustment* has two connotations, each of which must be considered separately. The first is the adjustment of the denture-bearing and occlusal surfaces of the denture made by the dentist at the time of initial placement and thereafter. The second is the adjustment or accommodation by the patient, both psychologically and biologically, to the new prosthesis.

After the resin bases have been processed and before recovery of the prosthesis and removal from the casts, the occluding teeth must be altered to ensure a good occlusal relationship between opposing artificial dentition or between artificial dentition and an opposing cast. The denture base sections of a removable partial denture must be finished to eliminate excessive bulk and perfect the contours of polished surfaces for the best functional and esthetic results. There should be minimal excess bulk of processed denture base resin material if the wax-up replicating soft tissues was accomplished prior to processing. In addition to correcting the occlusion using dental laboratory techniques, there usually exists a need for final adjustments intraorally and at chairside to improve the fit of the prosthesis to the intraoral tissue.

Final steps in finishing procedures necessary to produce a biologically acceptable prosthetic restoration require: (1) adjustment of the bearing surfaces of the denture bases (intaglio surfaces) to be in harmony with the supporting soft tissue, (2) adjustment of the occlusion to accommodate the occlusal rests and other metal parts of the denture, and (3) final adjustment of the occlusion on the artificial dentition to harmonize with natural tooth occlusion in all mandibular positions.

ADJUSTMENTS TO BEARING SURFACES OF DENTURE BASES

Altering bearing surfaces—the intaglio surface—to fit the denture base onto supporting tissues should be accomplished using an indicator paste (Fig. 21.1). The paste must be low viscosity such that the paste will be readily displaced by positive tissue contact and will not adhere to the tissue of the mouth. Several pressure indicator pastes are commercially available. An acceptable alternative is creating an indicator paste that consists of combining equal parts of a vegetable shortening and United States Pharmacopeia standard (USP) zinc oxide powder, thoroughly spatulated into a homogeneous mixture and stored in small ointment jars.

At the time of prosthesis insertion, use a pressure indicator paste on tissue-bearing areas of the prosthesis, rather than dismissing the patient with instructions to return when soreness develops. If adjustments are not corrected at the time of insertion, it is likely that the patient returns with hypersensitive areas, resulting in overcorrection of a traumatized area to restore patient comfort. Place a thin layer of pressure-indicating paste on

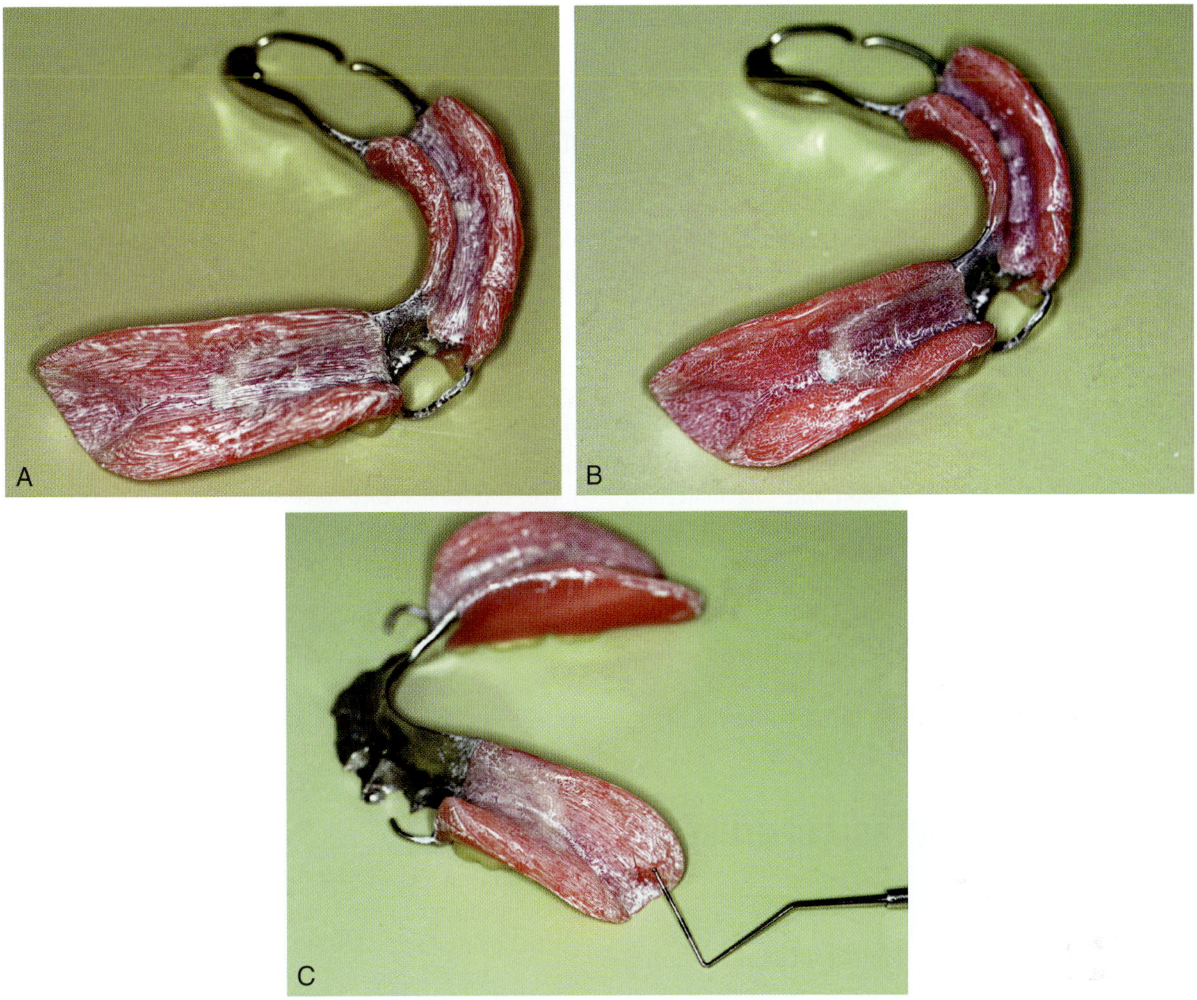

A B C

Fig. 21.1 **A,** Tissue side of finished bases of a Kennedy Class I, modification 1 removable partial denture, where paste indicates that pressure has been applied. The paste was applied following careful inspection of the tissue surface for irregularities or sharp projections, which must be eliminated before fitting in the mouth. The entire tissue surface of the bases was dried before it was coated with a thin coat of pressure indicator paste using a stiff-bristle brush. Brush marks are evident, and it is the change in the pattern of brush marks that guides adjustment. It is important to avoid thick application of indicator paste, which can hide the presence of significant pressure. **B,** The prosthesis can be dipped in cold water or sprayed with a provided release agent before placement in the patient's mouth to prevent the paste from sticking to oral tissues. After careful seating of the removable partial denture, the patient can close firmly on cotton rolls for a few seconds, or the dentist can alternately apply a tissue-ward pressure over the bases to simulate functional movement. The presence of tissue contact is evident in the pattern of the paste, which is different from the brushed pattern. There is no suggestion of excessive pressure in this tissue contact pattern. However, it is not uncommon to relieve the area adjacent to the abutment sparingly. Several placements of the denture with indicator paste are usually necessary for the evaluation of the accuracy of the bases. **C,** A different denture base recovered from the mouth after manipulation simulating function. The tissue contact reveals excessive pressure at the region lingual to the retromolar pad.

the intaglio surfaces; rinse lightly to help prevent the paste from sticking to the soft tissues. Apply digital pressure onto the prosthesis in a tissue-ward direction or have the patient chew on a moist cotton roll to apply a heavy enough functional force to the new denture bases to register pressure areas present. The dentist should apply both vertical and horizontal forces with the fingers in excess of what might be expected of the patient. The denture is then removed and inspected. Any areas where pressure has been heavy enough to displace a thin film of indicator paste should be relieved and the procedure repeated with a new film of the indicator until excessive pressure areas have been eliminated in order to demonstrate an even layer of displaced pressure-indicating paste. This procedure is more complex with patients with xerostomia such that a "show through" noted in displaced indicator paste may be erroneously interpreted as a pressure spot when actually the paste had adhered to the tissue in that area. Therefore only those areas that show through an intact film of indicator paste should be interpreted as pressure areas and relieved accordingly. The decision to relieve an area of pressure must consider whether the pressure is in a primary, secondary, or nonsupportive denture-bearing area. The primary denture-bearing areas should be expected to show greater contact than other areas.

Pressure areas most commonly encountered are as follows: in the mandibular arch—(1) the lingual slope of the mandibular ridge in the premolar area, (2) the mylohyoid ridge, (3) the border extension into the retromylohyoid space, and (4) the distobuccal border adjacent to the ascending portion of the mandibular ramus and the external oblique ridge; and in the maxillary arch—(1) the inside of the buccal flange of the denture over the tuberosities, (2) the border of the denture lying at the malar prominence, and (3) the point at the pterygomaxillary notch where the denture may impinge on the pterygomandibular raphe or the pterygoid hamulus. In addition, bony spicules or irregularities in the denture base will require specific relief which can occur in either arch.

The amount of relief necessary depends on the accuracy of the impression, the master cast, and the extent of the denture base. Despite the accuracy of impression and cast materials, many denture base materials leave much to be desired in this regard, and the element of technical error is always present. It is therefore essential that discrepancies in the denture base are detected and corrected before the tissues of the mouth are subjected to the stress of supporting a prosthetic restoration. Therefore the appointment time for the initial placement of the denture must be adequate to permit necessary adjustments to avoid causing soft and/or hard tissue trauma.

OCCLUSAL INTERFERENCE FROM DENTURE FRAMEWORK

Any occlusal interference from occlusal rests and other parts of the metal framework should be eliminated before or during the establishment of occlusal relations. Ideally, the metal removable partial denture framework should be tried intraorally prior to recording the final jaw relation records to eliminate occlusal interference with the remaining natural dentition. If planning for tooth preparations is made in consideration of the design of the removable partial denture framework and the treatment plan is well executed, it may not be needed. If planned well, occlusal interference from the metal framework may not require further adjustment at the time of prosthesis insertion. If the dentist had all laboratory procedures completed without an appointment for a framework try-in, there will be a need for fitting at the time of delivery.

ADJUSTMENT OF OCCLUSION IN HARMONY WITH NATURAL AND ARTIFICIAL DENTITION

The last step in the adjustment of the removable partial denture at the time of initial placement is the adjustment of the occlusion to harmonize with the natural dentition in all mandibular excursions. When delivering opposing removable partial dentures, it is advisable to fit one removable partial denture at a time to adjust the fit within the arch and then correct the occlusion for each separately. If the sequence is followed for each removable partial denture, then placement of opposing removable partial dentures simultaneously may reveal occlusal interferences that occur between the two removable partial dentures. In this manner, occlusal adjustment can be accomplished in a systematic manner. Ultimately, the occlusal adjustments are similar to opposing complete dentures when there are few remaining natural teeth. When natural teeth are present and occlude, the final occlusal adjustment will result in opposing natural teeth that articulate in maximum intercuspation and during mandibular movements. It is necessary, therefore, that the artificial dentition on the removable partial denture be made to harmonize with whatever natural occlusion remains.

Occlusal adjustment of tooth-supported removable partial dentures can be performed using intraoral methods. Occlusal adjustment of distal extension removable partial dentures is accomplished more accurately with the use of an articulator than if attempted intraorally alone. Because distal extension denture bases will exhibit some movement under a closing force, intraoral indications of occlusal discrepancies, whether produced by articulating paper or disclosing waxes, are difficult to interpret. Distal extension dentures positioned on remount casts can conveniently be related in the articulator with new, nonpressure interocclusal records, and the occlusion can be adjusted accurately at the appointment for the initial placement of the dentures (Fig. 21.2).

The methods by which occlusal relations may be established and recorded have been discussed in Chapter 18. In this chapter, the advantages of establishing a functional occlusal relationship with an intact opposing arch have been discussed, along with the limitations that exist to perfecting harmonious occlusion on the finished prosthesis by intraoral adjustment alone. Even when the occlusion on two opposing removable partial dentures is adjusted, it is best that one arch be considered an intact arch and the other one adjusted to it. This is accomplished by first eliminating any occlusal interferences that occur with mandibular movement imposed by one prosthesis; eliminating occlusal interferences is usually adjusted on the prosthetic teeth and only limited adjustments to opposing natural dentition. The choice for adjusting one removable partial denture versus the other in the situation with opposing prostheses is arbitrary with the following exceptions: If one removable partial denture is entirely tooth supported and the other has a tissue-supported base, the tooth-supported denture is adjusted to final occlusion with any opposing natural teeth. That arch is then treated as an intact arch and the opposing denture adjusted to occlude with it. If both removable partial dentures are entirely tooth supported, the one that occludes with the most natural teeth is adjusted first and the second denture is then adjusted to occlude with an intact arch. Tooth-supported segments of a tooth- and tissue-supported removable partial denture are likewise adjusted first to harmonize with any opposing natural dentition. The final adjustment of occlusion on opposing tissue-supported bases is usually done on the mandibular removable partial denture because this is the moving member, and the occlusion is made to harmonize with the maxillary removable partial denture, which is treated as part of an intact arch.

Intraoral occlusal adjustment is accomplished using an indicator to mark the occlusal interferences and suitable mounted burs or polishing points. Diamond or other abrasive points must

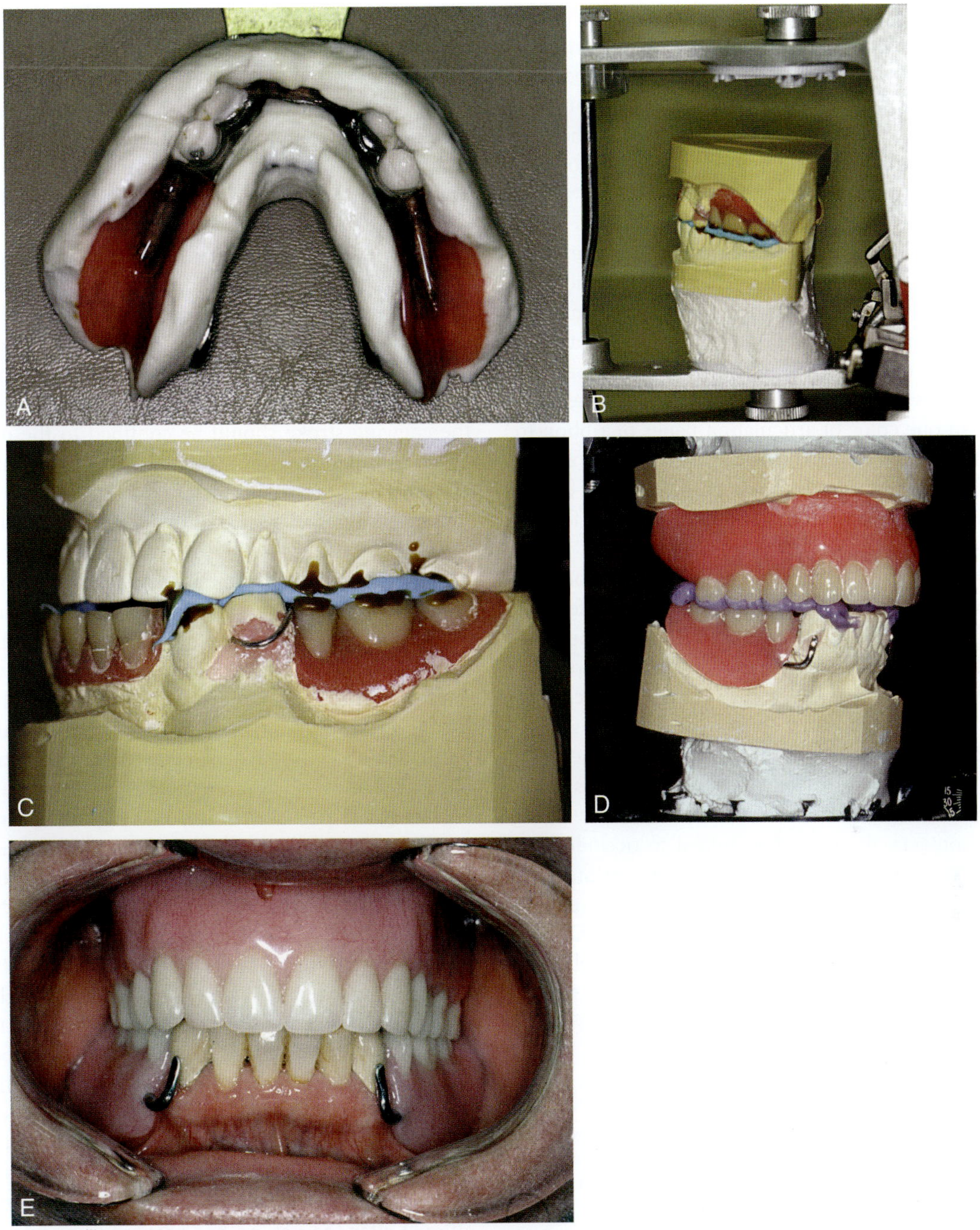

Fig. 21.2 Sequence of laboratory and clinical procedures performed for the correction of occlusal discrepancies caused by processing of removable partial dentures. The arch with the prosthesis will require a new cast and record to provide occlusal correction. If it is a maxillary prosthesis, this involves preserving the facebow record by replacing the processed maxillary removable partial denture and cast on the articulator and indexing the occlusal surfaces using a remount jig or making another facebow record at the try-in appointment. If it is a mandibular prosthesis, the opposing arch can be prepared before insertion. **A,** In this example, the opposing arch is a complete denture that is not to be altered. To produce a cast for use in correcting the occlusion on the articulator, a pick-up impression of the mandibular prosthesis is made. The prosthesis stays within the irreversible hydrocolloid impression; the clasps, proximal plates, and any undercut or parallel surface are carefully blocked out with wax before the remount cast is formed. **B,** The remount cast that is formed is then inverted and positioned with the use of an interocclusal record. **C,** The mounted mandibular cast and the interocclusal record showing that the record was made without tooth contact. This allows the position recorded to not be influenced by the teeth, which could alter the closure path and introduce error. **D,** This example shows a maxillary complete denture that was mounted before the patient visit with the use of a remount index (preserved facebow by indexing before recovery from the processed cast) and the mandibular remount cast and interocclusal record (as in **C**). The record is removed and occlusal correction accomplished to control the postprocess occlusion. The use of the completed prostheses provides the best chance to obtain an accurate and reliable interocclusal record, given the fact that the bases are very accurate and stable. **E,** The goal of the remounting procedure is to provide the occlusal position prescribed by the arrangement of prosthesis teeth. It would be inappropriate to allow the patient to attempt to accommodate a new prosthesis in which the occlusion is not optimized.

be used to reduce enamel, porcelain, and metal contacts, and burs may be used to adjust acrylic teeth. When using articulation paper or ribbon, heavy interocclusal contacts may become perforated, leaving only a light mark, while secondary contacts, which are lighter and frequently sliding, may make a heavier mark. Although the articulation ribbon is not easily perforated, the differentiation between primary and secondary contacts is difficult to ascertain.

In general, occlusal adjustment of multiple contacts between natural and artificial dentition with tooth-supported removable partial dentures follows similar principles as those for natural dentition alone. The similarity is because removable partial dentures are retained by design on the abutment teeth, whereas no mechanical retainers are present with complete dentures. The use of more than one color of articulation paper or ribbon to record and differentiate between centric and eccentric contacts is just as helpful in adjusting removable partial denture occlusion as natural occlusion, and this method may be used for the initial adjustment.

For final adjustment, the use of an occlusal wax may be necessary to establish points of excessive contact and interference when adjusting a removable partial denture; this cannot be done solely using articulation paper. An occlusal indicating wax (Fig. 21.3) that is adhesive on one side, or strips of 28-gauge casting wax or other similar soft wax, may be used. This should always be done bilaterally, with two strips folded together at the midline. Thus the patient is not as likely to deviate to one side as when wax is introduced unilaterally.

For centric contacts, the patient is guided to occlude into the wax. The wax is removed and inspected for perforations under transillumination. Premature contacts or excessive contacts appear as perforated areas and must be adjusted. One of two methods may be used to locate specific areas to be relieved.

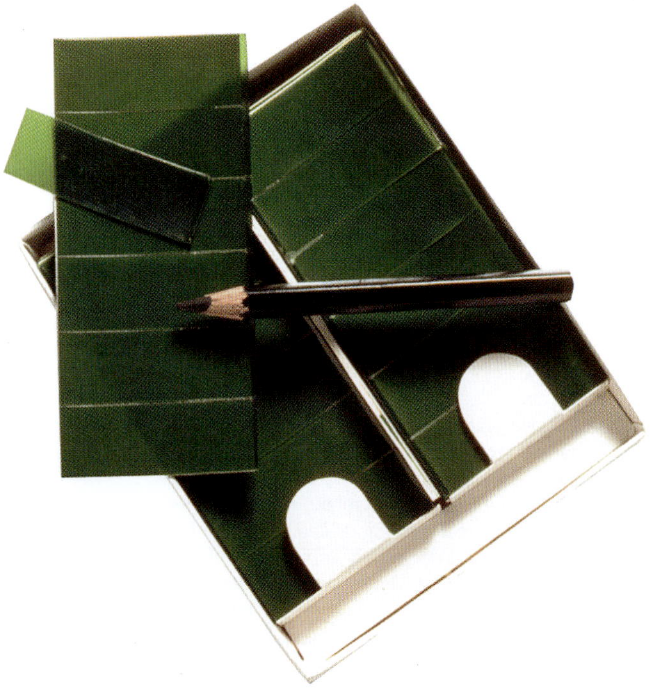

Fig. 21.3 Occlusal indicator wax. (Courtesy of Kerr Corp., Orange, CA.)

Articulation ribbon may be used to mark the occlusion; those marks that represent areas of excessive contact are identified by referring to the wax record and are relieved accordingly. A second method is to introduce the wax strips a second time, this time adapting them to the buccal and lingual surfaces for retention. After the patient has tapped into the wax, perforated areas are marked with a waterproof pencil. The wax is then stripped off and the penciled areas are relieved.

Whichever method is used, repeat the sequence until occlusal balance is achieved and uniform contacts without perforations are evident from a final interocclusal wax record. After adjustment has been completed, any remaining areas of interference are reduced, ensuring that there is no interference during the chewing stroke. Adjustments to relieve interferences during the chewing stroke should be confined to the buccal surfaces of mandibular teeth and lingual surfaces of maxillary teeth. This serves to narrow the cusps for a smooth movement into intercuspal contact. Occlusal interferences encountered during the chewing stroke are thus detected as perforations in the wax, which are marked with a pencil and relieved accordingly.

After occlusal adjustment is completed, the anatomy of the artificial teeth should be restored to maximize efficiency before restoring grooves and narrowing the teeth buccolingually, which increases the sharpness of the cusps and reduces the width of the food table. Mandibular buccal and maxillary lingual surfaces, in particular, should be narrowed to ensure that these areas will not interfere on closure; the selection of prosthetic teeth used on removable partial dentures that oppose natural or restored dentition should be a material that can be adjusted to create a harmonious occlusal surface. Final adjustment of the occlusion should always be followed by meticulous restoration of the most functional occlusal anatomy possible. Delay in refining the occlusion at the time of insertion can result in occlusal trauma and possibly create soft tissue injury due to occlusal overload on the removable partial denture. Therefore restoration of an efficient occlusal anatomy is an essential part of the denture adjustment at the time of placement. Again, this necessitates that sufficient time is allotted for the initial placement of the removable partial denture to permit the accomplishment of all necessary occlusal corrections.

Occlusal adjustments can be repeated at a reasonable time interval after the patient has adapted to wearing the prostheses. This second occlusal adjustment can be considered when tissue-supported denture bases no longer support the occlusion, and corrective measures—either reoccluding the teeth or relining the denture—must be used. However, a periodic recheck of occlusion at intervals of 6 months is advisable to prevent traumatic interference resulting from changes in removable partial denture support or tooth migration.

INSTRUCTIONS TO THE PATIENT

The patient should be reminded of the chronic nature of missing teeth and that treatment solutions, such as a removable partial denture, require monitoring to ensure optimum function without harming the mouth. Advise patients in the proper placement and removal of the removable partial denture and have the patient demonstrate insertion and removal. Clasp breakage can be avoided by instructing patients to remove the removable partial denture by the bases and not by repeated lifting of the clasp arms using their fingers or other means.

Patients should be advised that some discomfort or minor annoyance might be experienced initially. This may be caused by the perceived bulk of the prosthesis. Allowing time for the tongue to accommodate may resolve the issue. Also, advise the possibility of developing soreness despite the fitting procedures. Since patients vary in their ability to tolerate discomfort, noting that adjustments may be needed at a future time and recall appointments may be necessary. There are some patients who are unable to accommodate a removable prosthesis; however, the dentist should avoid any statements that might be misinterpreted or misconstrued by the patient. It is important to convey positive assurance that the patient will be able to use the prosthesis with comfort and acceptance.

Ensure the patient understands that the new prosthesis can influence speech and pronunciation. With few exceptions, which usually result from excessive and preventable bulk in the denture design, contour of denture bases, or improper placement of teeth, the average patient will experience little difficulty in wearing the removable partial denture. Most hindrances to normal speech will disappear in a few days.

Similarly, it may be best to avoid discussion about the possibility of gagging or inability to accommodate. Most patients will experience little or no difficulty in this regard, and the tongue will normally accommodate smooth contours without objection. Contours that are too thick, too bulky, or improperly placed should be avoided in the construction of the denture, but if present, these should be detected and eliminated at the time of placement of the denture. The dentist should palpate the prosthesis in the mouth and reduce excessive bulk accordingly before the patient has an opportunity to object to it. A common area that most often needs adjustment is the distolingual flange of the mandibular denture base. Here, the thickness of the denture flange should always be thinned during finishing and polishing procedures. The lingual flanges in distal extension removable partial dentures are reproduced as recorded in the impression, but distal to the second molar, the flange can be adjusted to be thinner. Then, when the denture is placed, the dentist should palpate this area to ascertain that a minimum of bulk exists that might be encountered by the side and base of the tongue. Additional reduction, if needed, should be accomplished and the denture flange repolished before the patient is dismissed.

Home care instructions are absolutely necessary to keep the removable partial dentures and the remaining natural teeth meticulously clean. If cariogenic processes are to be prevented, the accumulation of debris should be avoided as much as possible, particularly around the abutment teeth and beneath minor connectors. Furthermore, inflammation of gingival tissue is prevented by removing accumulated debris and substituting toothbrush massage for the normal stimulation of the tongue and food contact with areas that will be covered by the denture framework.

Routine hygiene procedures are needed both intraorally and in cleaning the removable partial denture after meals and at bedtime. Brushing before breakfast also may be effective in reducing the bacterial count, which may help to lessen acid formation after eating in the caries-susceptible individual. A removable partial denture may be effectively cleaned with a brush designed to clean prostheses. Debris can be removed effectively using nonabrasive dentifrices, but household cleaners and toothpaste should not be used because they are too abrasive for use on acrylic-resin surfaces. The patient—elderly or with disability in particular—should be advised to clean the denture over a basin partially filled with water so that denture impact will be less if the denture is dropped accidentally during cleaning.

Along with brushing with a dentifrice, additional cleaning may be accomplished with the use of an over-the-counter denture cleaning solution, noting instructions and whether the cleaning solution can be used on removable partial dentures with metal frameworks. Although hypochlorite solutions are effective denture cleansers, they tend to tarnish chromium-cobalt frameworks and should be avoided.

In some mouths, the precipitation of salivary calculus on the removable partial denture necessitates taking extra measures for its removal. Thorough daily brushing of the removable partial denture will help prevent calculus for many patients. However, any buildup of calculus noted by the patient between scheduled recall appointments should be removed in the dental office. This can be quickly and readily accomplished with an ultrasonic cleaner.

Since many patients may dine away from home, it is important to instruct the patient to rinse the removable partial denture and the mouth with water after eating if brushing is not possible.

There may be a question on whether a removable partial denture should be worn during sleep. Although generally speaking, the tissue should be allowed to rest by the removal of the denture at night; clinical conditions should determine the advice given to the patient. The prosthesis should be placed in a container and covered with water to prevent its dehydration and subsequent dimensional change; adding mouthwash to the water solution can help provide a sense of freshness and some may be antibacterial as well. The only situation that could justify wearing removable partial dentures at night is when stresses generated by bruxism would be more destructive because they would be concentrated on fewer teeth. Broader distribution of the stress load, plus the splinting effect of the removable partial denture, may make wearing the denture at night advisable. However, an individual mouth protector should be worn at night until the cause of the bruxism is eliminated.

Often the question arises whether an opposing complete denture should be worn when a removable partial denture is out of the mouth. The answer is that if the removable partial denture is to be removed at night, the opposing complete denture should not be left in the mouth. There is no more certain way of destroying the alveolar ridge, which supports a maxillary complete denture, than having it occlude with a few remaining anterior mandibular teeth.

The patient with a removable partial denture should not be dismissed as completed without at least one subsequent appointment for evaluation of the response of oral structures to the restorations and minor adjustment if needed. This should be made at an interval of 24 hours after the initial placement of the denture. It need not be a lengthy appointment but should be made as a definite rather than a drop-in appointment. This not only gives the patient assurance that any necessary adjustments will be made and provides the dentist with an opportunity to check on the patient's acceptance of the prosthesis but also avoids giving the patient any idea that the dentist's schedule may be interrupted at will and serves to give notice that an appointment is necessary for future adjustments.

PART III

Long-term Success: Patient and Prosthesis

22

Long-Term Care of the Patient

Fatemeh Afshari and Judy Chia-Chun Yuan

CHAPTER OUTLINE

Following the delivery of the definitive prosthesis, the patient must be advised as to future care of the mouth to ensure health and longevity of the remaining structures. Patients need to understand that the hard and soft tissue supporting a removable prosthesis will change with time. Additionally, regular "wear and tear," as defined by routine maintenance, and the associated minor or major complications must be professionally addressed. Thus the final and ongoing phase of removable partial denture (RPD) service is periodic recall and professional maintenance.

The recall appointment entails a thorough evaluation of the oral and paraoral structures, prosthesis, and its components, as well as the provision of maintenance care for the hard/soft tissues and prosthesis. Patient reeducation and professional recommendations for home care are also important components of the appointment. The frequency of the recall appointment depends on the oral health and physical condition of the patient. The success and survival of the prescribed prosthesis may be limited unless the patient returns for professional periodic oral evaluations and maintenance care.

Survival refers to any prosthesis presenting in situ (intraoral) at follow-up visits, no matter its condition. However, success is defined by set criteria and can be interpreted as a restoration that does not require any sort of modification or intervention during the observation period. The long-term outcomes of metal framework RPDs are well documented in the literature[1–3] with approximate survival rates of 50%[1] or as high as 90%[2] after 10 years of service. Similarly the long-term outcomes of implant-supported RPDs show high survival rates. Complications can be categorized as (1) biological and (2) mechanical in nature. The most commonly reported biological complications of removable clasp-retained partial dentures have been found to be caries (31.6%), periodontal disease (35.6%), or loss of abutment teeth (8.6%),[2] whereas the most frequently reported biological complications of implant-supported RPDs have been marginal bone loss around implants, implant mobility, bleeding on probing, or deep probing depths.[4] Typical mechanical complications of RPDs include fracture of clasps (16.1%), major connectors (5.1%), and minor connectors (3.4%); breakage of the denture base and acrylic teeth tends to be infrequent.[2] The following sections will provide a more in-depth view of the various major and minor complications and their associated maintenance care (Box 22.1).

BOX 22.1 Removable Partial Denture Complications

Biological Complications	Mechanical Complications
Caries	Loss of retention
Periodontal disease:	Loss of support/stability
Gingivitis	Clasp fracture
Attachments loss (recession, bone loss)	Minor connector fracture
Tooth mobility	Major connector fracture or distortion
Tooth loss	Denture teeth wear
Implant* complications:	Denture teeth fracture
Peri-implant mucositis	Acrylic fracture
Peri-implantitis	Implant* component loss/fracture/distortion
Implant failure	

Complications can be categorized as either (1) biological or (2) mechanical in nature.
*Denotes implant-supported removable partial dentures.

BIOLOGICAL MAINTENANCE NEEDS AND COMPLICATIONS

No assurance can be given to the patient that crowned or uncrowned abutment teeth will not decay at some future time. Several studies have shown an increase in caries risk with RPDs, most especially root caries, following gingival recession.[5,6] A randomized study found that even among annually recalled patients, there was a sixfold increase of caries in patients with

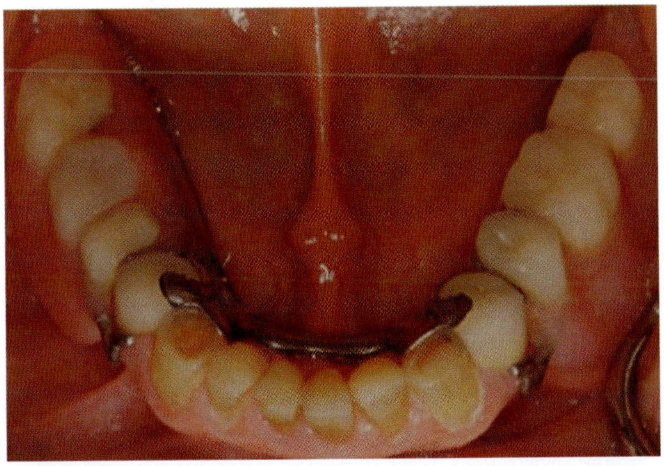

Fig. 22.1 Removable partial denture in service for 3 years. Tooth #29 fractured and was repaired twice, 2 years postdelivery. Patient presents with poor oral hygiene (plaque retention) and denture teeth wear.

mandibular RPDs as compared with cantilevered bridges within a 5-year time span.[7] The patient can be assured, however, that prophylactic measures in the form of meticulous oral hygiene, coupled with routine care by the dentist and chemotherapeutics (e.g., fluoride varnish, sodium fluoride toothpaste, and silver diamine fluoride), will increase the likelihood of improved oral health, a stable periodontium, and lowered risk for caries.

Due to the susceptibility of the prosthesis to plaque accumulation, several of the adverse oral health outcomes of RPDs are linked to poor oral hygiene (Fig. 22.1). A study found that within subjects who wore RPDs for over 10 years, only 36% of them were free of any hygiene-related problems.[8] One-third of the patients had accumulated calculus on the acrylic surface of the prosthesis. Increased retention of plaque and calculus could potentially increase susceptibility to periodontal diseases, especially of the abutment teeth. Gingival inflammation, increased probing depths, and gingival recession have been reported to be greater in those with RPDs. Excessive nonaxial occlusal loading force also may contribute to the mobility of abutment teeth. Long-term outcomes include loss of the abutment teeth and thus failure of the prosthesis. In addition, prostheses without proper opposing occlusal support tend to show greater areas of the mucosa pressure.[2] Nevertheless, "a well-constructed RPD with a hygienic design and favorable abutment teeth that is accompanied by a regular recall program and individually tailored oral hygiene instructions may lead to improved clinical outcomes."

An alternative treatment option of implant-retained or implant-supported RPDs provides additional retention and limits lateral and vertical displacement of the prosthesis, which disseminates the masticatory forces more uniformly. Patients with implant-retained RPDs will need additional evaluation of the implant mobility/survival, marginal bone loss around implants, and bleeding on probing around the implants. A high survival rate of implants (91.6%–100%) from the 22-month to 10-year observation period has been reported.[3] The mean marginal bone loss around implants has been reported to be between 0.64 and 2.11 mm, and the mean deep pockets ranged from 2 to 4 mm. Maintaining good home care for the implants is paramount. Regular professional appointments are essential to monitor the implant and its surrounding hard and soft tissues, ensuring their health and addressing any issues before major complications arise (Fig. 22.2).

MECHANICAL MAINTENANCE NEEDS AND COMPLICATIONS

Due to the physiological changes of the hard and soft tissue as well as the mechanical properties of the dental materials, RPDs tend to lose retention, stability, and support over time (Fig. 22.3). The need to increase retention on clasp arms to make the denture more secure depends on the type of clasp that has been used. Increasing retention should be accomplished by contouring the clasp arm to engage a deeper part of the retentive undercut rather than by forcing the clasp toward the tooth. The latter creates only frictional retention, which violates the principle of clasp retention. As an active force, such retention contributes to tooth and/or restoration movement in a horizontal direction, disappearing only when the tooth has been moved or the clasp arm has returned to a passive relationship with the abutment tooth. Unfortunately, this is almost the only adjustment that can

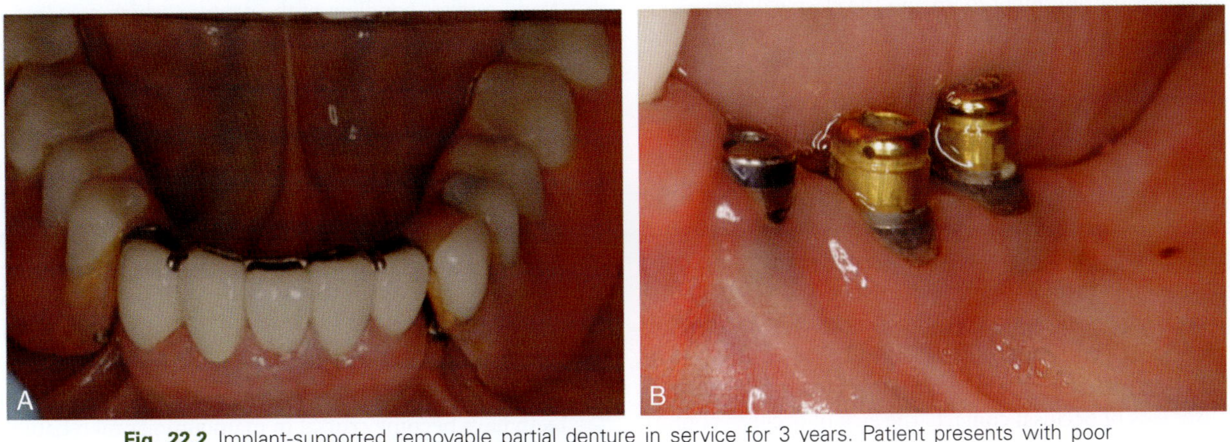

Fig. 22.2 Implant-supported removable partial denture in service for 3 years. Patient presents with poor adaptation of framework to supporting teeth, denture teeth wear **(A)**, bone loss, and plaque retention around dental prosthesis and implant abutments **(B)**.

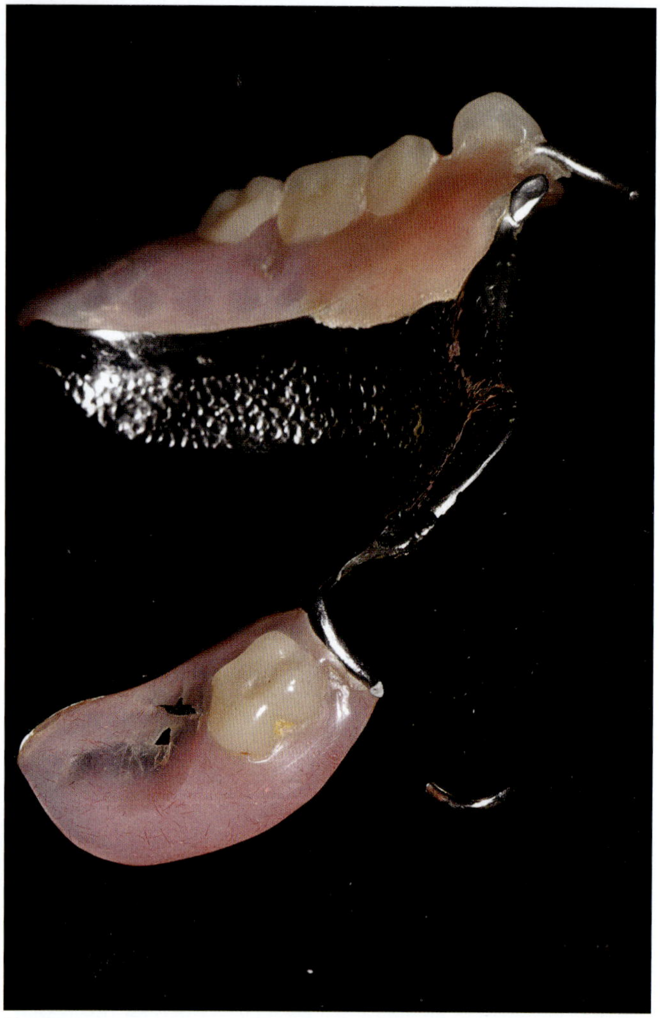

Fig. 22.3 Removable partial denture in service for 8 years. Patient presents with fractured retentive clasp, and wore acrylic resin.

be made to a half-round cast clasp arm. On the contrary, the round wrought-wire clasp arm may be cervically adjusted and brought into a deeper part of the retentive undercut (Video 22.1). Thus the passivity of the clasp arm in its terminal position is maintained, but retention is increased, because it is forced to flex more to withdraw from the deeper undercut. The patient should be advised that the abutment tooth and the clasp will serve longer if the retention is held minimally, which is only that amount necessary to resist reasonable dislodging forces.

The future development of denture rocking or looseness, due to loss of stability and support, may be the result of a change in the form of the supporting ridges rather than a lack of retention. This should be detected as early as possible after it occurs and corrected by relining or rebasing the partial denture. The loss of tissue support is usually so gradual that the patient may be unable to detect the need for relining. The dentist typically determines this during follow-up examinations, as indicated by the rotation of the distal extension denture base around the fulcrum line. If the RPD is opposed by natural dentition, the loss of base support causes loss of occlusal contact. The lack of occlusal contact may be detected by having the patient close on a medium such as dental wax placed bilaterally. If, however, a complete denture or a distal extension RPD opposes the RPD, the interocclusal wax test is not dependable. Posterior closure, changes in the temporomandibular joint, or migration of the opposing denture may have maintained occlusal contact. Alternatively, a low-viscosity impression material (e.g., light-body polyvinylsiloxane and vinyl polyether silicone) can be used to evaluate the intaglio surface of the denture base. Evidence of loss of ridge support may also be determined by the indirect retainer leaving its seat as the distal extension denture base rotates about the fulcrum.

Wear resistance of the denture teeth is also paramount for the longevity of dental prostheses (see Fig. 22.1). Patient-related factors, including the condition of the opposing arch (antagonist), may also affect the occlusal wear of denture teeth. Wear of the acrylic teeth has been the most prominent with antagonist ceramic prostheses.[9] Wear of posterior acrylic teeth may affect the vertical dimension of occlusion, resorption of the anterior ridge, masticatory efficiency, muscular function, esthetics, and fracture resistance and ultimately lead to the need for replacement of the teeth or prosthesis.[9] Studies have shown that occlusal wear of the denture teeth varies with individuals due to a combination of factors such as parafunctional habits, erosion, abrasion, and friction. Selecting the double-crosslinked and high-crosslinked polymethylmethacrylate denture teeth and keeping the glazed layer of the denture teeth have been shown to improve wear resistance.[10,11]

Periodic recall maintenance on the implant-associated components of implant-supported RPDs is also needed. Routine checks and replacement of these supporting components and surrounding acrylic relines help maintain the fit and retention of the prosthesis (see Fig. 22.2). Implant-supported RPDs have similar mechanical complications. However, additional maintenance needs include replacement of attachments, tightening of screws, and repair of the acrylic denture base.[12] Polymer-based framework partial dentures are relatively new and not typically prescribed; future study is needed to provide more insight into complications and maintenance needs of these prostheses.[13]

GENERAL RECALL RULES

The patient should be advised that maximal service may be expected from the RPD if the following rules are observed:

- Avoid careless handling of the denture, which may lead to distortion or breakage. Damage to the RPD can occur outside the mouth, often due to being dropped during cleaning or an accidental mishap when not being worn. Fractured teeth and denture bases and broken clasp arms can be repaired, but a distorted framework can rarely if ever be satisfactorily readapted or repaired. Furthermore, if the removable partial denture is not worn continuously for an extended time, a patient may have difficulty reseating the prosthesis because of tooth migration.
- Protect teeth from caries with proper oral hygiene, proper diet, and frequent dental care. An RPD denture will not protect the teeth from caries; instead caries susceptibility may increase due to plaque retention. Additionally the remaining teeth have become crucial in maintaining oral rehabilitation. Abutment teeth are especially valuable due to their importance in the success of the RPD. Therefore a rigid regimen of

oral hygiene, diet control, chemotherapeutics, and periodic clinical observation and treatment is essential for the future health of the entire mouth. The patient must be more conscientious about returning periodically for examination and necessary treatment at prescribed intervals.

- Prevent periodontal damage to the abutment teeth by maintaining tissue support of any distal extension bases. This can be detected via periodic oral evaluations and corrected by relining or other indicated procedures.
- Maintain implant health with routine dental visits. Implants are susceptible to peri-implant mucositis, bone loss, and peri-implantitis, requiring regular evaluation and maintenance. Components may need to be replaced or modified due to expected "wear and tear."
- Accept RPD treatment as something that cannot be considered permanent, but RPDs must receive regular and continuous care by both the patient and the dentist. The obligations for maintaining caries and periodontal control and for returning at stated intervals for treatment must be clearly understood.

PATIENT EDUCATION

Patients who are susceptible to caries, periodontal disease, or alveolar atrophy should be examined more frequently, thus necessitating the customization of the recall interval to the patient's risk level. Ideally check-ups should be conducted every 6 months if conditions are stable. A long-term study has supported the 6-month interval for periodontal maintenance to help prevent tooth loss.[14] Furthermore, patients with RPDs tend to lose motivation over time and are less inclined to adhere to hygiene instructions. Routine patient education and emphasis on oral hygiene habits must be continually reinforced during the regular recall visits. Innovative approaches, such as social media platforms as educational tools, may help improve patient health literacy and compliance in managing home care. The potential of recent advanced technologies can be harnessed to empower and engage patients in managing their own health.[15,16] Applications such as online videos, interactive apps, social media platforms, artificial intelligence, or a combination thereof can be utilized as tools to disseminate information to improve patient engagement. Investing time and effort in educating the patient to manage their care and making them a member of the health care team will ultimately help establish the importance of person-centered health care.

REFERENCES

1. Verma R, Joda T, Bragger U, Wittneben JG. A systematic review of the clinical performance of tooth-retained and implant-retained double crown prostheses with a follow-up of >/= 3 years. *J Prosthodont*. 2013;22(1):2–12.
2. Behr M, Zeman F, Passauer T, Koller M, Hahnel S, Buergers R, et al. Clinical performance of cast clasp-retained removable partial dentures: a retrospective study. *Int J Prosthodont*. 2012;25(2):138–144.
3. Longevity of Removable Prosthodontics: A Review of the Clinical Evidence [Internet]. Ottawa (ON): Canadian Agency for Drugs and Technologies in Health; 2015 Apr 10. https://www.ncbi.nlm.nih.gov/books/NBK304786/.
4. Bandiaky ON, Lokossou DL, Soueidan A, et al. Implant-supported removable partial dentures compared to conventional dentures: a systematic review and meta-analysis of quality of life, patient satisfaction, and biomechanical complications. *Clin Exp Dent Res*. 2022;8(1):294–312. https://doi.org/10.1002/cre2.521. Epub 2022 Jan 11. PMID: 35014207; PMCID: PMC8874059.
5. Steele JG, Walls AW, Murray JJ. Partial dentures as an independent indicator of root caries risk in a group of older adults. *Gerodontology*. 1997;14:67–74.
6. Jepson NJ, Moynihan PJ, Kelly PJ, Watson GW, Thomason JM. Caries incidence following restoration of shortened lower dental arches in a randomized controlled trial. *Br Dental J*. 2001;191:140–144.
7. Budtz-Jorgensen E, Isidor F. A 5-year longitudinal study of cantilevered fixed partial dentures compared with removable partial dentures in a geriatric population. *J Prosthet Dent*. 1990;64:42–47.
8. Wagner B, Kern M. Clinical evaluation of removable partial dentures 10 years after insertion: success rates, hygienic problems, and technical failures. *Clin Oral Investigations*. 2000;4:74–80.
9. Stober T, Bermejo JL, Rues S, Rammelsberg P. Wear of resin denture teeth in partial removable dental prostheses. *J Prosthodont Res*. 2020;64(1):85–89. https://doi.org/10.1016/j.jpor.2019.04.004. Epub 2019 May 10. PMID: 31085073.
10. Abbasi S, Nikanjam S, Shishehian A, Khazaei S, Fotovat F, Pana NH. A comparative evaluation of wear resistance of three types of artificial acrylic teeth after removing the glaze layer. *Dental Res J*. 2022;19(1):59.
11. Pham DM, Gonzalez MD, Ontiveros JC, Kasper FK, Frey GN, Belles DM. Wear resistance of 3D printed and prefabricated denture teeth opposing zirconia. *J Prosthodontics*. 2021;30(9):804–810.
12. De Freitas RF, de Carvalho Dias K, da Fonte Porto Carreiro A, Barbosa GA, Ferreira M. Mandibular implant-supported removable partial denture with distal extension: a systematic review. *J Oral Rehabilitation*. 2012;39(10):791–798.
13. Campbell SD, Cooper L, Craddock H, et al. Removable partial dentures: the clinical need for innovation. *J Prosthet Dent*. 2017;118(3):273–280.
14. Tada S, Allen PF, Ikebe K, Matsuda K, Maeda Y. Impact of periodontal maintenance on tooth survival in patients with removable partial dentures. *J Clin Periodontol*. 2015;42(1):46–53. https://doi.org/10.1111/jcpe.12320. Epub 2014 Dec 26. PMID: 25290913.
15. Zamora GT. Social media and the patient—on education and empowerment. *Rheumatol Immunol Res*. 2022;3(4):156–159. https://doi.org/10.2478/rir-2022-0028.
16. Jeyaraman M, Ramasubramanian S, Kumar S, et al. Multifaceted role of social media in healthcare: opportunities, challenges, and the need for quality control. *Cureus*. 2023;15(5):e39111.

23

Relining and Rebasing the Removable Partial Denture

Audrey Marie Selecman

CHAPTER OUTLINE

Changes in the oral mucosa and the underlying osseous structures are progressive, inevitable, and unpredictable. Time-dependent, pathological, or surgical alterations in the morphology of the supporting tissues may result in compromised support and stability of the removable partial denture, leading to prosthesis movement and further deterioration of these tissues. Therefore periodic recall and maintenance of the prosthesis are critical in prolonging the serviceable life of the removable partial denture (RPD). An acrylic removable partial denture base can be modified by a reline or rebase procedure to improve the fit and function of the prosthesis. Relining is the resurfacing of the intaglio side of a denture base with new material to improve adaptation to the underlying tissues. Rebasing is the replacement of the entire denture base with new material. Damaged, worn, or missing prosthetic teeth can also be replaced during the rebase procedure.

Relining and rebasing can be accomplished for a modification space or distal extension base. When support for a modification space is derived entirely from the abutment teeth or implants at each end of the edentulous span, these procedures will not alter the mechanics of the prosthesis. Relining or rebasing may be necessary to address denture base instability or base contours that allow food entrapment between the denture base and the residual ridge, fail to esthetically replace gingival tissues, or cause patient discomfort. When resurfacing or replacing the extension base of a Kennedy Class I, II, or IV removable partial denture, diagnosis is a crucial component to the resolution of framework movement. Clinical evaluation must assess the condition of the remaining teeth and associated restorations, design and fit of the existing framework, health, and morphology of the supporting tissues, and prosthetic and natural occlusion. Broken, bent, missing, or poorly adapted framework components, as well as unserviceable abutment teeth, might indicate the need for restorative therapy or extraction followed by replacement of the RPD. Evidence of pathology or irritation may require pharmacologic or surgical intervention before relining or rebasing. Evaluation of the base, prosthetic teeth, and underlying contours of the supporting tissues will determine if a reline or rebase procedure is indicated.

RELINE AND REBASE MATERIALS

The intaglio surface of the resin base segment of an RPD can be resurfaced with a resilient or hard liner. The choice of material is dependent on treatment goals, the health of the underlying tissues, and the expected duration of use of the liner and/or prosthesis. Prolonging the serviceable life of the RPD is best accomplished with hard, laboratory-processed acrylic resin material, whereas resilient materials are indicated for short-term use to promote tissue healing, provide comfort during a transitional period, or allow diagnostic assessment (Fig. 23.1). Resilient lining materials include plasticized acrylics and silicones that can be applied chairside or by laboratory processing. Plasticized acrylic resin liners are dispensed as a monomer liquid and polymer powder. The monomer-to-polymer ratio can be adjusted to the desired "softness" to suit the patient's needs.

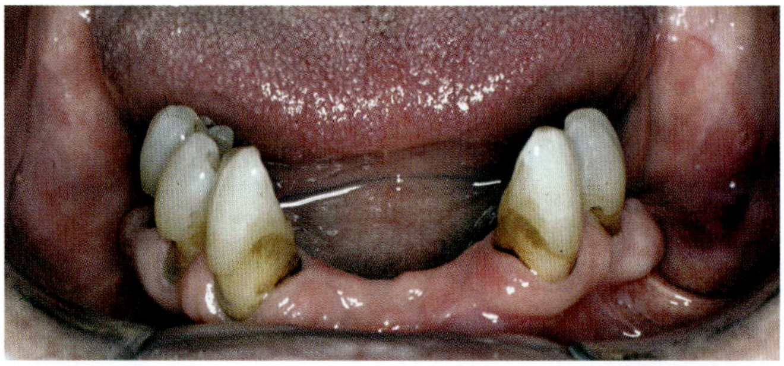

Fig. 23.1 Tissue abuse evident at the left buccal shelf region must be corrected before the reline impression is made. Management requires a period of function without the prosthesis or relief of the prosthesis in the affected region along with the placement of a resilient liner to reduce the traumatic effects of pressure while providing adequate support for the prosthesis.

This material will chemically bond to the acrylic resin base and to itself, permitting incremental layering to achieve the desired contour of the reline material. The loss of plasticizer over time hardens and distorts the material, making the serviceable life of a resilient acrylic resin liner approximately 2–4 weeks. Tissue conditioners are a specific type of plasticized acrylic resin liner formulated to be very soft to promote healing by allowing maximum tissue rebound but require replacement every 3–4 days.

Silicone liners are dispensed from an automix cartridge. While the catalyst-to-base ratio cannot be altered, some silicone liners offer a range of pliability or softness (e.g., soft and extra soft). The composition of a silicone liner allows the serviceable life to be extended up to 2 years. An adhesive layer must be applied to the surface of the base before the application of the liner because silicone does not chemically adhere to acrylic resin.

Hard acrylic resin is the material of choice for a definitive reline or rebase of an RPD, sometimes referred to as a "permanent" reline material but not referring to the longevity of the material. Both laboratory and chairside hard acrylic resin liners are available. However, the physical properties of chairside materials not cured under pressure are inferior to laboratory-processed liners in terms of strength, color stability, and porosity. Formulated from liquid methacrylate with prepolymerized poly(ethyl methacrylate) or poly(methyl methacrylate) (PMMA) powder or cartridge-dispensed diacrylate resin, the exotherm created during the self-cure process poses a substantial risk for mucosal burn. Caution must be exercised to block out all undercuts to prevent inadvertent binding of the relined base to the supporting oral structures. Therefore chairside hard acrylic resin liners are indicated only when expediency or cost is of the utmost priority.

Laboratory-processed hard acrylic resins include heat- and chemically activated PMMA. In contrast to resilient or chairside liners, laboratory-processed acrylic resin liners have superior physical properties and are the definitive material of choice for relining and rebasing procedures on otherwise healthy oral tissues.

To accomplish relining or rebasing, the original denture base segment of the RPD must be made of a resin material that can be relined or replaced. RPD bases made of metal as part of the cast framework generally cannot be relined appropriately. Thermoplastic resins such as polyamide or polypropylene do not chemically bond to acrylic resin, thereby requiring replacement by a rebase procedure when used in conjunction with a metal framework. Most resins used for digital manufacturing are methacrylate based, but the rapid development of new materials requires adhering to each manufacturer's instructions when choosing the appropriate material for a reline or rebase procedure.

RELINING

The need to reline a denture base is determined by evaluating the mechanics, occlusion, esthetics, and hygiene of the patient and prosthesis at reasonable intervals after delivery of the RPD. Before initial placement, the patient must be advised that (1) routine periodic examination is imperative to the health and longevity of the oral tissues and prosthesis, (2) the prosthesis and supporting abutment teeth are vulnerable to deterioration caused by normal daily use and may require further treatment, and (3) the patient will be financially responsible for all maintenance and recall treatment procedures. These procedures include relining, rebasing, repairs, or remaking a new partial denture. Repairs will be discussed separately in Chapter 24. A distal extension RPD base, which derives support from the tissues of the residual ridge, requires relining more frequently than a tooth-supported denture base to compensate for stress-related, physiologic changes of the soft and hard tissue-supporting structures. The primary reason for relining a distal extension base is to reestablish tissue support for the prosthesis. When opposing a complete denture, the destructive sequelae of Combination Syndrome (see Chapter 13) of the mandibular distal extension base partial denture can only be prevented by appropriate recall and maintenance procedures such as relining.

The loss of tissue support is evidenced by rotational movement of the prosthesis around the fulcrum line between the most posterior abutment teeth. A patient may indicate that the RPD "feels loose" because the retentive arms can no longer resist dislodgement when a force is applied to the distal extension base. To mistakenly tighten a retentive clasp in response to the patient's chief complaint would place undue stress not only on the retentive arm but also on the abutment tooth, resulting in possible catastrophic failure of the tooth and/or clasp assembly. The patient may also experience a decrease in chewing efficiency if the denture base tips away from the opposing occlusal contacts. Assess physiologic change by compressing the distal extension base; the lack of support will be evidenced by the lifting of the indirect retainer as the RPD rotates on abutment teeth. The resorption of the supporting tissues can be further measured by applying a thin wash of alginate or elastomeric impression material to the base and seating the framework to its terminal position without allowing the base to tip. After setting, the volume of residual impression material is inspected. Thin areas indicate tissue contact, while thick areas indicate space between the base and tissue and the need for a reline procedure.

Chairside Reline Procedure

The chairside reline procedure may be used for both resilient and hard reline materials. The procedure for applying a direct reline to an existing resin base is as follows:

1. Remove the acrylic from the tissue side of the denture base until the retention lattice is exposed. This will provide space for an adequate thickness of new material and eliminate the possibility of tissue impingement caused by the confinement of the material. Lightly relieve the borders to improve the bonding surface for the new material (Fig. 23.2).
2. If necessary, use rope wax to block out undercuts in the natural dentition or under extracoronal attachments to prevent the reline material from flowing into these areas. Elastic ring spacers can be used to provide relief around implant abutments.
3. Apply lubricant or tape over the polished surfaces from the relieved border to the occlusal surfaces of the teeth to prevent the adherence of excessive reline material that may extrude beyond the borders.

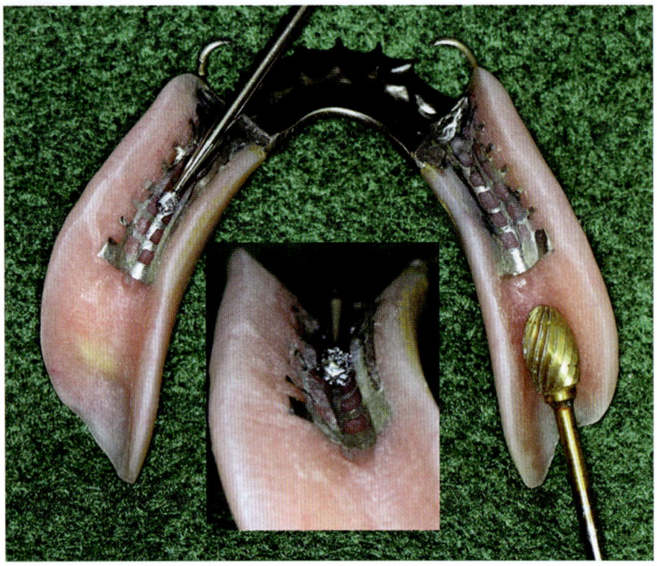

Fig. 23.2 Use of an existing Kennedy Class I removable partial denture base as a tray during a reline impression. The intaglio surface of the base is removed until the retention lattice is exposed, and all undercuts are removed to facilitate the removal of the cast after processing.

4. Following the manufacturer's instructions, mix (or dispense) and apply the chairside material to the prepared base, using a primer when indicated.
5. Within the appropriate working time, place the RPD in the mouth in its terminal position, maintain the framework in this position with finger pressure on the accessible components, and have the patient lightly close into the predetermined occlusal position. Avoid inserting the prosthesis too quickly, as the fluidity of the liner in the early stages will cause it to slump or flow out of the base. *Do not* have the patient close on cotton rolls, as this may destabilize or tip the base, impacting the final occlusion and/or functional fit of the prosthesis.
6. Muscle trim the border material in a manner similar to border molding in order to establish harmony with vestibular attachments. If a mandibular RPD is being relined, have the patient move the tongue into each cheek and then against the anterior teeth to establish a functional lingual border. To guard against framework displacement while molding of the borders with the tongue is accomplished, the framework is maintained in position with finger pressure on the accessible components such as occlusal rest seats.
7. Without disturbing the borders, excess material should be removed to facilitate finishing the final contour of the liner.
8. If using a hard acrylic resin material, remove the RPD multiple times during the curing phase to ensure that a path of draw is maintained and to prevent mucosal irritation or burn. When removed, excess acrylic resin can be trimmed with scissors and the patient's mouth can be rinsed with cold water to reduce discomfort. Otherwise, allow the liner to complete the curing phase.
9. After the curing time has elapsed, remove the RPD from the mouth and eliminate all excess material. Follow the manufacturer's instructions regarding postcuring procedures as complete polymerization may require additional curing in hot water in a pressurized vessel for a recommended amount of time. Hard acrylic resin liners can be finished and polished with conventional techniques used for an acrylic resin base. Excess resilient liner material can be trimmed using a blade, scissors, or burs designed to adjust soft liners and finished with polishing points per the manufacturer's recommended materials and techniques.

Laboratory-Processed Reline Procedure

Laboratory-processed reline materials are typically comprised of autopolymerizing or heat-cured resin material. However, resilient materials can be processed using the same clinical and laboratory techniques to control the contours, achieve maximum physical properties, and effectively refine the finish lines of the resilient reline material. The laboratory reline procedure is as follows:

1. Similar to the direct method, remove the acrylic from the tissue side of the denture base until the retention lattice is exposed. This will provide space for an adequate thickness of the impression material and facilitate cast retrieval during processing. Remove enough of the flange border to provide room for the border molding material. If the borders are deficient in length, simply roughen the surfaces.
2. Choose the appropriate impression material(s). Impression material selection is discussed at length in Chapter 16. Higher viscosity materials will compress the tissues, resulting in a functional form of the residual ridge. Conversely, lower viscosity materials result in minimal tissue displacement.
3. To extend the border to maximum extension, apply heavy body vinylpolysiloxane or compound to the border, insert the framework to its terminal position, and muscle trim the material while maintaining the position of the framework. When using elastomeric impression materials, the corresponding adhesive is necessary to adhere the impression to the base.
4. The base and its borders must be washed in the impression material of choice to obtain the surface quality and form of the soft tissue in the impression. Insert the framework again to its terminal position, and muscle trim the wash impression material while maintaining the position of the framework to prevent overextension of the previously contoured borders. While the occlusion should be briefly verified, the impression is made in an open-mouth position to allow the clinician to maintain the position of the rests in the rest seats with finger pressure (Fig. 23.3). Allowing the patient to close when relining a distal extension may cause the framework to tip distally, losing posterior occlusal contacts and rotating the framework components out of their intended location.
5. When the impression material has set, the prosthesis can be removed and the impression is inspected for accuracy, extension, and surface quality. The excess impression material should be removed from the adjacent clasp assembly, major connector, and/or polished and occlusal surfaces of the base. The prosthesis should be returned to the patient's mouth for the final inspection. The impressed contours of the denture base should fulfill its mechanical, occlusal, esthetic, and hygienic requirements.

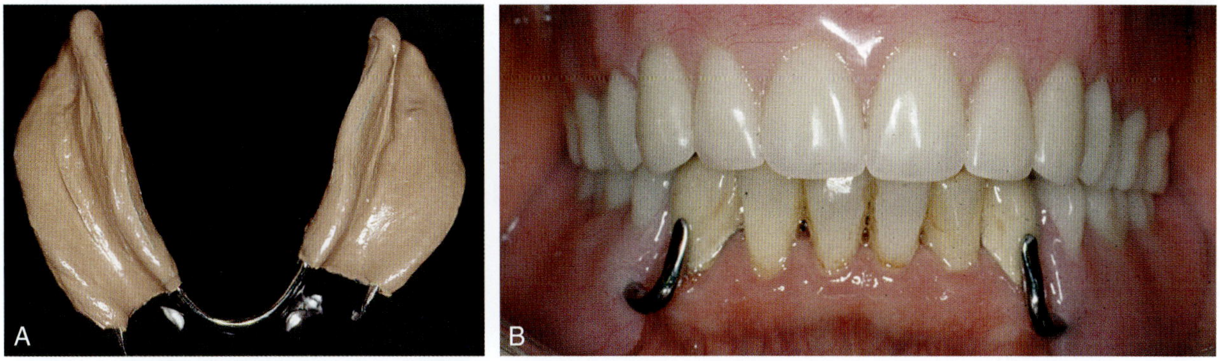

Fig. 23.3 A, Mandibular reline impression accomplished with an open-mouth impression technique. **B,** Following processing of the reline and occlusal correction with a clinical remount procedure (see Chapter 21), the occlusion is restored to the original relationship.

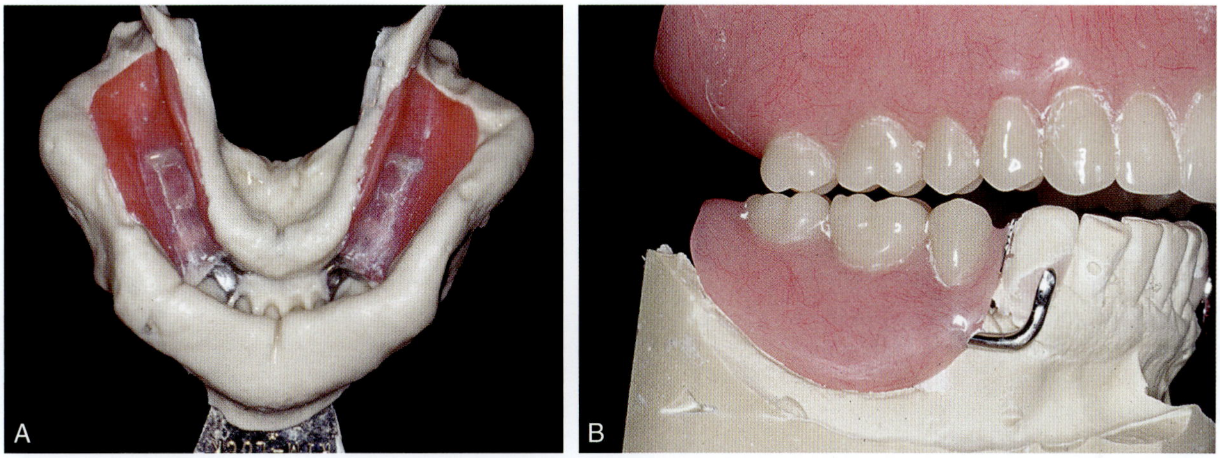

Fig. 23.4 A, An alginate pick-up impression is taken to capture the framework (with impressed bases) relative to the natural dentition. **B,** The resultant cast is mounted to the opposing occlusion, the base and prosthetic teeth are completely removed, and new prosthetic teeth are waxed to full contour for processing.

6. The prosthesis is then flasked and processed in the appropriate material. Laboratory procedures are discussed in Chapter 20. The finished removable partial denture is inserted and evaluated with the same techniques as a new removable partial denture (see Chapter 21).

REBASING

A rebase procedure requires removing the processed base in its entirety from the removable partial denture for reasons such as changing the acrylic base shade, improving the base contours, or replacing acrylic resin processed with porosity. If the prosthetic teeth are worn, damaged, or missing, replacement is indicated during the rebase procedure. This procedure follows the same steps as a laboratory-processed reline to prepare and make an impression of the underlying tissues in the base. During laboratory processing, the position of the remaining prosthetic teeth will be preserved by the flask. However, if the teeth are to be replaced, a pick-up impression is necessary to capture natural dentition relative to the prosthesis location (Fig. 23.4). To make a pick-up impression, the framework with the trimmed impression(s) of the supporting tissues is seated at its terminal location. A second impression tray is fitted, filled with alginate, and seated over the framework and natural dentition. When removed, the prosthesis should remain in the alginate impression when poured in stone. The cast can then be hand articulated or mounted using an occlusal registration to the opposing cast. If hand articulation is not possible, an occlusal registration is made after the impression step to ensure the final position of the prosthetic teeth is accurate and well supported. Once mounted, the framework is carefully removed from the cast and acrylic resin base(s) and prosthetic teeth are completely removed. The framework is returned to the cast, and the new teeth and contours of the denture base(s) are waxed to the framework and processed using conventional techniques.

24

Repairs and Additions to Removable Partial Dentures

Audrey Marie Selecman

CHAPTER OUTLINE

Removable partial denture (RPD) base materials, prosthetic teeth, and the components of the framework are vulnerable to time-dependent deterioration, distortion, and damage. Some problems require remaking the prosthesis while other complications can be managed with a repair procedure. Conventional repair techniques can be accomplished in-office with a limited amount of equipment when repairs apply to poly(methyl methacrylate) (PMMA) and metal denture bases utilizing PMMA, urethane dimethacrylate (UDMA), or porcelain teeth, and the repair can be accomplished with PMMA or poly(ethyl methacrylate) (PEMA) repair resin. Complicated repairs and modern resins such as ethoxylated bisphenol A–dimethacrylate (Bis-EMA) or UDMA may require the expertise, materials background, and equipment of a certified dental laboratory technician. Before attempting any repair, the RPD and supporting structures require a thorough examination to identify the material composition, as well as any additional problems, that may have contributed to the damage. For example, a broken clasp arm may be the result of sudden impact from dropping the prosthesis or the result of repeated, excessive flexure caused by rotational movement of an unsupported denture base. Thus an accurate diagnosis of the cause of the damage is essential to achieving a successful repair while patient education and routine recall are essential to preventing damage to both the RPD and the intraoral tissues.

DENTURE BASE REPAIR

If the fractured piece can be accurately realigned, a PMMA partial denture base can be repaired using chemically activated PMMA repair resin. Dispensed as a monomer liquid and polymer powder, chemically activated PMMA is the material of choice because of its low cost, short cure time, varied shade selection, long shelf life, and reliable physical properties. The following steps describe the repair procedure for a broken denture base segment:

1. Align the broken fragment with the denture base and secure the pieces together using sticky wax.
2. Using dental stone or putty, fill the intaglio surface—tissue side of the denture base segment—using dental stone, or a putty mixture extended to the border of the flange. Essentially, this creates a matrix to preserve the relationship of the base with the fragment. To facilitate matrix retrieval, using the putty is recommended if the intaglio surface has undercuts or appears narrow at the ridge crest.
3. Once the matrix is set, remove the prosthesis, disassemble the fragment from the base, and then remove and clean residual wax.
4. At this time, reduce the thickness of the denture base intaglio surface by approximately 1 mm of resin from the base and the fragment at the fracture line to make space for the repair resin. Additional retentive features such as a dovetail can be added to the fragment or base to improve the bond strength and retention of the repair.
5. Replace and secure the base and the fragment onto the matrix.
6. Using the salt-and-pepper technique, slightly overfill the repair gap site by adding autopolymerizing acrylic resin monomer and polymer alternately. Targeted application of repair resin can be achieved by creating a small bolus of material by dipping a sable brush into the monomer liquid and then gently contacting the polymer powder, placing it directly into the designated site. If using a cartridge-dispensed repair resin, the repair surface typically requires the application of a light-activated bonding agent to the repair surface before injection of the material into the gap site.
7. To prevent porosity caused by monomer evaporation, promptly place the repaired prosthesis and matrix into a positive pressure vessel containing water heated to 110°F and cure for 30 minutes at 20 PSI. Chemically activated cartridge-dispensed acrylic resins are formulated to cure very quickly, eliminating the need to cure under pressure.
8. Once cured, the repair material can be finished and polished with conventional techniques.

PROSTHETIC TOOTH REPAIR, REPLACEMENT, OR ADDITION

Damaged or delaminated prosthetic teeth can be repaired or replaced. If fabricated with PMMA or UDMA, a small chip in the prosthetic tooth can be repaired with a matching shade of chemically activated acrylic resin (PMMA or PEMA) or bonded composite resin. The mechanical retention, strength, and esthetics of an acrylic or composite repair resin are enhanced by abrading the surface abrasion, creating a mechanical undercut such as a diatoric or slot preparation, and adding a cavosurface bevel at the repair site in the remaining tooth structure. Chemical retention of acrylic resin is maximized by wetting the prepared surface with monomer to clean away debris and soften acrylic resin bonds while a light-activated bonding agent is necessary to bond composite resin to an acrylic resin prosthetic tooth. Once the repair resin has been added to replace the fractured segment, finishing and polishing can be achieved with carbide acrylic burs followed by polishing points, wheels, or buffs used with polishing paste.

The replacement or addition of a prosthetic tooth using repair acrylic or composite resin will require similar preparation and processing techniques used to repair the denture base material. When the patient returns with a delaminated tooth, the position of the tooth can be captured using a putty matrix adapted to the occlusal and buccal or lingual surfaces before preparing the base and tooth for repair. The addition of a tooth (or teeth) to a metal framework is more complex and may necessitate creating and/or soldering a retentive component to the framework to facilitate the attachment of the tooth and resin substructure (Fig. 24.1). When adding a new prosthetic tooth a cast of the opposing occlusion and a stable occlusal registration record are needed to position the tooth/teeth into a predictable occlusal relation.

When a natural tooth is lost, the remaining direct and indirect retainers must be evaluated to determine if the appropriate biomechanics are provided by the resultant repair design, especially if the tooth functioned as an abutment for the RPD. If the design is compromised, replacing the natural tooth with a prosthetic tooth is contraindicated and the prosthesis must be remade using a new design determined by the remaining natural teeth positions. The addition of a wrought-wire retentive clasp can be a viable modification if the remaining framework components provide the mechanical requirements of a clasp assembly on the new abutment tooth as well as for the design of the prosthesis.

Upon delivery of the repaired restoration, the occlusion must be evaluated for interfering contacts. In addition, the denture bases should be evaluated for fit on the supporting tissues. Signs of rotational movement in a distal extension base indicate the need for a reline or rebase, as the lack of support may have been the source of the initial failure of the tooth or restoration.

CLASP ARM REPAIR

Clasp arms are typically made from cast, sintered, or milled alloys; stainless steel wrought wire; or thermoplastic resins. To be retentive, the clasp arm must flex over the height of contour of the abutment tooth, into the appropriate depth of undercut. If the periodontal support is greater than the fatigue limit of the clasp arm, permanent deformation or fracture of the clasp arm occurs first. Otherwise, this could result in increased abutment tooth mobility and ultimately result in extraction. To prevent tooth loss, the terminus of the clasp arm must be precisely positioned into the undercut to provide minimal retention, as determined by an accurate survey of the master cast. Repeated flexure over time results in fatigue or permanent deformation.

Depending on the material and type of damage, the clasp arm can be repaired or replaced. Minimal modification of the metal clasp arm position or shape can be accomplished with two- or three-prong pliers as described previously (see Chapter 17). However, bending a clasp arm may result in fatigue fracture. Repeated flexure of the clasp arm occurs during insertion and removal. Exacerbated by prosthesis movement during function, excessive adjustments, poor structural integrity, and/or accidental damage, it is impossible to know the fatigue life of the clasp arm. Hence any manipulation of the metal arm may result in fracture and the patient should be advised of this risk. In addition, the patient must be educated to carefully insert and remove the prosthesis by the base and/or major connector using the appropriate path of insertion and avoiding the clasp arms as a point of leverage.

Thermoplastic clasp arms that have been adjusted or deformed beyond a serviceable position require replacement accomplished by a rebase procedure as described in Chapter 22. Replacement of a broken metal clasp arm is a suitable solution when the design of the prosthesis is not compromised (Fig. 24.2). Seated at its terminal position, an impression is made to "pick up" the removable partial denture relative to the natural dentition. The impression containing the prosthesis is poured in dental stone. The prosthesis is then carefully removed from the resultant cast to prepare the repair site. A new wrought-wire retentive arm is trimmed and contoured to be adapted to the abutment tooth in the appropriate position as determined by surveying. Sufficient space must be created to allow the replacement clasp arm to be secured to the denture base by repair acrylic, often necessitating the removal and replacement of an adjacent prosthetic tooth. Therefore including the opposing cast and relative bite registration will facilitate the repair procedure.

OCCLUSAL REST REPAIR

Fracture of an occlusal rest most often occurs at the junction to the proximal plate or minor connector. This result is usually due to insufficient depth preparation of the corresponding marginal ridge or rest seat as well as excessive occlusal adjustment to the rest itself to eliminate interferences with the opposing arch. The dimensions of the rest seat are determined by tooth morphology (see Chapter 6) as well as the material in which the framework is fabricated. The suggested thickness of a titanium rest to resist fracture is approximately 1 mm while most other cobalt-chromium alloys recommend 1.5 mm. Rests are fabricated or adjusted to an insufficient thickness risk fracture. Fracture of the rest may also be attributed to structural defects in the metal created during fabrication or sudden impact by accidental dropping.

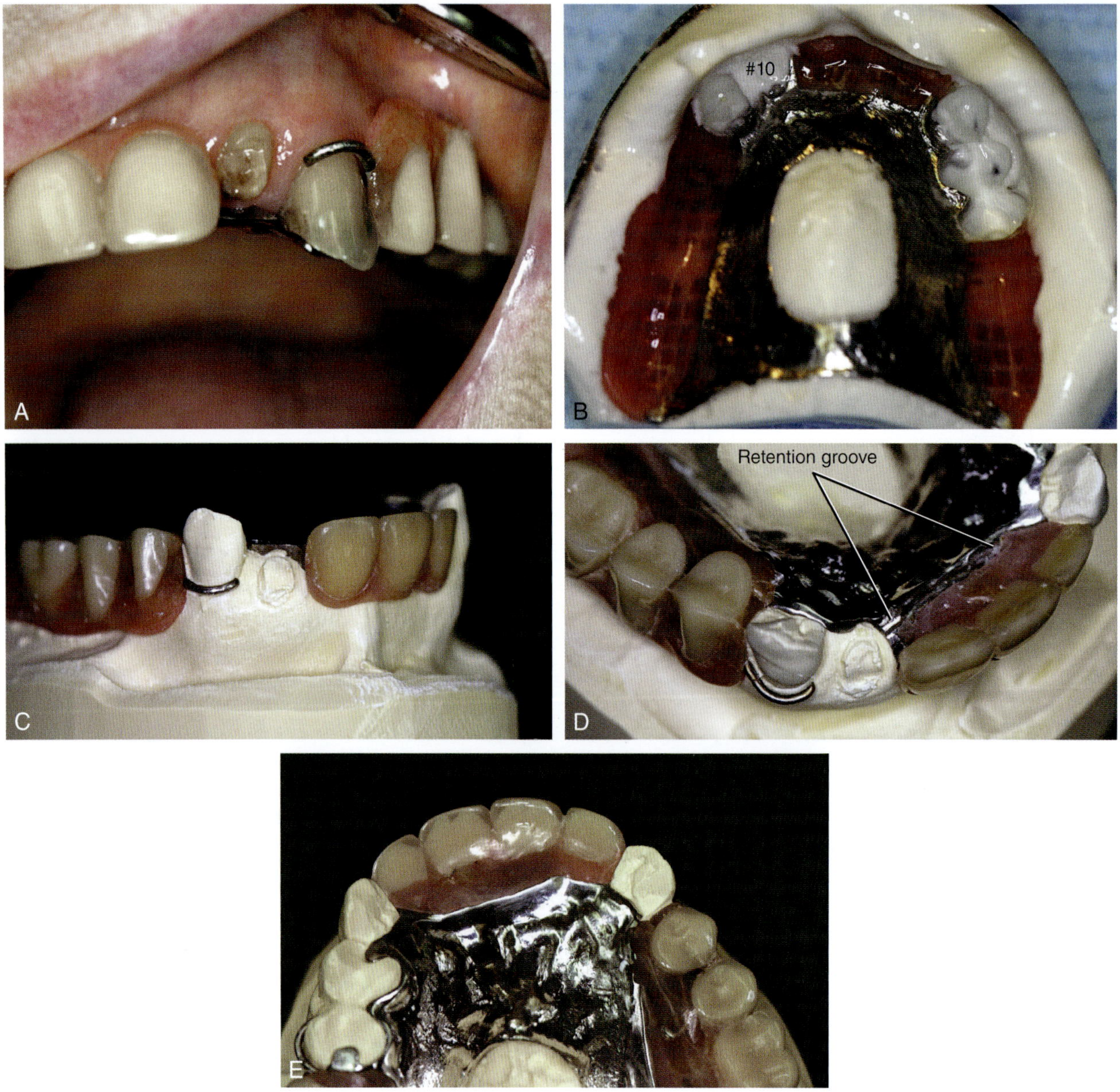

Fig. 24.1 Addition of a lateral incisor. **A,** Clinical presentation of the fractured tooth and prosthesis. Evaluation of the prosthesis revealed it to be adequately fitting, stable, and retentive. **B,** Pick-up impression of the prosthesis. **C,** Cast formed from the pick-up impression, showing a fully seated prosthesis. **D,** Preparation of the prosthesis included a mechanical means for retention (which was provided by creating a recess in the resin adjacent to the missing tooth) and creating a trough at the external finishing line to repair an area of marginal breakdown. **E,** The finished repair, which will be taken to the mouth and checked for occlusal clearance lingual to the maxillary anterior teeth.

A damaged or missing rest is best managed by the replacement of the removable partial denture. However, a new rest can be soldered to the framework as an alternative to the replacement of the prosthesis. In preparation for the rest repair the corresponding rest seat depth must be evaluated and adjusted if necessary to the appropriate dimensions. An overimpression (see Chapter 22) is then made in alginate to capture natural dentition and the RPD in its terminal position. This impression is poured in Type III vacuum-mixed dental stone. Once the stone is set, the RPD is removed from the cast, and platinum foil is adapted to the rest seat, marginal ridge, and guiding plane. The partial denture is then returned to the cast. A gold solder with the addition of flux is electrically fused to the platinum foil and the minor connector in sufficient bulk to form an occlusal rest. Industrial brazing alloy solder is a viable alternative. Although it has a higher fusing temperature, brazing alloys respond well to electric soldering and do not tarnish.

SOLDERING

Soldering is a technique by which two substrate metal surfaces (basis metal) are joined together with a molten metal filler

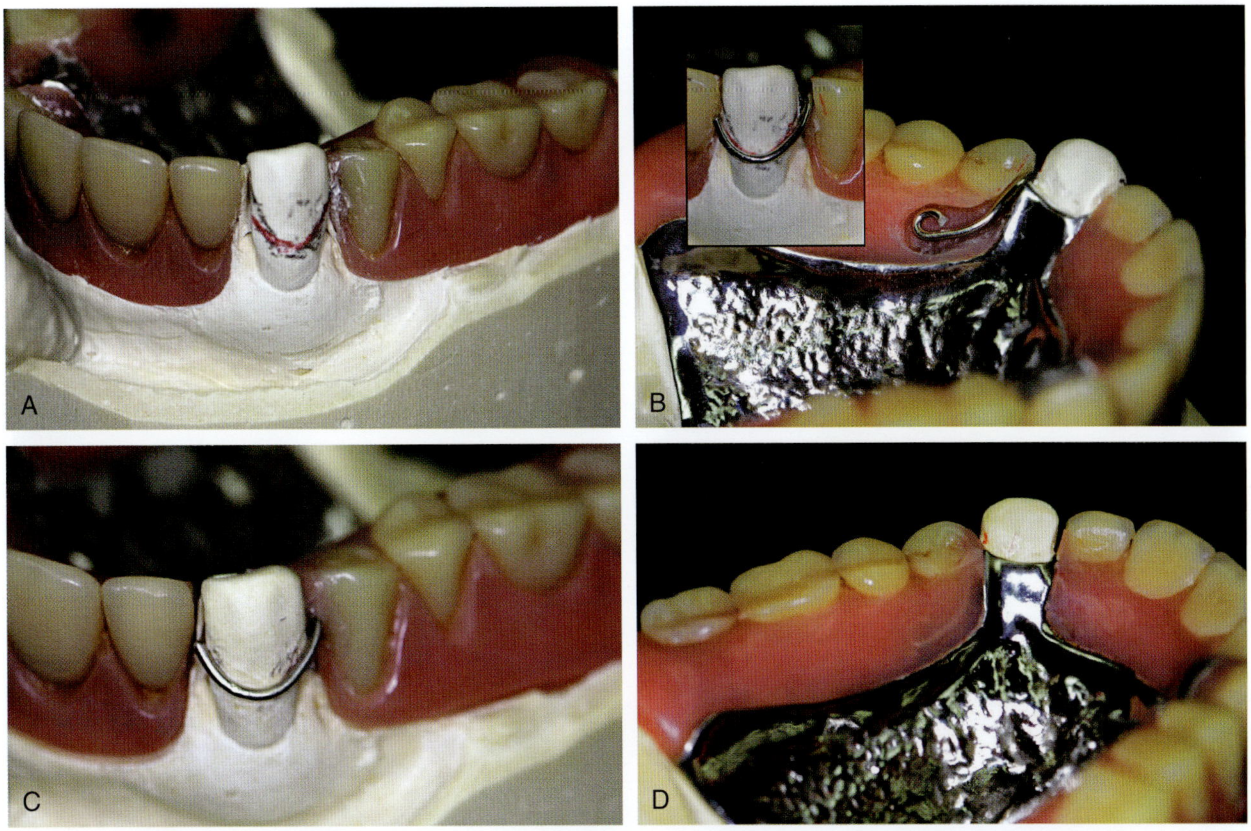

Fig. 24.2 Fractured direct retainer on canine abutment caused by long-term repeated flexure from movement associated with this 8-year-old distal extension prosthesis. Evaluation for a reline procedure is in order after the repair of the clasp arm. **A,** The cast produced from an alginate pick-up impression. The height of contour is shown in pencil, with a *red line* illustrating to the laboratory the location of the repair wire (18 gauge). **B,** Clasp adapted to the designated line on the canine and fitted into the resin trough distal to the canine and palatal to the first and second premolars. Note the curvature placed at the end of the wire to prevent movement within the polymerized resin. **C,** Finished and polished wire repair from the buccal. **D,** Palatal view.

called solder. The substrate metals are typically a component of a removable partial denture framework or wrought-wire clasp arm fabricated from a wide variety of metals and alloys containing gold, titanium, cobalt, chromium, nickel, palladium, copper, gallium, aluminum, and/or vanadium while the solder material composition can be equally diverse. The substrate metal and filler composition need not be the same, but they must be compatible. Compatibility of filler requires it to have an appropriate flow temperature, fluidity at the flow temperature, and the ability to wet the substrate metal.

The soldering process requires heating the filler material to a flowable temperature of approximately 100°F less than the solidus temperature (the temperature at which a metal or metal alloy begins to melt) of the substrate metals. The successful wetting of the substrate metal surface with the molten filler requires the elimination of an oxide coating with flux. In addition, flux acts to protect and dissolve any oxides or other structures that may contaminate the quality or decrease the strength of the soldered joint. Noble metal alloys work well with boric acid, boric anhydride, and borax fluxes whereas stable metal oxides of base metal alloys are better dissolved by fluoride flux.

Solder is typically heated using an electric soldering unit which permits rapid localization of heat at the electrode and the source of the repair as to avoid damage to other components of the removable partial denture, namely, resin base(s) or teeth. Torch soldering is used when the solder joint is long or unusually bulky and a larger quantity of solder is required. Torch soldering cannot be undertaken to repair a framework with resin components such as a base or teeth, which would be damaged by the flame.

PART IV

Maintenance

25

Considerations for the Use of Dental Implants With Removable Partial Dentures

Tamer El-Gendy and Russell J. Crockett

CHAPTER OUTLINE

The utilization of dental implants has expanded significantly in the realm of tooth replacement. When feasible, implant-supported fixed prostheses for the replacement of missing teeth are often the preferred choice. Should a patient be unable to pursue comprehensive implant-supported prostheses, they should not be deterred from considering implants altogether. In such instances, strategic use of dental implants can offer crucial clinical advantages when opting for removable partial dentures (RPDs). Moreover, implant placement in RPD cases can be planned to allow for future transition to fixed implant-supported treatment. This flexibility underscores the multifaceted benefits of integrating implants into dental prosthetic solutions.

This chapter presents basic considerations in the selection of dental implants to improve removable prosthesis performance by increasing functional stability and final esthetic results. Prosthesis instability is a commonly stated problem with RPDs.

When developing a comprehensive treatment plan for a patient's tooth loss, clinicians must carefully consider the range of prosthetic options available. Amidst choices such as tooth-supported fixed partial dentures (FPDs) and implant-supported FPDs, the RPD emerges as distinctly unique and often poses unique challenges. Effectively conveying this distinctiveness to our patients is essential in guiding them toward the most appropriate prosthesis. Furthermore, a deep understanding of this uniqueness provides valuable insights into the optimal integration of dental implants alongside RPDs.

Incorporating implants into RPD therapy serves to enhance the support, retention, and stability of the removable prosthesis, all while preserving the height of the alveolar ridge in the implant region. The successful utilization of implant-assisted RPDs (IARPDs) has shown significant improvements in the oral health-related quality of life for patients.[1,2] IARPDs are often recommended as a cost-effective and advantageous rehabilitation option, resulting in notable enhancements in patient satisfaction.

Numerous studies, including a 2012 systematic review, have documented a marked increase in patient satisfaction and exceptional survival rates of implants associated with mandibular RPDs featuring distal extensions.[3]

PHYSIOLOGIC DISTINCTION BETWEEN PROSTHESES

The most apparent contrast among RPDs, FPDs, and implant-supported prostheses (ISPs) treatment options lies in their mode of support. Conventional FPDs are supported by teeth with periodontal ligaments, implant prostheses utilize osseointegrated implants, and RPDs are reliant on teeth or a combination of teeth and mucosa for support. Another differentiating factor is the rigidity associated with the connection between the prosthesis and supporting structures—cemented prostheses rigidly connected to teeth, screw-retained implant prostheses rigidly linked between implants and bone, versus clasp-/attachment-retained RPD prostheses.

Given this variance in support and rigid connection, it becomes evident that a major distinguishing feature between fixed prostheses (whether tooth or implant supported) and tooth-tissue–supported RPDs is the potential for movement during function. The impact that such movement will have on related oral sensory and oral functional expectations of patients is potentially critical to understand. These patient-specific perspectives are variable because some patients are better at distinguishing oral sensory input than others, and some are more functionally capable than others. The importance of sensory-functional considerations is evident when it is realized that the oral cavity is unique from a sensory perception standpoint, because the sensory input from the mouth regions involved in the task of mastication represents one of the largest collections of sensory information processed for a single functional act in the body,[4] rivaled closely by the multifunctional hand (Fig. 25.1).

REPLACING ANATOMY AND FUNCTIONAL ABILITY

With the relative importance of oral sensory function associated with mastication in mind, it is helpful to consider what clinicians are attempting to replace when discussing with their patients the management of missing teeth. This involves both the physical tools for mastication and the oral ability for precise and stable neuromuscular functions to manipulate a bolus of food. Analysis of chewing studies shows that the oral receptor feedback that guides movement of the mandible comes from various sources. The most sensitive input (i.e., the input that provides the most refined and precisely controlled movement) comes from the periodontal mechanoreceptors (PMRs), with additional input coming from the gingiva, mucosa, periosteum/bone, and temporomandibular joint complex. Loss of teeth leads to loss of guidance precision, which may be caused by the deficit in PMRs.[5] No artificial replacement reestablishes the same ability inherent in the PMR guidance. Osseoperception, defined as tactile sensibility transmitted through osseointegrated implants, has been shown to restore some of the deficit caused by tooth extraction.[6] Yet prostheses may vary in their ability to affect the deficit based on sensory-related dynamics. This notion of variable prosthesis impact suggests that either the prostheses are not the same or patients may vary in terms of neuromuscular ability.

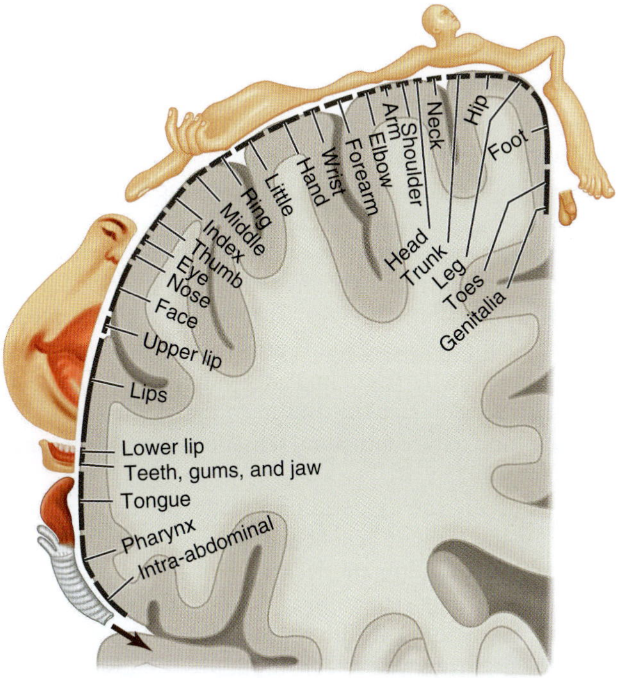

Fig. 25.1 Somatosensory cortex.

The term *neuromuscular ability* is the task-specific sensory-motor performance "ability" that a specific patient possesses for the task/act of mastication. It involves multiple factors, including the selection of a prosthesis that may vary in qualitative neuromuscular ability compared with the gold standard—natural teeth. The prosthesis influence can be favorable when replacements are more like teeth (in their neuromuscular sensory input nature), or it can be unfavorable if they are unlike teeth and potentially cause confounding sensory input that diminishes function (e.g., implant FPD vs. denture base). This therapeutic variability suggests that prostheses differ in the influence they have on oral sensory receptors; therefore this may affect a patient's perspective on how much a treatment has improved the rehabilitation of oral function (i.e., neurophysiologic ability rehabilitation).

Stability under function is critical for limiting confounding sensory input because instability is a significant confounder of normal function. Whether a prosthesis is stable or unstable influences whether it provides a positive or a negative contribution to an already reduced peripheral receptor influence. This is compounded by the inherent neuromuscular variability seen between patients. Consequently, in some of our patients, replacement teeth may have less of a "margin" for sensory contribution without creating functional impediments.

ADVANTAGES OF IMPLANT-ASSISTED REMOVABLE PARTIAL DENTURES

1. Improved stability: IARPDs offer enhanced stability, reducing movement during speaking and chewing.
2. Enhanced chewing function: Patients have reported better chewing function with IARPDs, as evidenced in several studies.
3. Aesthetic improvement: The aesthetics of IARPDs are often superior when compared with conventional RPDs (Fig. 25.2).
4. Bone preservation: Implants used in IARPDs can help maintain bone levels (Fig. 25.3).

Disadvantages of Implant-Assisted Removable Partial Dentures

1. Increased cost: The overall cost of an IARPD rises due to the addition of implants and attachments.
2. Surgical procedure: Patients must undergo a surgical procedure for implant placement, which can involve some level of discomfort and recovery time.
3. Maintenance requirements: IARPDs and their attachments require regular maintenance and care to ensure longevity and proper function.

Patient Selection for Implant-Assisted Removable Partial Dentures

Patients who are partially edentulous and interested in replacing missing teeth, yet unable to qualify for a fixed ISP, may find IARPDs to be an ideal solution. The Kennedy classification system categorizes RPD scenarios based on the location

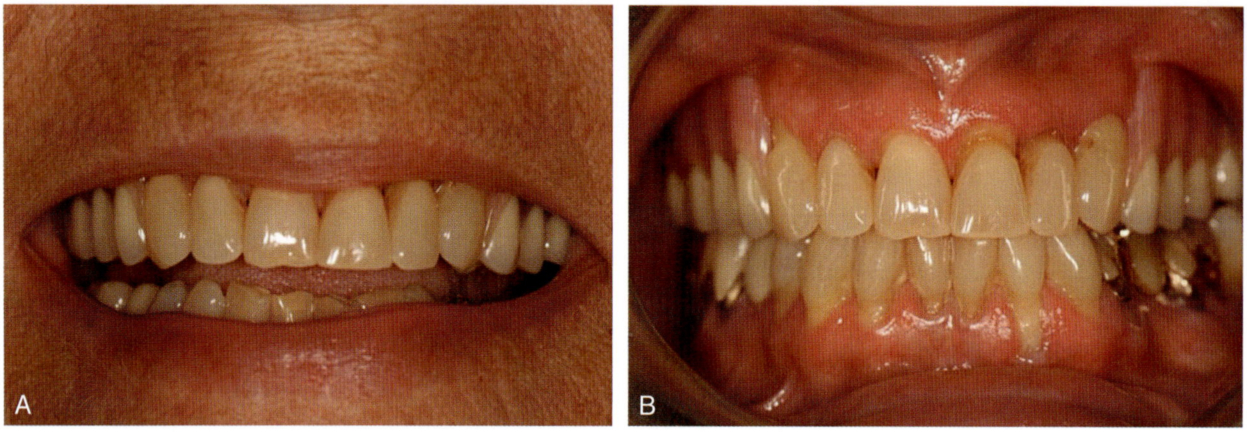

Fig. 25.2 The esthetics of implant-assisted removable partial dentures *(RPDs)* are often superior when compared with conventional RPDs. Because of the use of implant abutment attachments, no visible clasps are required. **A,** Frontal view of a patient with implants placed in the location of the maxillary premolars acting as direct retention. **B,** Same patient in repose.

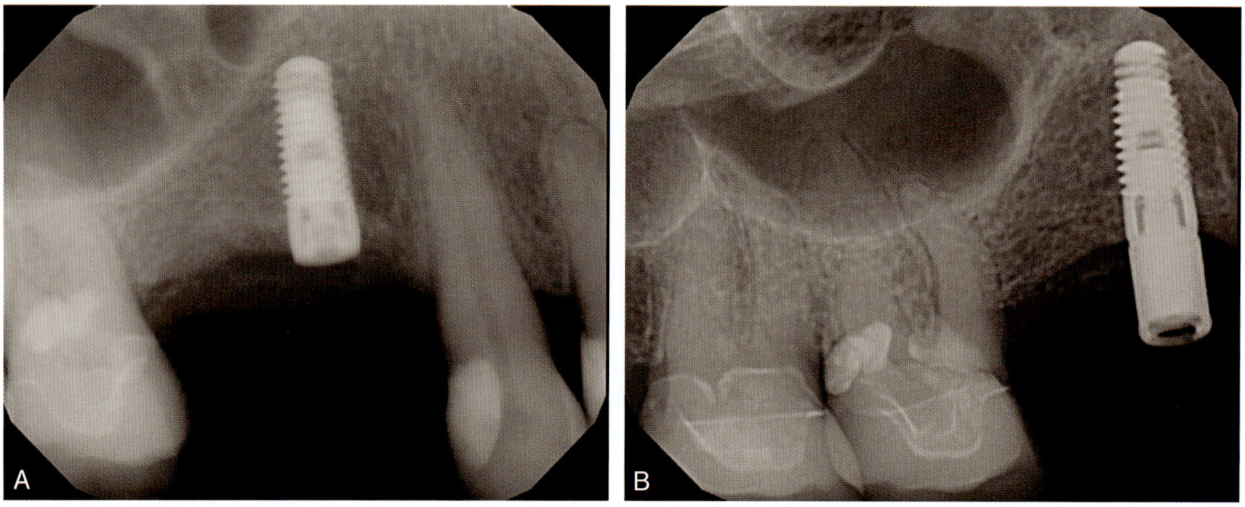

Fig. 25.3 Radiograph of dental implant in same location over time (**A** and **B**). **B,** Implants used in implant-assisted removable partial dentures can help maintain bone levels (4 years).

of the edentulous region, aiding in treatment planning and decision-making.

1. Kennedy Class I: This classification designates bilateral edentulous areas located posterior to the remaining natural teeth. IARPDs are particularly beneficial in Kennedy Class I scenarios as they can efficiently enhance support, stability, and retention. Implants placed in these regions assist an RPD through the use of various types of attachments. These attachments can improve support, stability, retention, and overall function (Fig. 25.4). In many cases the use of implants can create a situation similar to a tooth-supported Kennedy Class III rehabilitation, minimizing the potentially damaging class I lever forces exerted on the distal abutment teeth during function (Fig. 25.5, *A*). This can contribute to the longevity of the prosthesis and the overall oral health of the patient.
2. Kennedy Class II: In Kennedy Class II scenarios, a unilateral edentulous area is located posterior to the remaining natural teeth. Implants can play a significant role in improving support, stability, and retention here as well, leading to enhanced functionality and comfort for the patient as discussed in the previous paragraph regarding Kennedy Class I cases.

The most beneficial use of an implant with an RPD is to reduce the negative impact of any sensory input resulting from prosthesis movement. The greatest potential for movement is seen with Kennedy Class I and II prostheses. Consequently, the greatest benefits in the use of implants with Kennedy Class I and II RPDs are to gain stability and retention, control prosthesis movement, and reduce unnatural sensations that are movement related (see Fig. 25.5, *B*).

The clinician who is deciding exactly where to place an implant for the greatest benefit should take many factors into consideration. The ultimate decision will be influenced by a combination of important clinical issues. Basic considerations include factors associated with support, stability, and retention; residual ridge anatomy; strategic tooth loss; opposing occlusal influence; and the condition of a terminal tooth.

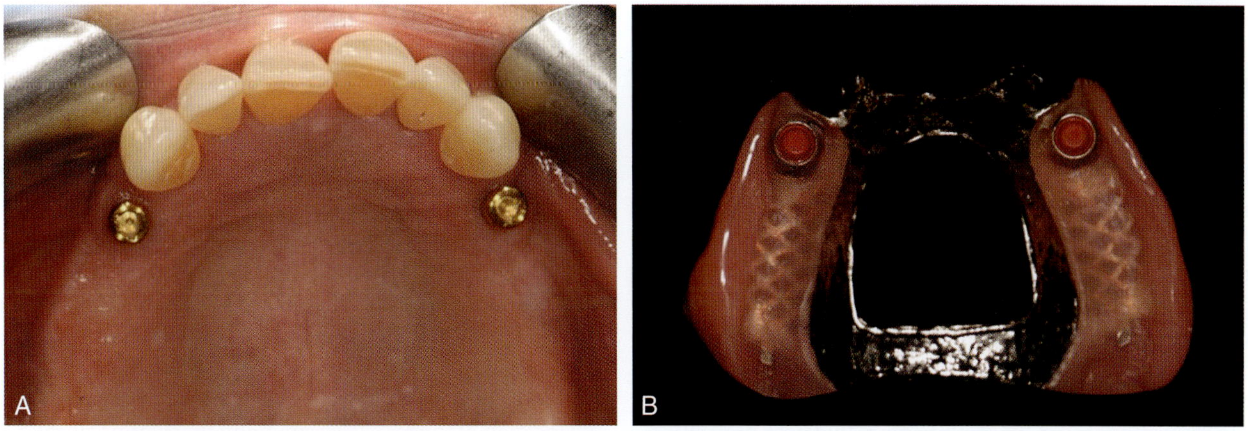

Fig. 25.4 Attachment used to provide retention to the maxillary removable partial denture *(RPD)* without the need for any traditional clasps. **A,** Occlusal view of maxillary arch with locator attachment for prosthesis retention. **B,** Intaglio surface of the corresponding maxillary RPD. Note the patriarchal attachments/housings in the region of the premolars.

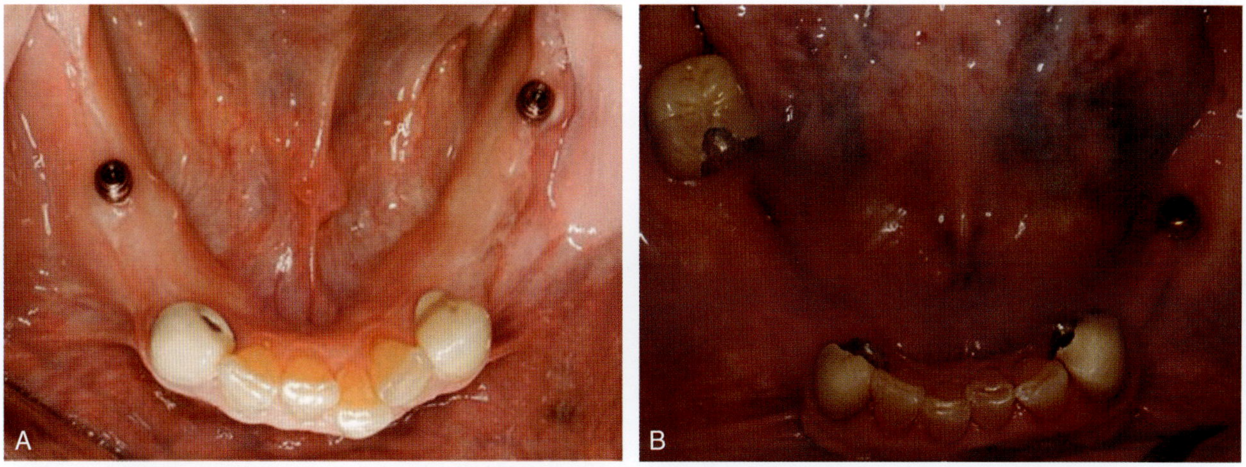

Fig. 25.5 **A,** Placement of dental implants in the molar region allows for conversion of a Kennedy Class I to Kennedy Class III to minimize the potentially damaging class I lever forces exerted on the distal abutment teeth during function. **B,** Similarly, a Kennedy Class II may be converted to a Kennedy Class III. (B, Courtesy of Dr. Carlos Jurado and Graduate Prosthodontics at the University of Alabama.)

IMPLANT POSITION FOR IMPLANT-ASSISTED REMOVABLE PARTIAL DENTURES

In recent years, IARPDs have emerged as a recognized treatment option for converting a Kennedy Class I or II partially edentulous arch to a Kennedy Class III rehabilitation.[7] The use of IARPDs is known to limit both vertical and lateral displacement, thereby reducing bone resorption under the distal free-end denture base. IARPDs serve as a viable alternative to conventional RPDs and implant-supported fixed partial prostheses, especially in cases where limited bone height and thickness restrict the placement of implants. In such scenarios, implants can be strategically placed to stabilize the RPD vertically. This approach not only enhances patient comfort but also contributes significantly to improved masticatory efficacy. By utilizing these implants, the RPD gains the necessary support and retention to function effectively, thereby providing patients with enhanced chewing ability and overall satisfaction.

The optimal location of the implant along the distal edentulous residual ridge has been a topic of controversy in both clinical practice and in vitro studies. This location is considered crucial as it can significantly impact the stress distribution within IARPDs, which may ultimately influence the clinical outcomes of this treatment.

Finite element analysis (FEA) has been a widely utilized method for predicting the biomechanical behavior of dental implants.[8] In an in vitro FEA study conducted by Ortiz-Puigpelat et al.,[9] various implant positions were analyzed using a three-dimensional mandibular model derived from a human patient. The study involved creating several test models where implants were placed in the first and second molar areas and the premolar area. A control model without implant support was included for comparison. The study evaluated overall displacement values, von Mises stress distribution maps, and nonlinear deformations in these different models.

The findings of the study indicated that placing an implant with a locator abutment significantly improved the biomechanical behavior of RPDs. Analysis of implant location revealed that an implant in the first molar area yielded superior biomechanical results compared with other positions. These enhanced results were observed in terms of general displacements, maximum stress values, distribution within the peri-implant bone, the RPD metal framework, and the implant itself. Based on these findings, the study suggests that the first molar area may be an advantageous location for implant placement when considering the biomechanical aspects of IARPDs.[9]

Keltjens et al.[10] highlighted that the use of IARPDs as a treatment alternative can offer several benefits:

1. Prevent bone resorption: IARPDs have been shown to prevent bone resorption under the denture base, therefore preventing the need for repeated relines to restore posterior support.
2. Enhanced retention and support: The incorporation of attachment systems with implant support can further improve the retention of the RPD, ensuring a secure fit and stability during use.
3. Reduced stress on supporting teeth: By distributing forces more evenly, implant support reduces the stress on the remaining natural teeth used as abutments for the RPD.
4. Reduced number of retainers: The need for additional coronal retainers, such as clasps, can be minimized with the use of implants, leading to a more streamlined and aesthetically pleasing prosthesis (Fig. 25.6).
5. Improved comfort: Patients often experience increased comfort with IARPDs, as the prosthetic is more stable and less likely to shift or move during daily activities.

These advantages collectively contribute to the overall success and satisfaction of patients. According to a systematic review done by de Freitas,[3] implant survival rates ranged from 95% to 100% with patient satisfaction ranging from 4.12 to 5.0 on a five-point questionnaire with 1 as the least favorable situation. The author stated that the load should be applied on the long axis of implants to guarantee long-term success.

DIMENSIONS OF DENTAL IMPLANTS USED IN IMPLANT-ASSISTED REMOVABLE PARTIAL DENTURES

The placement of implants within the alveolar ridge necessitates sufficient bone height and width, which can be evaluated during treatment planning. The residual ridge often undergoes resorption after tooth loss. In the posterior jaws, this resorption can lead to vertical loss of bone. This becomes particularly complex due to the location of the maxillary sinus and the inferior alveolar nerve. These anatomical considerations necessitate careful planning of surgical procedures by using cone-beam computed tomography (CBCT) and optical scans to fabricate an implant surgical guide.

In a multicenter prospective study investigating mandibular distal extension IARPDs by Payne et al.[11] 6 of 72 implants failed. All failed implants were short (6 mm), and the failures occurred more than 5 years after loading.[11] Although the survival rate of short implants was 93.4%, with mean bone loss of 1.04 ± 1.88 mm around implants in patients wearing distal extension IARPDs, Bellia et al.[12] found that 2 of 35 implants with a length of either 5 or 6 mm were lost in follow-up of 4 years.

An FEA study investigated the effects of implant length and diameter on von Mises stress by simulating the implants below hemimandibular IARPDs.[13] Results showed a decrease in von Mises stress associated with an increase in length or diameter of the implants. Another FEA study simulating mandibular distal extension IARPDs investigated the effects of implant length on stress distribution to the periodontal ligament of direct abutment teeth and concluded that longer lengths of dental implants decreased the stress distribution to the periodontal ligament of abutment teeth.[14]

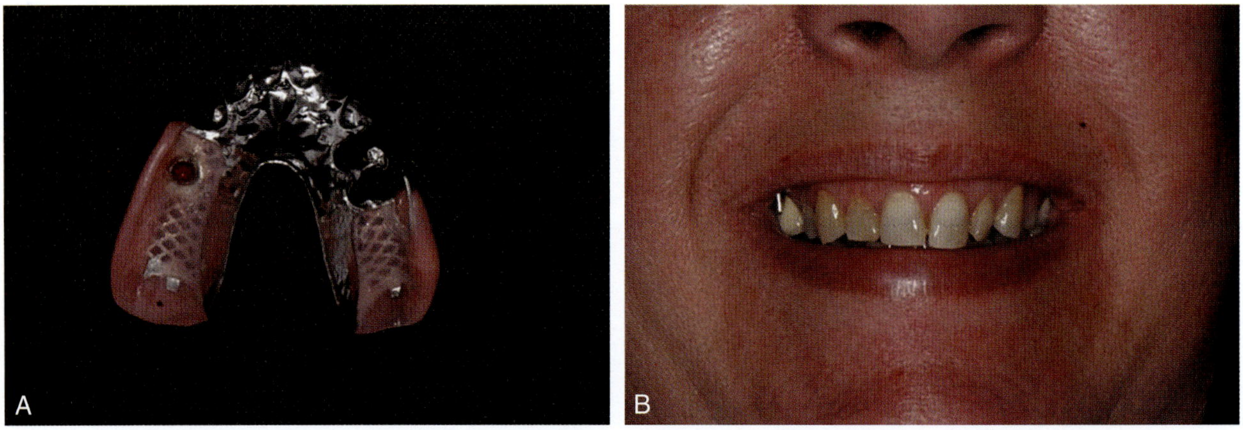

Fig. 25.6 A Kennedy Class I, with a long-spanning modification space crossing the mandibular midline. Without the use of dental implants, the lateral incisor would need to be clasped. The implants provide support and retention, thereby reducing the number of clasps needed. The implants improve function and comfort while reducing functional stress on the mandibular incisors. (Courtesy of Ahmed Mahrous Copyright © 2024. All rights reserved.)

CLINICAL EXAMPLES OF WHEN TO USE IMPLANT-ASSISTED REMOVABLE PARTIAL DENTURES

1. Kennedy Classes I and II: A patient presents with bilateral or unilateral posterior edentulous areas. Implant placement in the first molar areas can significantly enhance retention, stability, and support for the RPD. This will lead to improved chewing function, reduced stress on abutment teeth, and prevention of bone resorption under the denture base (see Fig. 25.5).
2. Avoiding clasp placement in the esthetic zone: If the patient prefers a more esthetic solution without visible clasps, the implant attachment can serve as a retentive feature for the RPD, eliminating the need for visible clasps. This will improve esthetics and enhance patient confidence.
3. Vertical ridge resorption: If the patient has significant vertical bone loss in the posterior maxilla or mandible due to long-term tooth loss, short implants can be used strategically to support the RPD vertically and prevent further bone resorption. This will enhance masticatory efficacy and improve retention and comfort for the patient.
4. Enhanced retention and stability: If a Kennedy Class I patient struggles with RPD retention and stability due to lack of posterior support, adding two implants strategically on each side will distribute forces and improve overall stability of the RPD. This will enhance patient comfort, reduce movement of the prosthesis, and improve masticatory function.
5. Loss of a critical tooth (canine): A patient missing a critical tooth, such as a canine, which is crucial for the stability and support of the RPD, can significantly diminish the prognosis of an RPD. Rather than extract the remaining teeth to accommodate a conventional complete removable prosthesis, an implant can be strategically placed to retain the RPD using an attachment. This is a conservative approach as the natural dentition is preserved. An implant with an attachment may provide stable anchorage for the RPD, which will enhance its retention (Fig. 25.7).

These clinical examples highlight the versatility and effectiveness of using implants to assist RPDs in various patient scenarios. Careful consideration of patient-specific factors with proper treatment planning and implant placement is crucial for successful outcomes.

CONSIDERATIONS WHEN TREATMENT PLANNING AN IMPLANT-ASSISTED REMOVABLE PARTIAL DENTURE

1. Bone quality and quantity: Adequate bone volume and density in the implant sites are essential for successful implant placement.
2. Evaluation and measurement: Clinical examination, radiographic assessment (CBCT scans), and articulated diagnostic casts are essential to assess the interocclusal space.
3. Surgical guide: It can be helpful to fabricate a surgical guide to assist in the placement of implants in critical areas.

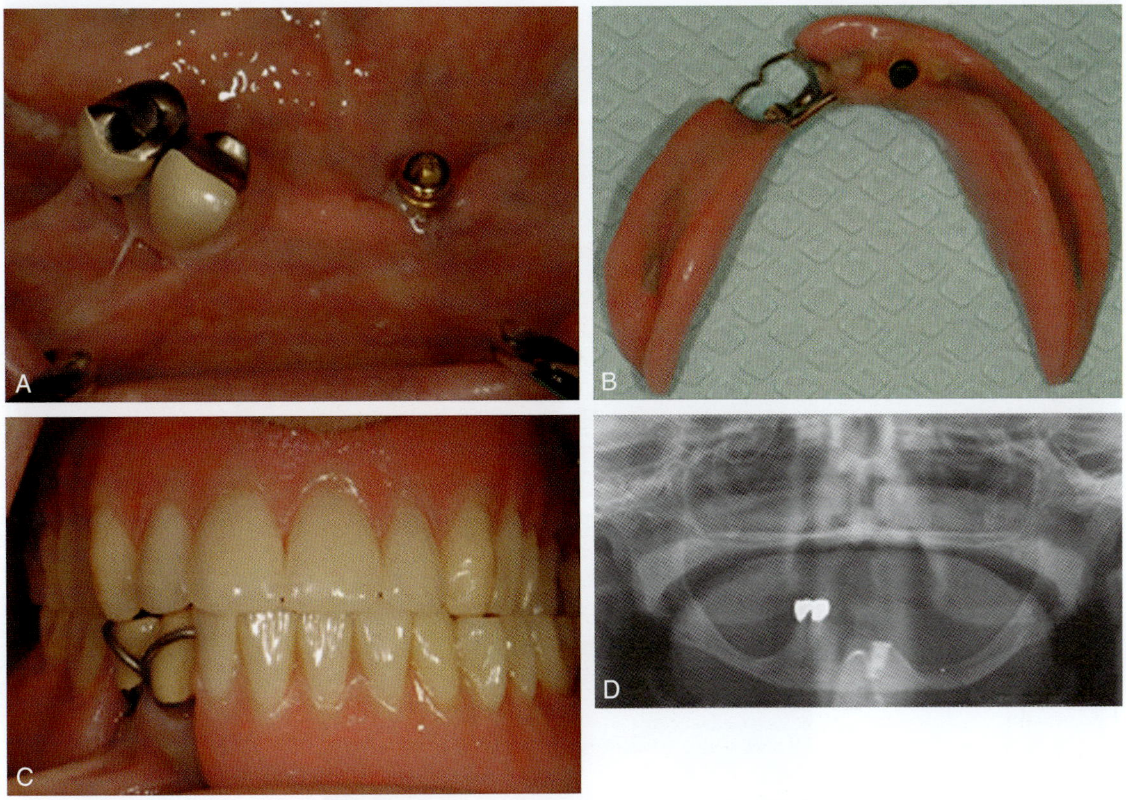

Fig. 25.7 Loss of a critical tooth (canine) leaving no abutment tooth on the contralateral side of the mandibular arch with significant residual ridge resorption. **A,** The implant replaces the strategically missing tooth #22. The implant provides sufficient support to improve functional comfort and occlusal function. **B,** intaglio surface of the mandibular IARPD. **C,** IARPD in place intraorally with opposing complete denture. **D,** Panoramic radiographic image of patient with remaining teeth and dental implant.

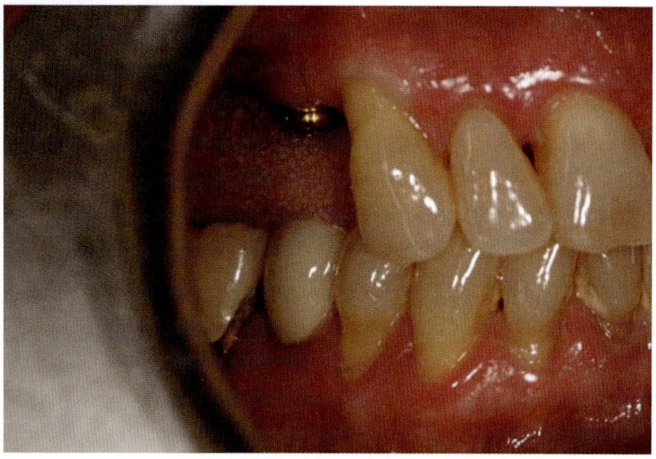

Fig. 25.8 Adequate interocclusal clearance: proper restorative space is essential to accommodate different attachments along with the implant-assisted removable partial denture framework, denture base acrylic, and denture teeth. Interocclusal clearance of 12 mm is needed.

Surgical guides can be used to control the depth, angulation, and location of the implants.

4. Interocclusal clearance: To assist an RPD without detriment, the patient must have adequate interocclusal clearance for the restorative components. The amount of space needed varies depending on the type of attachments used. Proper restorative space is essential to accommodate different attachments along with the IARPD framework, denture base acrylic, and denture teeth. If interocclusal clearance is inadequate, alternative implant positions or bone reduction may be necessary (Fig. 25.8).
5. Type of attachment: There are numerous types of attachments each with differing space requirements, indications, resilience, and effects on retention, support, and stability.
6. Strict follow-up and monitoring: Regular follow-up appointments are essential to monitor the fit, function, and stability of the IARPD.

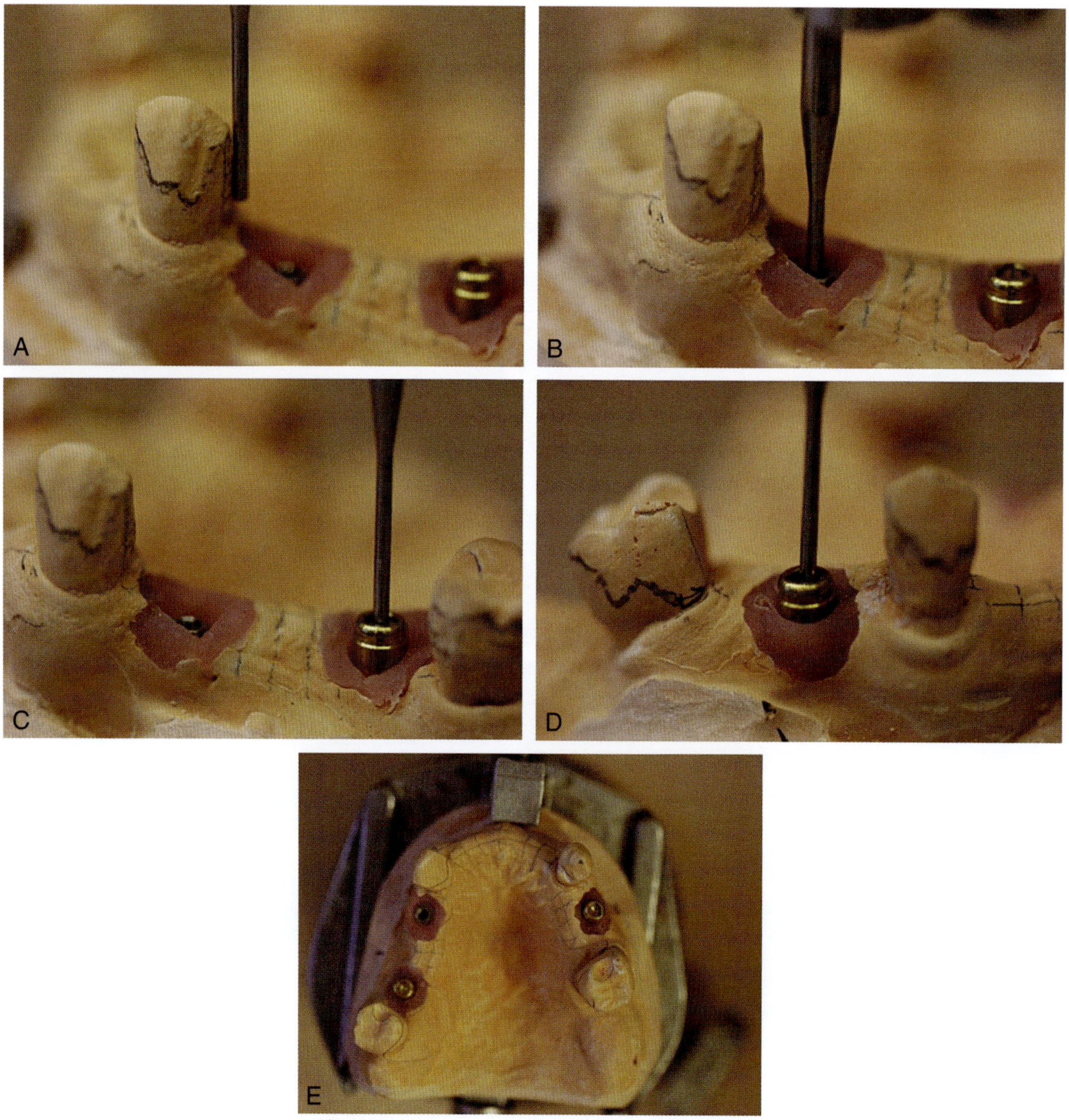

Fig. 25.9 A–D, Verification of parallel path of insertion established with tooth guide planes (distal of the canines and mesial of the molar) and long axis of adjacent implants. E, Occlusal view of maxillary cast.

7. Need for survey crowns: The need to use survey crowns is still a consideration for abutment teeth even when using implants to assist an RPD.
8. Path of insertion of the IARPD: The prosthesis path of insertion is critical for the success of this treatment (Fig. 25.9). There must be a common path of insertion between natural teeth and dental implant attachments. Nonparallel paths of insertion between implants or implants and abutment teeth can negatively affect the long-term prognosis of an IARPD and cause premature wear of the implant attachments.

Careful evaluation, treatment planning, communication, and ensuring sufficient interocclusal clearance are crucial for the successful placement and function of an IARPD.

REFERENCES

1. Gates WD, Cooper LF, Sanders AE, et al. The effect of implant-supported removable partial dentures on oral health quality of life. *Clin Oral Implant Res.* 2014;25:207–213.
2. Jensen C, Raghoebar GM, Kerdijk W, et al. Implant-supported mandibular removable partial dentures; patient-based outcome measures in relation to implant position. *J Dent.* 2016;55:92–98.
3. de Freitas RF, de Carvalho Dias K, da Fonte Porto Carreiro A, et al. Mandibular implant-supported removable partial denture with distal extension: a systematic review. *J Oral Rehabil.* 2012;39:791–798.
4. Haggard Patrick, de Boer Lieke. Oral somatosensory awareness. *Neurosci Biobehav Rev.* 2014;47:469–484.
5. Trulsson M. Sensory-motor function of human periodontal mechanoreceptors. *J Oral Rehabilitation.* 2006;33(4):262–273.
6. Mishra SK, Chowdhary R, Chrcanovic BR, Brånemark PI. Osseoperception in dental implants: a systematic review. *J Prosthodontics.* 2016;25(3):185–195.
7. Zancopé K, Abrão GM, Karam FK, Neves FD. Placement of a distal implant to convert a mandibular removable Kennedy Class I to an implant-supported partial removable Class III dental prosthesis: a systematic review. *J Prosthet Dent.* 2015;113:528–533.
8. Geng JP, Tan KB, Liu GR. Application of finite element analysis in implant dentistry: a review of the literature. *J Prosthet Dent.* 2001;85:585–598.
9. Ortiz-Puigpelat O, Lázaro-Abdulkarim A, de Medrano-Reñé JM, Gargallo-Albiol J, Cabratosa-Termes J, Hernández-Alfaro F. Influence of implant position in implant-assisted removable partial denture: a three-dimensional finite element analysis. *J Prosthodontics.* 2019;28:e675–e681.
10. Keltjens HM, Kayser AF, Hertel R, Battistuzzi PG. Distal extension removable partial dentures supported by implants and residual teeth: considerations and case reports. *Int J Oral Maxillofac Implant.* 1993;8(2):208–213.
11. Payne AGT, Tawse-Smith A, Wismeijer D, De Silva RK, Ma S. Multicentre prospective evaluation of implant-assisted mandibular removable partial dentures: surgical and prosthodontic outcomes. *Clin Oral Implant Res.* 2017;28:116–125.
12. Bellia E, Audenino G, Ceruti P, Bassi F. Clinical assessment of short implants retaining removable partial dentures: 4-year follow-up. *Int J Oral Maxillofac Implant.* 2020;35:207–213.
13. Verri FR, Pellizzer EP, Rocha EP, Pereira JA. Influence of length and diameter of implants associated with distal extension removable partial dentures. *Implant Dent.* 2007;16:270–280.
14. Fayaz A, Geramy A, Memari Y, Rahmani Z. Effects of length and inclination of implants on terminal abutment teeth and implants in mandibular CL1 removable partial denture assessed by three-dimensional finite element analysis. *J Dent.* 2015;12:739–746.

26

Interim Removable Partial Dentures

Wendy Clark and Patricia Swanson

CHAPTER OUTLINE

At times a temporary or transitional tooth replacement may be necessary for a relatively short period of time. These situations may precede definitive care. Examples of indications for temporary tooth replacement are when providing emergency or urgent care or during healing from tooth extractions or implant surgery. When such applications require the temporary use of removable partial dentures (RPDs), their fabrication and use must be incorporated into a total prosthodontic treatment plan. An interim RPD is a provisional prosthesis designed for use over a limited period of time, after which it is to be replaced by a more definitive restoration. This prosthesis may be delivered at the time of extraction (immediate interim) or after the sites have healed. Interim prostheses are frequently used for patients with a poor prognosis for maintaining one or all the remaining teeth; it can be designed to have teeth added over time as they are lost. If necessary it may be converted in the future to an interim complete denture.

Interim prostheses for the partially edentulous patient should ideally be fabricated with minimal time and expense. Consequently these prostheses are typically acrylic resin, with or without wire retention, and may include components to provide tooth support. Polymethyl methacrylic (PMMA) in part allows these prostheses to be easily modified. This includes adding teeth, adding clasps, and relining the prosthesis predictably and without much difficulty. It should be noted that these prostheses typically do not provide the same support, stability, and retention as a conventional alloy frame RPD. As tissue changes they can lose stability, unpredictably loading the soft and hard tissues. Patients with these prostheses should be monitored closely for prosthesis fit; they should understand that this is considered a short-term solution, to be replaced by a more definitive restoration or a new, well-fitting interim partial if necessary. The difficulty in achieving and maintaining strategic tooth support and stability may jeopardize the integrity of adjacent teeth and the health of supporting tissue if worn for extended periods without supportive care.

Such a restoration is usually made of various types of resin, which may be produced by any number of methods (sprinkling/sprinkle-on technique, visible light-cured resin method, waxing, flasking, and processing with autopolymerizing or heat-polymerizing resin or digitally with additive or subtractive manufacturing). It may be retained by circumferential wrought-wire clasps, Crozat-type clasps, interproximal spurs, or wire loops.

Alternatively, interim prostheses can be fabricated from thermoplastic materials, such as nylon, which have flexible bases. These flexible base prostheses can have flexible clasps which are clear or pink, making them less noticeable in the esthetic region. However, these flexible bases do not meet the ISO standards for a denture base and cannot be relined. The difficulty in adjusting flexible denture bases results in higher surface roughness, which can contribute to biofilm accumulation over time. Despite these pitfalls, many patients enjoy wearing flexible denture base partials and it may prove difficult to transition them to a cast metal base in the future, despite their superior mechanical properties and benefit to the remaining dentition.

Interim prostheses may be indicated as a part of total treatment for the following:

1. Preserve the esthetic appearance of a patient.
2. Maintenance of a space to prevent tooth movement.
3. Reestablishment of occlusal relationships.
4. Conditioning of teeth and residual ridges.
5. Interim restoration during treatment.
6. Conditioning the patient for wearing a prosthesis.

APPEARANCE

Often, anterior teeth need to be removed and patients desire immediate replacement. For the sake of appearance an interim RPD may replace one or more missing anterior teeth, or it may replace several teeth, both anterior and posterior. When replacing a single missing anterior tooth, these restorations are often made without clasps. This can improve esthetic outcomes and

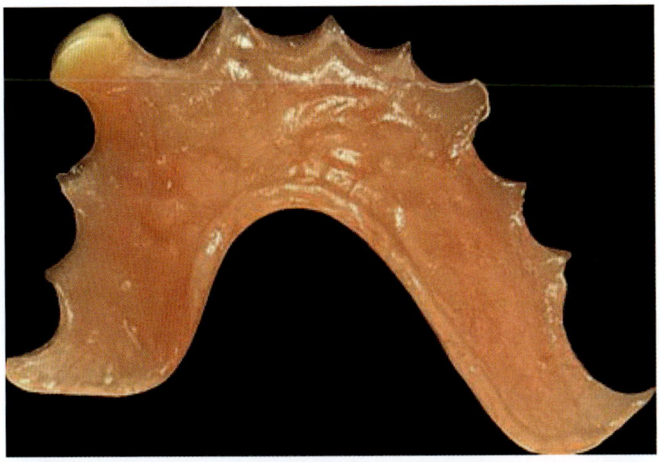

Fig. 26.1 When an anterior tooth is lost, an immediate or interim replacement is commonly desired by the patient. Interim removable partial dentures replacing a single tooth often do not require clasping. This decreases cost and complexity of fabrication and improves esthetics.

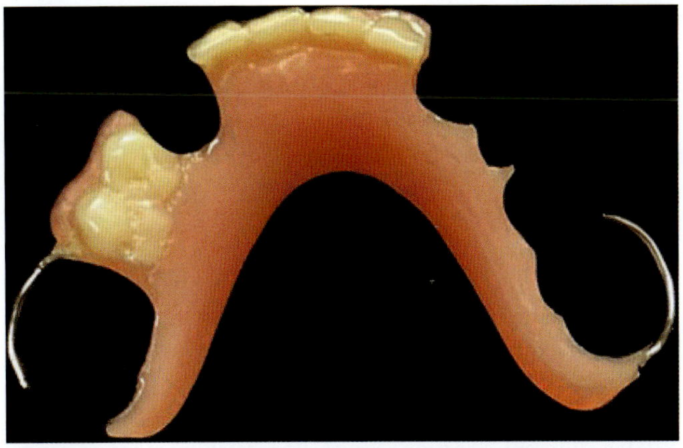

Fig. 26.2 In this case, mandibular anterior teeth required extraction due to periodontal disease. Following a period of healing, the patient will decide on a definitive treatment option, which may include a removable partial denture or an implant-supported prosthesis. Because the length of time until definitive care will be provided is not known, a temporary interim prosthesis not only replaces esthetically important teeth but provides stabilization of adjacent and opposing dentition as well.

can decrease the cost. These are typically retained by engaging dental undercuts with the denture base on the lingual and the path of insertion with the adjacent teeth (Fig. 26.1).

SPACE MAINTENANCE

When an edentulous space results from recent extractions or traumatic loss of teeth, it is usually prudent to maintain the space while the tissue heals. Maintenance of the space can prevent undesirable migration and extrusion of adjacent or opposing teeth until definitive treatment can be accomplished. In younger patients the space should be maintained until the adjacent teeth have reached sufficient maturity to be used as abutments for fixed restorations or for implant placement and restoration. In adult patients space maintenance during the course of treatment may be needed due to lapse of time required for adjunctive therapy during periods of healing (Fig. 26.2).

REESTABLISHING OCCLUSAL RELATIONSHIPS

Interim RPDs may be used to reestablish occlusal relationships for the following reasons: (1) to maintain the interocclusal relationship post tooth extraction, (2) to establish a new occlusal relationship or modify occlusal vertical dimension, and (3) to condition residual ridge tissue for optimum support of the definitive RPD that will follow.

At times a patient may lose teeth or wear tooth structure in a way that a stable occlusal position is lost. In other words, when a patient occludes, their teeth no longer have contact in their ideal vertical and/or horizontal relationship. For example, when posterior teeth are extracted, the clinical condition remaining may result in a lack of posterior support. In such situations, where there is no longer contact of opposing natural dentition to stabilize the interocclusal dimension, an interim RPD may be fabricated to maintain the interocclusal relationship. The prosthesis will ensure the patient's vertical dimension of occlusion is maintained, and it will help the patient to become accustomed to wearing a removable prosthesis.

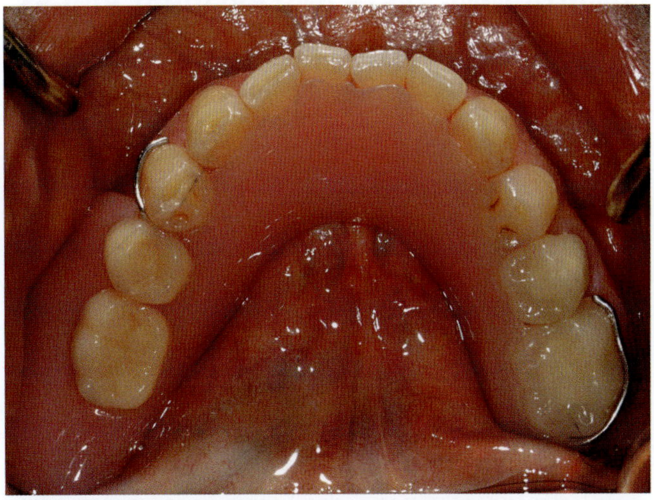

Fig. 26.3 When reestablishing occlusal vertical dimension, centric occlusion, or occlusal plane in the definitive treatment phase, an interim prosthesis can help confirm the patient's functional position. This makes the definitive care more predictable while stabilizing the patient during the interim phase.

When one functions in an unstable position for an extended time, it can be difficult to establish centric relation and the patient may experience any number of symptoms (including difficulty functioning, angular cheilitis, masticatory muscle, or temporomandibular joint symptoms). Interim RPDs may be fabricated to help determine and test a functional position and improve patient comfort.

Interim acrylic RPDs are often used as a precursor to establish this position before proceeding with a definitive treatment plan that may include cast frame RPDs (with or without implant support), fixed implant restorations, tooth-supported fixed partial dentures, or any combination of the above. This allows the patient to test a position or proposed treatment before a more significant cost or time investment by the clinician and patient (Fig. 26.3).

Interim RPDs also may be used as occlusal splints in much the same manner as resin occlusal splints are used on natural teeth. When total tooth support is available, there is little difference between the functionality of a fixed and a removable occlusal splint. However, a removable splint is more likely to be left out of the mouth unless the patient is made more comfortable by its presence. An example of such a situation is when wearing an occlusal splint alleviates a temporomandibular joint condition. Similar to a tooth-supported occlusal splint, an interim RPD may be eliminated in sections as restorative treatment is being done, thus maintaining the established jaw relation until all restorative treatment has been completed.

When one or more distal extension bases exist in the interim RPD, a different situation occurs. The establishment of a new occlusal relation depends on the quality of support and stability that the splint receives from the denture support. Both broad coverage and functional basing of tissue-supported bases are desirable, along with some type of occlusal rest on the nearest abutments.

CONDITIONING TEETH AND RESIDUAL RIDGES

Applegate[1] discusses the choice of partial or complete denture treatment and emphasized the advantages of conditioning edentulous areas to provide stable support for distal extension RPDs. This is accomplished by having the patient wear an interim RPD for a period of time before the final base is fabricated. In the absence of opposing occlusion, stimulating the underlying tissue by applying intermittent finger pressure to the denture base is advised. Whether the stimulation results from occlusal or finger pressure, there seems to be little doubt that the tissues of the residual ridge become more capable of supporting a distal extension RPD when they have been previously conditioned by wearing of a restoration.

Abutment teeth also benefit from wearing of an interim restoration when such a restoration applies an occlusal load to those teeth, either through occlusal coverage or through occlusal rests. At times a tooth planned for use as an abutment for an RPD may have been out of occlusion for a period of time. Immediately on applying an occlusal load to that tooth sufficient to support any type of removable prosthesis, some intrusion of the tooth will occur. If such intrusion occurs after initial placement of the final prosthesis, the occlusal relationship of the prosthesis and its relation to the adjacent gingival tissue will be altered. This may account for gingival impingement, which occurs after the prosthesis has been worn for some time, even though seemingly adequate relief was provided initially. When an interim RPD is worn, such abutment teeth can become stabilized under the loading of the temporary restoration and intrusion occurs before the impression for the master cast is made. There is sufficient reason to believe that both abutment teeth and supporting ridge tissue are more capable of providing continued support for the RPD when they have been previously conditioned by the wearing of a temporary interim restoration.

At times patients may have unhealthy tissues in support-bearing areas, due to a fractured or otherwise ill-fitting existing RPD. A well-fitting interim RPD can serve as a carrier for tissue conditioning material to prepare the tissues for a definitive prosthesis.

INTERIM RESTORATION DURING TREATMENT

In some instances an existing RPD can be used with modifications as an interim RPD. Such modifications may include relining and adding teeth and clasps to an existing denture. In other instances, an existing RPD may be converted to a transitional complete denture for immediate placement while the tissue heals, and an opposing arch is prepared to receive an RPD. Sometimes a temporary interim RPD must be made to replace missing anterior teeth in a partially edentulous arch, which ultimately may be replaced with fixed restorations. When using an interim RPD in this type of situation, the anterior portion of the restoration is cut away when the fixed restorations are placed; this leaves the remainder of the denture to be worn while the posterior area is in progress (Fig. 26.4).

CONDITIONING THE PATIENT FOR WEARING A PROSTHESIS

A temporary restoration may be made to aid the patient in making a transition to complete dentures when the total loss of teeth is inevitable. Such an RPD also may be considered a valid part of the treatment because the patient is at the same time being conditioned to wear a removable prosthesis. This type of RPD may be worn for prolonged periods; here it may periodically undergo revision to changes in the underlying supporting residual ridge, modification to include additional tooth lost, or relining when it becomes necessary or advisable due to changes in the underlying supporting residual ridge.

The dentist should agree to provide such an RPD only under the following conditions: (1) that a definite fee for the treatment is appropriate and that the fee will depend on the servicing necessary and (2) that when further wearing of the transitional denture is unwise and jeopardizes the health of the remaining tissue, the transition to complete dentures will proceed. Regardless of the purpose of the interim RPD, it is imperative that a distinction is made between temporary restorations and a definitive RPD service and that the patient is advised of the purposes and limitations of such restorations.

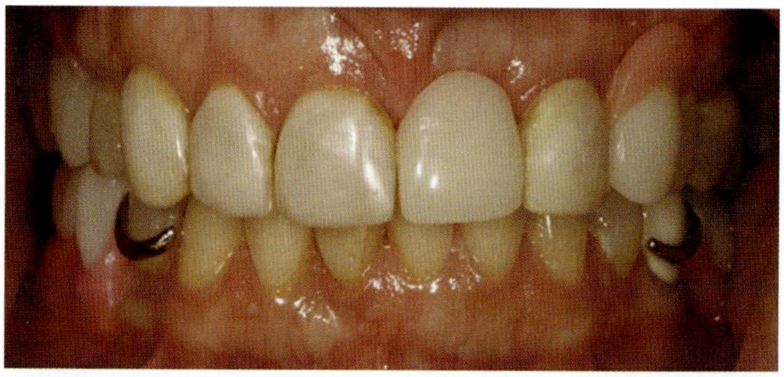

Fig. 26.4 A patient presented needing anterior and posterior teeth extracted. An interim removable was fabricated to replace the maxillary right molars and left central incisor and canine.

To fabricate an interim RPD, impressions must be made that capture all the relevant soft tissue and remaining dentition. Often, irreversible hydrocolloid (alginate) is the material of choice—particularly when teeth are mobile or compromised. When teeth are severely compromised, tissues are healing, or prostheses are tooth supported, a digital impression with an intraoral scanner may be a more ideal choice. Whether digital or conventional techniques are utilized, the appropriate tissue capture to allow tissue extension is critical. An interocclusal record is necessary before proceeding with prosthesis fabrication as well. The casts should be positioned in maximum intercuspation or centric relation, depending on diagnostic findings (Chapter 13). The interocclusal record should be made in this determined position, as close to occlusal vertical dimension as possible.

There are many materials and techniques to fabricate interim RPDs. Conventional methods for fabrication include heat polymerization, autopolymerizing acrylic resins (sprinkle on technique), and pour-type base resins. The sprinkle on technique is commonly used due to its low cost. Conventional carded denture teeth can be used, or teeth may be printed or milled out of resin. Digital methods are becoming more common as well. There are many software systems available that allow for interim RPD design (Fig. 26.5). The designs can then be milled or printed at the discretion of the clinician and technician. The bases can be milled or printed with denture teeth bonded, or they can be fabricated monolithic (Fig. 26.6). When milled, the prostheses are generally fabricated from pucks of PMMA. With this material the base can be readily relined or modified, including the addition of more denture teeth in the future. Alternatively, when prostheses are additively manufactured (3D printed), they are made of different types of resins. This can make repair and tooth addition less predictable. It is, however, a lower cost option and a much more practical process for in-office fabrication (Fig. 26.7). If desired, wrought-wire clasps can be embedded after fabrication for extra retention, no matter the fabrication method.

CLINICAL PROCEDURE FOR PLACEMENT

It is important to consider proper fitting of the prosthesis to ensure comfortable use during the temporary phase of treatment. Careful attention to planned use of the teeth for support, stability, and retention without undue stress from gingival tissue contact or improper occlusal loading will ensure more comfortable use.

To ensure proper use of the remaining natural teeth, the prosthesis must be completely seated in the arch. Common areas requiring adjustment to ensure complete seating include interproximal extensions, regions where clasps exit from the acrylic-resin base, tissue undercuts (labial undercuts from recent extractions or the lingual/retromylohyoid region), and any portion of the prosthesis that lies inferior to the height of contour, especially if bilaterally opposed (Fig. 26.8).

Once seated it is important to check that no undue pressure to the marginal gingival region is present. To facilitate this step and help with the complete seating requirement, it is possible to have the laboratory block out the marginal gingival region and infrabulge regions to reduce seating problems (Fig. 26.9). Infrabulge regions may include lingual and palatal tooth surfaces, as well as modification space regions. Because temporary prostheses are generally fabricated on unprepared teeth, these regions often require correction. However, if the blockout is not accomplished carefully, the prosthesis may seat easily but it may

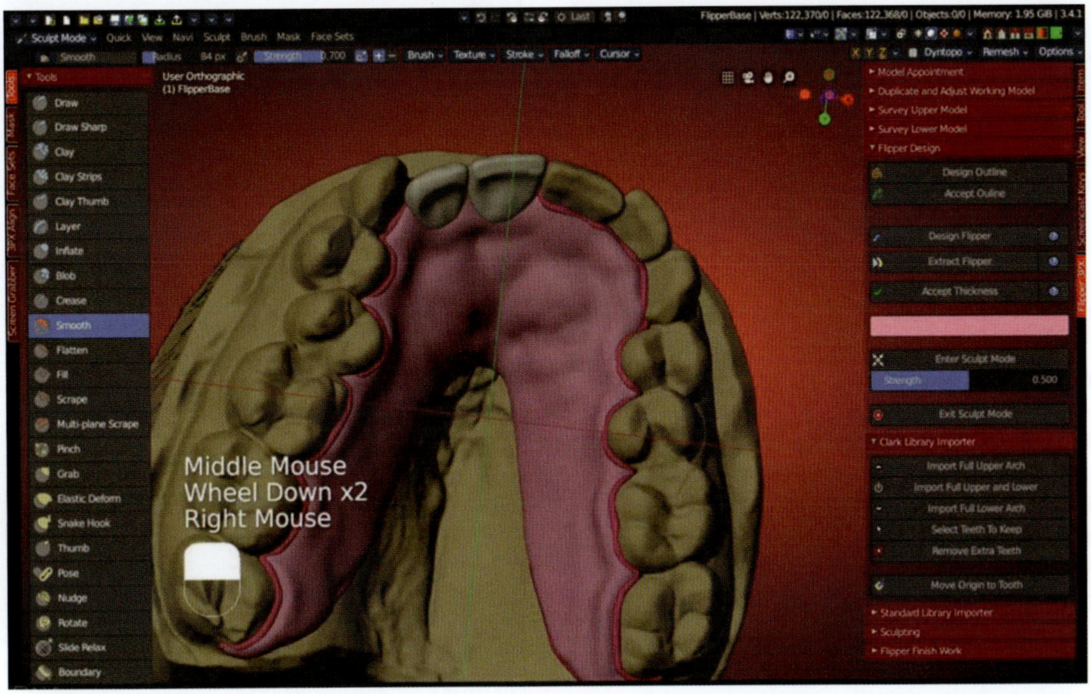

Fig. 26.5 There are numerous software systems available that allow users to design removable partial dentures. This example shows a freeware program being utilized to design a two-piece interim removable partial denture. The teeth and base will be printed separately and bonded together during postprocess.

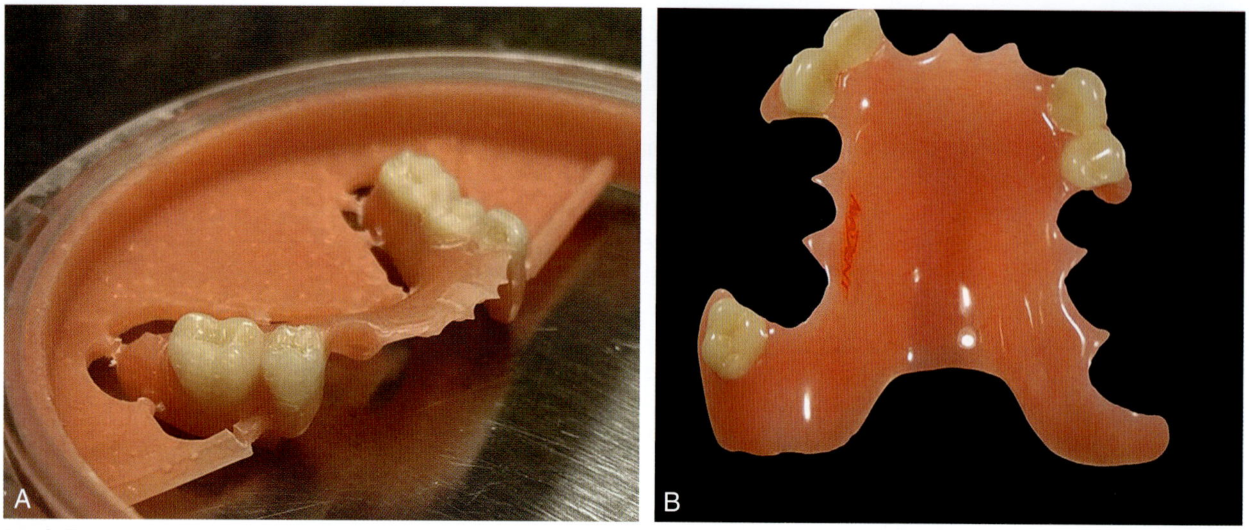

Fig. 26.6 A, There are a multitude of ways to fabricate interim removable partial dentures with computer-aided manufacturing. In this case the base was milled out of a custom puck polymethyl methacrylic, with conventional carded denture teeth processed in place. **B,** A different kind of custom puck was fabricated for this milled removable partial denture case. The acrylic resins for the denture teeth and denture base were incorporated into the puck before milling. This results in a monolithic prosthesis, with no separate denture teeth. This eliminates the risk of debonded teeth and capitalizes on the material strength. (A, Courtesy of 3 Point Dental Lab, Cleveland, OH; B, Courtesy of Avadent Digital Dentures, Scottsdale, AZ.)

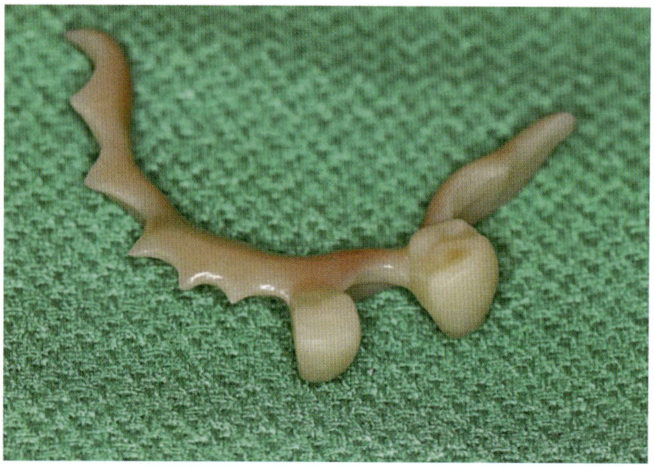

Fig. 26.7 A printed interim removable partial denture can be a quick and cost-effective solution. The preservation of design data makes it easy to modify and refabricate as needed throughout treatment. In this case, pink composite resin was added to improve esthetics.

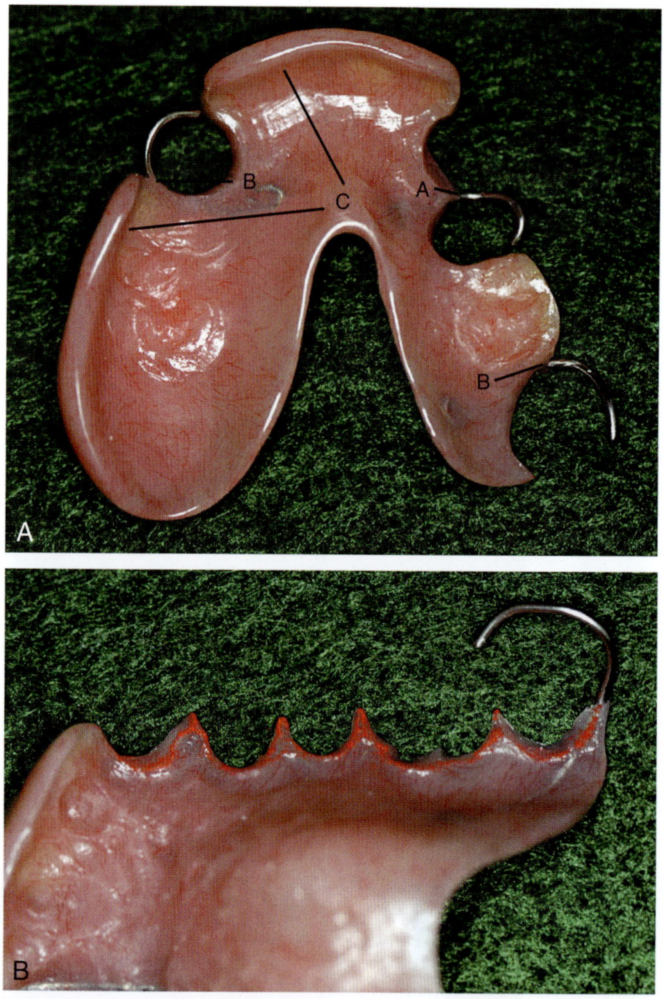

Fig. 26.8 A, Maxillary interim removable partial denture. Areas that require adjustment commonly include interproximal extensions *(A)*, the region where the clasp exits from the resin *(B)*, and tissue undercuts of prosthesis extensions *(C)*. **B,** Interproximal tooth extensions and regions where marginal gingival is crossed by the prosthesis should be carefully adjusted *(outlined in red)*.

not be as stable as possible because of insufficient tooth contact. Stability and retention are improved when it is possible to have the prosthesis contact portions of the teeth superior to the height of contour because of tooth-dictated control of movement.

It is possible to create occlusal imbalance if the lingual/palatal portion of the prosthesis is too bulky. Consequently an opposing cast should be provided to allow placement of clasps and acrylic-resin contours that do not cause occlusal interference (Fig. 26.10). Once fully seated and relieved appropriately, the occlusion should contribute to the remaining natural dentition (as in a definitive prosthesis) and harmonize with natural tooth–dictated function. Typically the prosthesis should not be the sole source of occlusal contact. In such situations the functional forces are concentrated at the acrylic resin-to-tooth junction, and predictably a change in orientation occurs, allowing tissue-ward movement and a change in occlusion with an increase in soft tissue contact.

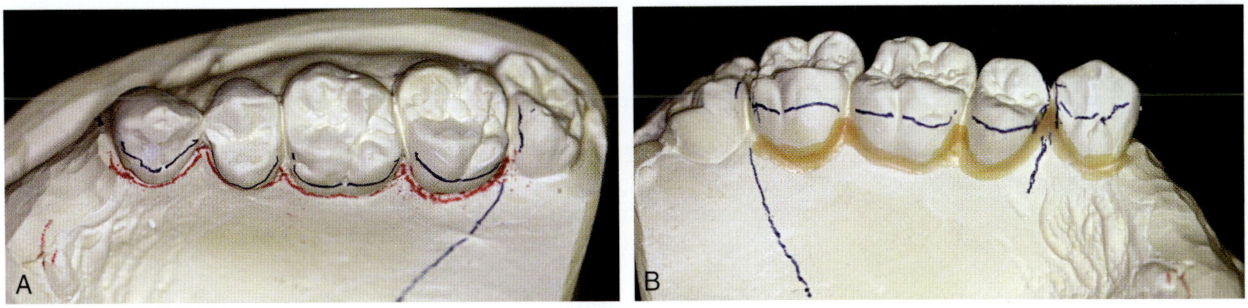

Fig. 26.9 **A,** Maxillary cast with an outline of the prosthesis design and with the region at the marginal gingival crossing outlined. If the cast is not relieved at the marginal gingival, the prosthesis should be corrected before insertion. **B,** Cast showing gingival regions relieved with baseplate wax. A duplicate of this cast will provide the necessary relief for use as a processing cast. If interproximal regions have undercuts, these can also be blocked out to allow easier insertion of a temporary prosthesis.

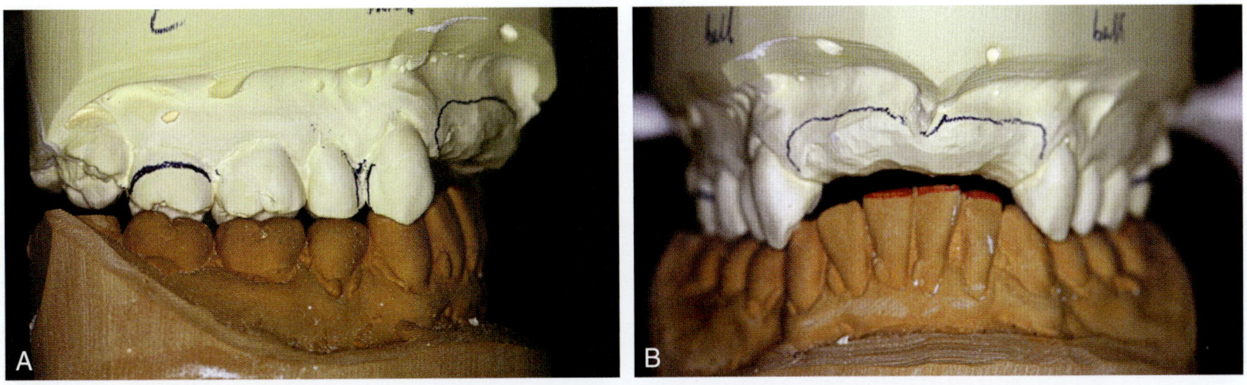

Fig. 26.10 **A,** Evaluation of mounted casts allows determination of the occlusal impact on maxillary temporary prosthesis clasp selection and placement. Interocclusal space allows placement of a ball clasp distal to the canine and a circumferential clasp from the distal of the second molar, both without occlusal interference if the clasps are carefully contoured. **B,** Anterior cast modification in anticipation of postextraction ridge contours for this immediate temporary prosthesis. Diagnosis of the limited space at the anterior region before surgery allows presurgical discussion of the possible need for mandibular incisor modification to improve the interim and final prosthesis occlusion.

REFERENCE

1. Applegate OC. Conditions which may influence the choice of partial or complete denture service. *J Prosthet Dent*. 1957;7:182–196.

INDEX

Page numbers followed by *b*, *t*, or *f* refer to boxes, tables, or figures, respectively.

A

B

C

D

E

F

G

H

I

J

K

R

S

X

Y

Z